Treatment Options Before and After Edentulism

Yasemin Özkan

Editor

Treatment Options Before and After Edentulism

Tooth Supported Overdentures

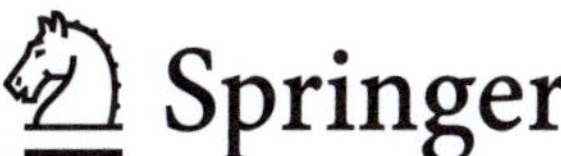 Springer

Editor
Yasemin Özkan
Faculty of Dentistry, Department of Prosthodontics
Marmara University
Istanbul, Türkiye

ISBN 978-3-031-37584-2   ISBN 978-3-031-37582-8   (eBook)
https://doi.org/10.1007/978-3-031-37582-8

This Springer imprint is published by the registered company Springer Nature Switzerland AG
The registered company address is: Gewerbestrasse 11, 6330 Cham, Switzerland

Preface

This book is the first book in a series of three books:

1. Tooth-supported overdentures
2. Implant retained overdenture applications in edentulous patients
3. Implant retained fixed restoration applications in edentulous patients

The book consists of 9 chapters and more than 600 colorful pictures of our own clinical cases. The book will help clinicians offer the most proper treatment options to patients who will soon be edentulous and also provide practical information about the solutions to problems that occur when using tooth-supported overdentures. This book also offers options for patients who will soon be edentulous, allowing them to consider tooth-supported dentures as a means to increase physical and psychological confidence before rehabilitating them with implants.

I would like to thank RHEIN 83, CEKA PRECI-LINE, and PREAT CORPORATION for allowing me to share clinical and laboratory cases. Again, I would like to thank Optimal Dental Laboratory for their continuous support in the laboratory stages of our clinical cases and to all who contributed during the writing and publishing of the book.

Also, I would like to thank everyone who contributed during the writing and publishing of the book.

Istanbul, Turkey

Yasemin Özkan

Acknowledgments

I would like to thank all my friends who contributed to the writing of this book. I would also like to thank RHEIN-83 and CEKA company for allowing me to publish all their cases and pictures for the book. Again, I would like to thank dear Ulrich Heker, who shared his cases with me and contributed to my book.

Contents

Theoretical and Technical Background and Clinical Considerations for Tooth-Supported Overdentures

1

Yasemin Ozkan and Rifat Gozneli

1.1 Introduction

Loss of teeth causes impairment in the oral tissues. Adaptation to conventional complete denture (CCD) requires a complex learning process based on a somatic and psychological foundation. Approximately 30% of the patients wearing CCD have complaints. They suffer from various problems related to their dentures, generally for the lower denture, such as lack of stability, retention, and pain during mastication. Patients adapted to CCD can also experience loss of adaptation in time due to alveolar crest resorption and physiologic, intraoral, and muscular modifications. Psychosocial problems are the result of diminished facial appearance, difficulties with speech, and avoidance of social contact. Tooth-supported overdenture (TSO) is an excellent alternative to a CCD because of its many advantages.

1.2 Historical Development of the Overdentures

The history of overdenture goes back to the 1800s. The idea of retaining some teeth/roots was described nearly 150 years ago. In the 1950s, clinicians reported that when teeth were extracted, the residual alveolar bone was resorbed; and due to continuous resorption, very little support was used for CCD resulting in wearing difficulty. The research for root-supported dentures to stabilize the denture was started in 1856. Ledger was the first one to propose the use of natural teeth supporting a removable denture. In 1861, Barker reported that keeping roots under the denture contributed to retention. Then the concept of TSO was presented at the World Dental Congress in 1861 by Butler, Roberts, and Hays, exhibiting 12 years of treatment results. In 1896, Easing described the telescopic dentures made with copings. The

Y. Ozkan (✉) · R. Gozneli
Faculty of Dentistry, Department of Prosthodontics, Marmara University, Istanbul, Turkey
e-mail: ykozkan@marmara.edu.tr

© The Author(s), under exclusive license to Springer Nature Switzerland AG 2023
Y. Özkan (ed.), *Treatment Options Before and After Edentulism,*
https://doi.org/10.1007/978-3-031-37582-8_1

use of roots/teeth as a support to improve the functional effect of prosthetic rehabilitation was encouraged by Rehm, Brill, and Miller in 1958. In 1969, Morrow et al. stated that a reduction of natural teeth length to a few millimeters (keeping roots as TSO abutments) increases the support to dentures, and furthermore they described the concept as "preventive prosthodontics." In 1969, Lord and Teel published an article titled "The Overdenture" and thus the term "overdenture" has taken its place in the literature. The current concept of overdenture was presented at the American Dental Association's annual meeting in Las Vegas in 1970. Later on, the "overdenture" concept was supported by two long-term studies published by Crum and Rooney [1], and Van Waas et al [2].

For many years, CCD designs have been modified to obtain additional support and stability from a few retained and conveniently prepared natural teeth. In 1994, Mericske-Stern et al. [3] stated the effectiveness of such tooth-supported complete dentures (CDs) and proposed that they are an alternative to CCD. They reported that the roots, which are maintained under the denture base, preserve the alveolar ridge, provide sensory feedback, and improve the stability of the dentures. In recent years, successful results have been obtained in overdenture treatments that used implants as teeth/roots for support. Morais et al. [4] reported that overdenture treatment with the use of implants has become popular for edentulous elderly patients suffering from their CCD.

1.3 Advantages of Tooth-Supported Overdentures

1.3.1 Preservation of the Alveolar Bone

Preservation of the alveolar bone should be considered before the beginning of the resorption problem. It should be noted that the application of TSO is essential to prevent bone loss. Patients should be informed about the importance of keeping the roots since they offer support and retention.

Crum and Rooney [1] described bone loss in CCD and TSO-treated patients after 5 years using various radiographic examinations. In 16 male patients (aged between 46 and 67), eight patients treated with TSO and eight patients treated with CCD were investigated. In TSO patients, the supporting teeth were designed as mandibular canines (canine preparation was planned to be 1.5 higher than the alveolar bone). In an evaluation after 5 years, the vertical bone loss in the mandible was determined to be 0.6 mm in TSO patients and 5.2 mm in CCD patients. Van Waas et al. [2] also reported a similar study. They investigated 23 CCD patients and 26 TSO patients for 4 years. They reported less bone loss in TSO patients than in CCD patients. They stated that "the difference in the bone loss was present not only in the anterior region—near the remaining canines but also in other regions."

Long-term studies reported 0,4 mm bone loss annually in the edentulous anterior mandible due to physiologic changes. It was reported that average bone loss was 0.5 mm in 5 years, which equals 0.1 mm annually with TSO (Figs. 1.1 and 1.2).

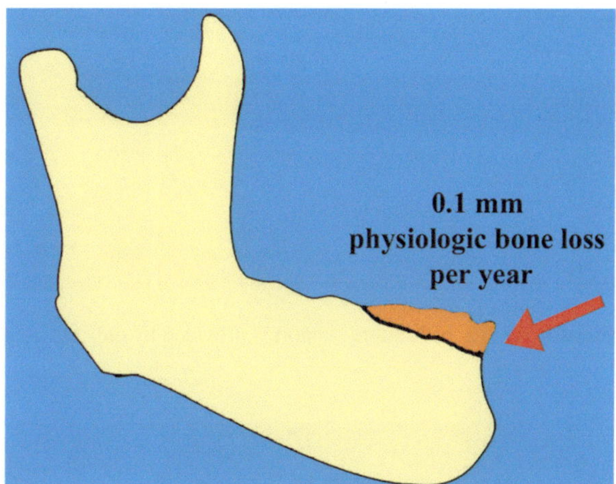

Fig. 1.1 Alveolar crest resorption pattern at mandibula

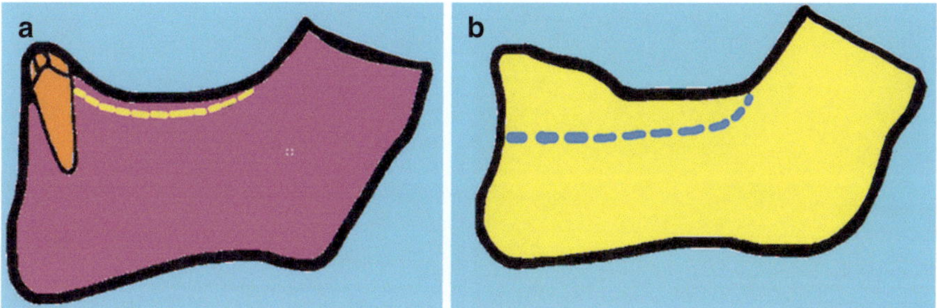

Fig. 1.2 Resorption patterns of edentulous crests: (**a**) before extraction and (**b**) after extraction

Resorption of the edentulous crest is a complicated biophysical condition that includes functional factors (e.g., density and duration of received forces), prosthetic factors (techniques and materials used in denture fabrication), and metabolic factors (systematic reasons effects on osteogenesis and resorption).

In edentulous patients, biomechanical factors such as support, stability, and retention of dentures affect the success of prosthetic treatment. A significant loss in the alveolar bone with the loss of teeth leads to a more complicated prosthetic treatment (Fig. 1.2). Despite the different factors' effects on alveolar bone resorption, changes in the alveolar bone and soft tissues in CCD patients are inevitable in the presence of loss of natural teeth, occlusal factors, and long-term denture use.

Alveolar bone resorption affects mainly the mandible rather than the maxilla because the mandible has a narrower space for a denture, which causes uneven occlusal load distribution to the mandible. [5] measured an average of 9–10 mm vertical height loss in the mandible and 2.5–3 mm vertical height loss in the maxilla in CCD patients who used their dentures for more than 25 years. Tallagren also described that the resorption level in the mandible is four times bigger than the resorption level in the maxilla.

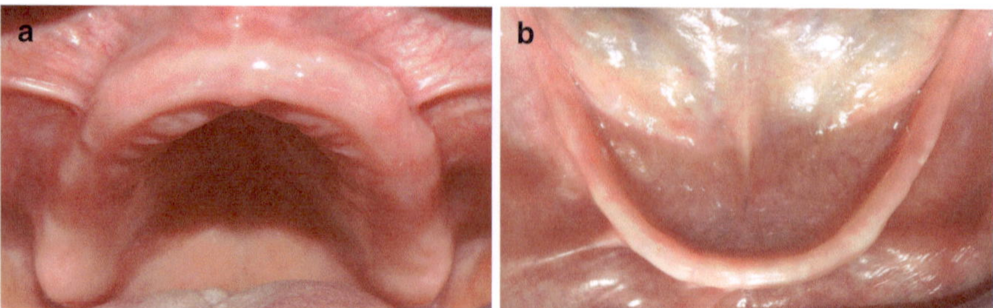

Picture 1.1 (**a**, **b**) Denture support is provided by only the edentulous mucosal surface when all teeth are lost

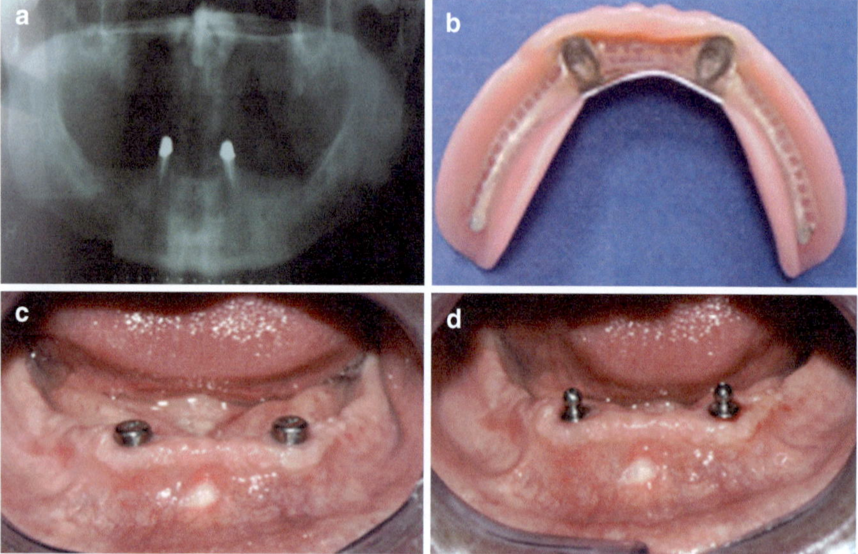

Picture 1.2 Preservation of the anterior teeth: (**a**) Radiographic view of two canines used for abutment of TSO, (**b**) intaglio surface of TSO, (**c**) implant placement after the abutment extractions (after seven years of usage of TSO), and (**d**) ball attachments in situ

In the absence of supporting teeth (complete edentulous situation), all support is only received from mucosal surfaces (Picture 1.1). However, if the patient has some remaining teeth, it is suggested that the anterior teeth should be protected, if possible, in order to increase patients' satisfaction. Furthermore, the preservation of teeth also prevents bone resorption and enhances a sufficient bone mass for future implant treatments (Pictures 1.2 and 1.3; Fig. 1.2).

Edentulous crest resorption in the mandible can be classified into four categories (Fig. 1.3).

Class 1: This type of crest is just present in 11% of total edentulous cases. Resorption is not much. There is a sufficiently long and wide crest for implants.

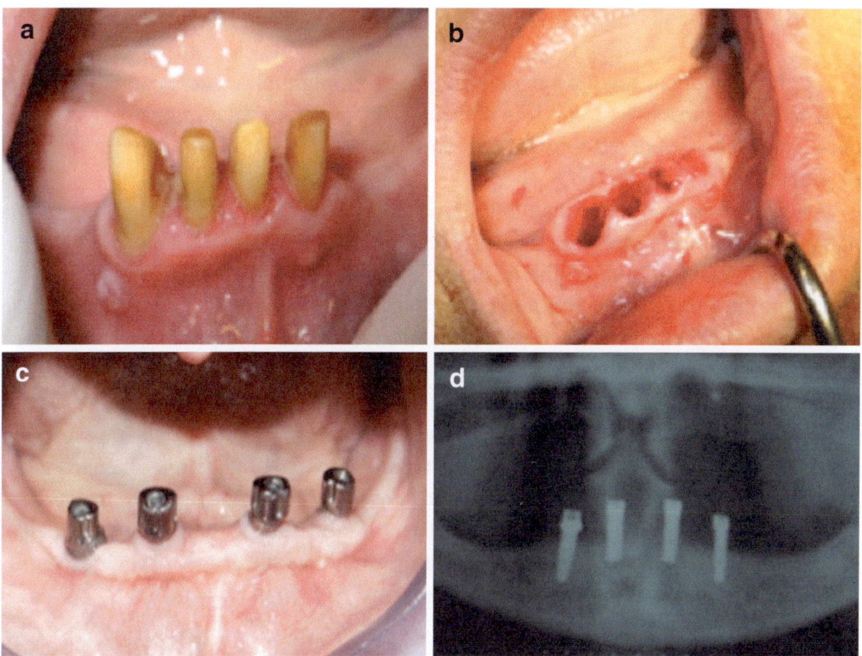

Picture 1.3 (**a**) Mandibular anterior teeth in situ, (**b**) extraction of the teeth (after five years of usage of TSO), (**c**) immediate placement of four implants, and (**d**) periapical X-ray view of the immediately placed implants

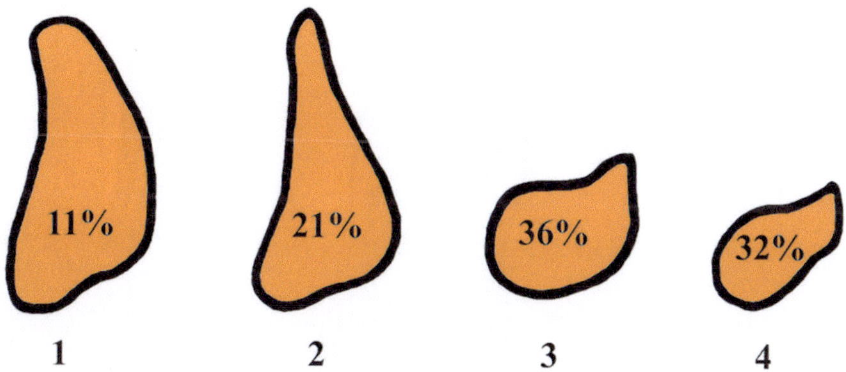

Fig. 1.3 Edentulous crest resorption classification in the mandible

Class 2: (knife-edge crest): This type of crest is seen in 21% of total edentulous cases. In this class, bone resorption occurs mostly buccolingually rather than vertically in the mandible. This type of crest is not suitable for implant placement despite its crest height.

Class 3: (low and round crest): It is present in 36% of total edentulous cases. The crest is low and round. The atrophy in this class includes reduced crest height. Through the application of proper configuration implant placement can be possible.

Class 4: (depressive crest): It is present in 32% of total edentulous cases. In this class, there is severe atrophy in all dimensions. It is not suitable for implant placement.

After resorption of the remaining alveolar crest, there are a few treatment alternatives for denture-supporting tissues. These alternatives are alveolar crest augmentation using natural and synthetic materials, and tissue extension procedures for revealing intraoral tissues and relocating muscle attachments. Unfortunately, these procedures have complex treatment sequences leading to the possibility of various complications that might occur, and the cost of treatment significantly increases because of the extra treatment procedures.

To keep the remaining weakened teeth, it is essential to prevent resorption (Pictures 1.2 and 1.3). A tooth, which is considered weak, that cannot be used as an abutment for the removable denture might be suitable for TSO. Besides, the vertical walls of the remaining roots offer additional stabilization for the denture; also, decreasing the height of the abutment tooth right above the gingiva provides stability, and using attachment provides retention for TSO (Figs. 1.4 and 1.5).

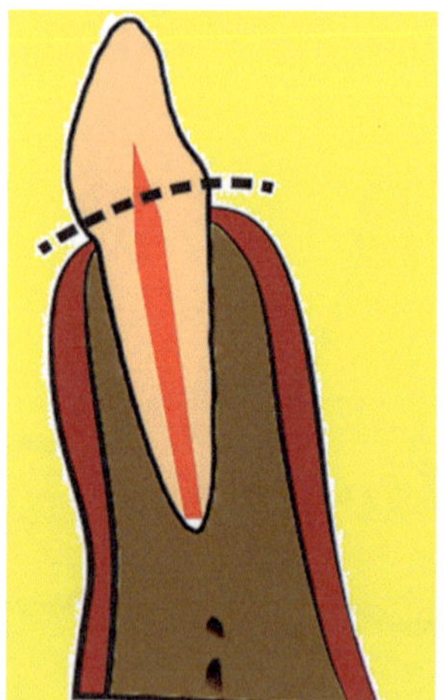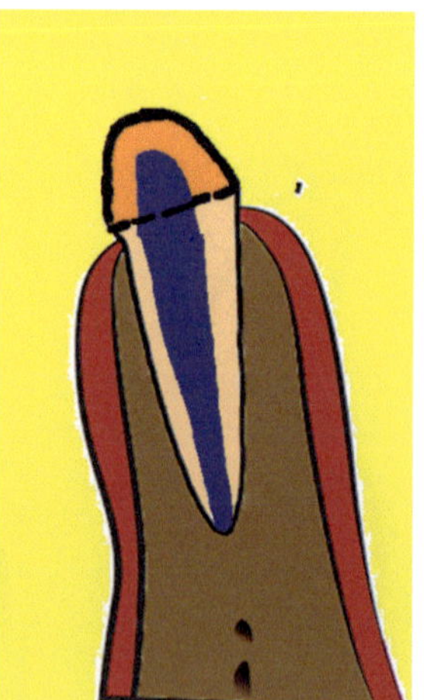

Fig. 1.4 Reduction of tooth crown height just above the mucosal level provides the ideal crown/root ratio and endodontic treatment

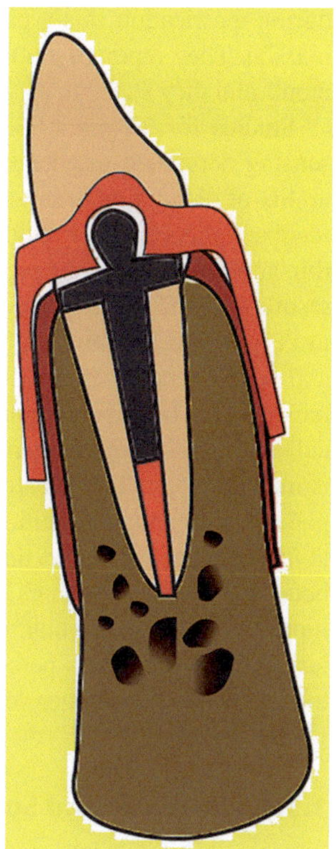

Fig. 1.5 Additional retention is gained by providing parallel vertical walls of copings or attachments

1.3.2   Tactile Sensing

After the loss of a tooth, which is the most essential component of the masticatory system, the nerve transmission that offers a proprioceptive effect on the alveolar bone does not provide feedback to the central nervous system. The reason for TSO being more successful in demonstrating a proprioceptive effect compared to CCD patients is the presence of the remaining roots. Sposetti et al. [6] studied masticatory efficiency by measuring the maximum biting force and Electromyography (EMG) activities during mastication in six patients who used TSO in the mandible and CCD in the maxilla. They reported a 50% increase in biting force after placement of the attachments and they stated that TSO had improved stability with increased biting force.

Studies for 30 years have demonstrated that dentate patients have much more sensing compared to edentulous patients. However, because of a slight loss in the ability of distinction even when the teeth are under anesthesia, it is believed that this feedback mechanism extends to posterior areas. Enkling et al. [7] demonstrated the thin test foils placed between the artificial teeth of the TSO gave more sensitive results than the implant-supported overdenture (IOD). Receptors in the mucosa, proprioception in the muscles, and Temporomandibular joint (TMJ) affect distinction, and periodontal receptors play a significant role in this result. It was reported that patients had better mastication activity and saliva flow through the proprioceptive cells in the periodontal ligament. Also, sensory feedback of the periodontal receptors is maintained, and masticatory performance is enhanced. The chewing efficiency of patients with natural dentition was measured at 90%, CCD wearers at 59%, and TSO at 79%. Pacer [8] found that TSO patients discriminate measured occlusal forces better than patients with CCD. The discrimination was enabled through the sensory input from the periodontal receptors. Also, Fenton [9] stated that a TSO patient had less occlusal thickness perception than a patient with CCD. Therefore, the natural tooth/root provides better vertical support than the CCD.

1.3.3 Stability and Support

The stability and support of the TSO also can be better in comparison to CCD. Roots maintained under the denture base improve the stability of the dentures. Furthermore, the use of copings and attachments on the remaining teeth enhances the retention of the denture. Retained root abutments can give better retention, support, and stability to a TSO and also provide proprioception, which would have been lost at CD treatment.

1.3.4 Psychological Relaxation

The loss of the last remaining teeth and the replacement with CCD have many adverse effects. The patient must accept edentulousness, and this may lead to psychological and social problems. It has been stated that the retention of some teeth for TSO abutments prevents the negative feeling of total loss and allows the patient to adjust to denture wearing.

1.4 Disadvantages of Tooth-Supported Overdentures

Endodontic and periodontal treatments are necessary for the supporting teeth (Figs. 1.4, 1.5, and Picture 1.4).

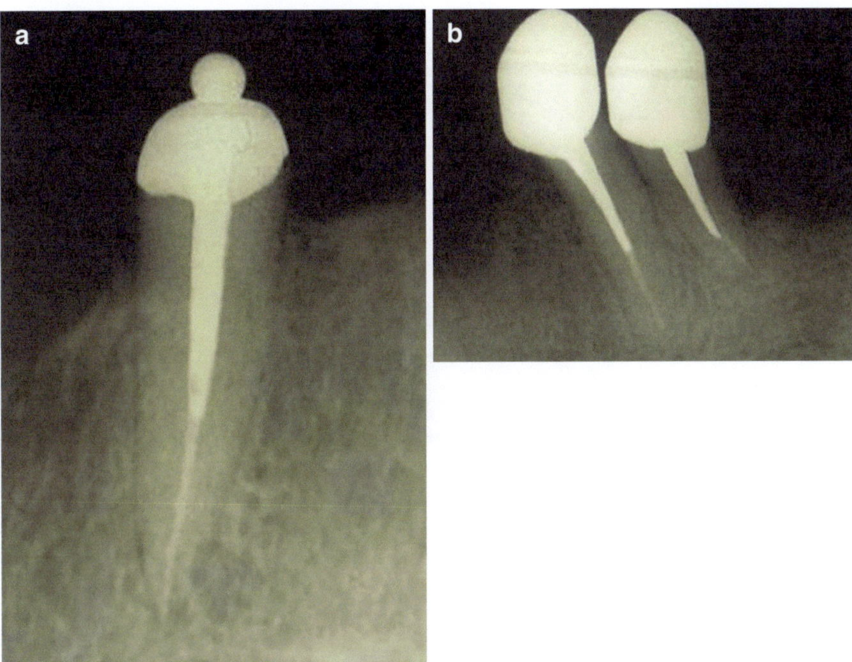

Picture 1.4 (**a**, **b**) Root canal treatment should be applied on teeth used as an abutment

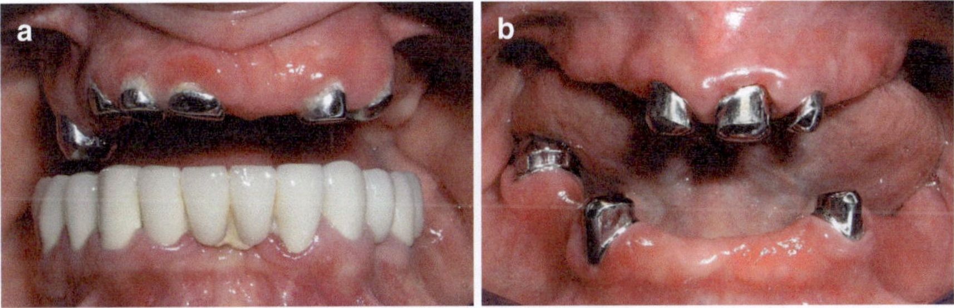

Picture 1.5 It is difficult to obtain plaque control and hygiene at TSO: (**a**) Gingival recession and hygiene problems on supporting teeth and (**b**) periodontal problems at supporting teeth and root area

- It is difficult to prevent plaque accumulation and provide hygiene. Periodontal problems and caries may be seen around the abutments (Picture 1.5).
- It is bulkier than the CCD and removable partial dentures (Picture 1.6).
- The thickness of the acrylic resin around the supporting tooth may be insufficient, which may cause a lack of resistance to fracture (Picture 1.7a, b). The metal framework should be used for TSO to prevent fracture (Picture 1.7c).
- If there is a deep undercut around the abutments, aesthetic problems may occur (Picture 1.8).

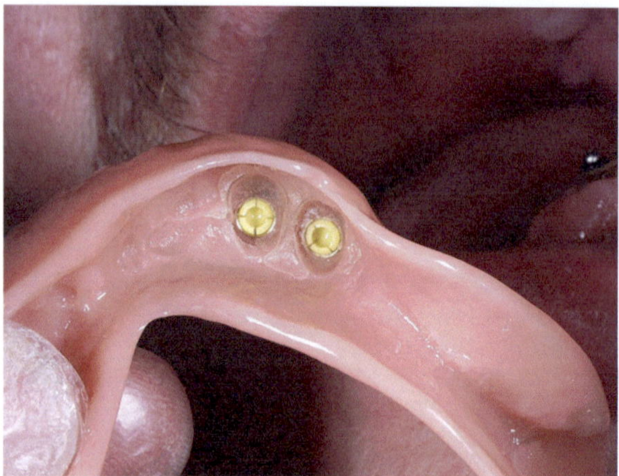

Picture 1.6 TSO is bulkier than the CCD and removable partial denture

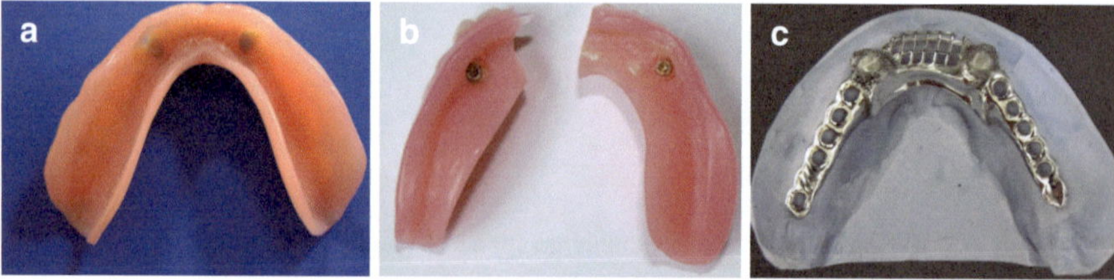

Picture 1.7 (**a**, **b**) Unsupported, thin acrylic base material may be fractured under occlusal forces and (**c**) the metal framework should be used for TSO

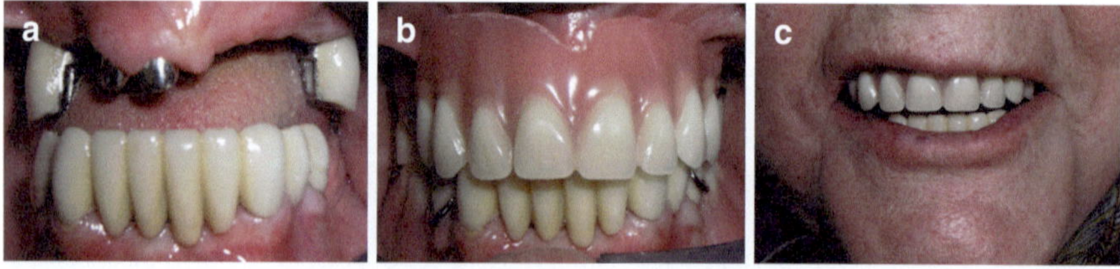

Picture 1.8 (**a**, **b**) Aesthetic problems occur when there is a deep undercut around the supporting tooth (a telescopic crown made on a supporting tooth, which has a deep undercut) and (**c**) aesthetic problems occur in the smiling position. The dominant root shape of canines should be carefully considered in TSO rehabilitation

- This treatment modality is an expensive approach with a more frequent recall of the patient than a CCD and also it takes time during the fabrication process. Since it is difficult to insert and remove the TSO, it is not recommended for mentally or physically disabled patients.

1.5   Indications of Tooth-Supported Overdentures

1.5.1   Better Support and Aesthetics

When a removable partial denture is planned, the remaining weakened teeth that are distributed unevenly in the opposing arch may cause difficulties in providing stability, retention, and occlusion. If there are a few remaining teeth, it is better to use them as supporting teeth under the denture in order to avoid this problem. Furthermore, if possible, leaving one or two remaining teeth will be useful for the opposing supporting teeth (Picture 1.9).

It is considered that the patient would have adaptation problems because of the fabrication procedures of CCD. To keep the weakened teeth/roots under TSO, the patient can be rehabilitated easily. These cases are classified as:

- Deeper palatine vault and higher alveolar ridge slope cases.
- Insufficient sublingual gland space cases.
- Class III tongue-shaped cases.
- Knife-edge alveolar ridge cases.
- Congenital deformity cases.

1.5.2   Severe Attrition Cases

Tooth-supported overdenture treatment is an effective method for rehabilitating the loss of vertical dimension of occlusion and aesthetics, which is caused by age, bruxism, or a high acidic diet (Picture 1.10).

1.5.3   Remaining Teeth Protection

When the remaining teeth are mobile or the crown-root ratio is not appropriate for removable partial denture support, TSO rehabilitation is a better alternative for prosthetic treatment.

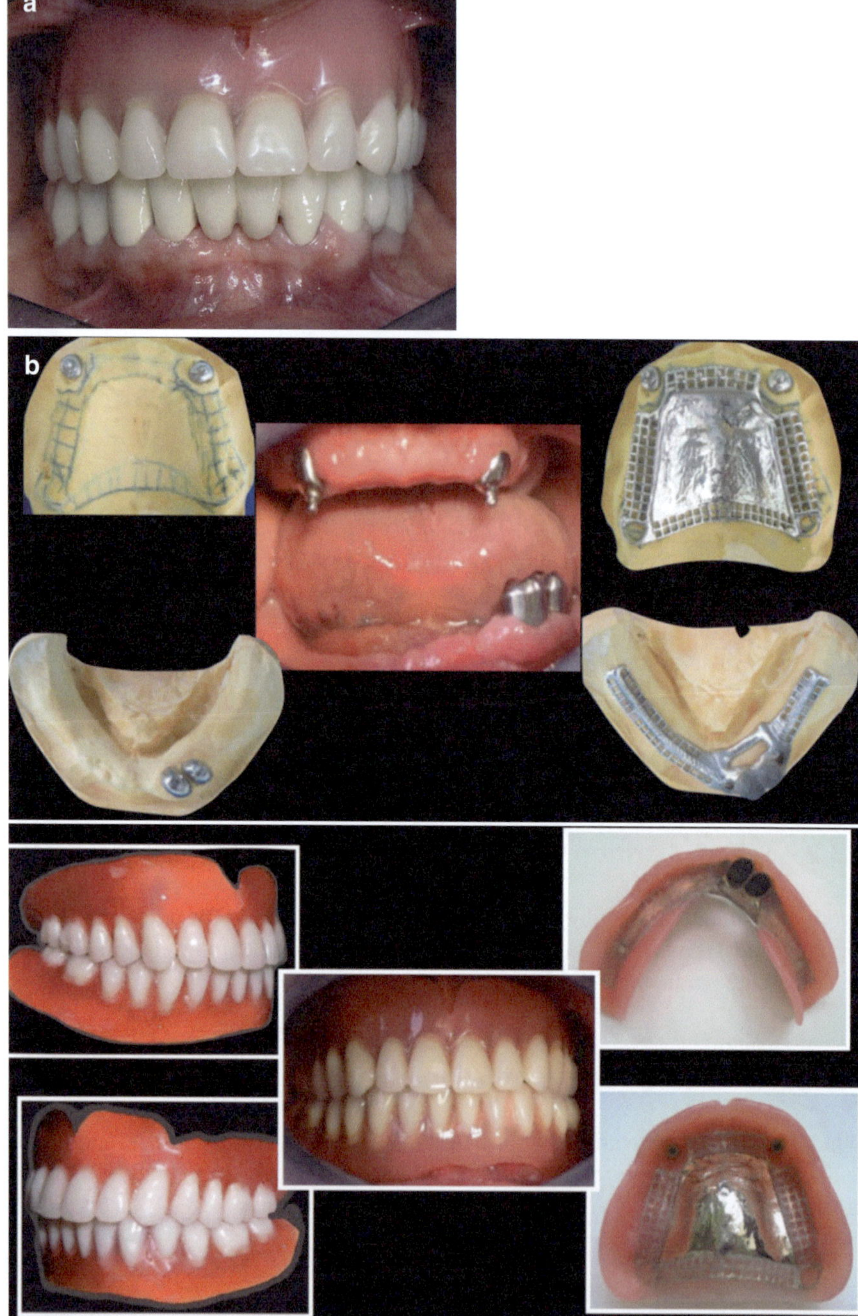

Picture 1.9 (**a**) It is more advantageous if both jaws' abutment teeth are used for TSO and (**b**) maxillary TSO is more advantageous than the CCD when opposing natural dentition

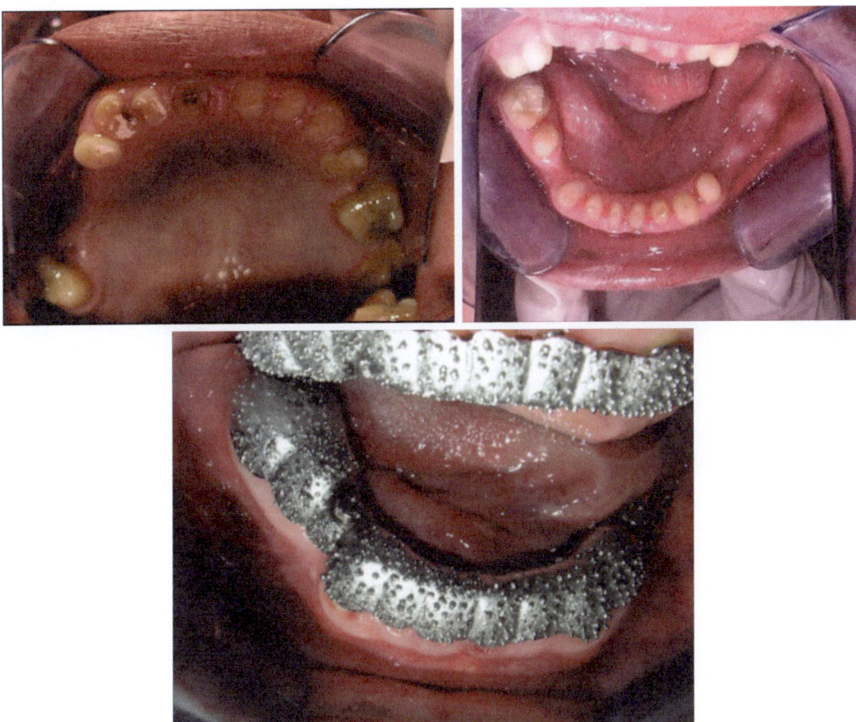

Picture 1.10 TSO treatment is an effective method for rehabilitating the lost vertical dimension using the worn teeth for support

Picture 1.11 TSO should be used in the treatment of congenital and non-congenital defects

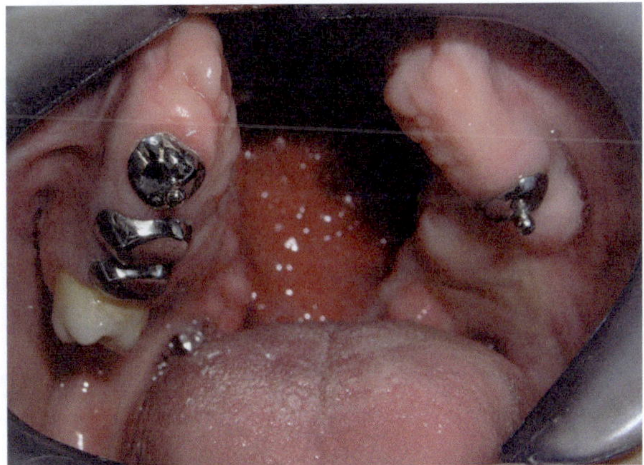

1.5.4 Congenital and Acquired Jaw Defects

Tooth-supported overdenture rehabilitation is preferred in cleft lip and palate, hypodontia, micrognathia, amelogenesis imperfecta, dentinogenesis imperfecta, and partial anodontia cases (Picture 1.11).

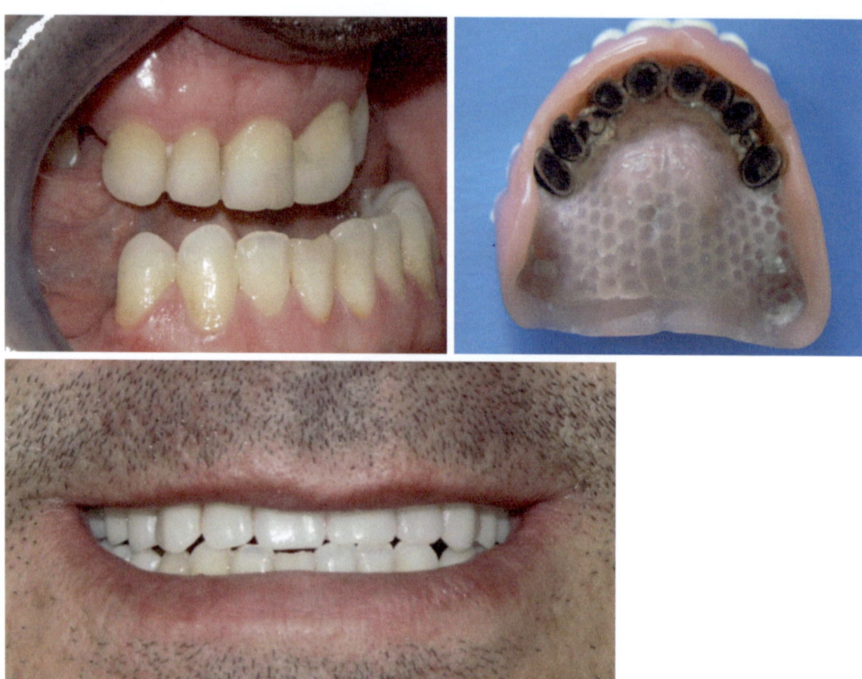

Picture 1.12 Severe Class III patients should be treated by TSO if they do not want orthognathic surgery

1.5.5 Class III Cases

In such cases, orthodontic and/or orthognathic surgical treatment is required to rehabilitate the aesthetic. Patients may reject these treatment alternatives due to economic or other reasons. TSO should be preferred to rehabilitate these cases instead of surgical procedures (Picture 1.12).

1.5.6 Transitional Denture

During the adaptation period of the CCD, the case can be rehabilitated by a TSO initially. However, the high cost of TSO should be considered in these cases.

1.5.7 Contraindications of Tooth-Supported Overdenture

- Tooth-supported overdenture patients have difficulties in maintaining intraoral hygiene, especially mentally or physically disabled patients.

- When endodontic and periodontal treatments are considered not to be successful. Unsuccessful endodontic treatment may cause increased alveolar bone loss, insufficient crown-root ratio, vertical fractures, mechanical root perforations, and horizontal root fractures under crest level. On the other hand, unsuccessful periodontal treatment may cause bone defects, insufficient attached gingiva, and the presence of Class III mobility.
- When the vertical dimension of occlusion is not suitable to include all the height of artificial teeth, acrylic base, and attachments, it is difficult for the patient to use the TSO. In such cases, the vertical dimension should be checked by using a temporary TSO.

Tooth-supported overdenture can be categorized as tooth-supported and tooth- and tissue-supported.

Tooth-Supported (Rigid) Type: This type depends on the support of the suitable roots to provide all the support for the prosthesis. This can be achieved through either root cap forms alone or in combination with a non-resilient precision attachment (the Conod Anchor, the Dalla Bona Cylindrical Anchor, the Gmur Anchor, the Baer Cylindrical anchor, the Rothermann Eccentric Anchor, the Gerber Retention Cylinder, the Ceka Attachment, the Quinlivan Attachment, the Regulex anchor, and the Ancrofix). This type of TSO acts as a rigid bridge and a lot of teeth/roots should be used in this type of teeth-supported removable dentures.

Tooth- and Tissue-Supported Type: This type involves an equal amount of load application to the tissues and the teeth that bear the loading. In other words, the load is shared, thus, overloading of the abutments is prevented.

The TSO can function in this manner if space is provided in the denture to allow movement vertically over the root cap. Precision attachments are designed to allow this vertical movement and better control over the root cap. Attachments designed for "resilience" include the Rothermann Cylindrical Resilience Anchor, the Dalla Bona Resilient Ball Anchor, the Dalla Bona Resilient Cylindrical anchor, the Bona Buffer Anchor, the Battesti Resilient Anchor, the Gerber Retention Buffer, the Biaggi Resilient Anchor, the Zest Attachment and the Mini Zest Attachment, the Ceka Attachment, the Kurer Stud Attachment, the Ginta attachment, the B & F Resilient Anchor, and the Ancrofix Attachment.

1.6 Classification of Tooth-Supported Overdenture

1.6.1 Tooth-Supported Overdenture Classification According to Types

1. Temporary TSO.
2. Transition or interim TSO.
3. Immediate TSO.
4. Permanent TSO.

Their purpose is determined based on the prognosis of the remaining teeth. Through its concept, TSO offers a flexible solution.

1.6.1.1 Temporary TSO

Temporary TSO can be used if the patient already uses a removable partial denture. Temporary TSO is applied through the modification of the removable partial denture after the reduction of the teeth by covering the roots.

1.6.1.2 Transition or Interim TSO

It is a conservative approach, which allows the clinicians to apply a tooth-supported OD before CCD. This denture type offers flexibility while planning the treatment to meet the changing needs of patients. Transition TSO is easily converted to CCD after using weakened teeth/roots as abutments for a specified period. It allows the patient to adapt to the new posterior dentition and the maxilla to the closure of the palate. Adaptation also includes speech, mastication, and swallowing of the patient.

1.6.1.3 Immediate TSO

Immediate dentures are fabricated immediately following the extraction of the natural teeth and the other necessary surgical procedures. The prosthesis may even be a modification of the existing one. In this type of treatment option, which is one of the most common treatment options, retaining the root of one tooth or more teeth for overdenture offers patients advantages such as improved stability, better proprioception, and a feeling of naturalness. Unfortunately, the state of complete edentulism is inevitable for immediate TSO patients, so the principle of immediate TSO is to delay this inevitable end as long as it is possible.

1.6.1.4 Permanent TSO

This type is called tooth-supported overdenture (with or without coping) or precision retained overdentures (Pictures 1.9, 1.10, 1.11, and 1.12). These dentures can include metal bases and attachments. A metal base increases denture resistance. It is especially recommended for patients who previously broke their dentures, have strong muscle tonus, or have natural teeth or fixed restoration on the opposing arch. Cr-Co is preferred for the maxilla and Type IV gold for the mandible.

1.6.1.5 Tooth-Supported Overdenture Classification According to Supporting Teeth Preparation

TSO Without Coping (Bare Tooth/Root) (Fig. 1.6)

TSO with Coping (Figs. 1.6 and 1.7)
- Short coping.
- Medium coping.
- Long coping.

Attachment-Retained TSO (Fig. 1.8)
1. Attachments directly placed in the root.
2. Attachments used with the coping
   (a) Stud attachment.

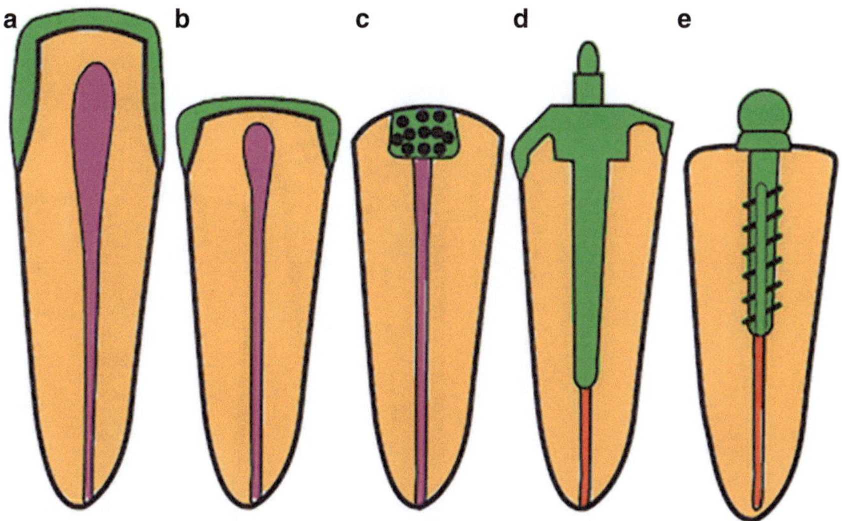

Fig. 1.6 Support/retention tooth types according to restoration type: (**a**) Medium coping (retention), (**b**) short coping (support), (**c**) bare tooth (support), (**d**) attachment with coping (retention), and (**e**) only attachment on prepared teeth (retention)

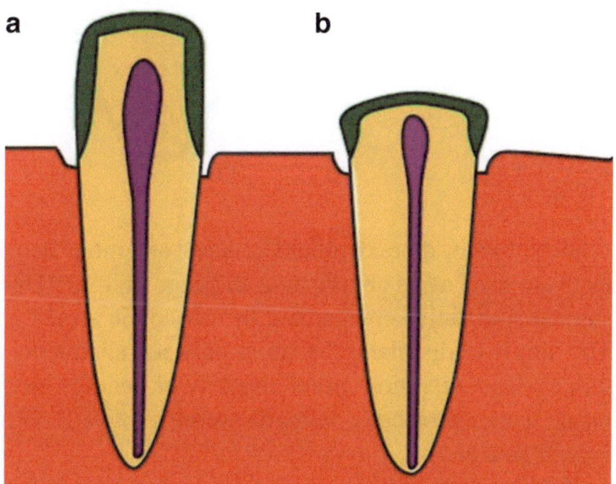

Fig. 1.7 (**a**) Medium coping and (**b**) short coping

(b) Bar attachment.
(c) Magnet attachment.
(d) Telescopic attachment.

1.6.1.6 Tooth-Supported Overdenture Without Coping (Bare Tooth/Root)

Tooth-supported overdenture treatment concept is not a new concept, and clinicians have successfully used weakened tooth/root structures for support for more than a

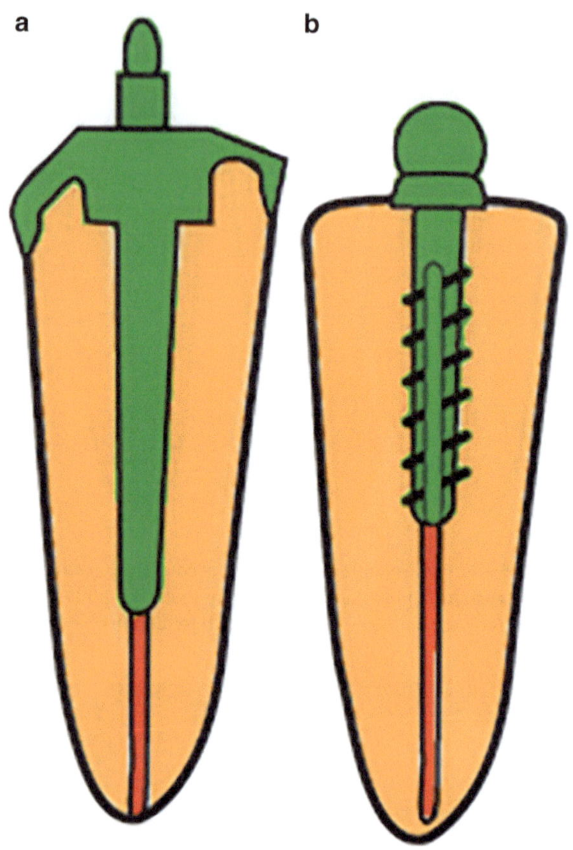

Fig. 1.8 (**a**) Attachment on coping and (**b**) attachment on the root

century. Two or more coronally reduced and more frequently endodontically treated teeth are used as an abutment in this type of TSO. This type of denture is the most suitable alternative considering the economic aspect among the treatment options. The aim is to distribute the stress between abutments and denture-supporting soft tissues. Root retention offers a variety of benefits including alveolar bone maintenance, better prosthetic support, proprioceptive feedback, aesthetics, and psychological benefits.

Supporting teeth's crown height is reduced by 2–3 mm and prepared in a convex or dome form. Endodontic treatment is mostly necessary for these abutments (Fig. 1.9). The shortened crown improves the crown-to-root ratio, thereby decreasing the mobility of the abutment tooth under the TSO. Renner et al. [10] showed that 50% of roots used as TSO abutments remained immobile after 5 years. Also, 25% of roots that were initially mobile became less mobile. They suggested that teeth that are generally compromised can be used for TSO after root canal therapy and coronal reduction.

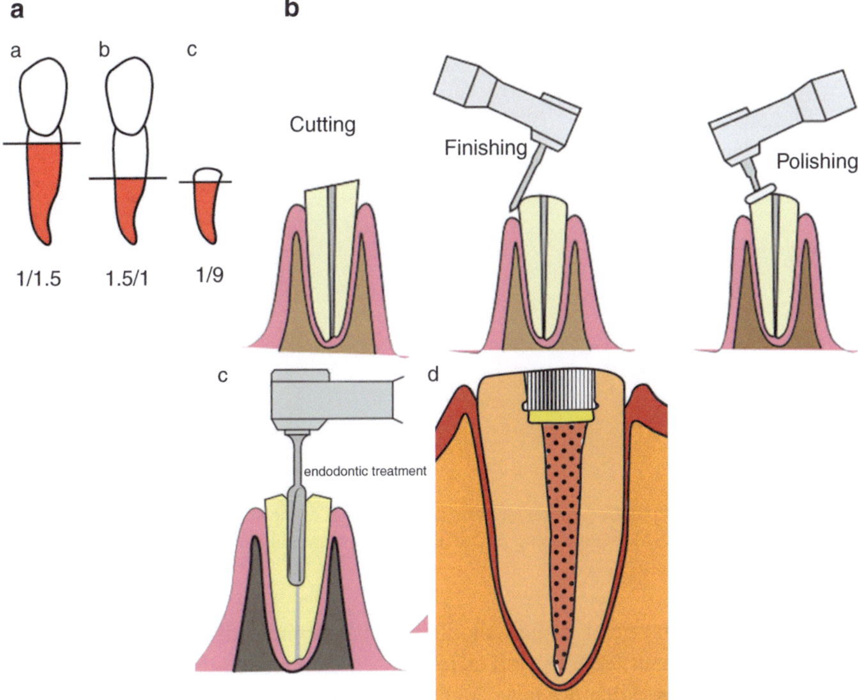

Fig. 1.9 (**a**) The shortened crown improves the crown-root ratio, thereby decreasing the mobility of the abutment teeth under TSO; (**b**) abutment teeth are prepared without coping; (**c**) endodontic treatment; and (**d**) entrance of the pulp cavity is sealed

Indications
- Remaining uncompromised roots
- Elderly patients
- Patients with poor health
- Caries-free roots
- Low caries index
- For transition dentures

Disadvantages
- It provides only stabilization
- Exposed dentin is susceptible to carries

1.6.1.7 Tooth-Supported Overdentures with Coping

While planning this type of TSO, copings made from the metal cast are cemented on the prepared tooth surface. The preparation for the copings can include modifications that are necessary for gaining retention from the tooth. There are three types of copings: short, medium, and long (Figs. 1.6, 1.7, 1.10, 1.11, 1.12 and Pictures 1.4b, 1.13, 1.14, 1.15, 1.16). The preparation of a tooth depends on which type of

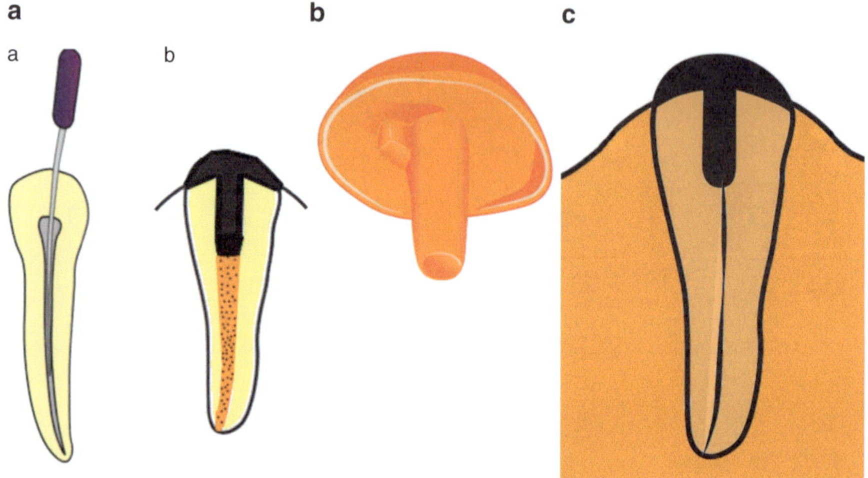

Fig. 1.10 (**a**) Root preparation for endodontic treatment and dome shape coping with post placed on the abutment tooth, (**b**) metal coping post with an anti-rotational element, and (**c**) the cemented dome shape coping in situ

coping is used. The metal coping should provide optimal distribution of loading forces to the abutment teeth as well as to adjacent supporting tissues. A coping for a TSO is covered by a denture base, and the placement of a crown margin does not have any importance for aesthetic reasons. The decision on the placement of the TSO coping should be made in terms of providing retention, stability, adequate height for prosthesis, and providing an optimal cleansing area in order to prevent caries and maintain periodontal health.

In general, it is proposed to use precious alloys (primarily Au-Cu, and possibly Au-Pt alloys and other metals), but for economic reasons, semi-precious alloys (Ag-Pd) or non-precious alloys are acceptable as an alternative.

In cases with limited interarch space, reinforcement of the denture base with a metal framework would be useful to prevent denture fracture due to the reduced thickness of acrylic resin. Thus, stress, concentrated in the midline of the denture and around the copings, was reduced and functional rigidity was improved. Furthermore, the occlusal stress to the underlying denture-bearing areas was distributed evenly.

Advantages
- Retains roots and conserves bone
- Remaining teeth/roots provide support (often retention)
- Better stability

It is cheaper than the attachment-retained TSO.

Fig. 1.11 Coronal preparation is made less on supporting teeth for the long coping

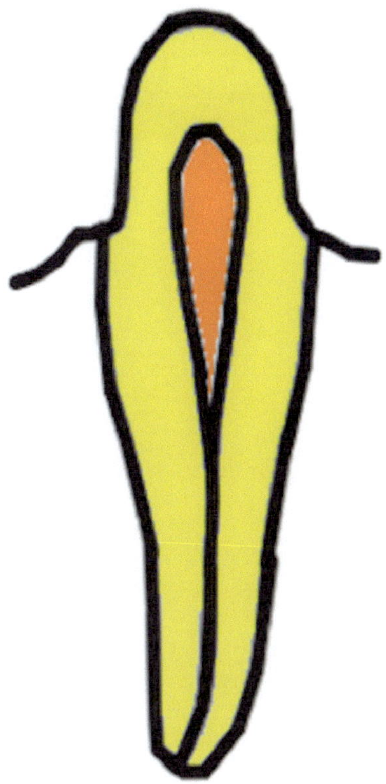

Disadvantages

- Retention is not stable
- The prosthesis can be bulky and less aesthetic than the attachment-retained TSO
- Short copings provide minimal retention
- Only friction type of retention exists
- Long or medium copings cannot be used when the vertical dimension is limited

Fig. 1.12 Tapered metal coping

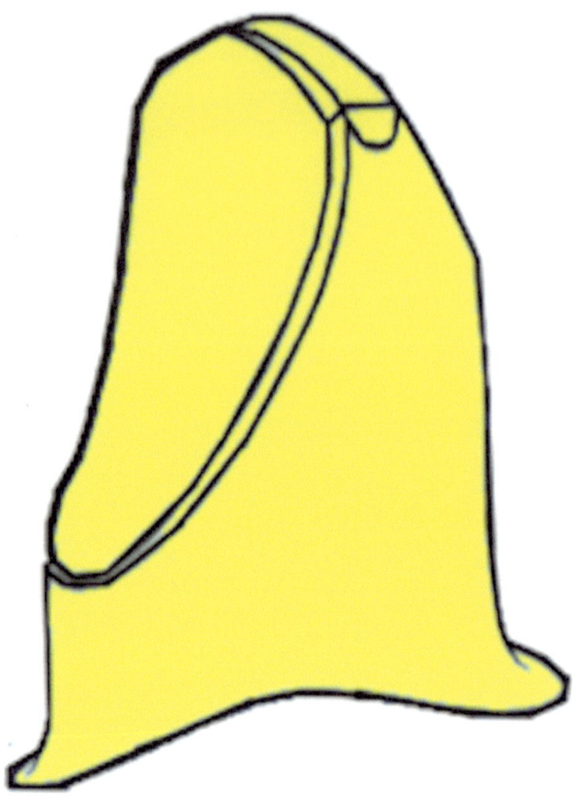

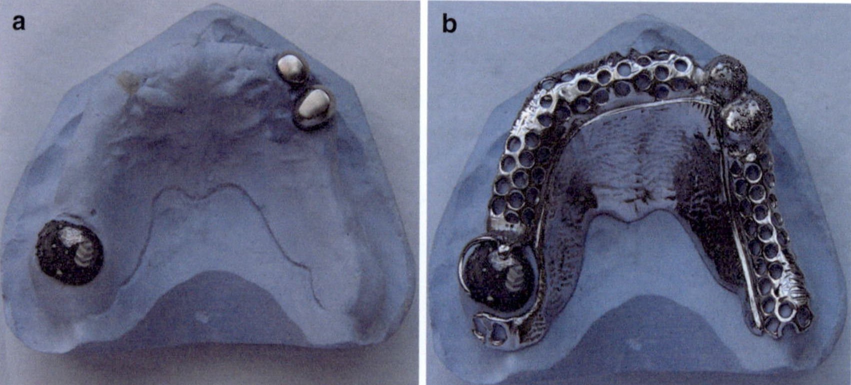

Picture 1.13 Coping for TSO: (**a**) Primary coping (medium copings) and (**b**) the metal framework over the copings on the model

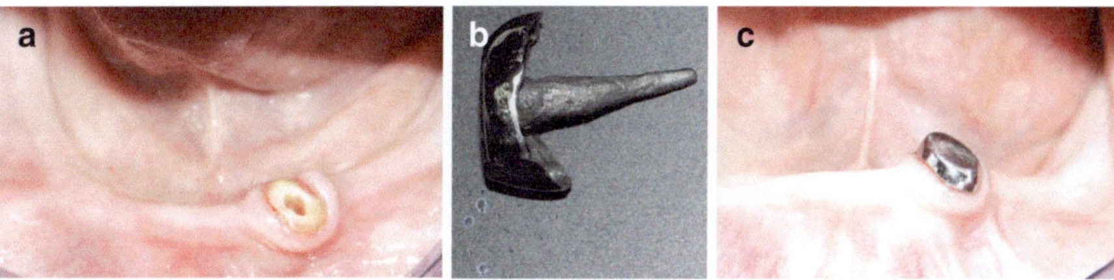

Picture 1.14 Short copings. (**a**) Tooth and post preparation for short copings, (**b**) short copings with post, and (**c**) short coping cemented on the abutment tooth

Picture 1.15 Medium copings on the model

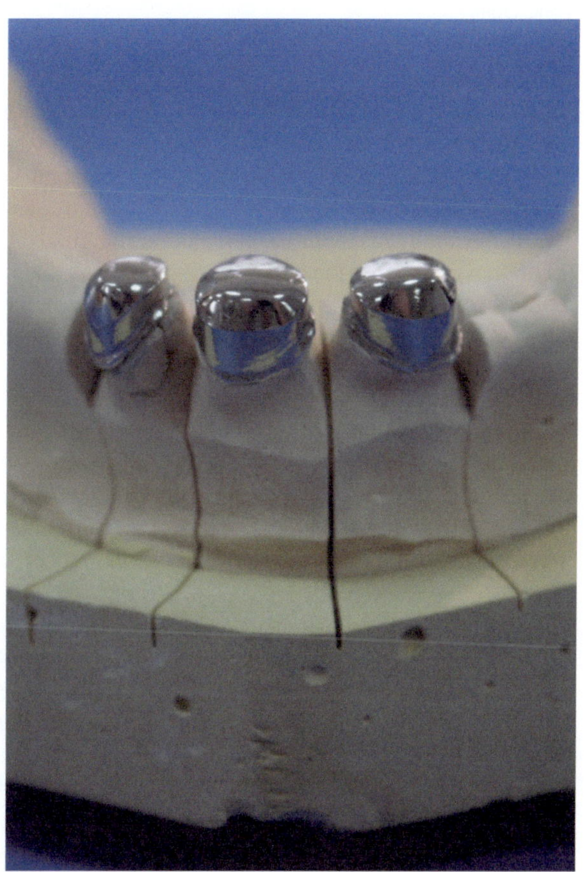

- The failures of root copings are considered as complications, such as gingival deterioration (periodontal pocketing, gross gingival recession, gingival proliferation); root caries; tooth mobility (functional, periodontal); and decementation of coping (Picture 1.5).

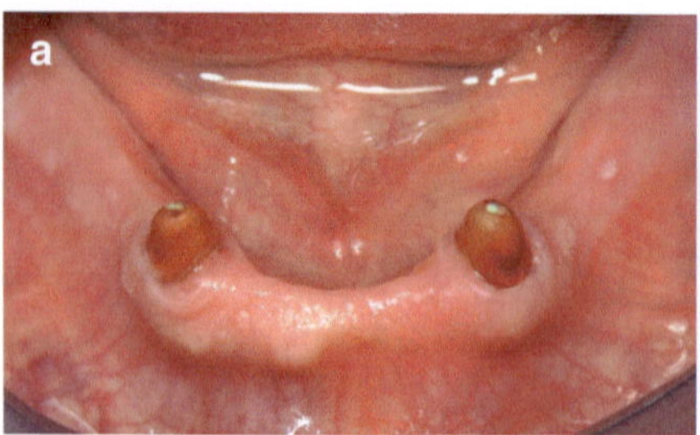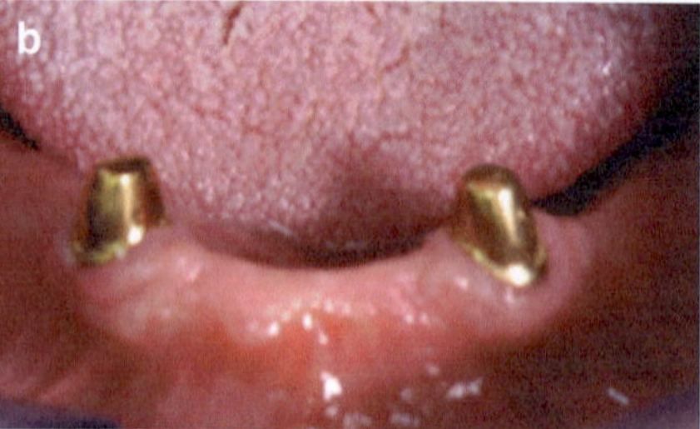

Picture 1.16 Long coping (telescopic coping). (**a**) Tooth preparation and (**b**) gold telescopic coping

Short Coping

Short copings are 2–3 mm in length and should be in dome form (Figs. 1.6, 1.7, and 1.10; Picture 1.14). Since coronal tooth reduction can expose the pulp, it usually needs endodontic treatment. Short copings transmit the mastication forces to the periodontium, increase the stability of the denture, and have little effect on retention. If the abutment tooth is shortened to the gingival level, problems concerning retention will occur in the coping during insertion and removal of the denture due to shortness of coping. It is more convenient for these copings to be used with a post. The short coping is indicated if the vertical dimension is inadequate, and the tooth is going to be used as a supporting element.

Medium Coping

Generally, 4–6 mm length cast copings are used on the abutment teeth. Coronal preparation is done less on the supporting teeth, and a long ellipsoid-shaped coping is obtained (Fig. 1.11). Through this design, a significant improvement is achieved concerning retention and support from the abutment teeth (Picture 1.15).

Long Coping

The height of long copings is between 6 and 8 mm. The tapered angle of long copings should not exceed six degrees. These copings are generally used in vital teeth with an excellent periodontal condition (Fig. 1.12 and Picture 1.16) for telescopic TSO.

The copings should be resisted to vertical and rotational movement and show resistance in order to prevent root fracture.

References

1. Crum RJ, Rooney GE Jr. Alveolar bone loss in overdentures: a 5-year study. J Prosthet Dent. 1978;40:610–3.
2. Van Waas MA, Jonkman RE, Kalk W, Van't Hof MA, Plooij J, Van Os JH. Differences two years after tooth extraction in a mandibular bone reduction in patients treated with immediate TSO or with immediate CDs. J Dent Res. 1993;72:1001–4.4.

3. Mericske-Stern R, Steinlin Schaffner T, Marti P, Geering AH. Peri-implant mucosal aspects of ITI implants supporting overdentures. A five-year longitudinal study. Clin Oral Implants Res. 1994;5:9–18.
4. Morais JA, Heydecke G, Pawliuk J, Lund JP, Feine JS. The effects of mandibular two-implant overdentures on nutrition in elderly edentulous individuals. J Dent Res. 2003;82:53–5.
5. Tallgren A. The continuing reduction of the residual alveolar ridges in complete denture wearers: A mixed-longitudinal study covering 25 years. J of Prosthet Dent. 1972;27:120–32. https://doi.org/10.1016/0022-3913(72)90188-6.
6. Sposetti VJ, Gibbs CH, Alderson TH, Jaggers JH, Richmond A, Conlon M, et al. Bite force and muscle activity in overdenture wearers before and after attachment placement. J Prosthet Dent. 1986;55:265–73.
7. Enkling N, Heussner S, Nicolay C, Bayer S, Mericske-Stern R, Utz KH. Tactile sensibility of single-tooth implants and natural teeth under local anesthesia of the natural antagonistic teeth. Clin Implant Dent Relat Res. 2012;14:273–80. https://doi.org/10.1111/j.1708-8208.2009.00252.x.
8. Pacer FJ, Bowman C. Occlusal force discrimination by denture patients. J Prosthet Dent. 1975;33:602–9.
9. Fenton AH. The decade of overdentures: 1970–1980. J Prosthet Dent. 1998;79:31–6.
10. Renner RP, Gomes BC, Shakun ML, Baer PN, Davis RK, Camp P. Four-year longitudinal study of the periodontal health status of overdenture patients. J Prosthet Dent. 1984;52:593–8.

Further Reading

Allen PF, McKenna G, Creugers N. Prosthodontic care for elderly patients. Dent Update. 2011;38:460–2.
Awed MA, Lund JP, Dufresne E, Feine JS. Comparing the efficacy of mandibular implant-retained overdenture and conventional dentures among middle-aged edentulous patients: satisfaction and functional assessment. Int J Prosthodont. 2003;16:117–22.
Bassi F. Comparing overdenture therapies with teeth and implant abutments. Int J Prosthodont. 2009;22:527–8.
Brewer AA, Morrow RM. Overdentures made easy. 2nd ed. St. Louis, MO: CV Mosby Co; 1980.
Brill N. Adaptation and the hybrid prosthesis. J Prosthet Dent. 1955;5:811–24.
Carlson GE. Implant and root supported overdenture – a literature review and some data on bone loss in edentulous jaws. J Adv Prosthodont. 2014;6:245–52.
Chao YL, Meijer HJ, Van Oort RP, Versteegh PA. The incomprehensible success of the implant stabilized overdenture in the edentulous mandible: a literature review on the transfer of chewing forces to the bone surrounding implants. Eur J Prosthodont Restor Dent. 1995;3:255–61.
Chikunov I, Doan P, Vahidi F. Implant-retained partial overdenture with resilient attachments. J Prosthodont. 2008;17:141–8.
Dong J, Ikebe K, Gonda T, Nokubi T. İnfluence of abutment height on strain in a mandibular overdenture. J Oral Rehabil. 2006;33:594–9.
Doundoulakis JH, Eckert SE, Lindquist CC, Jeffcoat MK. The implant-supported overdenture is an alternative to the complete mandibular denture. JADA. 2003;134:1455–8.
Ettinger RL, Jakobsen JR. A Comparison of patient satisfaction and dentist evaluation of overdenture therapy. Community Dent Oral Epidemiol. 1997;25:223–7.
Alfred GH, Kundert M, Charles KC. Complete denture and overdenture prosthetic. New York: Thieme Medical Publishers Inc.; 1993.
Jacobs R, van Steenberghe D. Role of periodontal ligament receptors in the tactile function of teeth: a review. J Periodontal Res. 1994;29:153–67.
Klineberg I, Murray G. Osseoperception: sensory function and proprioception. Adv Dent Res. 1999;13:120–9.

Krawczykowska H, Panek H. Applying the overdentures in the geriatric patients with residual and reduced dentition. Dent Med Prob. 2004;41:255–61.

Lord JI, Teel S. The tooth-supported overdenture. Dent Clin N Am. 1969;13:871–8.

Meijer HJ, Raghoebar GM, van't Hof MA, Geertman ME, van Oort RP. Implant-retained mandibular overdenture compared with complete dentures: a 5-years follow-up of clinical aspects and patient satisfaction. Clin Oral Implants Res. 1999;10:238–44.

Menicucci G, Lorenzetti M, Pera P, Preti G. Mandibular implant-retained overdenture a clinical trial of two anchorage systems. Int J Oral Maxillofac Implants. 1998;13:851–6.

Mericske-Stern R, Piotti M, Sirtes G. 3-D in vivo force measurements on mandibular implants supporting overdenture. Clin Oral Implants Res. 1996;7:387–96.

Morrow RM, Feldman EE, Rudd KD, Torvillion HM. Tooth-Supported complete dentures: an approach to preventive prosthodontics. J Prosthet Dent. 1969;21:513–22.

Pavlatos J. Root-supported TSO. CDS Rev. 1998;91:20–5.

Preiskel HW. TSO made easy: A guide to implant and root supported prostheses, vol. 1. Berlin: Quintessence Publishing; 1996. p. 38–56.

Quirynen M, Naert I, van Steenberghe D, Dekeyser C, Callens A. Periodontal aspects of osseo-integrated fixtures supporting a partial bridge. An up to 6-years retrospective study. J Clin Periodontol. 1992;19:118–26.

Rissin L, House JE, Manly R, Kapur K. Clinical comparison of masticatory performance and electromyographic activity of patients with Complete Dentures, overdentures and natural teeth. J Prosthet Dent. 1978;39:508–11.

Rutkunas V, Mizutani A, Takahashi H. Wear simulation effects on TSO stud attachments. Dent Mater J. 2011;30:845–53.

Rutkunas V, Mizutani H, Takahashi H. Evaluation of stable retentive properties of TSO attachments. Baltic Dent Maxillofac J. 2005;7:115–20.

Sadowsky SJ, Caputo AA. Effect of anchorage systems and extension base contact on load transfer with mandibular implant-retained TSO. J Prosthet Dent. 2000;84:327–33.

Samra RK, Bhide SV, Goyal C, Kaur T. Tooth supported TSO: a concept overshadowed but not yet forgotten! J Oral Res Rev. 2015;7:16–21.

Schuch C, Pinheiro de Moraes A, Onofre RS, Cenci TP, Boscato N. An alternative method for the fabrication of a root-supported TSO: a clinical report. J Prosthet Dent. 2013;109:1–4.

Shah FK, Gabriel A, Elshokouki A, Habib AA, Porwal A. Comparison of the immediate CD, tooth and implant-supported TSO on vertical dimension and muscle activity. J Adv Prosthodont. 2012;4:61–71.

Tallagren A. The continuing reduction of the residual alveolar ridges in CD wearers: a mixed-longitudinal study covering 25 years. 1972. J Prosthet Dent. 2003;89:427–35. https://doi.org/10.1016/0022-3913(72)90188-6.

Thayer HH, Caputo AA. Occlusal force transmission by TSO attachments. J Prosthet Dent. 1979;41:266–71.

Trulsson M. Sensory and motor function of teeth and dental implants: a basis for osseoperception. Clin Exp Pharmacol Physiol. 2005;32:119–22.

Attachment-Retained Overdentures

2

Yasemin Ozkan and Rifat Gozneli

2.1 Attachment-Retained Overdentures

Attachment-retained overdentures help in the distribution of masticatory forces, minimize trauma to abutments and soft tissues, attenuate ridge resorption, improve aesthetics, and retain proprioception. Overdenture attachments have similar functions to conventional clasps in removable partial dentures. Attachment in tooth-supported overdenture (TSO) is generally used by directly placing it in the root or used with the coping (Figs. 2.1, 2.2, 2.3, 2.4, 2.5, 2.6, 2.7, 2.8, 2.9, and 2.10, Pictures 2.1, 2.2, and 2.3).

Attachments should provide:

- More aesthetically pleasing outcomes
- Stability and ease of use
- Alveolar bone preservation
- Proprioception
- Psychological satisfaction
- Improved chewing efficiency
- However, to use this type of attachment system, the patient must provide;
- Low carries risk
- Increased hygiene
- Excellent periodontal health

Y. Ozkan (✉) · R. Gozneli
Faculty of Dentistry, Department of Prosthodontics, Marmara University, Istanbul, Turkey
e-mail: ykozkan@marmara.edu.tr

© The Author(s), under exclusive license to Springer Nature Switzerland AG 2023
Y. Özkan (ed.), *Treatment Options Before and After Edentulism*,
https://doi.org/10.1007/978-3-031-37582-8_2

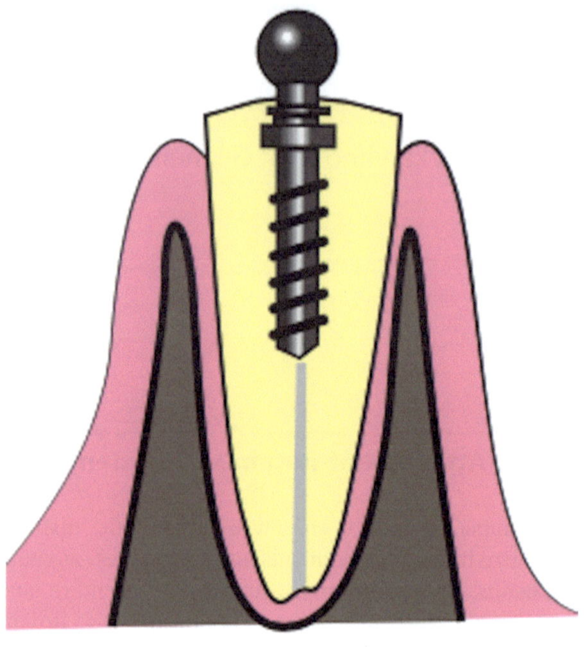

Fig. 2.1 Direct attachments placed on the root

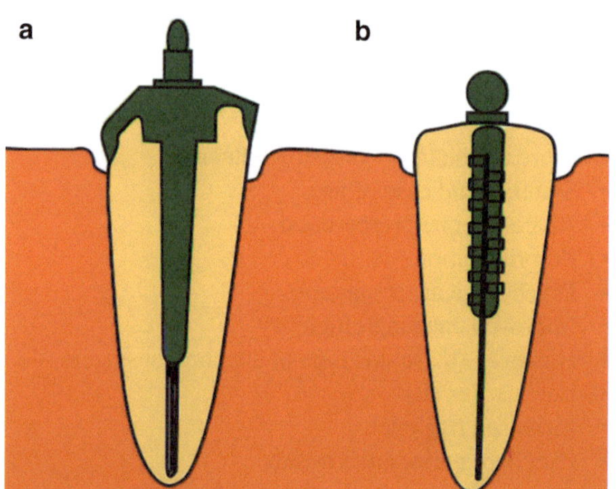

Fig. 2.2 (**a**) Attachments placed on copings, (**b**) attachments placed on the root

2.1.1 Advantages of Attachments

Bone loss is prevented by the supporting root.
Caries is prevented by coping coverage.
Splinting can be used to strengthen weak abutments.
The level of retention can be changed.
The attachments can bear extra forces and change the direction of the load due to their ability to increase retention.

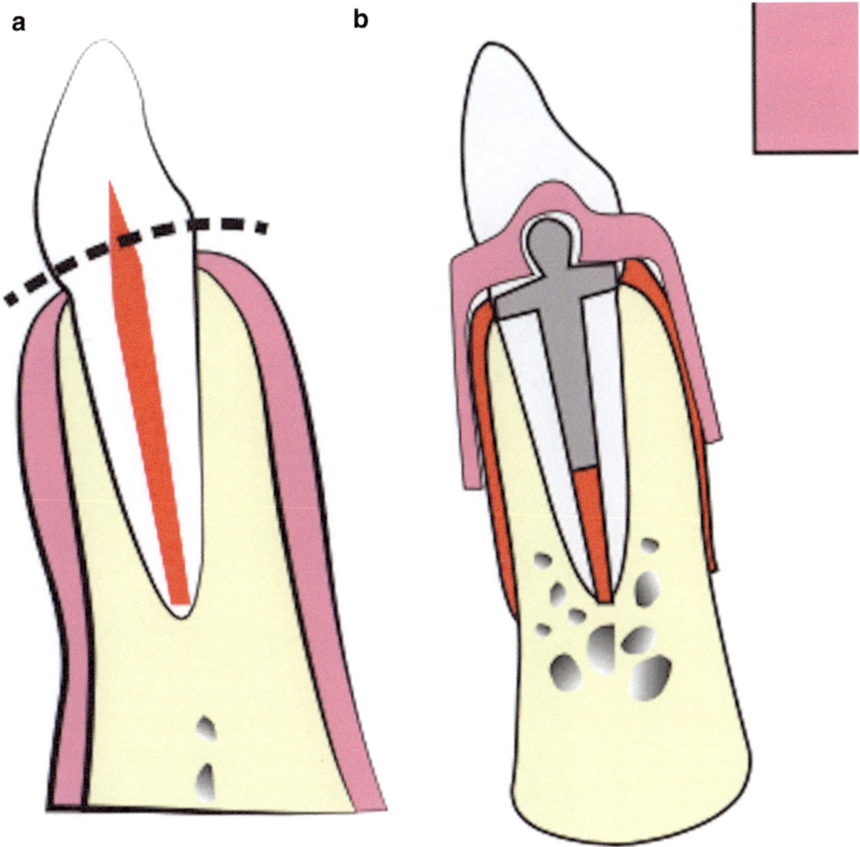

Fig. 2.3 (**a**) Tooth reduction is important for decreasing the leverage ratio, (**b**) the attachment casting with coping

The attachments exhibit rigid or resilient characters
Enhances the aesthetic
Improves patient acceptability and comfort
Improved force distribution between the abutment and soft tissues

2.1.2   Disadvantages of Attachments

Extends the chair time
Extra forces on the supporting tooth may result.
More difficult to manipulate and necessitates patient caution.
Repairing the denture is difficult.
Difficult to maintain oral hygiene (poor oral hygiene may increase the risk of periodontal disease and caries)

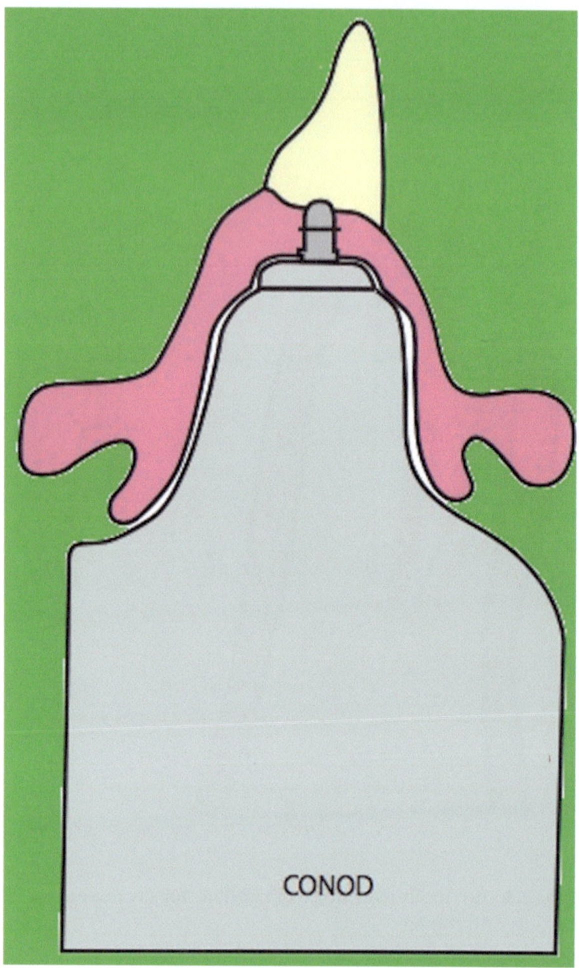

Fig. 2.4 The Conod attachment

More expensive than copings

Repair may be required regardless of the type of attachment used.

Because the height of some attachments is long and requires enough interarch space to avoid aesthetic issues

Manipulation is difficult for patients who are mentally and physically disabled.

The repair and maintenance should be difficult compared to the simple TSO

Fig. 2.5 The Gerber attachment

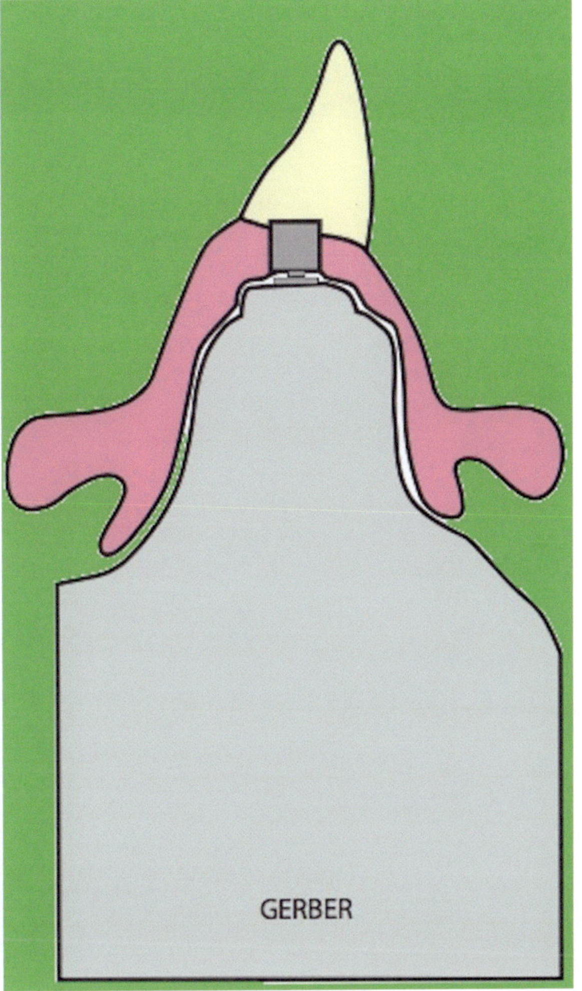

Fig. 2.6 The Ball attachment

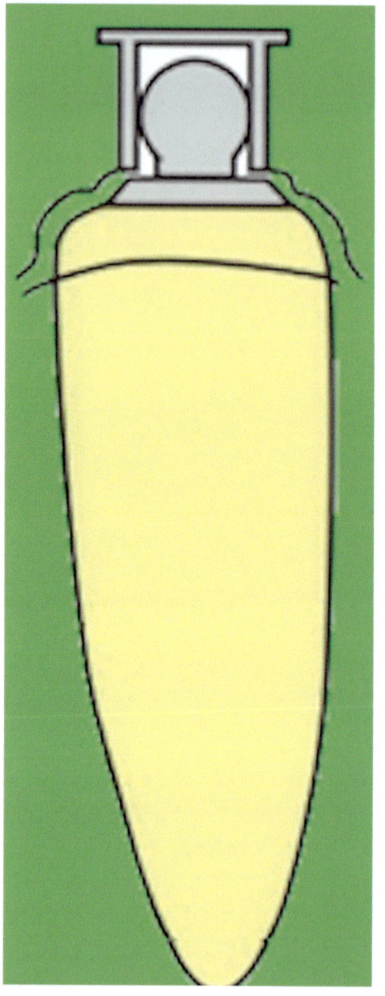

Fig. 2.7 The Locator attachment

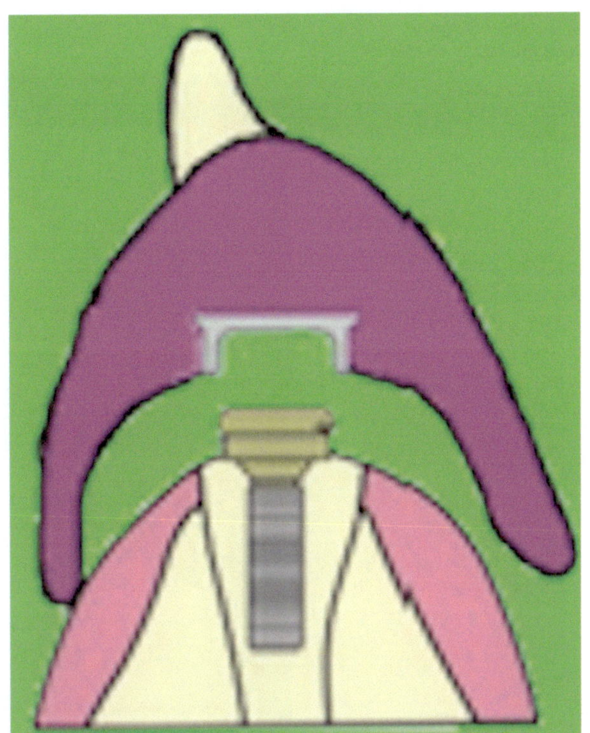

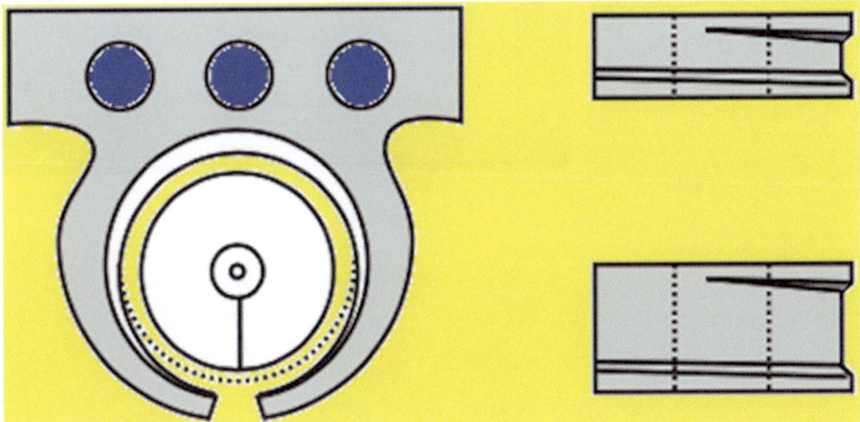

Fig. 2.8 The Rothermann attachment

Fig. 2.9 The Zest attachment

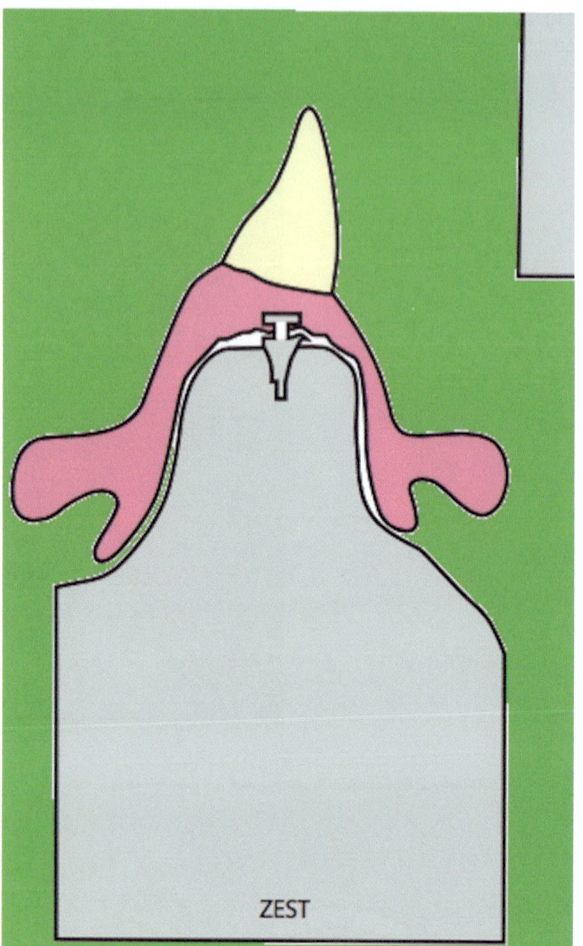

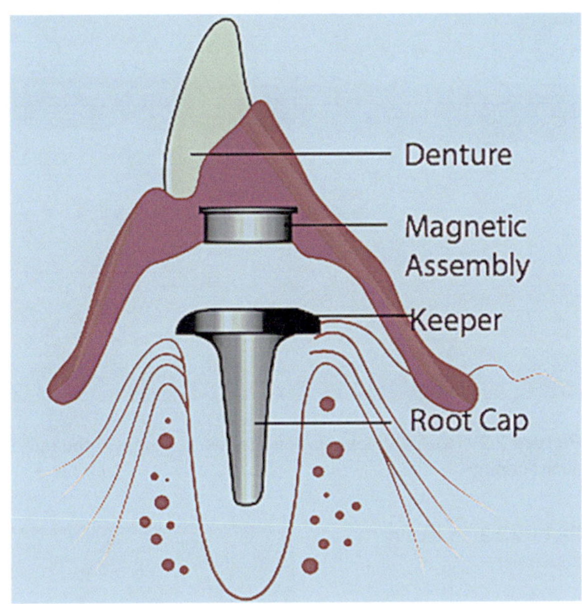

Fig. 2.10 The Magnetic attachments

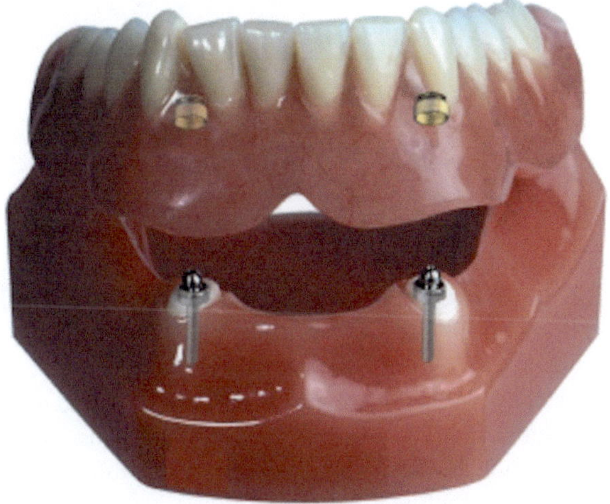

Picture 2.1 An attachment directly placed in the root canal without using a coping

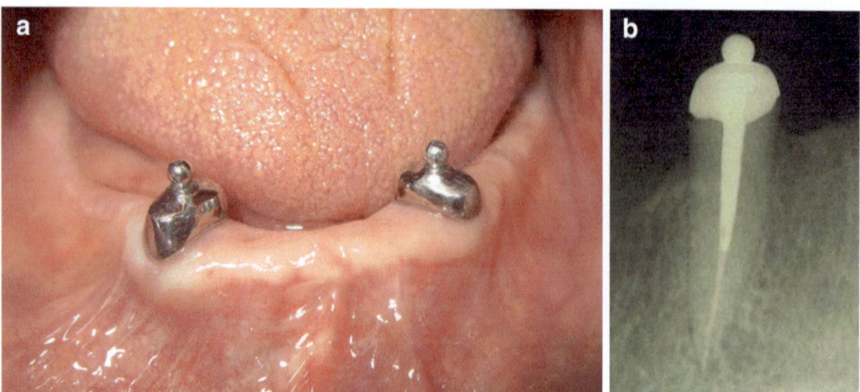

Picture 2.2 (**a**) An attachment on the cast coping, (**b**) the radiologic view of an attachment with a cast coping

Picture 2.3 A locator attachment

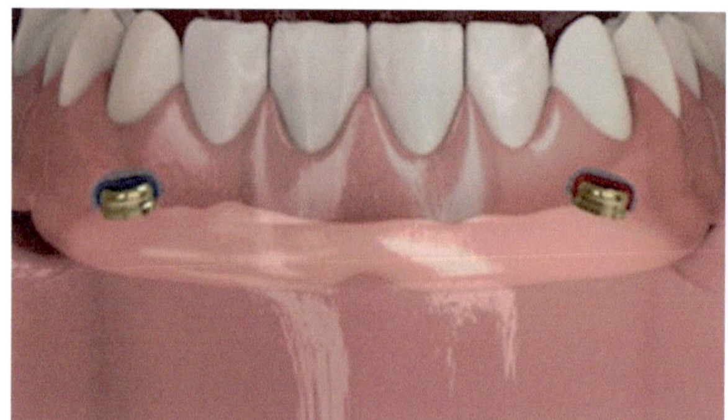

2.2 Attachments Inserted Directly into the Root Canal

These attachments are directly attached to the tooth or the root to improve retention and stability. When teeth are devitalized and used as abutments, periodontal fibers transmit occlusal forces to the underlying bone structure, stimulating periodontal regeneration and bone repair and reducing or delaying alveolar bone loss (Figs. 2.1, 2.2, and 2.3; Picture 2.1).

2.3 Attachments Placed on Copings

Attachments can also be used to add retention to the cast copings. Attachments must be precisely positioned on the coping casting. Before deciding to use this system, the interarch space should be determined. The diagnosing casts should be mounted on the articulator, and the attachment's appropriate height should be determined.

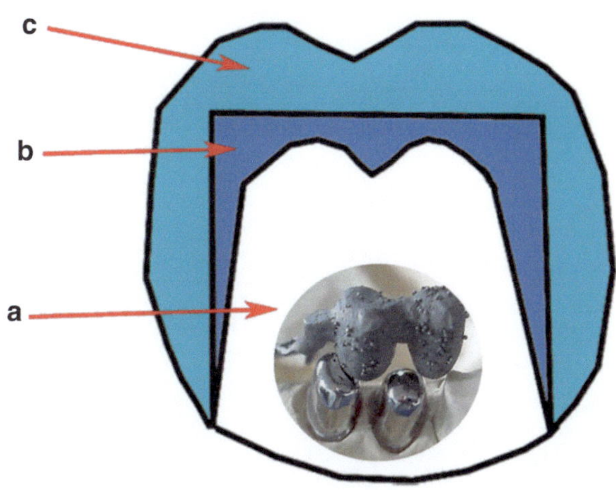

Fig. 2.11 The telescopic crown. (**a**) prepared tooth, (**b**) telescopic cap, (**c**) crown

These extra components complicate the design of the prosthesis and raise the treatment cost (Figs. 2.2 and 2.3; Picture 2.2).

Overdenture attachments are typically composed of two major components: female and male parts. There are various attachment designs available, including studs (ball and O-ring), bar and clip, magnet, and telescopic crown attachments (Figs. 2.4, 2.5, 2.6, 2.7, 2.8, 2.9, 2.10, 2.11, 2.12, 2.13, 2.14, 2.15, 2.16, 2.17, 2.18, and 2.19).

When choosing the appropriate attachment, the leverage ratio should be considered. When the leverage ratio is already high, it is critical to use a low-profile attachment system to avoid significantly increasing the leverage ratio (Fig. 2.3).

Even though the majority of overdenture cases have a small interarch distance, the availability of vertical space frequently indicates the appropriate attachment system. Because of the reduced vertical dimension, choosing high attachment systems is usually limited. The interarch distance should be sufficient for both the attachment height and the denture thickness when selecting the appropriate size for the attachment. However, a common mistake made in the clinic is to only check if the vertical space is sufficient for the attachment itself when there is also supposed to be extra space for the final denture thickness.

When using multiple attachments in an arch, choose attachments with an easy path of insertion. Many patients are unable to manipulate the complex path of insertion created by various attachments in an arch during denture insertion and removal. Because most attachment wear occurs during denture insertion and removal, designing an easy path of insertion will reduce the potential wear of the attachment selected.

The attachment retention should be kept to a minimum when an overdenture is delivered. The retention may be increased when the patient is comfortable with the denture and has experience with the path of insertion and removal. As a general rule, give patients no more retention than they request. When only one or two attachments are used in an arch, it is critical to choose attachments with higher retention.

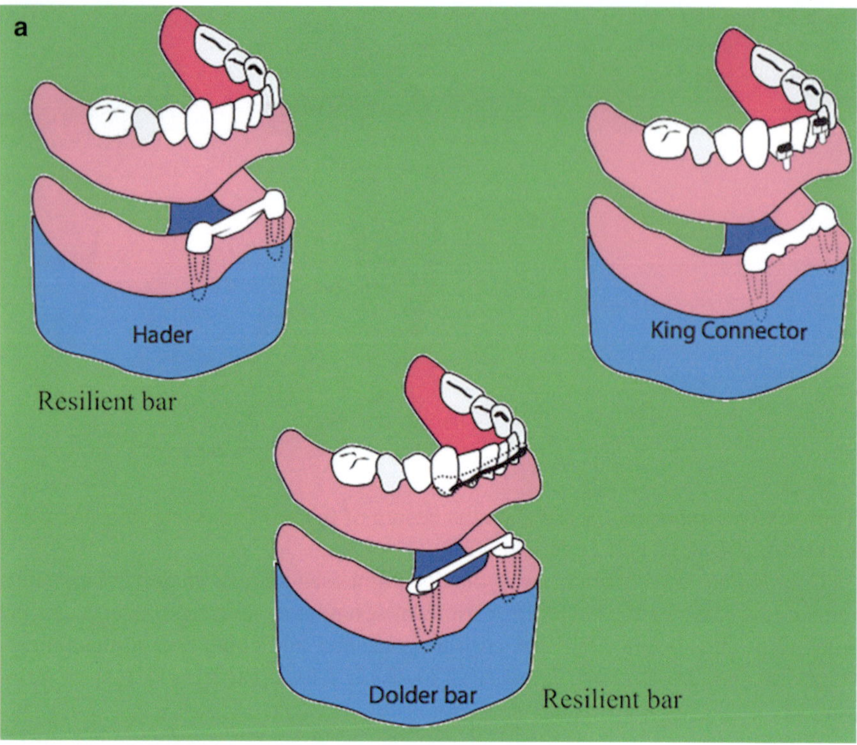

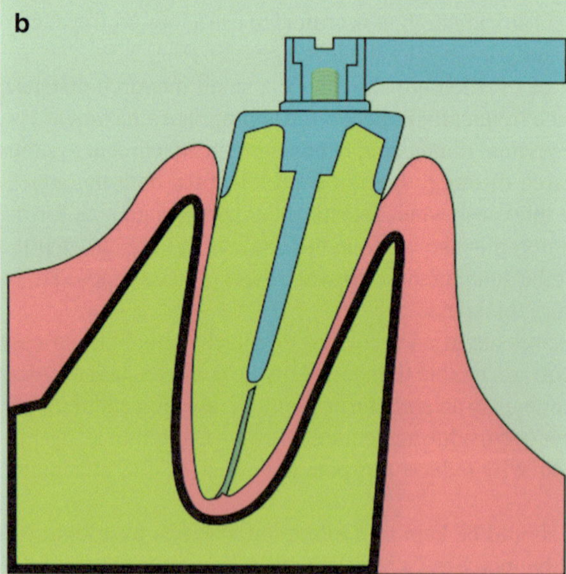

Fig. 2.12 (**a**) The bar attachments. (**b**) The Schubiger screw block system

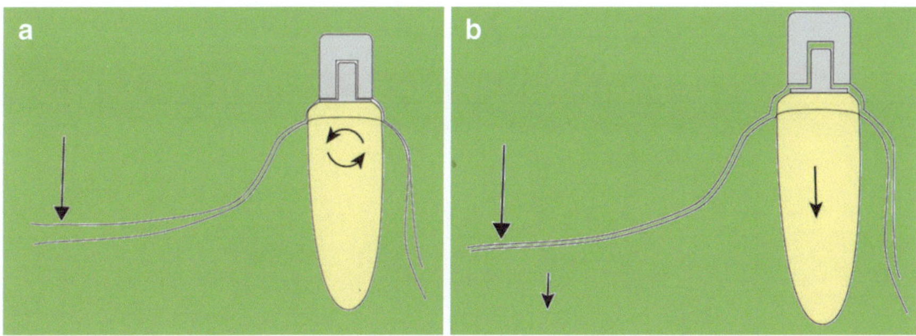

Fig. 2.13 (**a**, **b**) The theoretical concept of resilient design. The movement of dentures when using resilient attachment

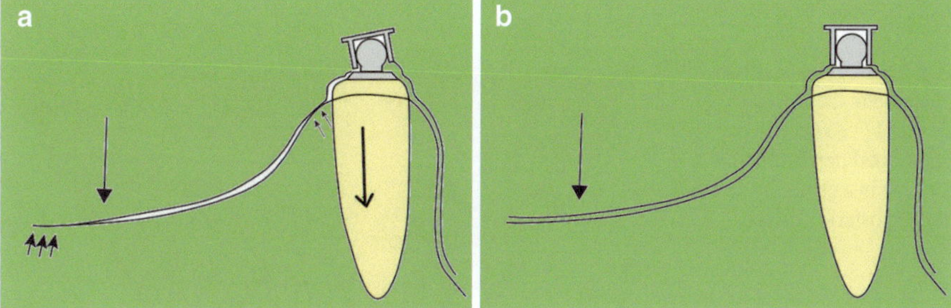

Fig. 2.14 (**a**) The effect on the abutment and tissues of a purely rotational attachment under load, (**b**) resilient design allows more even distribution of forces

Fig. 2.15 Magnetic attachment adjacent to a free end saddle under load

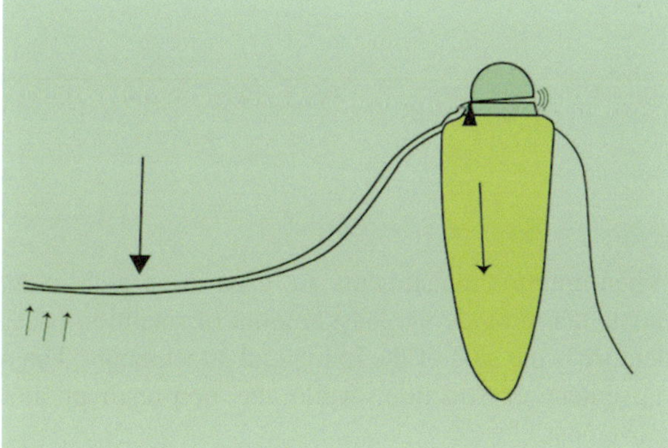

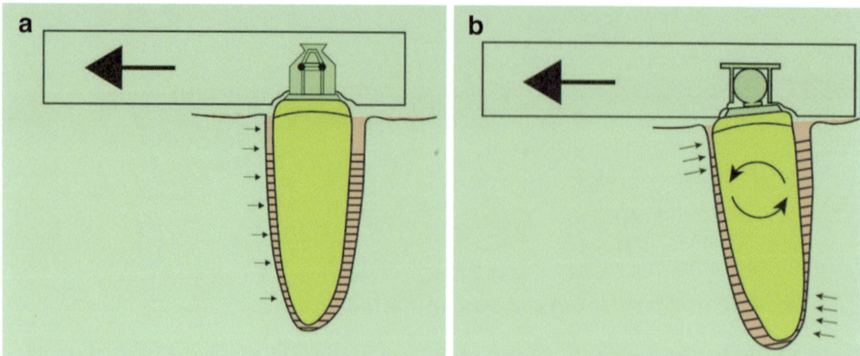

Fig. 2.16 (**a**) The effect of horizontal loading on abutment with cylindrical attachment. (**b**) The effect of horizontal loading on abutment with Ball attachment

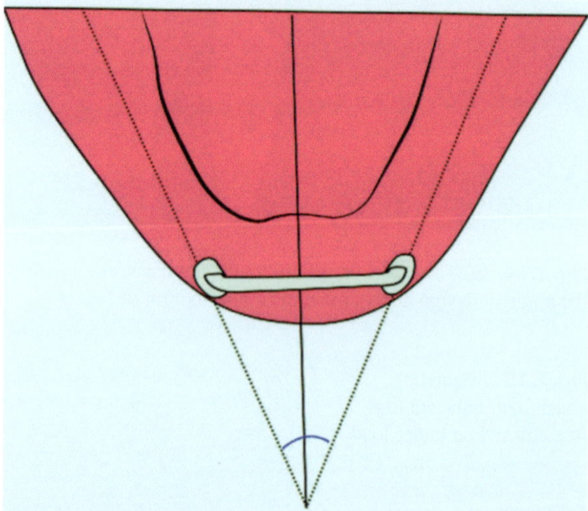

Fig. 2.17 The ideal bar placement according to Prieskel (1967). The bar is positioned perpendicular to the line bisecting the angle at the posterior ridges

When multiple attachments are used in an arch, clinicians should choose attachments that provide the least amount of retention because the total retention of the denture is the sum of the individual attachments. The resilient attachments provide movement or function, while the non-resilient attachments offer little or no movement.

Fig. 2.18 The magnetic attachment system for root

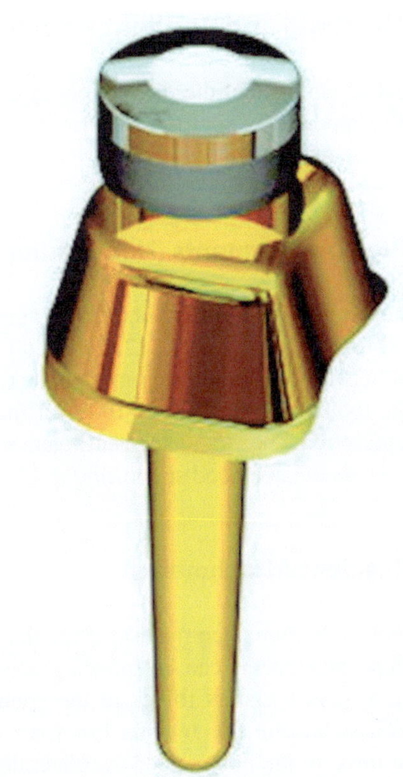

Fig. 2.19 Alloys used for fabricated overdenture attachment

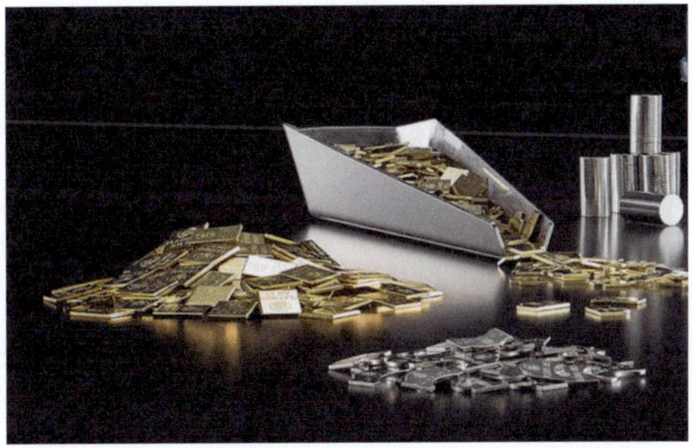

2.4   The Rigid and Resilient Attachment Concepts

It is critical to understand the distinctions between rigid and resilient restoration. Only tooth-supported restorations are rigid, whereas tooth- and tissue-supported restorations are resilient.

2.4.1   Rigid Attachments (Non-resilient)

Vertical movement is not permitted by rigid attachments used in removable bridges and TSO (Figs. 2.4, 2.5, 2.11, 2.12, 2.13, and 2.16a). These attachments prevent movement between the supporting tooth and the denture. When a rigid attachment is used, the tooth/implant receives 100% of the mastication forces. These attachments are preferred when there are a sufficient number of supporting teeth/implants and when the teeth have good supporting quality.

2.4.2   Resilient Attachments

The concept of resilience compensates for the effects of vertical loads. Dentures with resilient attachments can be moved precisely. The movement amount in the attachment system transfers forces to the edentulous crest along with the teeth/implants. These attachments transfer less force to the supporting tooth and a large part of the force to the bone under the edentulous mucosa. These attachments are usually used when only a few weak abutments are remaining, or tissue support is required (Figs. 2.6, 2.7, 2.8, 2.9, 2.10, 2.12, 2.14, 2.15, 2.16b, and 2.18).

The movements of resilient attachment are as follows:

2.4.2.1 Vertical Movement
It is the movement of the denture toward the mucosal tissue. The denture can only move upward and downward. The movement stops when the denture gets into contact with the crest and exceeds the soft tissue resilience. Typically, the movement stops with the supporting feature of the residual crest. In attachment systems with limited vertical flexibility, while 5–10% of mastication forces are provided by supporting tissues, the remaining forces are directly transmitted onto the teeth/implants. The locator-type attachment can be given as an example (Fig. 2.7, Picture 2.3).

2.4.2.2 Hinge Movement
The denture makes a hinge movement around an axis between the most posterior attachments on both sides of the arch. Hinge-resilient attachments show resistance to lateral, rotational, and sliding forces and provide 30–35% force relief in supporting teeth/implants. When a resilient hinge attachment uses vertical components of the mastication forces shared among attachments and posterior parts of the residual crest such as the buccal shelf and retromolar areas, the Hader bar or round section bars provide hinge resilience movement (Fig. 2.12).

2.4.2.3 Combination Movement

The denture moves in combination with all the movements mentioned above. The attachment systems with combination resilience allow for unlimited hinge and vertical movements. They transmit all the vertical loads of the mastication uniform to the residual crest. When this kind of attachment is used, the tissue support from the denture during mastication increases. Irrespective of the position of the mastication force on the denture, the vertical component of the force is transmitted to the crest. These attachments provide 45–55% force relief in supporting the teeth/implants. The Dolder bar (egg section) is an example of this kind of attachment (Fig. 2.12).

2.4.2.4 Rotational Movement

Rotation is the movement around the axis in the anterior-posterior direction. When the mastication movement is concentrated on one side, it is the upward movement from the crest on the other side of the denture. These attachments exhibit vertical hinge and rotation movements. They allow the denture to move vertically and in the direction of the hinge and a rotational movement on the sagittal axis. The rotational resilient attachments transfer vertical and horizontal components of mastication forces to the residual crest. The movement of the denture is determined by the location, direction, and intensity of the forces transmitted to the denture. The rotational resilient attachment systems allow for rotation movements, and the forces received by the teeth/implants, reducing 75–85% of forces depending on the intensity of the movement. Some stud (stud coping) attachments have rotary resilience (Fig. 2.6, Picture 2.2).

2.4.2.5 Translation Movement

The movement of the denture in the buccal-lingual direction without rotation is referred to as translation.

2.4.2.6 Universal Movement

This attachment system allows for movement in all directions. Vertical hinge, translation, and rotation movements are demonstrated by these attachments. The attachments merely prevent the denture from moving away from the tissues. These attachments provide 95% force relief in supporting the teeth/implants. Magnetic attachments are the most common type of universal resilient attachment (Fig. 2.10).

2.5 The Vertical Load Behavior of a Resilient and Rigid Attachment Design

The resilient attachment, in theory, allows the denture to be supported equally by the tissues and the abutments (Fig. 2.13a, b). Most resilient attachments provide approximately 0.4 mm vertical translation (Fig. 2.13b). The Rothermann attachment has a thickness of 0.6 mm, while the Dalla Bona attachment has a thickness of 0.8 mm. The Gerber and Dalla Bona attachments provide a returning steel spring impact and allow for functional loading of the supports under light loads. The aluminum spacer rings adapted to the root surface during movement compensate for the flexibility of tissues and attachments. The Dalla Bona attachment makes use of a double spacer. When compared to teeth, tissues are more compressible (0.5–1 mm). When the denture is inserted, the supporting tooth is subjected to increased load. When a spacer is used, the resilient attachments allow for a vertical movement of 0.4 mm (Fig. 2.14a, b).

The relationship between the denture base and the support is obtained through the lining in this technique, and the denture fits the tissue well.

When the denture is tooth-supported, the attachment has the potential to rotate. It should be noted that when using rotary attachments, the denture base will rotate and torque force will occur on the abutment, and the ideal situation cannot always be maintained. However, the forces generated by a completely rotational allowance are not always favorable.

Thayer and Caputo (1980) [1] used photoelastic stress analysis to investigate various overdenture attachments. Non-attachment design (amalgam plug, dome coping, and coping with an occlusal concavity are examples); extracoronal stud attachments (Ceka, Rothermann, Gerber, and Ancrofix); intracoronal attachment (Zest); and bar attachments are examples (Dolder bar, King connector, and Hader bar). When applying vertical forces, they reported that stud attachments exerted forces on the abutments as designed. The more rigid the attachment, the greater the force. This is also true for the Zest attachment, which demonstrated more torque than the Ancrofix, most likely due to its tight fit in the matrix when the matrix is new. Furthermore, they reported that bar restorations appear to be beneficial due to their splinting effect, but only if they are resilient in design. On vertical loading, the resilient Dolder bar design produces less torque on the teeth than Zest attachments. The same cannot be said for non-resilient designs such as the King connector and, to a lesser extent, the Hader bar, which allows only rotatory movement.

Magnetic attachment with a rounded dome shape of the keeper was preferable for allowing maintenance of the contact during vertical loading. However, in a distinct form, a resilient design magnetic attachment is for the tooth-supported denture, and, thus, the rotatory design may allow the tissue pressure around the abutments (Fig. 2.15).

2.6 Horizontal Load Effects on Attachments

The effect of horizontal forces on the abutments is the main point of consideration in the force distribution analysis. The horizontal loads are transmitted by occlusal forces created in lateral movements and can be the cause of mobility of the abutments. The lateral stabilization of the denture can differ between patients depending on their anatomy as residual crest height and muscle attachment depth. All possible advantages should be taken from the oral structure in a denture design. The horizontal loads have an impact on the health of the supporting tissues. When the denture base is exposed to shearing, it was reported that the impact is similar to tipping forces on the supports under horizontal loads.

According to Gerber, the effect of simulating shearing forces on the denture base demonstrated the tipping forces that can occur on abutments under horizontal loading (Fig. 2.16a, b). The horizontal loads can cause ball attachment tipping on their own or in conjunction with occlusal forces (Fig. 2.16b). Furthermore, tipping forces under horizontal loads increase for rigid attachments that only allow for one-quarter movement. The orthodontic treatments demonstrated that the force required for bodily tooth movement is significantly greater than the force required to incline a tooth. Even on rigid attachments, a force of more than 3 kg applied for a specific duration can result in a precise movement.

The more rigid the attachment, the higher the load transmitted to the support under forces from all directions. It is believed that rotational resilient attachment prevents overload of the supporting tooth by allowing more load on the denture rather than causing tipping. Splinting the supporting teeth, doubling the surface area of the root with a resilient and rotational attachment (e.g., Dolder bar), and transferring a significant portion of the load to the tissues can all help to improve this effect. To provide the greatest mechanical advantage, the bar attachment should be positioned vertically to the bisector of the angle formed by the posterior crests (Fig. 2.17). Dolder hypothesized that the bar sleeve attachment prevented alveolar crest atrophy by preventing conversion into lateral forces. True, these forces exist during mastication, but they can also be created by the supports. According to Dolder, the bar attachments can be used as a square arch form when the remaining roots are straight. Because the bar is more rigid and does not allow for rotational movements, it will put more strain on the supports even when subjected to vertical forces. When the supporting teeth are splinted, the weak supporting tooth, rather than providing resistance, causes damage to the healthy tooth. If the supporting tooth has mobility for any reason including pulpal, periodontal, or functional, the bar will function as a long cantilever extension and cause severe rotational and tipping forces. As a result, by converting the case into a simple stud attachment, the Schubiger screw block system can be useful (Fig. 2.12b). It was reported that if the supports are strong enough, adding a cantilever in the form of one or two short bars to the support's distal end will ensure stability in all directions. Furthermore, the bar's distal extensions can significantly increase the movement of the supporting tooth in the event of a posterior force from the occlusal and lateral directions. When there are supports left on one side of the arch, a bar design like the one identified by Dolder can be useful in some cases. The bar attachment's movement capacity can largely remain unchanged, but the load may not be equal, and the resilient component of the bar attachment can allow for bilateral and even occlusal forces. It was shown that the rigid bar system generates more torque force on the supporting teeth. When compared to stud or conventional methods, all bar systems place more stress on the contralateral side.

Magnetic attachments exert the least lateral force on the supporting tissues of any precision attachment (Fig. 2.18). Theoretically, all magnet systems with a flat surface implement lateral resilience. Jackson magnets, on the other hand, allow for rotational movement and have a central pin that prevents lateral movement. Finally, the lateral stresses in these attachments are high enough to cause tipping forces. The best way to achieve lateral resilience is to use "cement in keepers" with a flat surface close to the gingival margin. Clinically, "cement on keepers" are more practical, but they lack lateral resilience. The lateral movements affect the contours of the periradicular structures, root and crest form, attached gingiva, and exposed root surface area (Figs. 2.10 and 2.18).

Excessive lateral movement is not desirable due to the overdenture occlusal diagram. If a balanced occlusion is not achieved, lateral forces will cause denture movement. The magnetic systems are only horizontally resilient; the position of the denture is defined by the tissue contour rather than the location of the precision attachment.

2.7 Force Evaluation of Overdenture Attachments

It is necessary to have information about attachment retention and materials before deciding which attachment to use in which case. For almost all retention methods, the value of the retention force decreases relatively quickly (clasps, attachments, bars, and telescopic crowns).

When the retention is examined from various aspects, it is clear that the retention level is primarily determined by the denture material used, particularly its retentive elements. The number of loading cycles in which the retention force is reduced by half can be used to predict the rate of wear. The contact of saliva-lubricated metal surfaces results in less alloy wear and a slower decrease in retention force.

Precision attachments' retentive properties are determined by:

1. Material retention.
2. Undercut retention.
3. Retention of frictional grip.
4. Magnetic retention.

2.7.1 Material-Related Retention

The material used in the fabrication of the attachment determines the ability to adjust elasticity, and other parts can offer sufficient resistance in case of failure of a particular part. As a result, the resistance of the attachment parts to corrosion and continuous distortion, as well as the survival rates of attachments, vary depending on the type and quality of the material (Figs. 2.19, 2.20, and 2.21). When attached and detached more than 1000 times, gold alloys (especially Grade 3 and 4) can be considered resistant to distortion and corrosion. Other attachments that use a nylon or rubber O-ring wear out faster and must be replaced. Depending on the mechanical resistance to separation, all precision attachments are prone to corrosion and distortion.

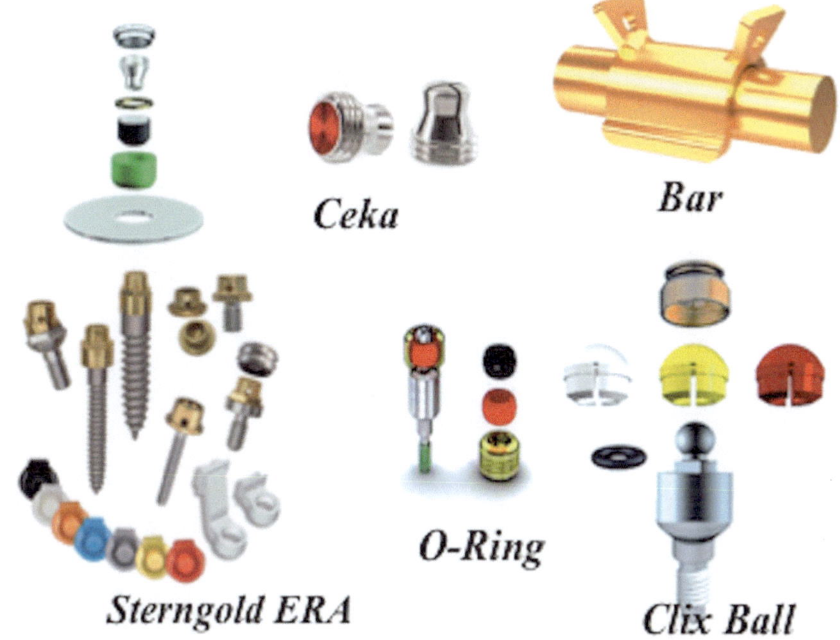

Fig. 2.20 Different types of attachments produced by different types of alloys

Magnetic retention tests, on the other hand, revealed that the time-dependent attraction force did not change for a long time. The retention does decrease as the magnet in the mouth corrodes. Unprotected SmCo5 corrodes, and magnetic distribution or retention decreases gradually as the air gap and magnet length increase. As a result, retention is determined by the material used.

2.7.1.1 Gold Alloys

Gold is a strong, long-lasting metal that expands and contracts at the same rate as natural teeth. Gold has numerous advantages, including its chemically static nature, which means it does not oxidize at any temperature in air or water and is unaffected by hot and strong acids. Gold has also been shown to be effective in the oral environment. It is gentle on soft tissues, and it does not react with food acids. Gold improves the workability, polishing ability, density, and ductility of the alloy to which it is added.

Type 4 gold alloys are typically used in the major connector. Gold alloys are strengthened by the addition of platinum and palladium, depending on the alloy's need for high rigidity and resistance to high load and weathering factors. Precision attachment producers use their own-patented alloys and do not share their entire content and proportions. On the other hand, efforts were made to develop different parts of attachments due to the specifications of these different alloys. However, due

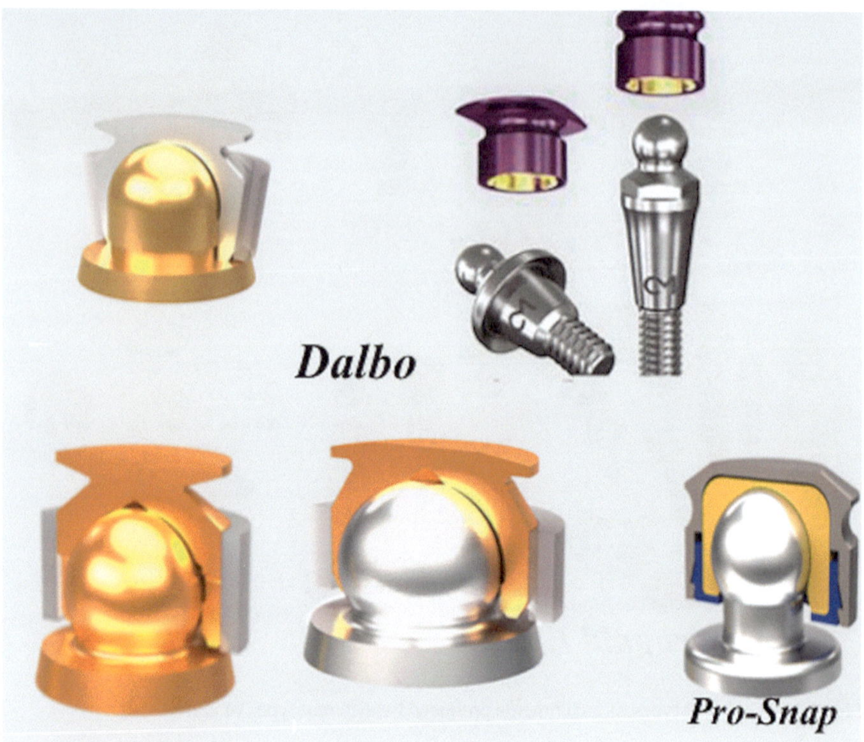

Fig. 2.21 The Dalla Bona attachment; male part and female part

to the specifications of these various alloys, efforts were made to develop new attachment parts.

In 1972, Cendres and Metaux categorized gold alloys utilized in precision attachments into four distinct categories.

2.7.1.2 Metal 1 (OSV)

OSV is a soldering alloy of precious metals with high strength. It consists of platinum, gold, and palladium and is utilized in the attachment's rigid structures. They can be utilized in both male and female attachments (Conod, Dalla Bona, Battesti, Gmur, Rothermann, Schneider, Schubiger, Biaggi, CM round bar, and Hruska screw). Except for the Dalla Bona system, the hardest metal alloys, which is the most difficult to replace, are utilized in all other cases. This metal is typically tempered and hardened for use with acrylic; however, for soldering, it is heated to 400 °C for 15 min and cooled in water.

2.7.1.3 Metal 2 (Elitor)

It is a hard gold and platinum alloy used when rigidity and resistance are required. Elitor is a yellow alloy of precious metals. It is less durable than OSV. It is utilized in the production of replaceable components (Dalla Bona cylindrical and resilient attachment male part, Gmur attachment, Gerber, Dolder bar, CM driver, Ipsoclip female part, and Hruska male part). If soldering, Elitor should be heated to 700 °C for 30 min.

2.7.1.4 Metal 3 (Elasticor)

Elasticor is used for components requiring resilience and elongation. Generally, it is used in the fabrication of wrought wire, orthodontic springs, and labial archwires. In only one attachment, the Rothermann cylindrical attachment is the female component utilized. It is a flexible, heated, and heat-treated alloy. The female component can be applied to the resin and soldered to the unit's moving component. After soldering, the unit should be maintained at 400 °C for 15 min.

2.7.1.5 Metal 4 (Ceramicor)

Ceramicor is a non-oxidizing, copper-free, precious metal alloy that can be cast at 732°C after preheating. Attachments used in conjunction with porcelain-fused-to-metal restorations are made from this metal. The melting point is high, and it contains a significant amount of platinum. It has less rigidity, offers low fracture strength and sufficient tensile strength, and has more elongation than OSV. It can be used as an alternative to Elitor in Gmur, Gerber, and Schneider. It is also utilized in the Conod attachment, the Battesti attachment, the female part, the retainer pins, and the female part container of the Schubiger screw block. When Ceramicor is to be soldered to platinum alloy, it is heated in a carbon pot at 700 °C for 30 min. It is hardened in the salt bath.

Materials usually used for male and female parts are: C = Ceramicor; O = OSV; K = Korak [Burnout plastic. Minimum proof stress (Rp 0.2%) required of the casting alloy: 500 N/mm^2]; V = Valor (a palladium- and copper-free, precious metal alloy); OR = Orax (Au 67 - Pt 8.6 - Ag 13.2 - Cu 11 - Zn 0.2); E = Elitor; D = Doral (a white precious metal alloy); T = Titanax (Ti 90 – Al 6 – V 4); and I = Irax (Au 60 - Pt 24 - Pd 15 - Ir 1).

Materials of Dalbo Attachment (Fig. 2.21)

The EC is the premier Mini-Dalbo® model. The male component can be cast onto the abutment tooth or soldered to it. The female component is made from the superior yellow alloy Elitor® and is easily adjustable. The Mini-Dalbo® EO can only be retained on the abutment tooth through soldering. As the male is composed of high-strength OSV, any above-average mouth loads can be compensated for. The female component is made from the superior yellow alloy Elitor® and is easily adjustable. The DK is the economical alternative to the Mini-Dalbo®. As the male component of the Korak is cast, any casting alloy may be used. This reduces the quantity of alloys utilized in the patient's mouth. The only limitation is the stated minimum strength of the casting alloy. The female component is made of the adjustable white alloy Doral.

Materials of Ceka Attachment (Fig. 2.20)

Producers of Ceka attachments recommend that retainer attachments be manufactured with suitable materials. They are:

Type 1 metal (Au, Ag, Pd) (Pallax 1): The white metal is utilized for soldering the post-retained coping.
Type 2 metal (AuPt) (Orax 1): It is employed to solder fine gold post-retained coping.
Type 4 metal (Cobalt cast alloy) (Ceremax 1): It possesses a high melting point. It is suitable for direct casting and adheres to all precious metals except porcelain gold. Similar to Ceramicor, it is applied by heating a carbon block in an oven at 700 °C for 30 min.

The reason for constructing Ceka components from entirely compatible materials may be to allow for corrosion between components and replacement as needed. When the female component is permanently attached to the bar, the hardest of these three metals should be used.

Alternatively, the attachment could be soldered to the post coping (precious or non-precious alloys). For direct casting with precious and palladium-based alloys, IRAX is a high-fusing alloy (white, Au-Pt-Ir) with a high melting point. The gold alloy is composed of Au 60%, Pt 19%, Pd 20%, Ir 1%, and NOPRAX (with non-precious alloys).

Ceka M3 Axial IR/TI: IRAX base ring for direct casting with precious metal and alloys containing palladium, or for soldering to the post coping. Female TITANAX retention in acrylic resin. Male on the post coping or bar for increased stability of the denture.

Ceka M3 axal PA/TI: PALLAX base ring intended for soldering to the post cap or bar. Female TITANAX retention in acrylic resin. Male on the post coping or bar for increased stability of the denture.

Stainless Steel Material

Stainless steel contains 73% iron, 18% chrome, 8% nickel, 1% molybdenum, 1% copper, 1% manganese, and 1% silica. When 18–8 stainless steel split rings and springs and gold parts cannot provide the necessary flexibility, it is used as a replacement component in certain attachment types. For instance, split rings made of stainless steel are utilized in Gerber cylinder and buffer attachments, whereas replaceable springs made of stainless steel are utilized in Gerber buffer and Ipsoclip. When heated above 400–900 °C, the corrosion resistance of stainless steel is lost. These springs are intended for assembly following the final soldering and heat treatment. Although stainless steel has a superior elongation rate compared to other materials, it can fail in applications involving corrosion and continuous forces. Therefore, it is suggested to replace it every year.

PVC Rings Material

These are utilized in Dalla Bona, Baer, and Ancrofix attachments to create a space for the outward extension of retention edges on the female component. This

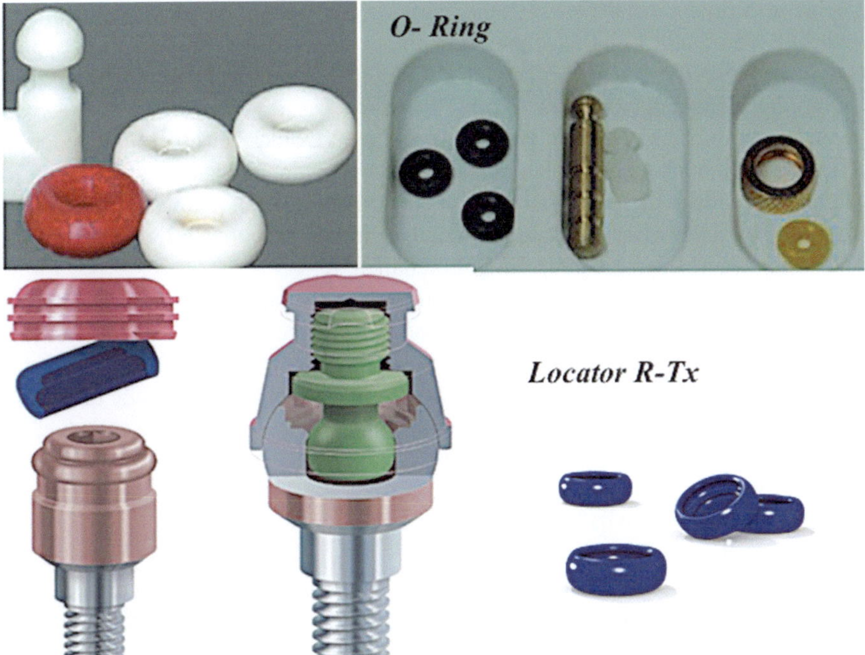

Fig. 2.22 Rubber plastic and nylon attachment (Locator and O-Ring attachment)

material is only necessary for construction and is not utilized during the attachment's operation.

Silicon Rubber Rings Material

Rubber rings are used to retain attachments cast in the Quinlivan, O-Ring, and certain attachment systems. As a result of deformation, corrosion, and organism infiltration, it is suggested that the rubber be replaced at specified intervals. With silicon becoming harder and less flexible over time, retention decreases significantly (Fig. 2.22).

Nylon Material

Nylon components in the Zest system are susceptible to rapid deformation and corrosion as a result of friction with the metal female component. Corrosive waste in the female part shortens the male part's retainer life (Fig. 2.9).

2.7.2 Undercut Retention

This retention relies on the attachment leaving a degree of flexibility in the undercut. Numerous attachments utilize a similar spring clip action because it provides a more secure and recognizable attachment seating. Rothermann attachment and

Gerber attachment are the attachments with undercut retention (Figs. 2.5, 2.6, 2.7, and 2.8). The Dalla Bona attachment combines undercut retention with frictional retention, while the Ancrofix, Ceka, and Schneider attachments combine undercut retention with lamella retention.

Ackermann bar, CM driver, Hader bar, and oval Dolder bar utilize the undercut area of the lamellar figure, which ranges from two retainer ends in the CM driver to six retainer ends in the Schneider attachment. Other undercut retainer methods consist of two parallel wires that pass through the denture, as with the B&C attachment, and wrap around the male undercut gold retainer.

Pressomatic and Ipsoclip both offer an undercut retainer with a spring-loaded retainer that can be configured for retention with a screw and locked to a vertical counter surface. Similar to the Quinlivan attachment, "O" ring retention provides retention comparable to that of lamella retention. The rubber's tendency to deform facilitates the settlement of the male component.

2.7.3 Frictional Grip Retention

This type of retention is facilitated by the contact of the spring lamella surfaces with the surfaces opposite the parallel surfaces (Figs. 2.23 and 2.24). Numerous cylindrical attachments are compatible with this retention. These include a cylindrical attachment from Dalla Bona, a cylindrical attachment from Conod, a cylindrical attachment from Battesti, a cylindrical attachment from Introfic Gmür, and a cylindrical attachment from B&F. Biaggi and Dalla Bona attachments feature a friction/extrusion coupling combination, and Dolder U-bars and other parallel-edged bars

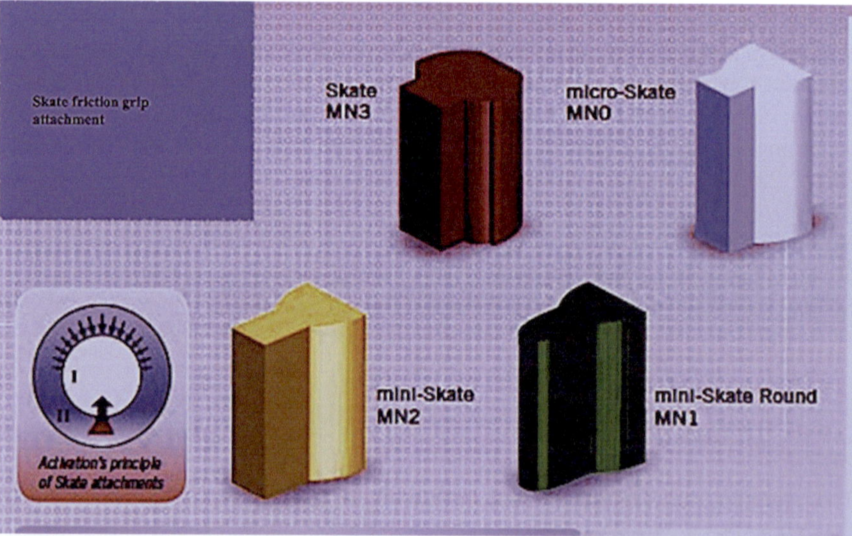

Fig. 2.23 Frictional grip attachment (Skate)

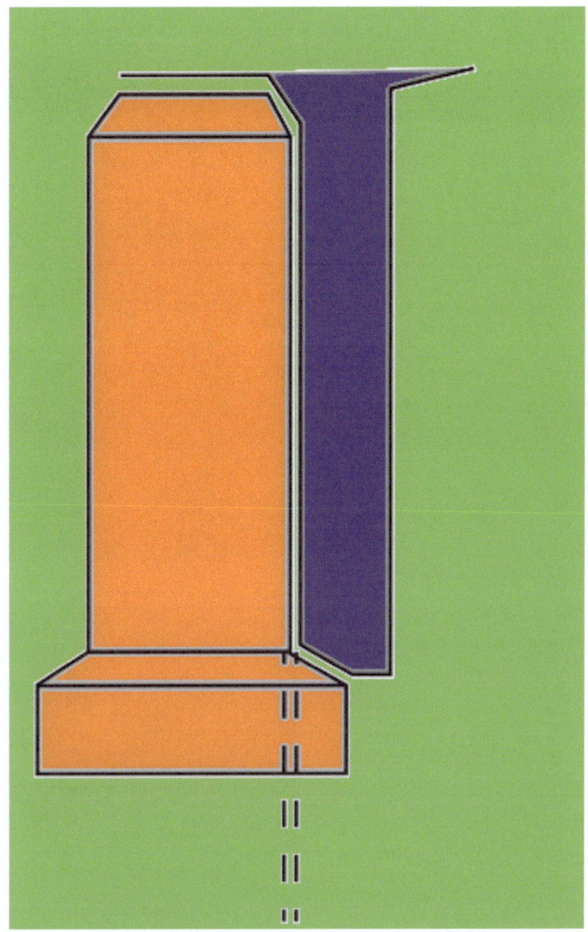

Fig. 2.24 Retention in a frictional attachment is achieved by increasing the surface area of contact at the expense of deflection

feature friction-coupling retention. Because not all friction-coupling attachments provide extrusion, they permit vertical flexion during retention. However, the rotation movement around the attachment is impossible. The light lamella design of the cylindrical attachment from Dalla Bona provides gentle retention. Attachments for the Conod, Biaggi, and Battesti have slit pin or slip knob attachments. It is located on the opposite side of Biaggi's slit ring, which has two configurable zones.

2.7.3.1 Adjustment of Attachment Retention

With wear and metal fatigue, the retention force diminishes significantly. It can be improved by adjusting the lamella's position or by pushing it to the undercut area so that it makes complete contact with the parallel surface. In the case of split pins or split ball attachments, tools such as the Battesti, a retention adjuster, are provided. For the retention setting, a slight detaching force is applied to lamellae with a screwdriver, or, if it is not a configurable attachment, the retainer part is entirely replaced (Figs. 2.25 and 2.26).

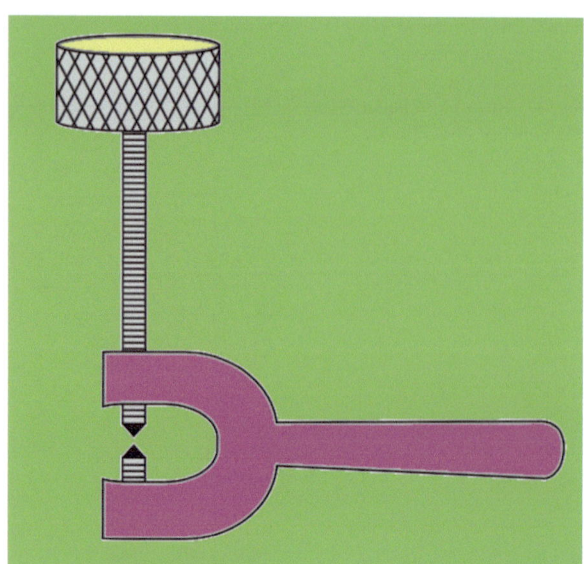

Fig. 2.25 The CM retention adjustor

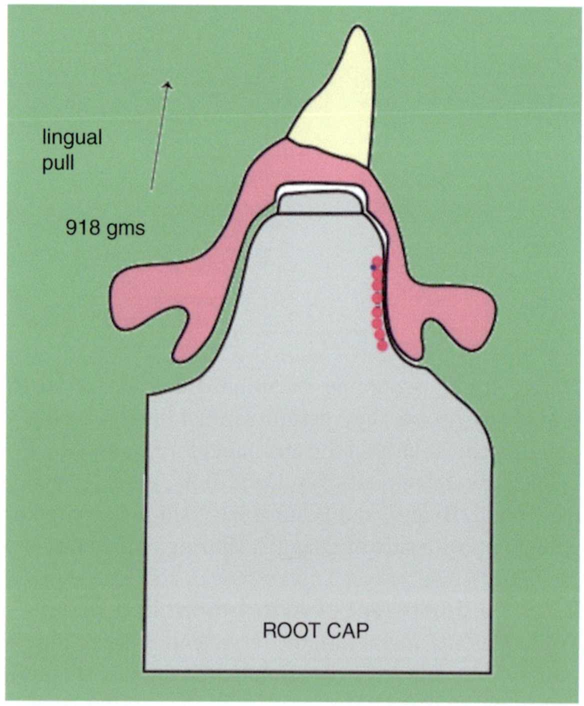

Fig. 2.26 Retention of standard root cap from the lingual direction

2.7.4 Magnetic Retention

The residual roots are positively indicated for retention of dentures by using magnetic attachments. By application of magnetic attachments, residual roots came to play a part in retentive effects as well as the support of dentures. The magnetic attachment (Fig. 2.27) appeared to have a substantially lower retentive force than the other attachments. The concept of "locking on," which occurs on the vertical faces of the root cap, can be used to explain this phenomenon. Due to the shape of the keeper, which prevents the denture from "locking on," there would certainly be no increase in retention. It seems crucial to have strong retention in precision attachments to make the denture "tight" in the mouth, thereby preventing plaque accumulation under the denture. Therefore, the breakaway load is essential for dentures

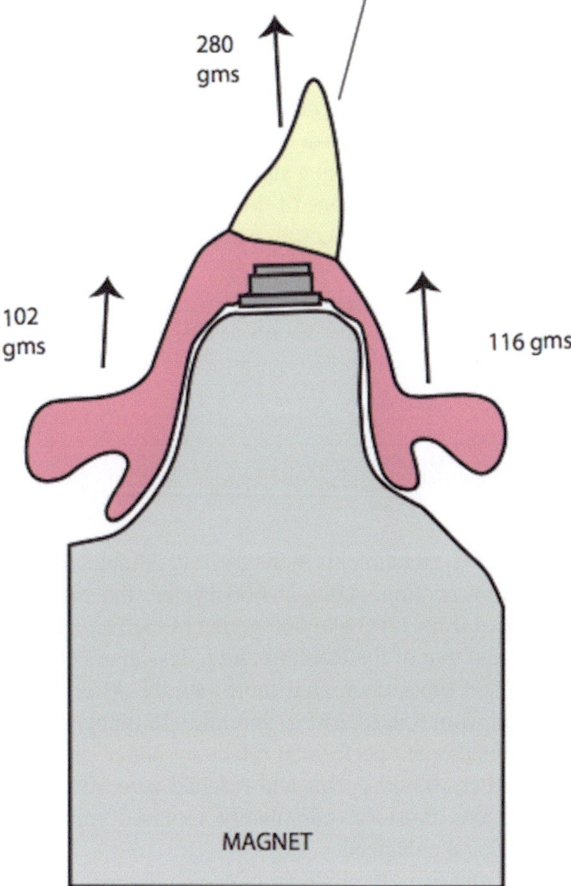

Fig. 2.27 Dislodgement forces with the magnetic attachment

with precision attachments. However, magnets have the unique characteristic of being "sticky" – they return to position after slight dislodgement. Hence a magnet could exert a fraction of the retention of a precision attachment, but still be useful as an aid to denture stability. It is stated that the breakaway load decreases when prostheses are withdrawn in directions other than axial. When the denture is removed, there is no risk of overloading the keeper or the labial or lingual tissue near the root. When the magnet is lifted eccentrically, the magnetic flux surrounding the keeper is reduced by half.

2.8   Retention Values of the Attachments

In the literature, the majority of photoelastic analysis studies evaluated load transfer through the root cap and other tooth root attachments. Based on the effect of loading different attachments, it is reported that in TSO, the torque load caused by a more positive attachment, such as the Ceka, was significantly higher than for a straight root cap, and that different post designs exerted different forces on the roots, causing stresses that could lead to root fracture. Nevertheless, loading tests may not be entirely relevant to overdentures in withdrawal movement. The patient's proprioceptive discrimination is a significant factor that can limit the load on the denture and abutments; this is one of the primary benefits of overdentures.

The approximate retention values of some precision attachments are as follows:

Ceka: 840–1000 g retention
Dalla Bona: 400–1000 g retention becoming less with time
Kurer: 300–1900 g retention
Gerber buffer: 1200 g retention
Zest: 750 g retention
Rothermann: 425 g retention
"O" ring /O-SO: 775 g retention
Magnets: 300–720 g retention at least and constant

However, attachments made entirely of metal lost their retention due to corrosion caused by friction. After 25,000 cycles, the retention of the Gerber attachment decreased from 1200 g to 600 g, that of the Dalla Bona to 550 g, that of the Ceka to 650 g, and that of the Rothermann to less than 200 g. The retention of non-metallic attachment types decreased more rapidly. After 5000 cycles, the Zest attachment dropped from 750 to 250 g, and after 18.00 cycles, it had no retention value. The O-SO attachment performed relatively better, as its weight decreased from 775 to 250 g after 10,000 cycles and reached zero after 22,500 cycles. While non-metal attachments must be completely replaced, metal attachment retention can be adjusted and enhanced.

In comparison to other attachments, the magnetic attachments had stable retention and were unaffected by cycles. The regular size Jackson attachment provided 720 g of retention, while the mini size provided 575 g. The Innovadent magnet had 600 g, Gillings slit pole 300 g, Magnedent 240 g, and Dyna magnet 200 g retention.

In addition, it is important to note that magnetic retention can manifest differently in the mouth. When exposed to occlusal forces in the mouth, cobalt-samarium magnets are affected by oral fluids, become susceptible to rapid corrosion, and lose their retention. If magnet attachments are well-preserved in a liquid-resistant case, as with Innovadent magnets, their long-term retention values are enhanced. Similarly, magnet size affects retention in certain magnet case design concepts. As the magnet grows in size, greater retention is achieved, but the compatibility between the denture and magnet may be compromised.

Almost any attachment is known to provide adequate retention for an overdenture when properly positioned, aligned, and seated upon initial placement. However, it is crucial to note how significantly each attachment type varies in function.

Also, it gives us an insight as to the possible cause of tissue damage and failure of attachment coping. It is fascinating that even the plain root cap exhibits retentive forces (Figs. 2.26 and 2.28). Surprisingly, there is an increase in this retention with the lingual angle of pull. This can be explained as locking on the vertical lingual surface of the root cap and the labial surface of the root prominence, and thus the exact shape of the root cap has a direct bearing on this effect. A dome-shaped root cap would have a significant difference. Factors that may affect plain root cap

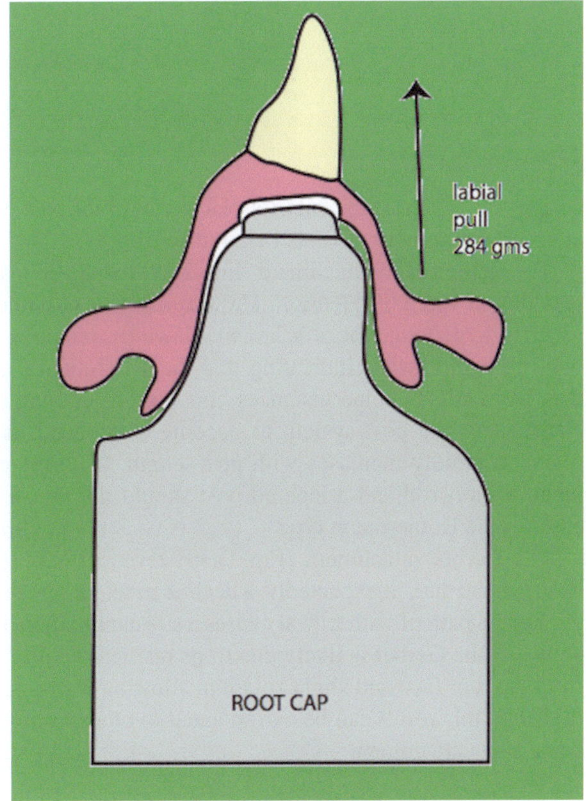

Fig. 2.28 Retention of standard root cap from the labial direction

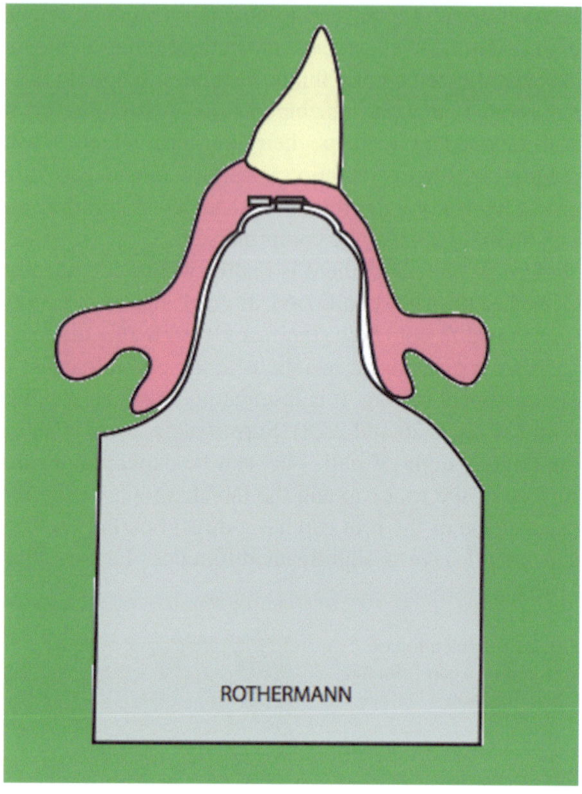

Fig. 2.29 Retention of Rothermann attachment

designs may include the anterior placement of the root, the degree of undercut labially, and the number of roots being utilized.

The Rothermann attachment (Fig. 2.29) displayed a straight path of withdrawal, resulting in 466 g of retention. The varying path of withdrawal over 2 kg of force is required to dislodge the attachment. However, retention dropped significantly after only 20 withdrawals, indicating that the attachment's arms were deformed rather than worn out. In some instances, this kind of dramatic increase in retentive force could cause the post system to become overloaded. It is demonstrated that post retention rapidly increases with post length. If torque can be applied to the abutment, a short rod and a tapered post should not be used for precision attachment cases of the Rothermann type.

The Gerber attachment (Fig. 2.30) revealed less retention diversity than the Rothermann and, unexpectedly, a decline in retention in the labial pull. Nonetheless, the lingual path of withdrawal causes a substantial increase in retention. The removability of the Gerber is likely due to its resilient nature, which permits lifting away from the root face and slight rotation, allowing it to emerge from a slight undercut. Probably, this result can be extrapolated to other resilient stud designs, such as the Dalla Bona attachment.

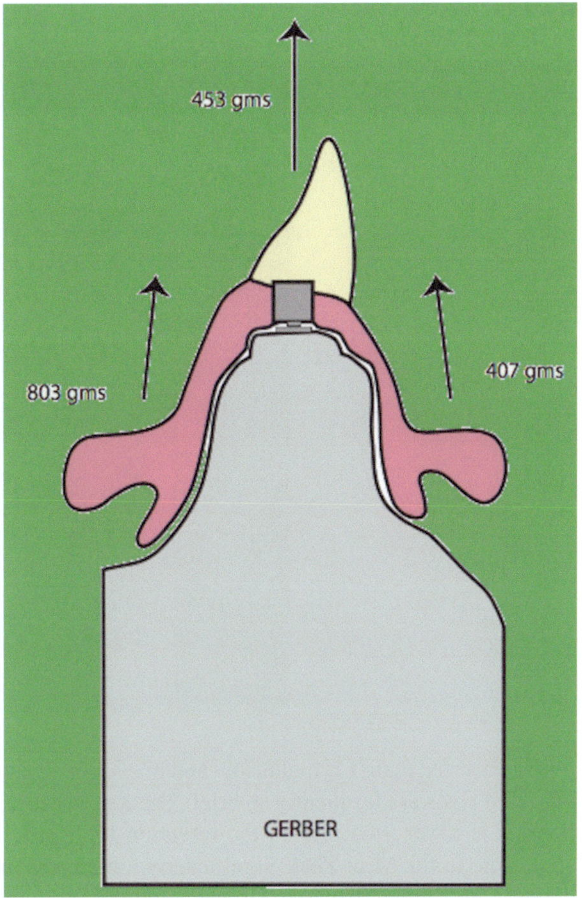

Fig. 2.30 Dislodgement forces with Gerber attachment

The Conod attachment (Fig. 2.31) is a rigid, tooth-supported attachment. In this instance, it denotes rigid contact with the model and the absence of elasticity. The insertion path occurs in only one direction. Consequently, any deviation from the straight pull should prevent appliance removal. In the case of a long abutment or two abutments where a fulcrum line exists, the rigid type of attachment not only causes torque on the roots during function but also exerts excessive force on the abutments during removal if the appliance is removed in any direction other than vertically.

The Zest attachment (Fig. 2.32) is significant in that a slight variation in the amount of force required to remove the denture is caused by a change in the direction of removal. This could be explained by the fact that the Zest attachment is flexible, bending to the insertion path and not "locking in." In addition, the preparation of the root face leaves a little vertical tooth surface above the gingival level. For this reason, the preparation of the root face is made minimal.

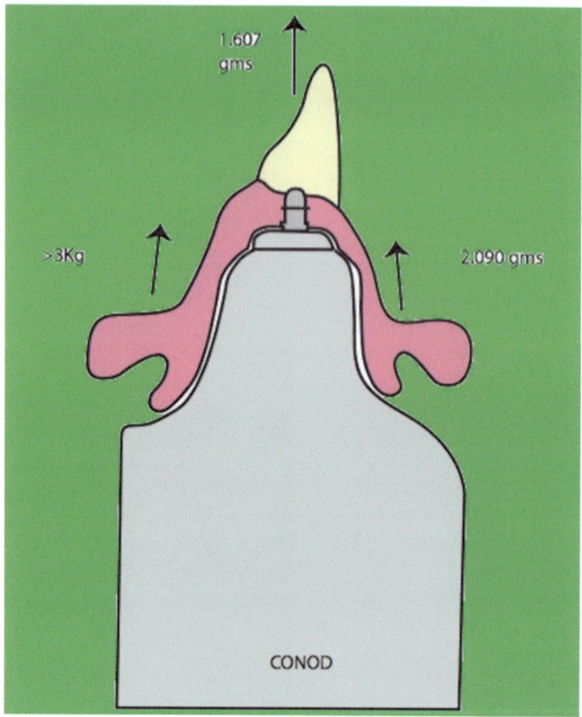

Fig. 2.31 Dislodgement forces with Conod attachment

The inserted matrix remains low and may even be countersunk. This may explain why Zest posts are frequently so brief. The force necessary to separate the two components is never greater than the retention limit provided by the post, especially applicable to the Mini Zest. Significantly, on the second pull after eccentric pulls, the Zest attachment displayed only a slight decrease in retentive force.

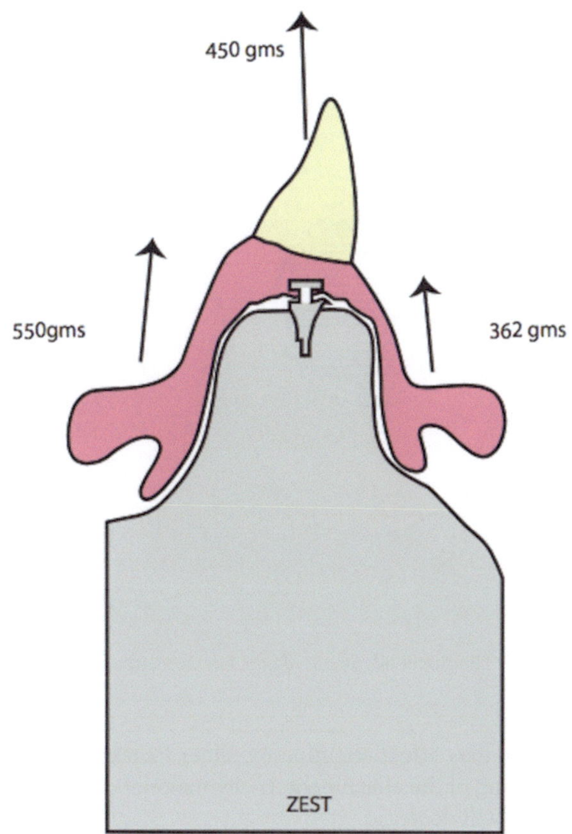

Fig. 2.32 Dislodgement forces with the Zest attachment

2.9   The Retentive Parameters Factors of Precision Attachments

The retention of precision attachments is dependent upon the amount of force required to resist the elasticity of the material, the amount of deflection, the surface roughness, and the surface area. While the initial retention of the Dalla Bona ball attachment was 400 g, the retention of the Dalla Bona cylinder attachment was 1000 g, which was explained by the increase in the surface area of the cylindrical attachment. Attachment retention is significantly influenced by the factors that influence individual attachment design, technical procedures, and care planning.

Other factors that influence retention include:

- The Functional Simplicity of the Attachment (Freedom to Function)
- Any attachment, which functions by deflection, should be allowed to function. Each material that maintains the function of attachment retainer areas increases retention. Acrylic or any other hard material removed from behind the retentive

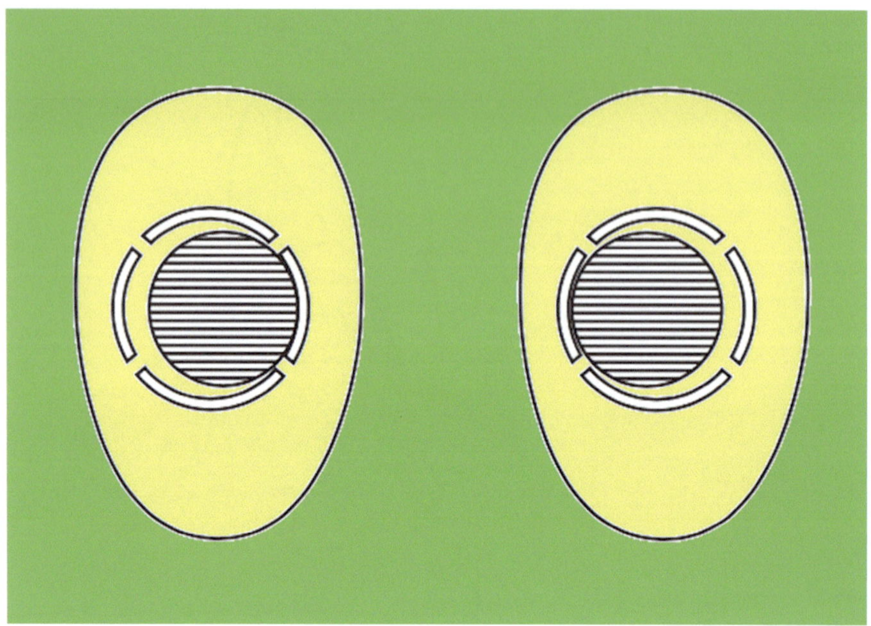

Fig. 2.33 Improper alignment of attachment matrixes distorts the attachment and/or damages the abutment

arms may affect retention by either increasing retention or preventing the functioning of the attachment. If any material covers the magnetic attachment, retention will decrease.

- Incorrect Attachment Alignment due to Incorrect Insertion Discrepancy
- In the case of multiple attachments, the abutment face should be milled, or soldering should be done in the correct path of insertion. It is also essential to set parallelism of longer and more cylindrical attachments. Rothermann, some Stud attachments, and Zest attachments allow for a slight angle in the path of insertion but are worn faster and cause rapid load transmission on the supporting teeth.
- Improper Placement of Female Body Parts on Male Body Parts
- In the acrylic processing phase, the wrong alignment may occur which can cause a change in retention amount. These problems may occur mainly as a result of insufficient relief being provided around the female part. Incomplete alignment causes stress on the abutments, eccentric wear patterns, and rapid loss of retention in the attachment (Fig. 2.33).
- Over-Adjusted Attachments
- Manufacturers advise that the initial configuration of attachment be optimized for minimal retention and then gradually increased to the patient's needs. Excessive increase in retention can result in excessive tilt between attachment levers, lamella, and other attachment components. This can lead to metal fatigue and eventual attachment failure.

Also, excessive retention can cause tissue damage. A healthy periodontium will not collapse when subjected to 1–2 kg of force while detaching attachments. In a distal extension case, it was able to generate 1.5–2 kg of repulsive force, according to reports. When a cylindrical attachment is used, this force does not occur vertically to the attachment, but rather in the direction of tipping to the anterior teeth and attachment. Rapid periodontal gingival recession in this area can provide insight into the forces transmitted. If the lower two canine teeth are significantly positioned in the crest, Dalla Bona Knob, Rothermann, or Kurer attachments permit rotational movement of the denture and prevent torque forces on the labial root surface.

When the attachment is used in an overdenture, clinicians must know how to classify attachments by application, function, and size. Furthermore, clinicians need to understand the attachment's specific design, degree of precision, and force distribution (Table 2.1).

In practice, it can be noted that almost any attachment should provide adequate retention for an overdenture when the attachment is first placed and is correctly aligned and seated. However, there are significant differences that demonstrate how greatly each type of attachment varies in function. Attachment retention should be considered in the following situations:

Table 2.1 Considerations when selecting the attachment

Considerations	Significance
The condition of periodontal support	When teeth are strong or can be made strong through splinting, non-resilient designs are the connectors of choice.
The condition of the residual ridge and other soft tissue support	A residual ridge showing evidence of rampant resorption generally contraindicates resilient designs.
	Two resilient prostheses should generally not oppose each other, as two mobile occlusal planes will impair chewing efficiency.
Opposing arch	Every attachment has a minimum height requirement; for example, most
Vertical height	intracoronal designs require at least 3.5 mm and preferably more.
Size of abutments	A large pulp chamber or very small mesiodistal dimension may
Strength of bite	contraindicate an intracoronal design.
Number of abutments	Virtually all attachments will withstand a normal bite. But when faced with strong bruxing, avoid small, dainty attachments.
Position of abutments	Double abutments distal extension cases are always a good idea; however, when not possible, resilient designs are preferred to
Patient dexterity	deemphasize the supportive role of the abutments.
Alloys	Attachments with a restricted hinging action, like the Dalbo, must be approximately parallel not only vertically but also along the ridge so the hinges can function in unison. If a hinging design is desired, and the position of abutments prevents parallelism along the ridge, a universal joint such as the Stern ERA or Octolink is preferred.
	Extracoronal attachments are generally a bit easier to insert than intracoronal. The intracoronal designs such as tapered attachments are easier than parallel-walled attachments.
	Some attachments must be used only with precious metals. Others should be used with non-precious alloys.

- Before separation, non-resilient (rigid) attachments exert a greater force on the attachment and root than resilient attachments.
- The shorter the root, the less pressure occurs in the labial or lingual tissue.
- If the shape of the attachment on the root surface shows short, vertical walls it is causing the clamping effect. In this situation, the patient is to reseat and remove the denture from the correct path of withdrawal or risk dislodging the root cap or distorting the arms of the attachment.
- If the root structure is protruding, tissue damage occurs during the removal of the prosthesis when resilient attachments are used.
- The magnetic attachment exhibits the least damaging force upon removal of all tested designs and is possibly the gentlest form of retentive fixation to the teeth of all attachments tested in this situation.

It can be seen that one simple factor can dramatically change the prognosis of a case. In TSO, it is necessary to design the attachment design in a way that the patient can use. Due to the difficulty of aligning the nylon matrix into the matrix, the Zest attachment, for example, requires good perception and manual dexterity to insert. Unaligned dentures can cause gingival damage or permanent deformation of the matrix.

Ball attachments and others allowing rotational movement may permit easier removal and transfer less force to the abutment under loading, but they also permit impingement on the labial tissues upon removal, which may result in gingival damage on the labial face of the root. Cylindrical designs also only allow one path of insertion and removal, as demonstrated by the Conod attachment, which could not be separated on a lingual pull even when the removal force exceeded 3 kg.

The Rothermann attachment provides a degree of adaptability around its cylindrical matrix. Clinically, however, it is the most probable connection to "lock-in."

Removal of the prosthesis and an incorrect path of insertion causes an inflexible portion of the matrix to damage the soft portion, resulting in wear of the elastic parts or dislocation of the male parts.

The Dolder type is mostly preferred in cases of bar joint mandibular dentures. If an abrasion of the outer edge of the root copings occurred, it was stated that the reason was the rotation of the denture at the sagittal or transverse axis which caused intermittent contact and friction between the copings and the base of the denture. This may be associated with the fact that 10% of these patients require amalgam restorations on anterior root surfaces following the gingival recession.

The decision between a resilient or non-resilient attachment is whether the vertical support is desired primarily from the abutments or tissue. The majority of vertical support from the abutments is provided by the non-resilient attachment, while the majority of vertical support from the tissue is provided by the resilient attachment. Overdenture using a rigid attachment feature equally distributes the masticatory loads vertically similar to the fixed prosthesis.

Reference

1. Thayer HH, Caputo AA. Photoelastic stress analysis of overdenture attachments. J Prosthetic Dentistry. 1980;43:611–7.

Further Reading

Bayer S, Grüner M, Keilig L, Hültenschmidt R, Nicolay C, Bourauel C, et al. Investigation of the wear of prefabricated attachments – an in vitro study of retention forces and fitting tolerances. Quintessence Int. 2007;38:229–37.

Besimo CE, Guarneri A. In vitro retention force changes of prefabricated attachments for overdentures. J Oral Rehabil. 2003;30:671–8.

Chikunov I, Doan P, Vahidi F. Implant-retained partial overdenture with resilient attachments. J Prosthodont. 2008;17:141–8.

Chung KH, Chung CY, Cagna DR, Cronin RJ Jr. Retention characteristics of attachment systems for implant overdentures. J Prosthodont. 2004;13:221–6.

Crum RJ, Rooney GE Jr. The alveolar Bone loss in overdentures: a 5-year study. J Prosthet Dent. 1978;40:610–3.

Cune M, van Kampen F, van der Bilt A, Bosman F. Patient satisfaction and preference with magnet, bar-clip, and ball-socket retained mandibular implant overdentures: a cross-over clinical trial. Int J Prosthodont. 2005;18:99–105.

Evtimovska E, Masri R, Driscoll CF, Romberg E. The change in retentive values of locator attachments and Hader clips over time. J Prosthodont. 2009;18;479–83.

Fromentin O, Lasssauzay C, Nader SA, Feine J, de Albuquerque RF Jr. Clinical wear of overdenture ball attachments after 1, 3 and eight years. Clin Oral Implants Res. 2011;22:1270–4.

Pacer FJ, Bowman C. Occlusal force discrimination by denture patients. J Prosthet Dent. 1975;33:602–9.

Pigozzo MN, Mesquita MF, Henriques GE, Vaz LG. The service life of implant-retained overdenture attachment systems. J Prosthet Dent. 2009;102:74–80.

Preiskel HW. Overdentures made easy: a guide to implant and root supported prostheses, vol. 1. Berlin: Quintessence Publishing; 1996. p. 38–56.

Jain R, Aggarwal S. Precision attachments–an overview. Ann Prosth Rest Dent. 2017;3:6–9.

Rutkunas V, Mizutani H, Takahashi H. Evaluation of stable retentive properties of overdenture attachments. Stomatologica. 2005;7:115–20.

Rutkunas V, Mizutani A, Takahashi H. Wear simulation effects on overdentures stud attachments. Dent Mater J. 2011;30:845–53.

Setz I, Lee SH, Engel E. Retention of prefabricated attachments for implant stabilized overdentures in the edentulous mandible: an in vitro study. J Prosthet Dent. 1998;80:323–9.

Sposetti VJ, Gibbs CH, Alderson TH, Jaggers JH, Richmond A, Conlon M, Nickerson DM. Bite force and muscle activity in overdentures wearers before and after attachment placement. J Prosthet Dent. 1986;55:265–73.

Pavlatos J. Root-supported overdentures. CDS Rev. 1998;91:20–5.

Stud Attachments Used in Tooth-Supported Overdenture

3

Yasemin Ozkan and Rifat Gozneli

3.1 Stud Attachments

Stud attachments, among other attachments, are the most popular and widely available type of attachment for overdentures and have been on the market for decades. For improved retention and stability, stud attachments are placed directly on the tooth or root or attached (indirectly) to the cast copings (Pictures 3.1, 3.2, and 3.3). They are simple to use and offer adequate retention and stability for implant overdentures. In addition, they have a low profile to reduce leverage on the abutments, are comfortable for the patient, permit independent physiologic movement of the abutments, and are simple to repair.

Stud attachments can be extraradicular (Fig. 3.1; Pictures 3.1 and 3.2) or intraradicular (Fig. 3.2, Picture 3.3), and they can be classified as either flexible or rigid (Fig. 3.3). The resilient attachments permit some vertical and rotational tissue movement to protect the abutments or implants from overload. In addition, the resilient attachments allow vertical movement during mastication, reducing stress transfer to the abutments (stress-breaking function) and transmitting forces to the residual ridge as stress transmitters. With a vertical movement of the denture, resilient attachments may cause posterior mandibular resorption and necessitate additional space. The non-resilient (rigid) type, on the other hand, did not permit any movement of the overdenture during the function.

There are a variety of stud attachments available on the market. Dalla Bona, Gerber, Stern ERA, Ball, Locator, Ceka, Rothermann, OT Equator, CM Lock, Bredent, Sterngold, and Zest are the following attachments (Figs. 3.4, 3.5, 3.6, 3.7, 3.8, 3.9, 3.10, 3.11, 3.12, 3.13, 3.14, 3.15, and 3.16).

Y. Ozkan (✉) · R. Gozneli
Faculty of Dentistry, Department of Prosthodontics, Marmara University, Istanbul, Turkey
e-mail: ykozkan@marmara.edu.tr

Y. Özkan (ed.), *Treatment Options Before and After Edentulism*,
https://doi.org/10.1007/978-3-031-37582-8_3

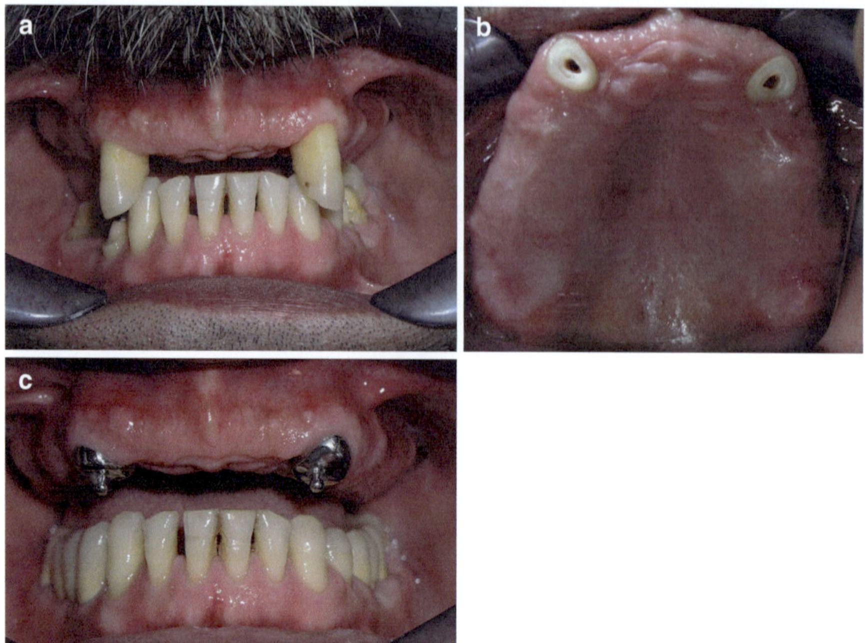

Picture 3.1 (**a–c**) Extra indirect radicular attachment: (**a**) patient has two canine teeth with poor support; (**b**) after endodontic treatment, teeth are prepared according to the preparation rules; and (**c**) extracoronal attachment/cap

3.1.1 Selection Criteria for a Suitable Stud Attachment

In general, the selection of the optimal system depends on many variables, including: inter-arch distance, crown/root ratio, number of supporting teeth, quantity and quality of bone support, location of the supporting teeth, opposing dentition, angulation of the root to the occlusal plane, chewing pattern, the patient's musculature, and the patient's desire. All these factors play a role in the decision-making process for the treatment procedure.

The inter-arch distance can be the most important factor when choosing an attachment. Always consider intraradicular attachments in cases of decreased inter-arch distance. Mounted on the articulator, diagnostic casts are necessary for a more accurate evaluation of the buccolingual and inter-arch spaces available for the attachment, as well as the remaining teeth and dentures. For the selected attachments to be surrounded by a consistent thickness of the denture without compromising the denture base, sufficient buccolingual and vertical space must exist.

3.1.1.1 Height
The minimum required distance between the prepared abutment root surface and the opposing occlusal surface.

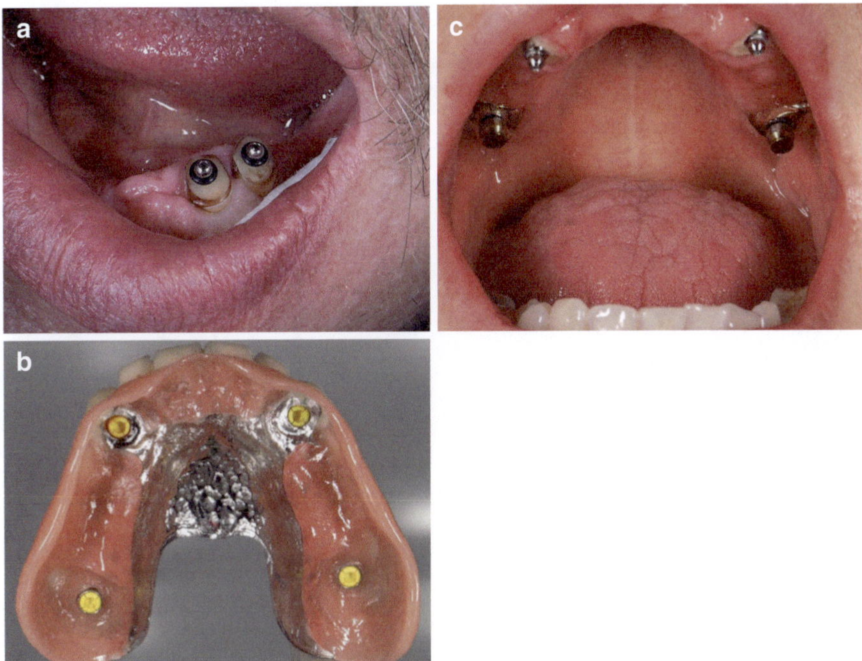

Picture 3.2 (**a–c**) Extraradicular direct and indirect attachments: (**a**) attachment directly placed on the root (direct); (**b**) extraradicular direct and indirect attachment used in same patients; and (**c**) inside view of denture

Picture 3.3 Intraradicular direct attachment

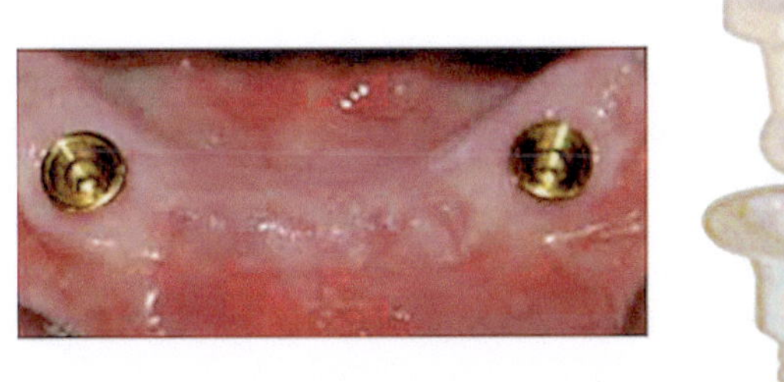

3.1.1.2 The Fixed Portion (FC) of the Attachment's Width

FC width is the minimum diameter of the space required for the component with a fixed attachment. Determine the smallest diameter of the surface of the root.

To ensure retention, the most stable and extensive attachment should be chosen. Therefore, the retention of the denture will increase, and the attachment will wear less. Therefore, the attachment should be chosen after determining the buccolingual distance and vertical dimension from the crest.

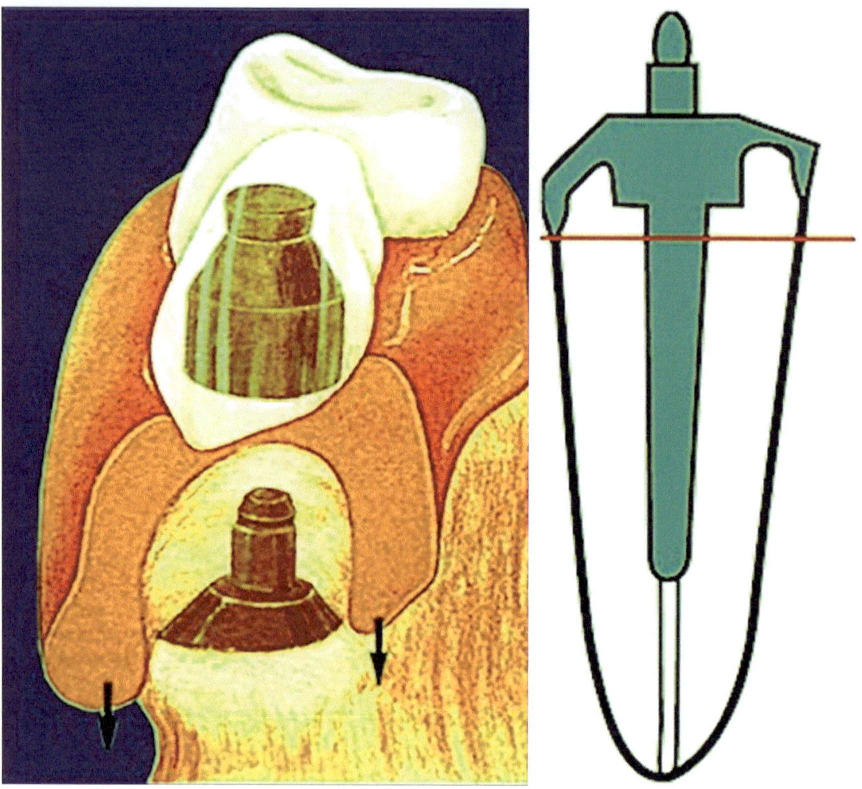

Fig. 3.1 Extraradicular attachment

3.1.1.3 The Width of the Detachable Component of Attachment (RC)

RC width is the smallest diameter required in the denture for the removable attachment component.

Preparation Depth

Preparation depth is the minimal amount of tooth structure required to prepare the attachment space (Fig. 3.17).

3.1.2 Stud Attachment Placement

The alignment of stud attachments should be 10°; all stud attachments must be parallel to one another. Some universal joints: Ball and socket attachments can be 5–7° out of parallelism and still function properly. However, these attachments are contraindicated when there is a significant inclination in the roots.

Fig. 3.2 Intraradicular attachment

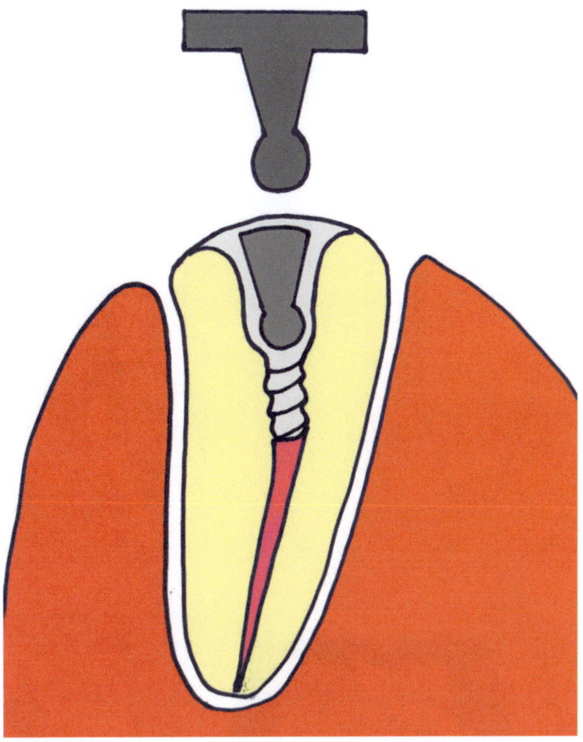

3.1.2.1 Relationship Between the Extracoronal Stud Attachment and the Insertion Path

Attachments should be parallel to one another and on the same plane as the insertion path; they should not obstruct the insertion path of the overdenture (Picture 3.4; Figs. 3.18 and 3.19). The use of a surveyor is required for soft and hard tissue undercuts (an alternative path for insertion or surgery). When there are competing undercuts, surgical intervention cannot be used to reduce them; instead, the base extension must be shortened. Stud attachment will compromise the base's rigidity and retention.

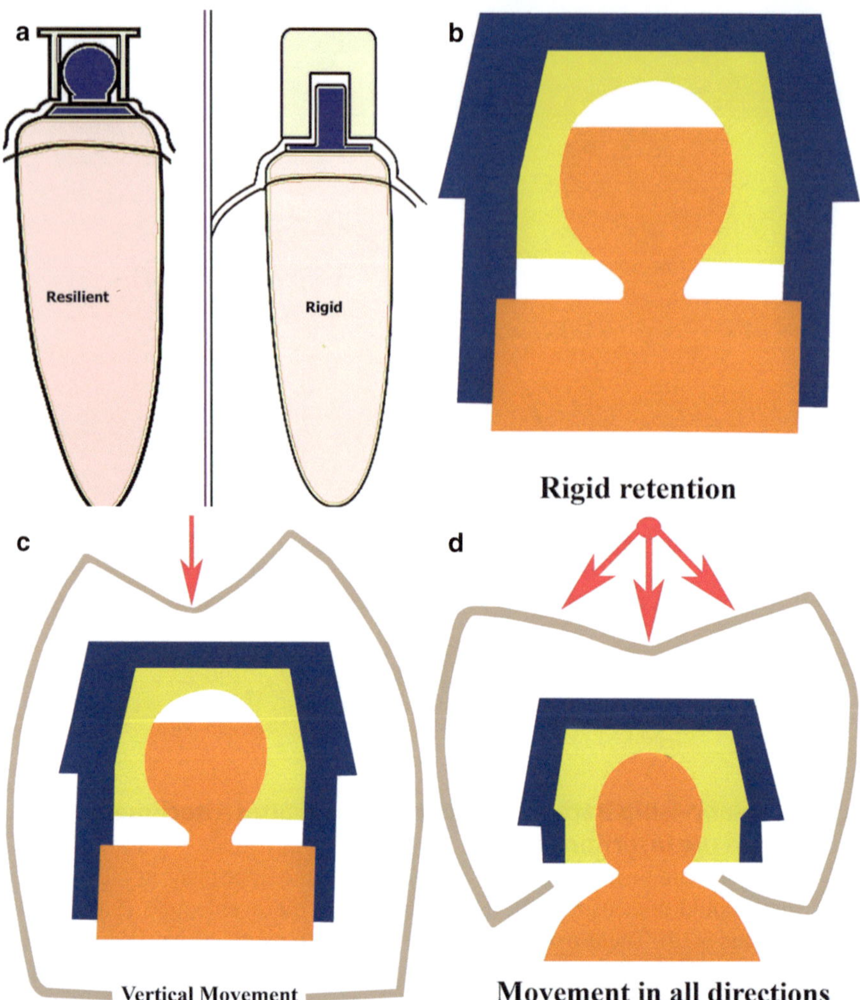

Fig. 3.3 (**a**) Rigid and resilient stud attachment, (**b**) rigid retention, (**c**) vertical movement, and (**d**) movement in all direction

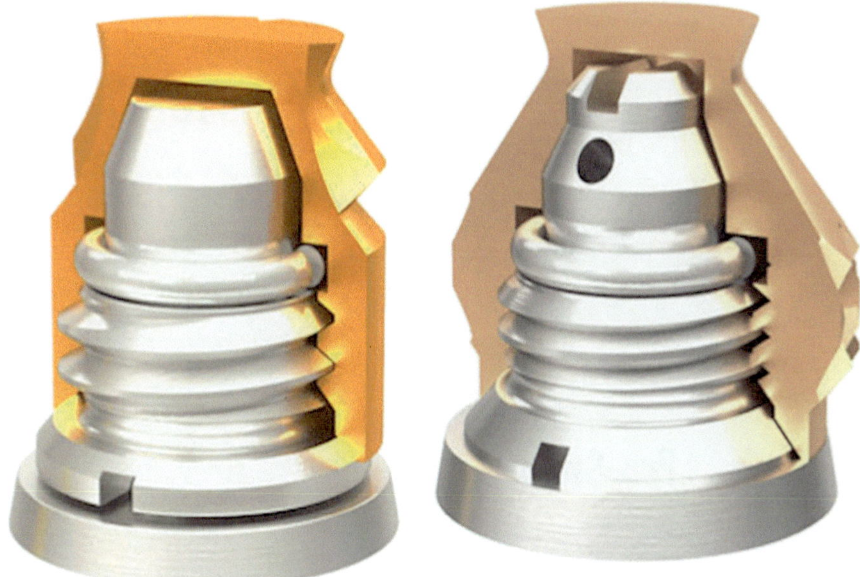

Fig. 3.4 The Gerber attachment

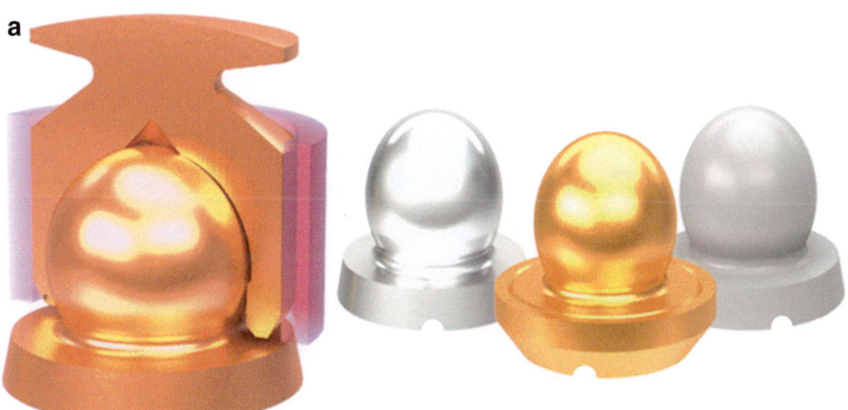

Fig. 3.5 The ball attachments: (**a**) Dalla Bona (Dalbo) attachment, (**b**) Pro-Snap and Profix attachment, and (**c**) Preci Clix and Preci Ball attachments

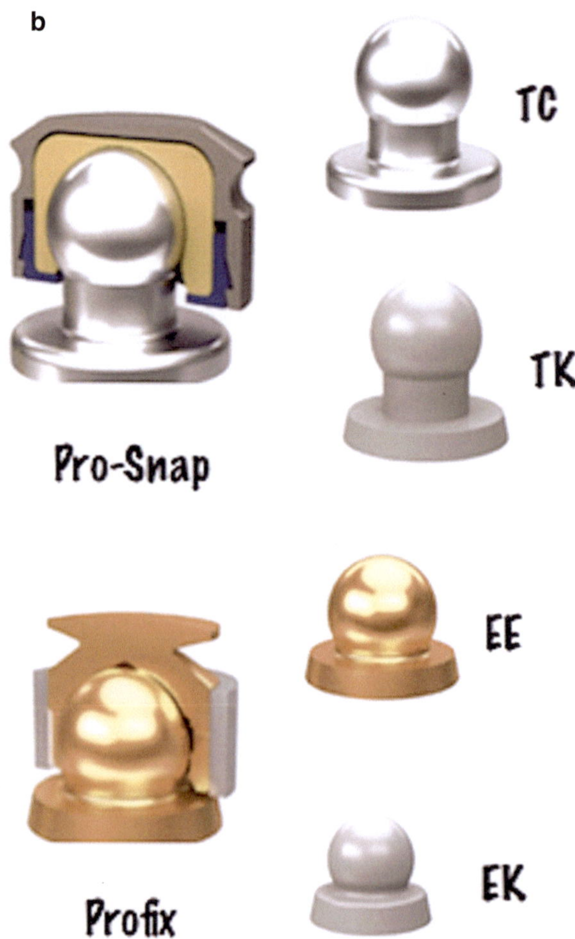

Fig. 3.5 (continued)

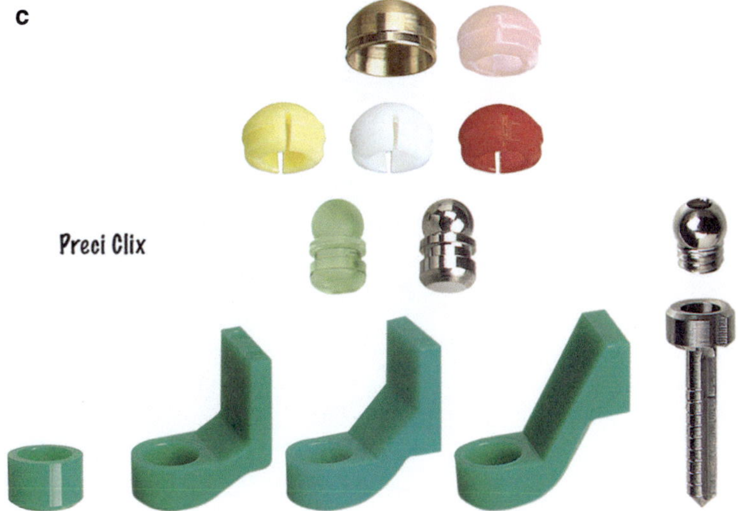

Fig. 3.5 (continued)

Fig. 3.6 The Stufenexzenter attachment

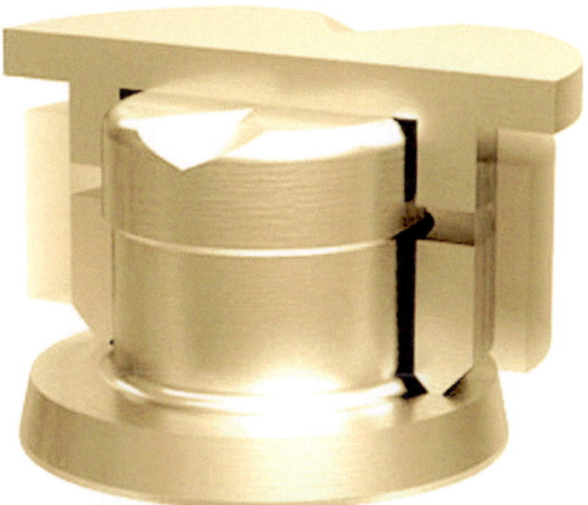

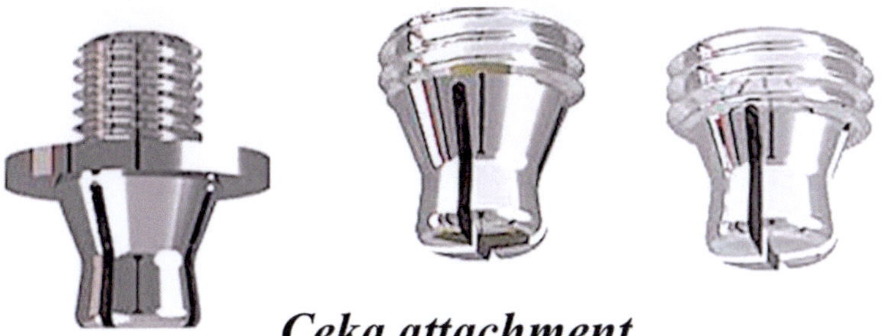

Fig. 3.7 The Ceka attachment

Fig. 3.8 The O-Ring attachment

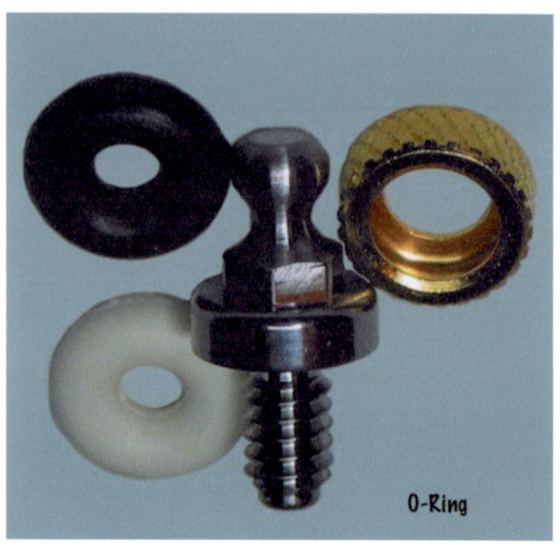

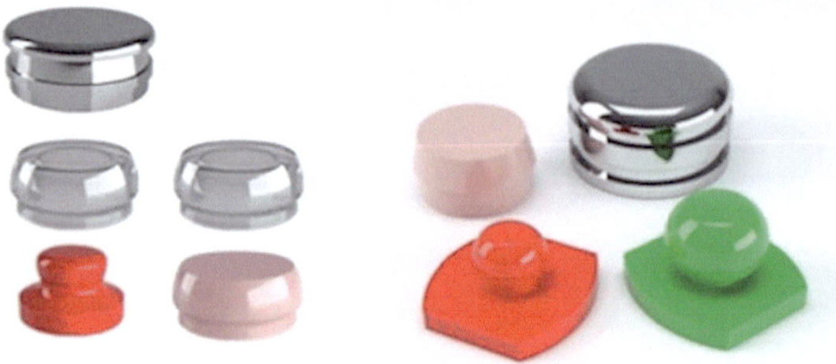

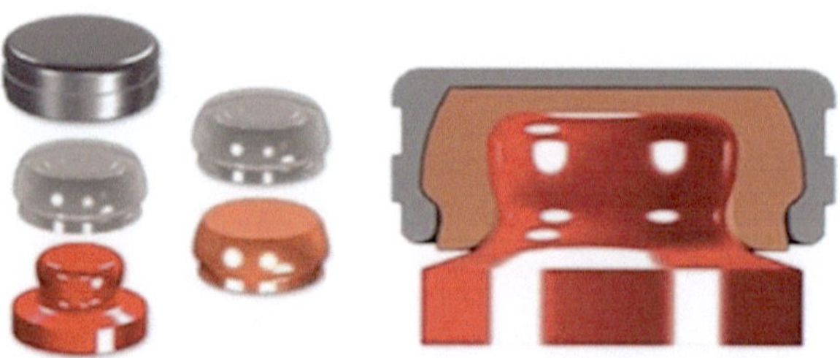

Fig. 3.9 The OT Equator attachment

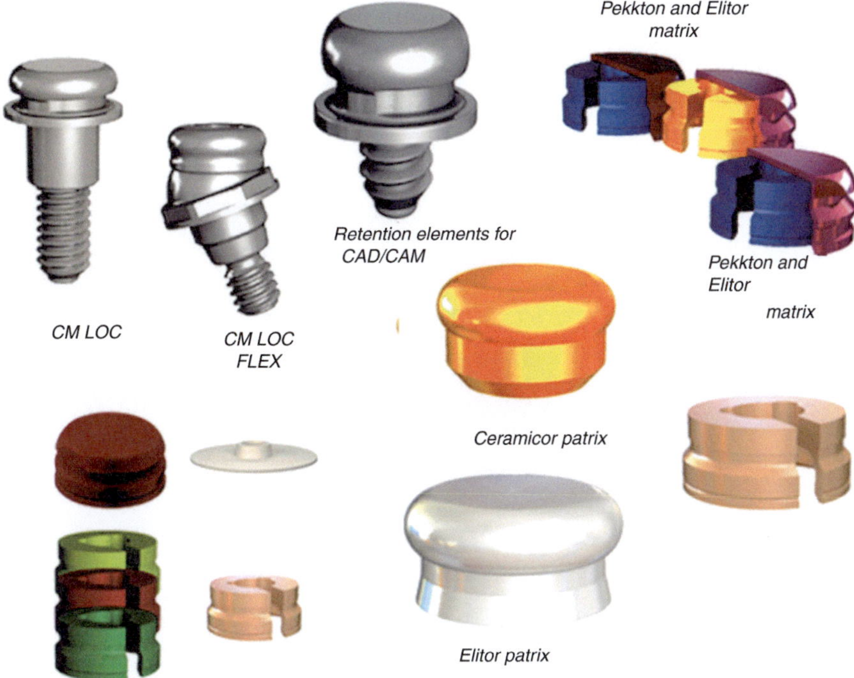

Fig. 3.10 The CM LOC attachment

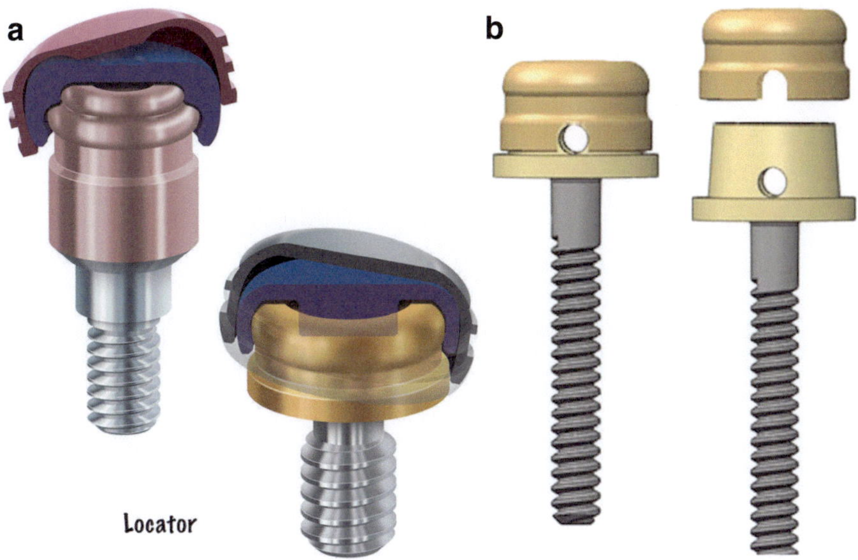

Fig. 3.11 (**a**) The Locator attachment and (**b**) Locator Retrofit-ERA root attachment

Fig. 3.12 The Stern ERA attachment

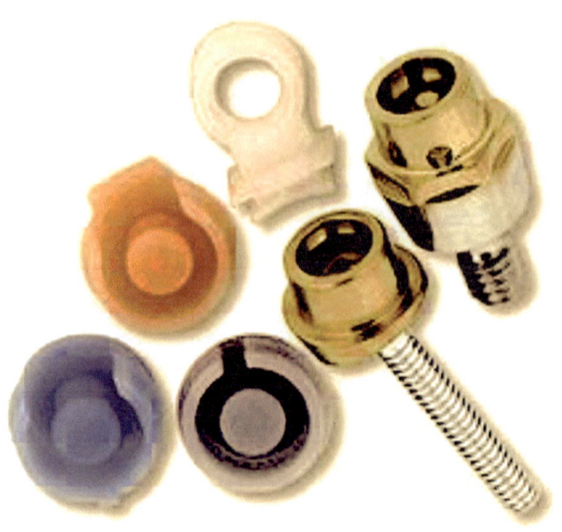

Fig. 3.13 The Rothermann attachment

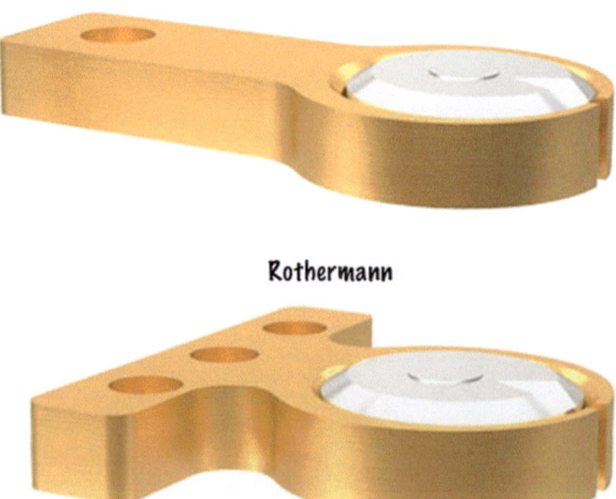

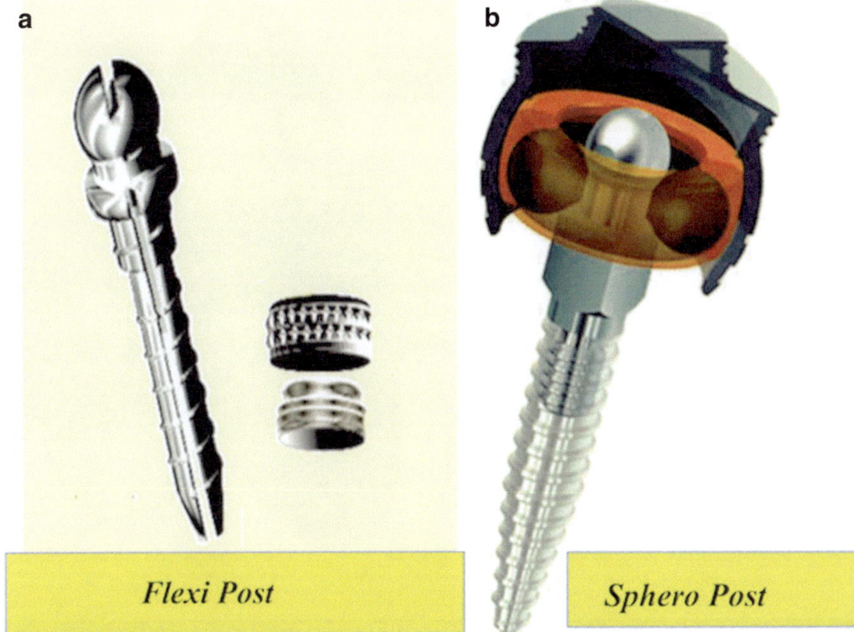

Fig. 3.14 (**a**) The Flexi Post attachment and (**b**) the Sphero Post attachment

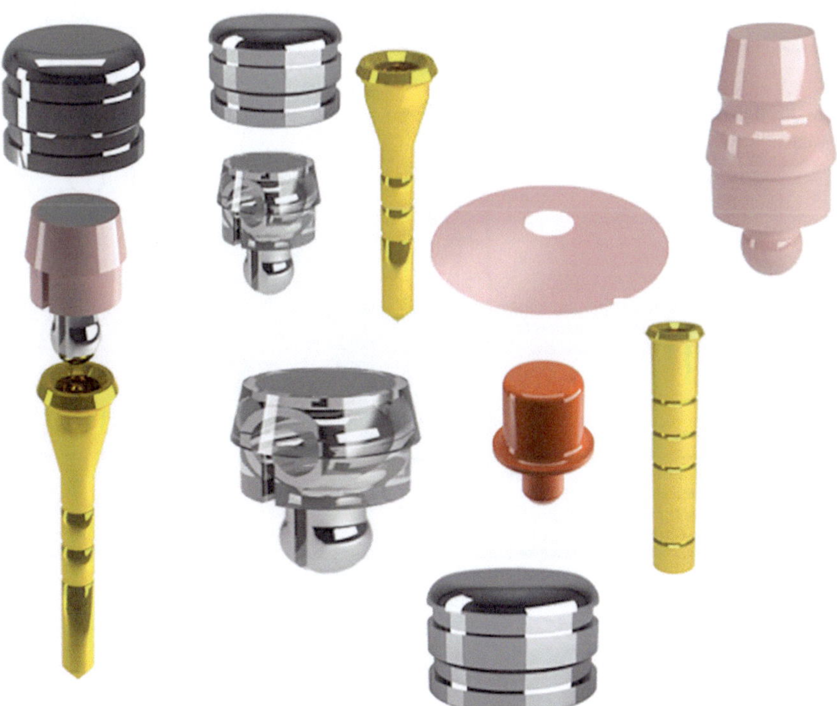

Fig. 3.15 Intraradicular attachment

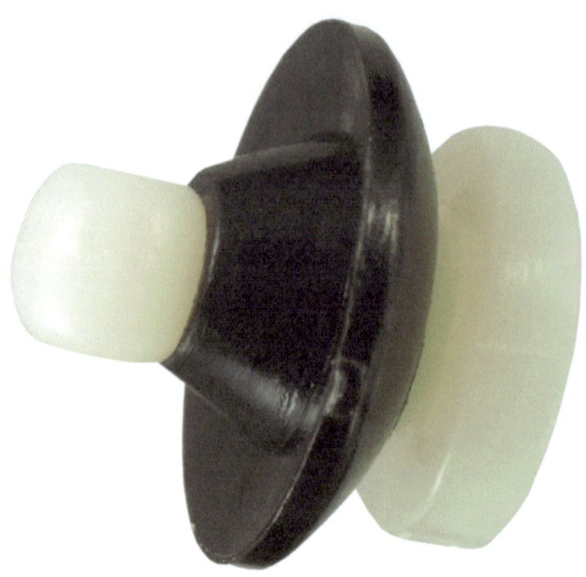

Fig. 3.16 Intraradicular Zest attachment

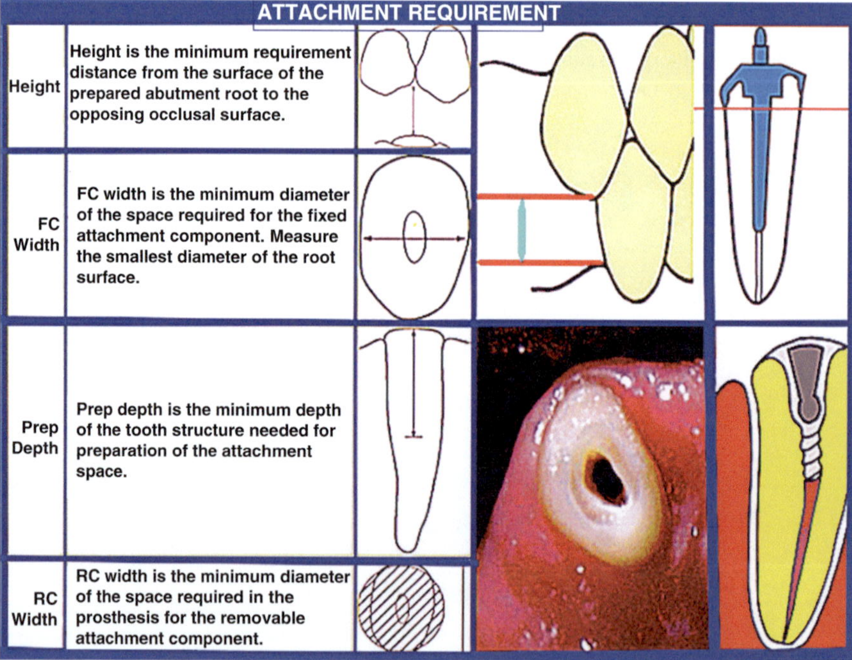

ATTACHMENT REQUIREMENT

Height	Height is the minimum requirement distance from the surface of the prepared abutment root to the opposing occlusal surface.			
FC Width	FC width is the minimum diameter of the space required for the fixed attachment component. Measure the smallest diameter of the root surface.			
Prep Depth	Prep depth is the minimum depth of the tooth structure needed for preparation of the attachment space.			
RC Width	RC width is the minimum diameter of the space required in the prosthesis for the removable attachment component.			

Fig. 3.17 The required criteria for attachments

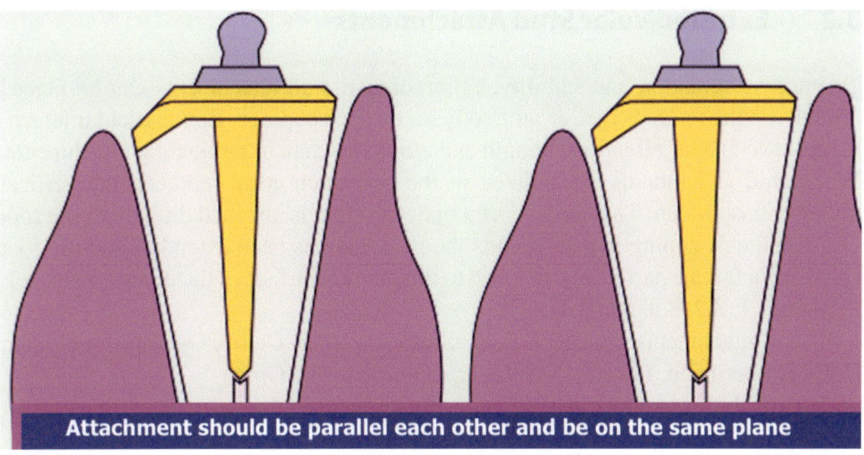

Fig. 3.18 The attachment should be placed in a right angle with the occlusal plane, and some angled attachment could be placed parallel to the long axis of the tooth with the surveyor

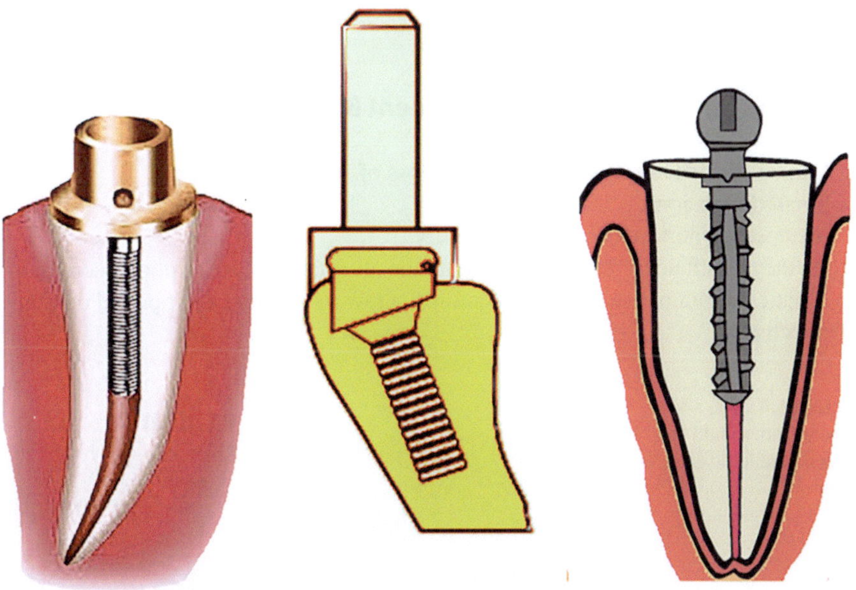

Fig. 3.19 The attachment should be placed in a right angle with the occlusal plane, and some angled attachment could be placed parallel to the long axis of the tooth with the surveyor

3.2 Extraradicular Stud Attachments

To improve retention and stability, extraradicular stud attachments can be placed directly on the tooth or root or indirectly on the cast copings. Extraradicular attachments have greater retention strength and efficiency than intraradicular attachments. When stud attachments are utilized in the construction of dentures, the vertical dimension is crucial. They consist of a male part that is attached directly to the root or a metal cast coping that surrounds the post that has been extended into the root canal and a female part that is attached to the interior surface of the denture (Fig. 3.1, Pictures 3.1, 3.2, 3.3, and 3.4).

These attachments include Gerber, Stufenexzenter, Dalbo, O-Ring, Preci Clix, Ceka, Rothermann, Introfix, Schubiger, Quinlivan, and Gmur.

The need for extraradicular stud attachments is specified.

- Healthful periodontal tissue.
- Sufficient region of attached gingiva.
- Meticulous dental and oral hygiene.
- Sufficient inter-arch and buccolingual space (adequate acrylic resin thickness around the attachment) (Picture 3.5).

3.2.1 Extraradicular Stud Attachment Benefits

- Can be applied to teeth with excessive loss of supporting tissue.
- Small dimensions.
- Increase support, retention, and stability.
- As they continue to regularly stimulate the alveolar bone, resorption decreases.
- If patients cannot use complete dentures, allow them to use their partial dentures effectively.

Picture 3.4 The attachments should be placed parallel to each other

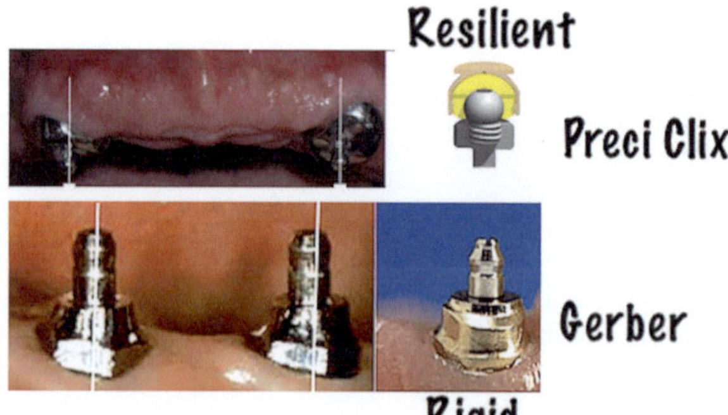

Picture 3.5 The reasonable thickness of acrylic resin should surround the attachment

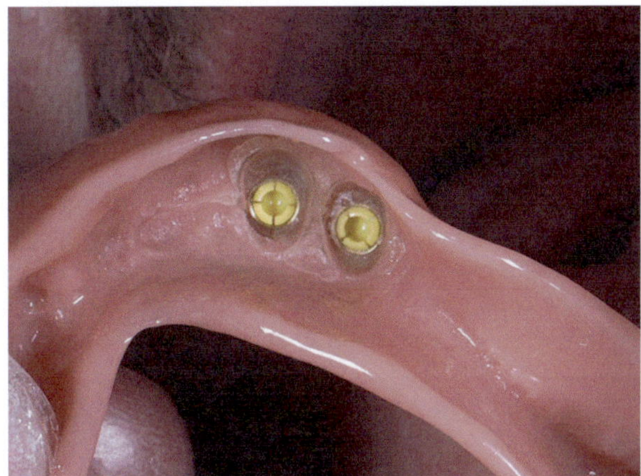

Picture 3.6 The stud attachment should support the metal framework

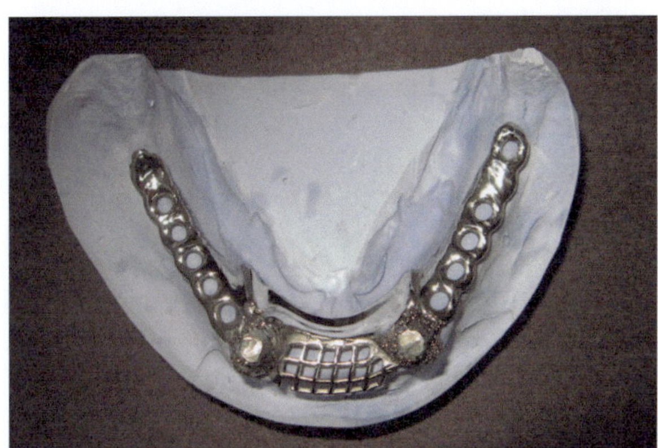

3.2.2 Negative Aspects of Stud Attachments

- The buccolingual and vertical distances should be sufficient for placement.
- They cover the gingival margins.
- They create areas where plaque accumulates.
- Can raise the probability of tooth decay.
- In cases of attachment relief, the base movement can cause gingival irritation; gingiva proliferates into the space.

While attachments improve the denture's stability and retention, they can also weaken it. Therefore, it is essential to surround the attachment with the correct thickness of acrylic resin. An attachment must be surrounded by a layer of acrylic resin at least 2–3 mm thick. To prevent denture fracture, the infrastructure must be supported by a metal frame (Picture 3.6).

3.3 Choosing Between Rigid and Flexible Extracoronal Attachments

Rigid attachments are used when:

- The supporting teeth have excellent supporting characteristics.
- During function and parafunction, less force will be applied to the edentulous area, and they require less maintenance than resilient attachments.
- If the coping post is too short and a rigid attachment is used, the post will dislodge from the root after uncontrolled movement.

Resilient attachments are used when:

- The teeth lack sufficient supporting quality.
- The geometric distribution of the remaining teeth is insufficient for the stability of a denture.
- If soft tissues have greater resiliency but less width, unintentional displacement and inclination movement will occur (Picture 3.4).

3.3.1 The Number of Attachments to Extracoronal Stud

One attachment per side of the arch is sufficient. More attachments do not necessarily improve retention; they strengthen the substructure while weakening the superstructure. If there are teeth on one side of the arch, you cannot use the attachment on adjacent teeth. This condition will make it difficult to maintain hygiene and will deteriorate the denture base. Covering the remaining roots with simple copings is possible. Connecting adjacent copings effectively resists rotational load but complicates plaque control and overdenture construction. However, inclined forces are resolved along the long axes of the roots (Picture 3.7).

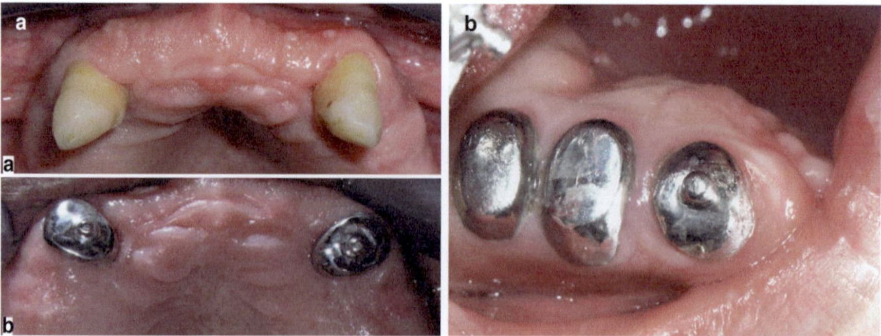

Picture 3.7 (**a**) The stud attachment should be placed on each side of the arch; (**b**) there are few teeth on one side of the arch and only one tooth/root placed on the attachment. The remaining roots can be covered with simple copings

An increase in the number of attachments may increase the denture's stability but at the expense of its strength.

Extraradicular stud attachments are utilized when there is sufficient vertical space and are robust. Multiple techniques can generate extraradicular indirect attachments. Either the tooth or its root must be vital or nonvital. The threaded base ring can be cast, soldered, or laser-welded into a coping or directly into a tooth. These attachments are utilized on cast copings of varying heights (short, medium, and long). The casting with a high-fusing base ring for the cast-on technique should be with a precious or a non-precious alloys or prefabricated. Also, some attachments have replaceable male and female components.

3.3.2 Gerber Attachment

The Gerber is a versatile attachment consisting of a male post embedded in the screw soldered to the base and a female part with a spring and ring for retention. Soldering connects the male unit to the denture, and components can be removed from the denture base.

There are two types: those that permit some vertical movement and those that are completely rigid (Picture 3.4; Figs. 3.20, 3.21, 3.22, 3.23, and 3.24). The retention of the Gerber stud attachment is achieved by inserting the female retainer spring into the male peripheral duct. If two or more teeth are to be used, the most distal

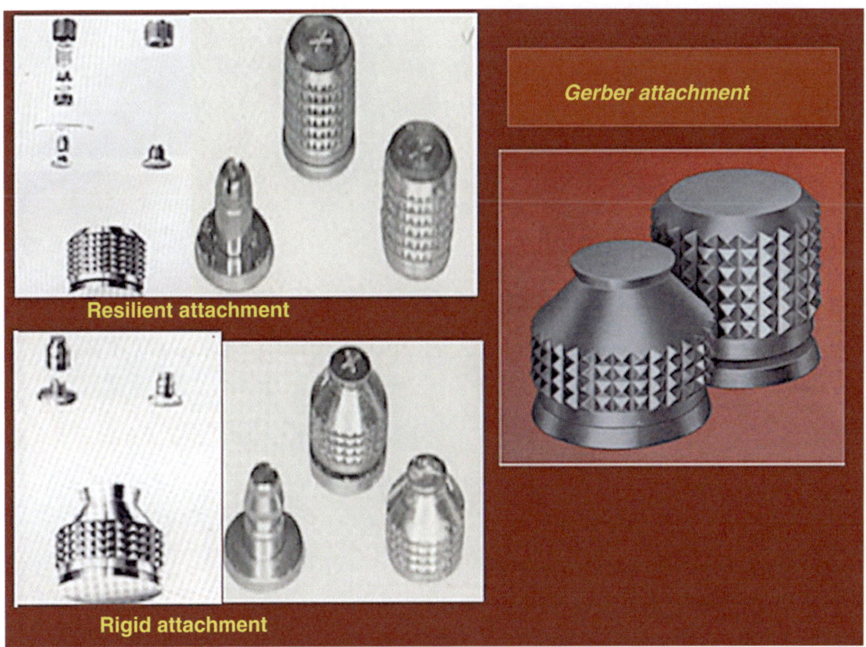

Fig. 3.20 Resilient and rigid Gerber attachment

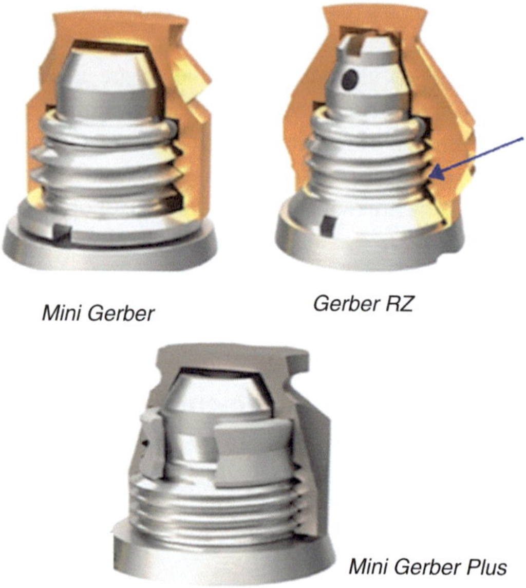

Fig. 3.21 Types of Gerber attachment

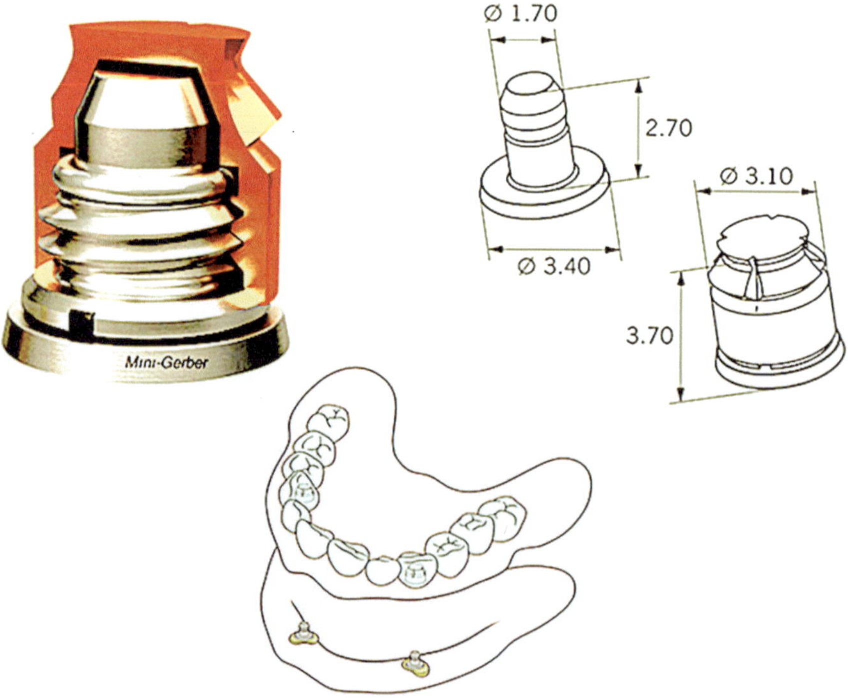

Fig. 3.22 Mini Gerber attachment

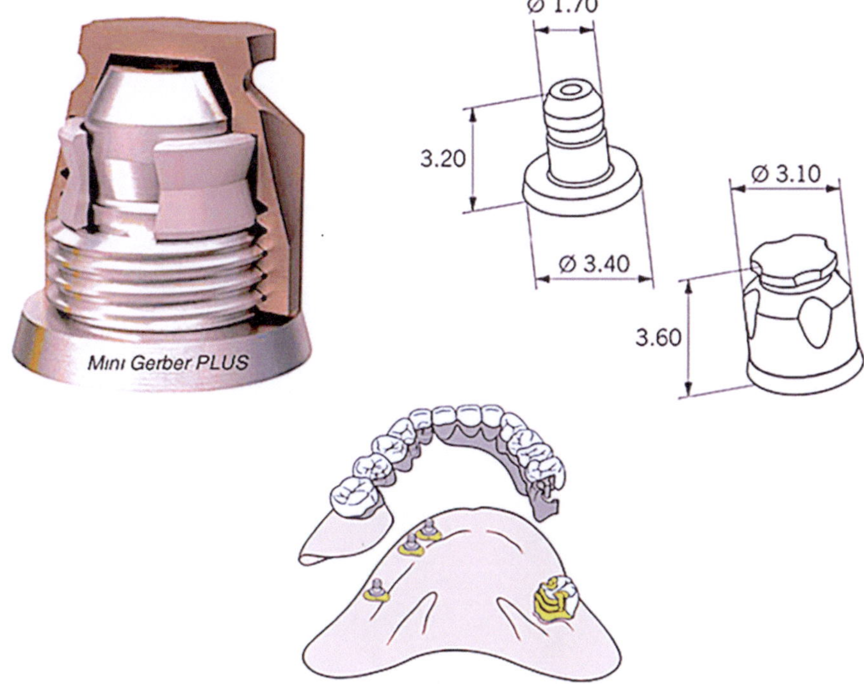

Fig. 3.23 Mini Gerber Plus attachment

attachment should allow for greater vertical movement than the anterior attachments, as the tipping forces on the molar mastication surfaces of dentures are greater. If the supports are canine and first premolar, the canine attachment should be square and rigid, whereas the premolar attachment should be resilient. A square, resilient attachment is preferred for posterior teeth, whereas a conical, rigid attachment is preferred for anterior teeth. Both attachments have the benefit of being easy to replace.

The spring-loaded, vertically resilient attachment known as the puffer is the resilient Gerber attachment. It consists of nine components and is one of the most complex and expensive stud attachments. A resilient attachment permits vertical movement and, as a result, reduces the torque force applied to the supporting tooth. The soldering base of the male stud has a different retention post (Fig. 3.20). If the base moves due to an incorrect impression or decreased adaptability, the rigid Gerber attachment applies torque to the tooth.

3.3.2.1 The Rigid Gerber Attachment

The Mini Gerber is an attachment for the anterior regions of the lower and upper jaw that is supraradicular and cylindrical with small dimensions. It is utilized for devitalized-root removable and rigid hybrid dentures (Fig. 3.22).

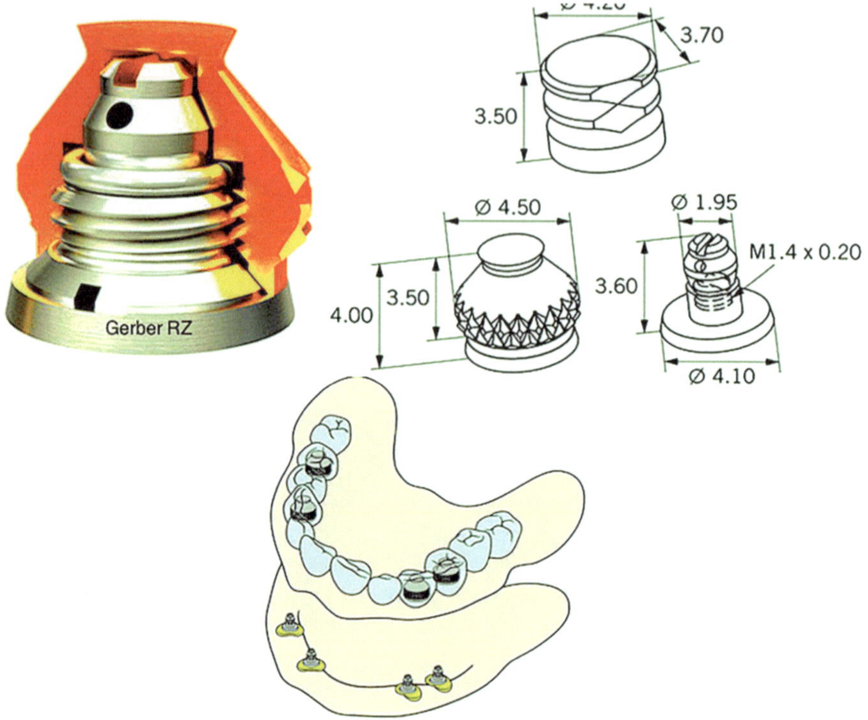

Fig. 3.24 Gerber RZ precision attachment (retention-grip and rigid)

Mini Gerber Plus is a supraradicular retention device with a friction grip. This cylindrical attachment can be utilized as a friction-grip attachment or a retention-grip attachment (Fig. 3.23).

Gerber RZ is a cylindrical supraradicular retention grip attachment. It functions as a cylindrical retention principle (Fig. 3.24).

3.3.2.2 Positive Aspects of a Gerber Attachment

- Rebasing is simple.
- The soldering base can be replaced (Gerber attachments are easily replaceable, male units can be removed by unscrewing the thread, and other attachments can be fixed).
- The spring-loaded function allows the base to adapt.

3.3.2.3 Negative Aspects of a Gerber Attachment

- It is heavy (more bulk is needed; more interocclusal space must be present).
- The design is complex.
- Torque can occur if denture base support is inadequate.

3.3.3   Stufenexzenter Attachment

The Stufenexzenter attachment is a friction-retentive supraradicular cylindrical attachment that can be activated (Figs. 3.25 and 3.26). The matrix constructed of

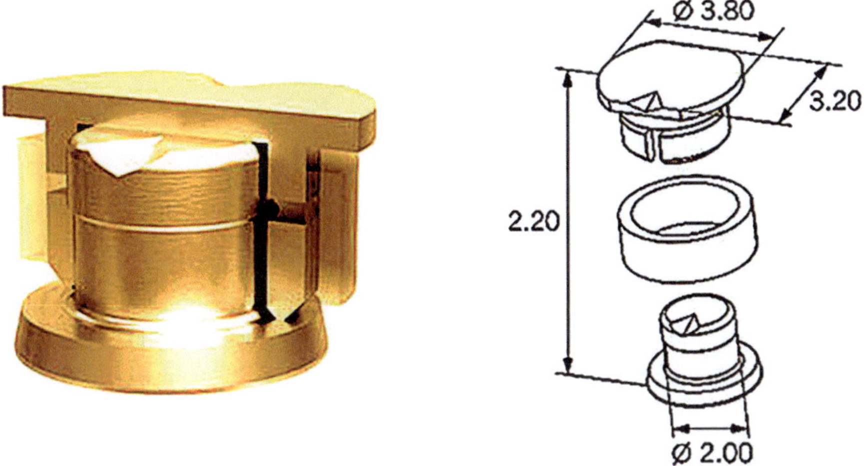

Fig. 3.25   Stufenexzenter attachment

Fig. 3.26   Stufenexzenter attachment placed in the denture

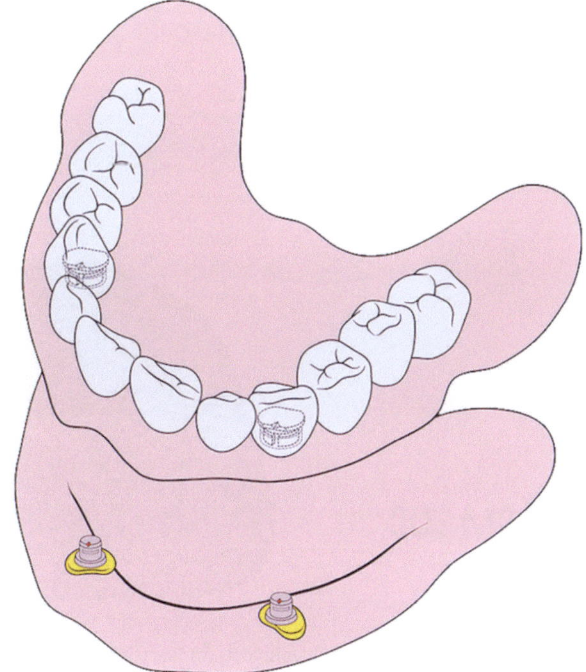

OSV, a high-strength precious metal alloy for soldering to cast root caps, does not present any difficulties for the technician. The function of the attachment is determined by the placement of the matrix on the male (frictive or retentive).

3.3.3.1 Specifications of the Stufenexzenter Accessory

- Attachments with multiple purposes.
- Compact and robust.
- Low profile.
- Due to its small size, it can also be used in confined areas.
- Change the matrix from fricative to retentive.
- Easy processing of the components and simple activation.

3.3.4 CM LOC Attachment

Additionally, the CM LOC attachment is a supraradicular, cylindrical attachment that improves rigid retentive attachments (Fig. 3.10, Picture 3.8). This system has the distinct advantage of compensating for divergence across the abutment, making it suitable for a wide variety of clinical applications. This system can correct divergences of up to 60° (30°) and significantly reduces wear. The matrices with various retention inserts and force levels are highly resilient.

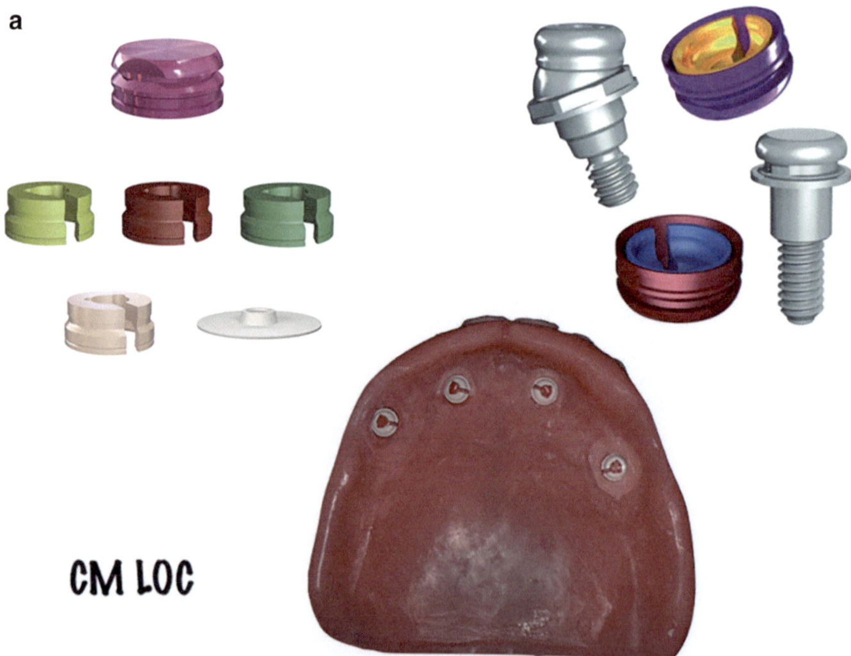

Picture 3.8 (**a, b**) CM LOC attachment; (**c**) Inserting male part of CM LOC

b

CM LOC

Laser welding

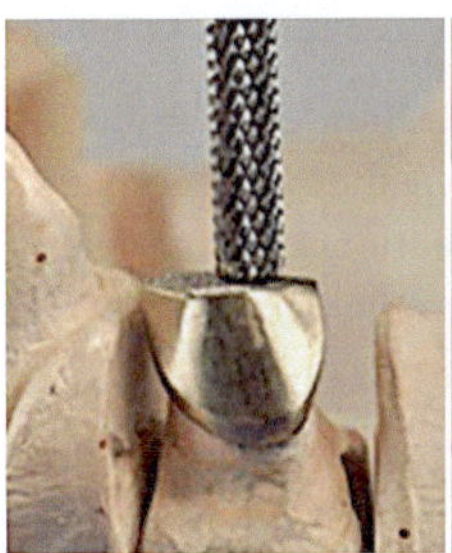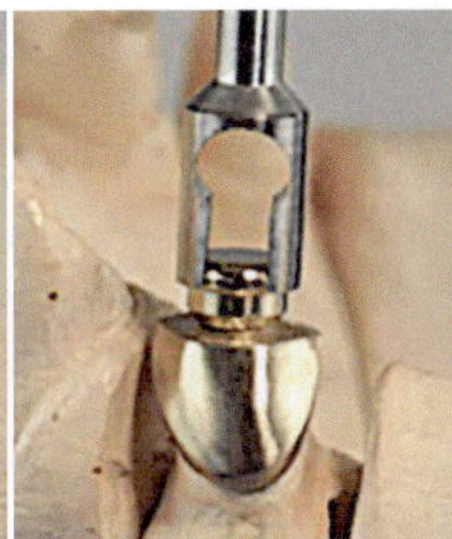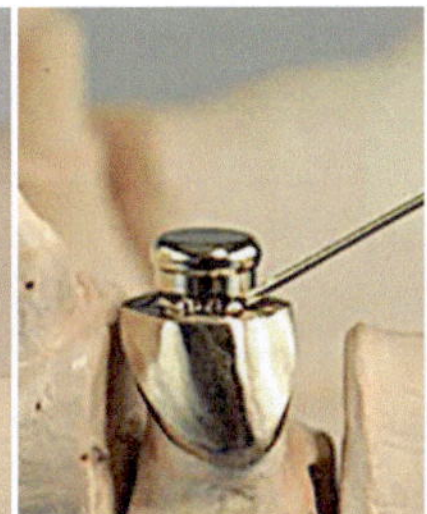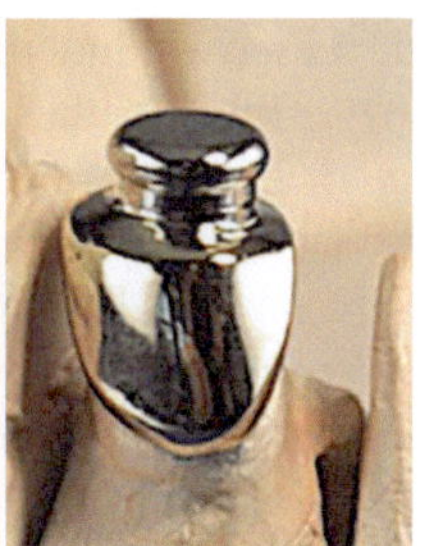

Casting

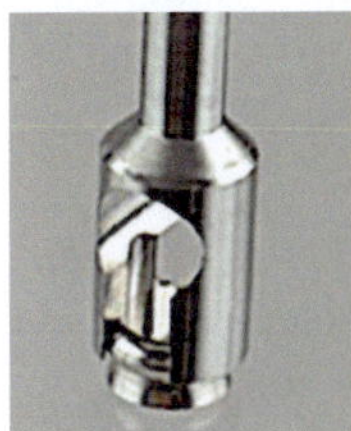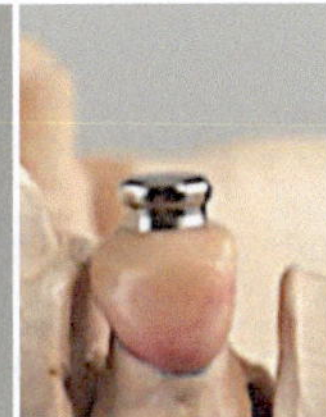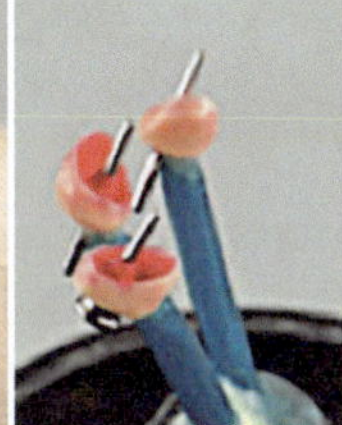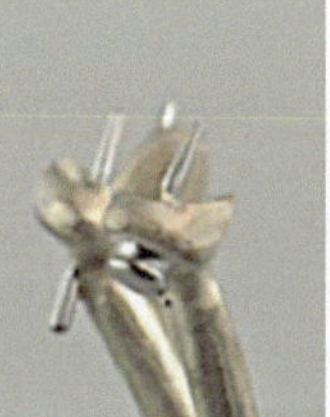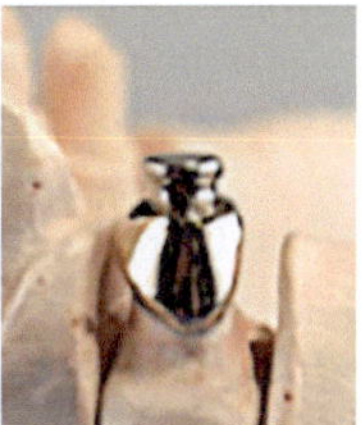

Soldering

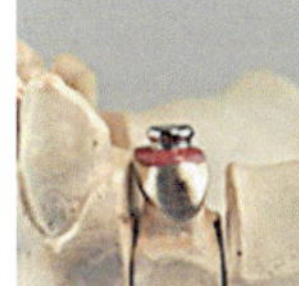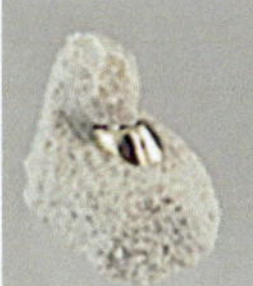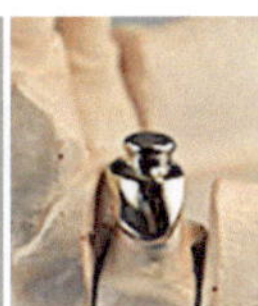

Picture 3.8 (continued)

The CM LOC male parts C and E can be used for hybrid-supported, root-removable dental prostheses. The CM LOC FLEX abutment components are also intended for complete or partial fixation of overdentures (complete dentures) or partial dentures using maxillary or mandibular endosseous implants. This attachment can be used in conjunction with hybrid-supported removable dental prostheses on implants and the specific CM LOC system for the female component.

Components employing CM LOC:

C = Ceramicor®, male component.
E = Elitor®, male component.
S = Syntax-Abettment (male part), CAD/CAM retention element (male part), Housing (female part).
Pekkton® = P and E = Elitor®, retention inserts part.

3.3.4.1 Dealing with the CM LOC Attachment (Picture 3.8b)

The three-way can accommodate the male organ.

1. Laser-welding the male component of Elitor into place.

   Initially, the root canal cap was milled at right angles, parallel to the direction of insertion, using a milling machine. The male component then positions and laser welds around the circumference, filling all undercuts with laser wire. Using a standard rubber wheel and a polishing brush, smooth down the laser welds. For male organ protection, the spacer should be placed on the male organ.

2. Installing the male ceramic component

   Casting

   The male part positions the surveyor as centrally as possible, waxes it to the root canal cap, and casts it according to the dental casting alloys' usage instructions. In addition, the spacers protect the male component during sandblasting and processing.

3. Insert the male component in Ceramicor

   Soldering

   Using a surveyor, a face-milled root canal cap, and wax, the male part is positioned as centrally as possible on the tooth that has already been cast. The solder gap should be continuous and between 0.05 and 0.25 mm wide. Then, design the soldering block so that the male component is held securely and good flame access is ensured after soldering, and cool the soldering block to room temperature gradually.

Attachments used in prosthetic dentistry are subject to a great deal of stress in the mouth, which is a constantly changing environment, and are consequently susceptible to wear over time. Normal deterioration cannot be avoided; it can only be reduced. The amount of wear is dependent on the system as a whole.

To reduce wear to an absolute minimum level, the manufacturer recommended using materials that are optimally matched whenever possible. The perfect fit of dentures on the mucosa must be evaluated annually and relined if necessary to prevent tilting movement (overload). Initially, check hybrid prostheses every 3 months and replace the retention inserts if necessary.

3.3.5 Ball Attachments

The ball attachments are among the simplest stud attachments due to their low cost, ease of handling, minimal chairside time requirements, and applicability with both root- and implant-supported prostheses. This attachment system is a practical and relatively inexpensive concept for prosthetics. Individual balls were said to be less expensive, less technique-sensitive, and easier to clean than bars. Furthermore, single-ball attachments reduced the risk of mucosal hyperplasia even further.

The ball and socket attachments consist of a metal ball (male portion) and a female component incorporated into the denture's fitting surface (Figs. 3.27, 3.28, 3.29, 3.30, 3.31, 3.32, 3.33, 3.34, 3.35, 3.36, 3.37, 3.38, 3.39, 3.40, 3.41, 3.42, 3.43, 3.44, 3.45, and 3.46). The female component could be one of the following varieties:

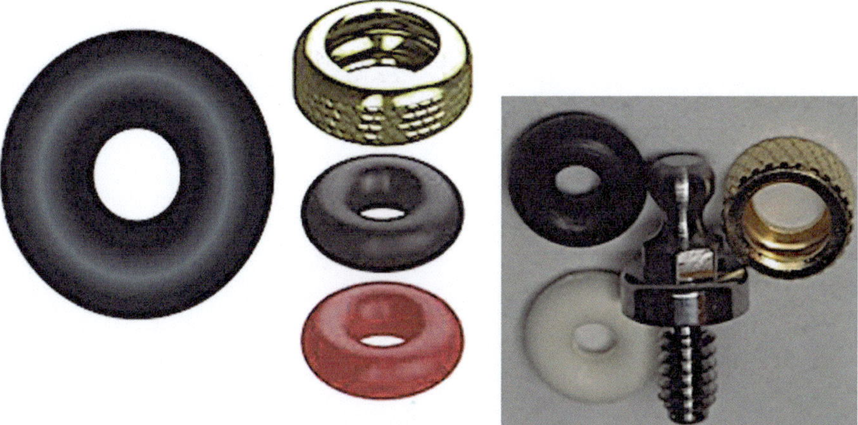

Fig. 3.27 O-ring attachment assembly

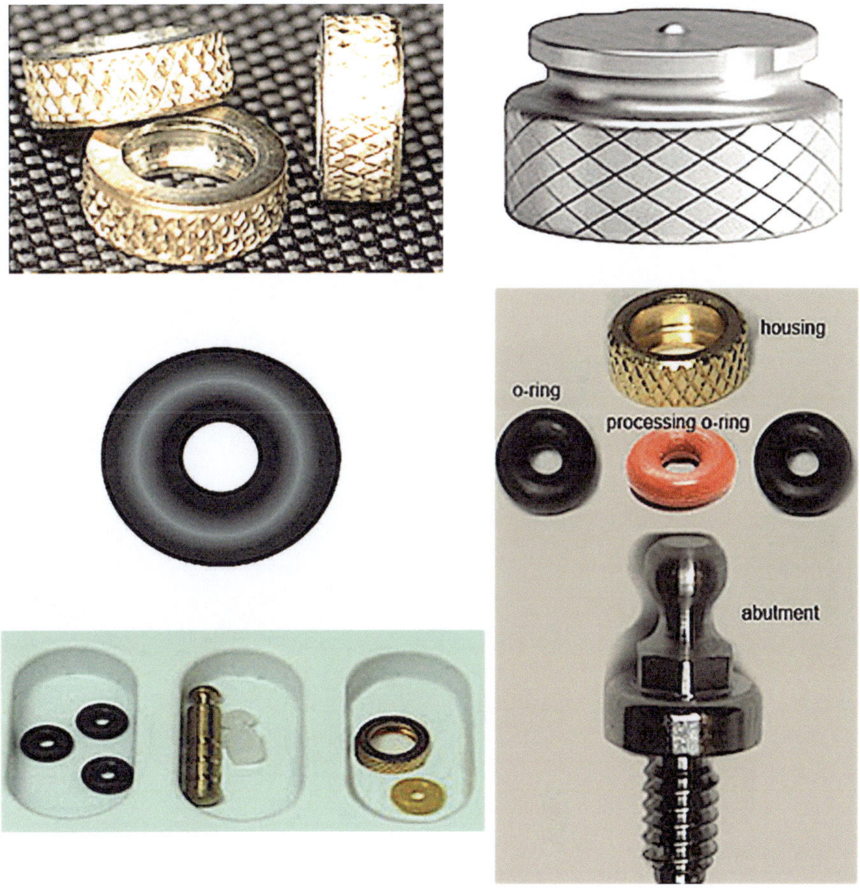

Fig. 3.28 Rubber O-ring and open and close metal housing

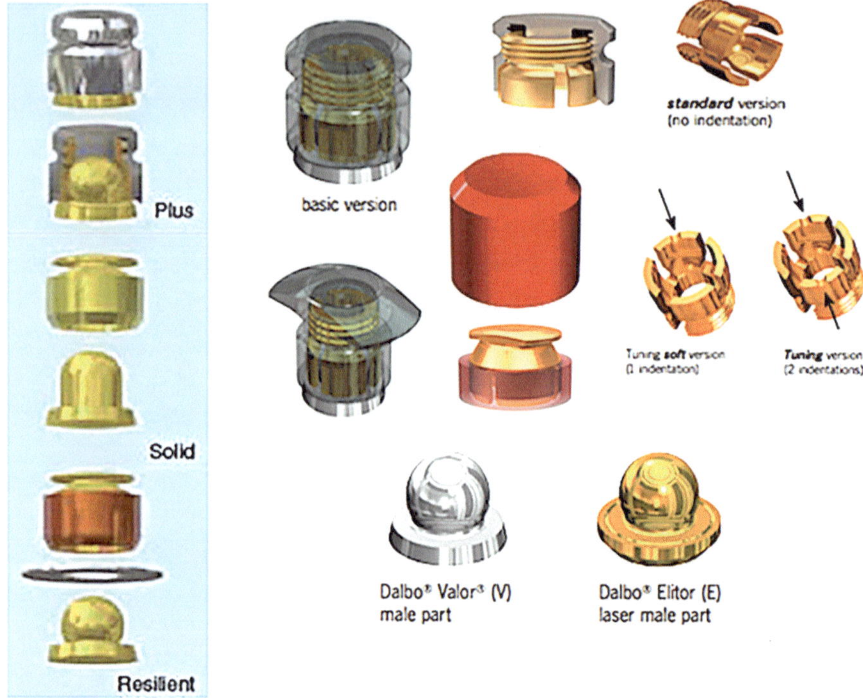

Fig. 3.29 Types of Dalbo (Dalla Bona) attachment

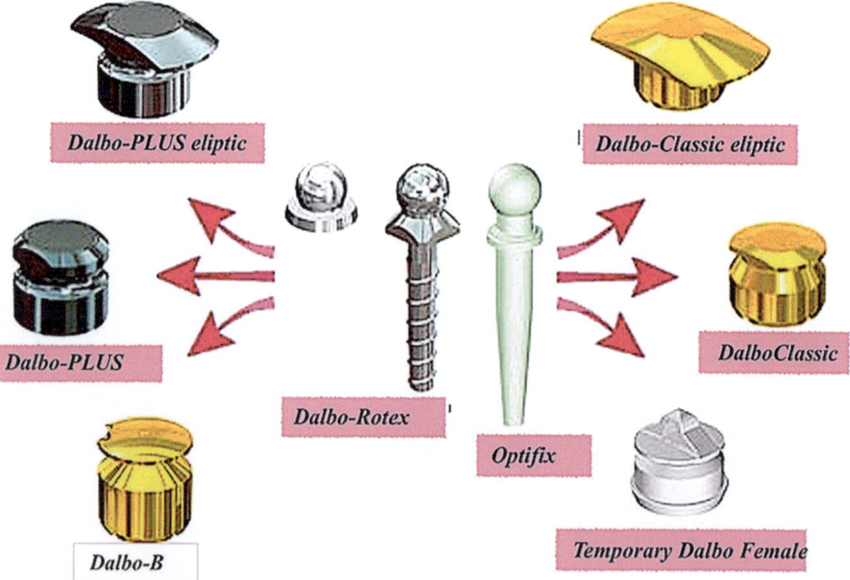

Fig. 3.30 Types of Dalbo (Dalla Bona) attachment

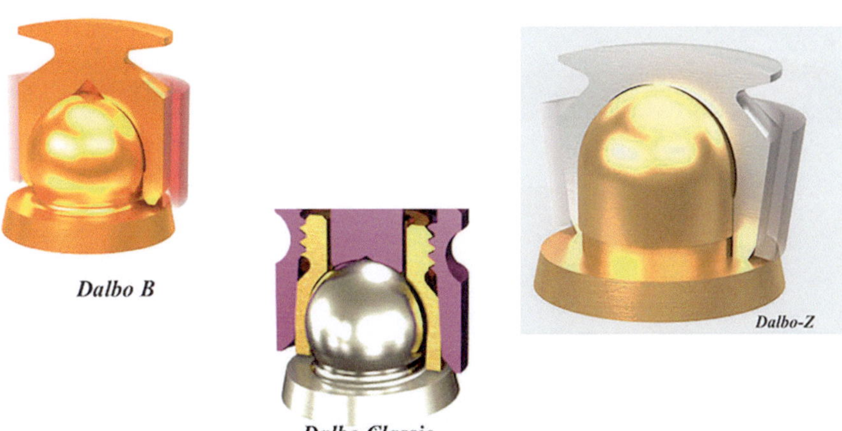

Fig. 3.31 The Dalbo B, Dalbo classic, and Dalbo Z attachment

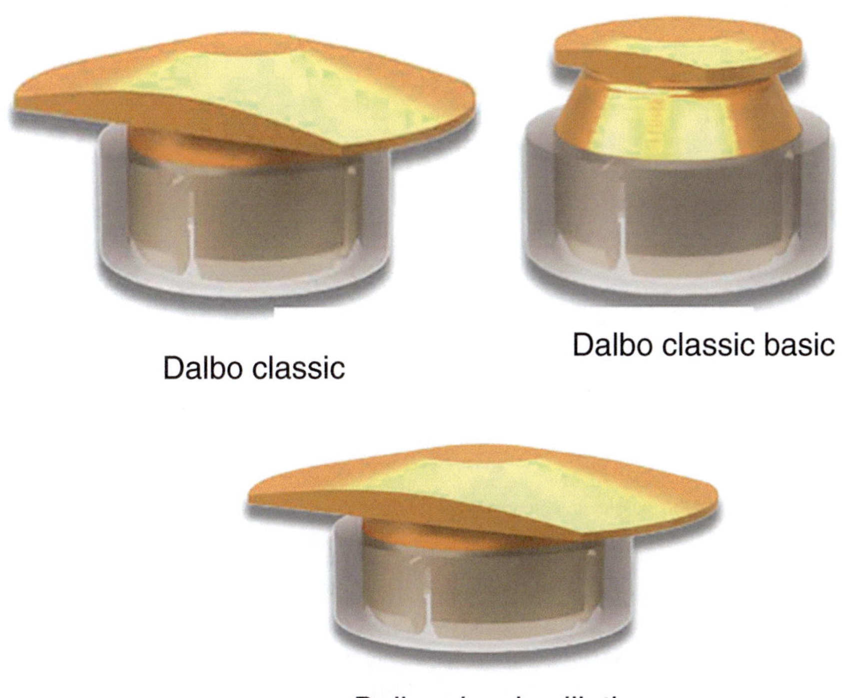

Fig. 3.32 The Dalbo female part has flexible precious metal lamellae

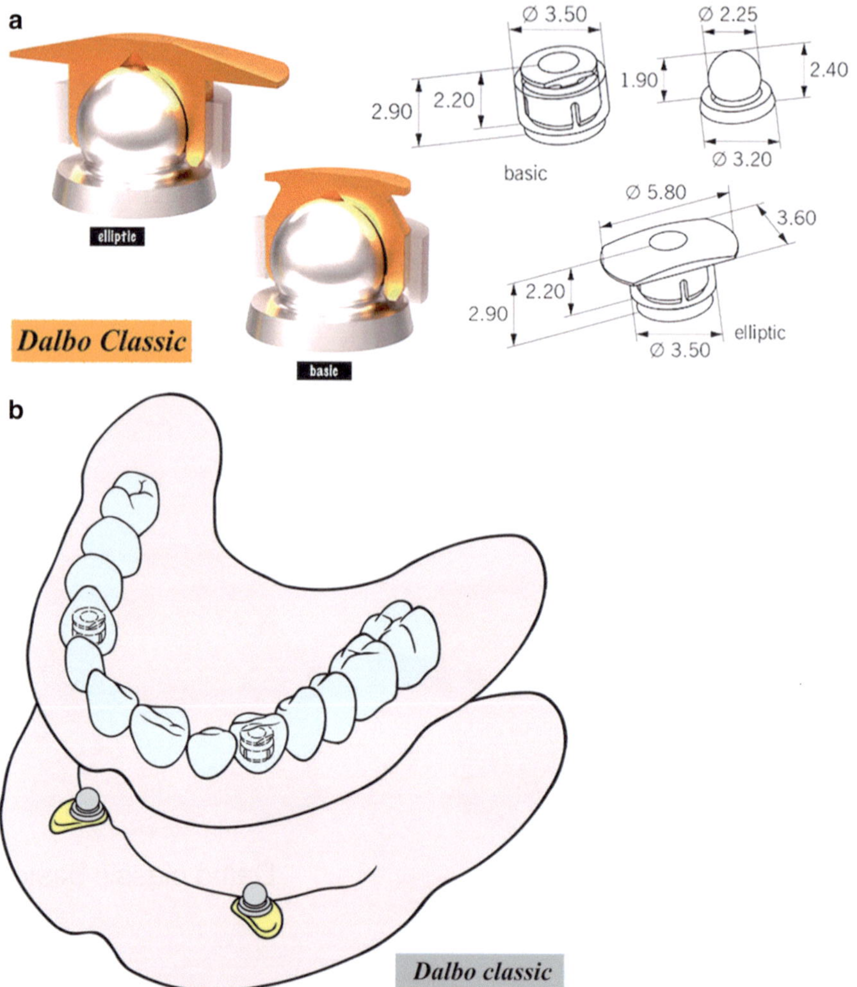

Fig. 3.33 The Dalbo classic attachment: (**a**) Schematic view and (**b**) schematic prosthetic view

(a) The O-ring, whose retainer is a rubber ring. If the roots are not parallel, the rubber ring will deteriorate within a few weeks (Picture 3.9, Figs. 3.27 and 3.28).

(b) This system is less resilient than an O-ring attachment. However, the retention forces are nearly double those of the O-ring system (Picture 3.10, Figs. 3.29, 3.30, 3.31, 3.32, 3.33, 3.34, 3.35, 3.36, 3.37, 3.38, 3.39, and 3.40).

(c) Different types and materials of spherical/equator attachments with various retentive caps on the female part (Pro-Snap/Profix ball attachment, Preci Ball/ Preci Clix attachment, Figs. 3.41, 3.41, 3.42, 3.43, 3.44, 3.45, and 3.46).

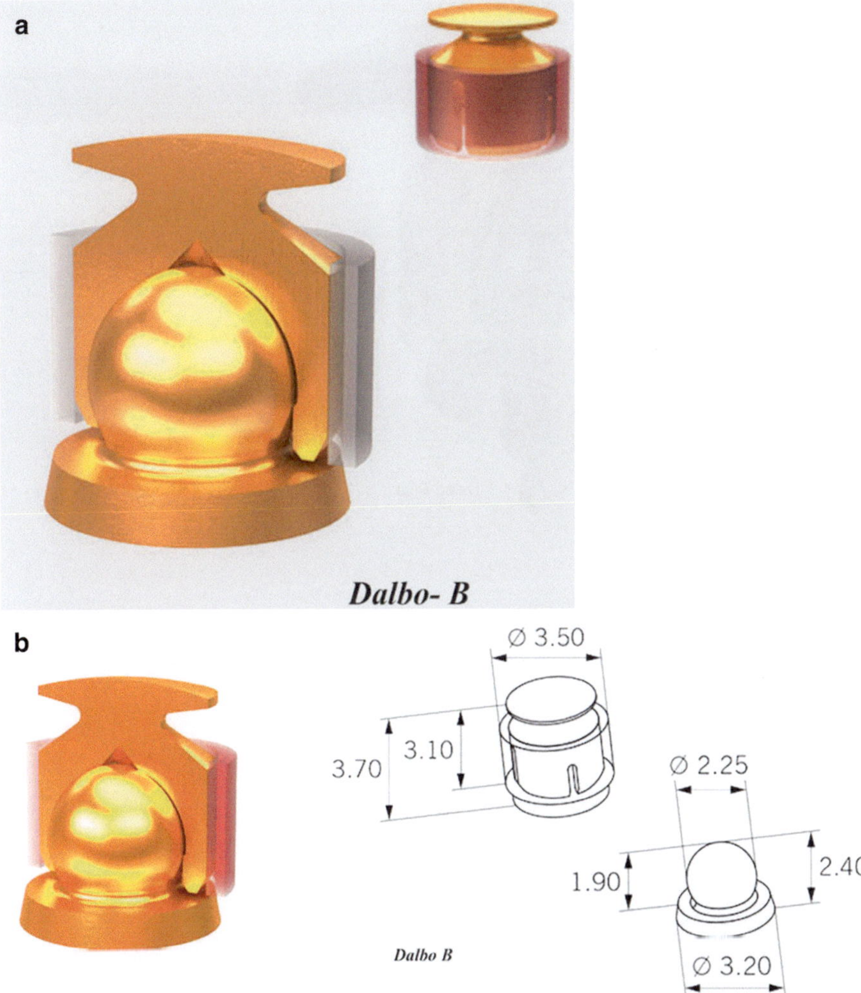

Fig. 3.34 The Dalbo B attachment: (**a**) male and female part and (**b**) schematic view

3.3.6   O-Ring Connection

O-ring attachments are the most common and convenient type of stud attachments (Picture 3.9; Figs. 3.27 and 3.28). The O-ring abutment is made of titanium alloy and is available in various cuff heights with coronal spherical geometry that snaps into a rubber. The O-ring is held in place by a metal retainer ring, and the housing is held in place by the denture. O-ring attachments are elastomeric attachments typically made of silicone that resemble the inner tire of a wheel. Rings of retention are

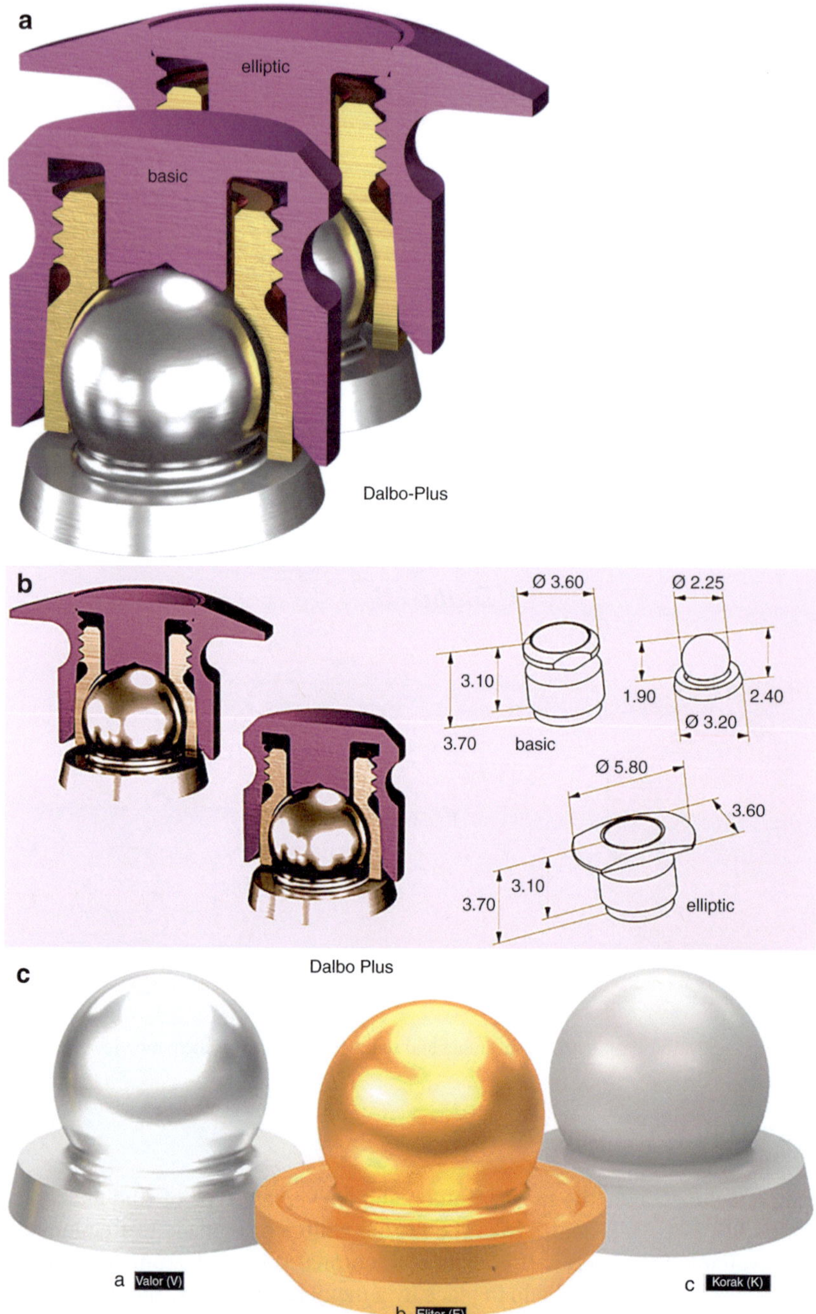

Fig. 3.35 The Dalbo–Plus attachment: (**a**) male and female part, (**b**) schematic view, (**c**) different materials of Dalbo male attachment, (**d**) Dalbo plus female attachment types, (**e**) the flexible precious metal lamellae, (**f**) the Dalbo–Plus basic, (**g**) the Dalbo–Plus elliptic, and (**h**) Dalbo plus schematic prosthetic view

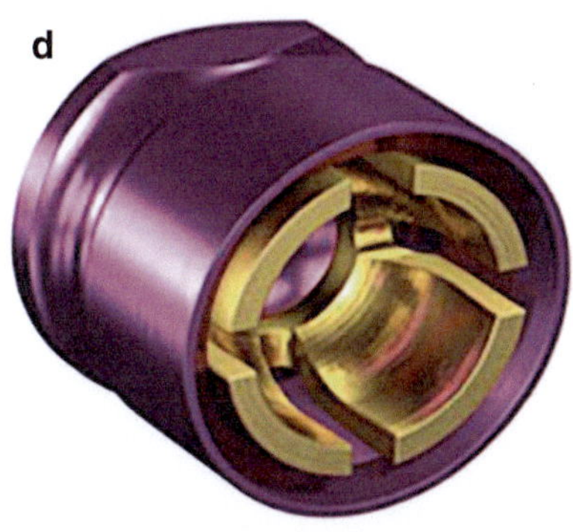

female part dalbo plus

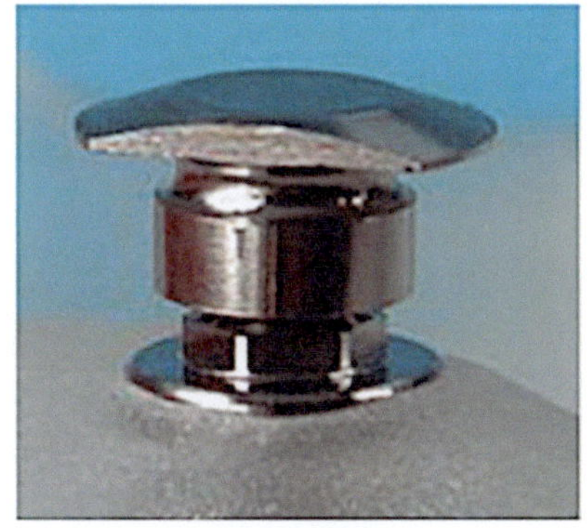

Dalbo plus female elliptic

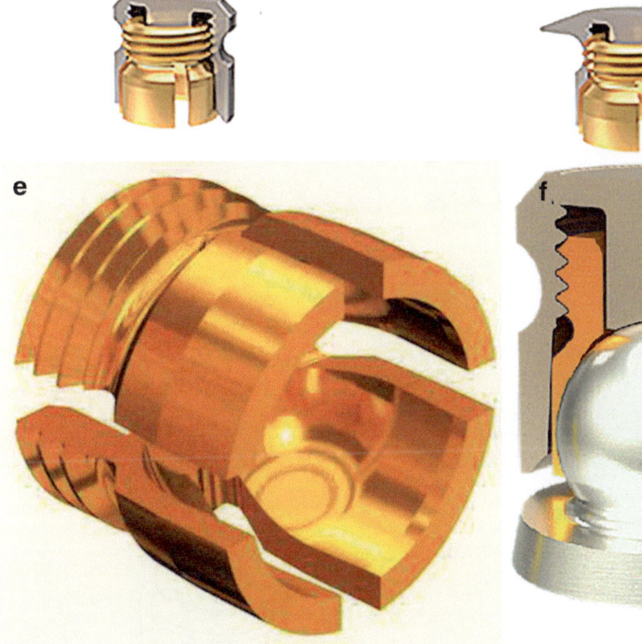

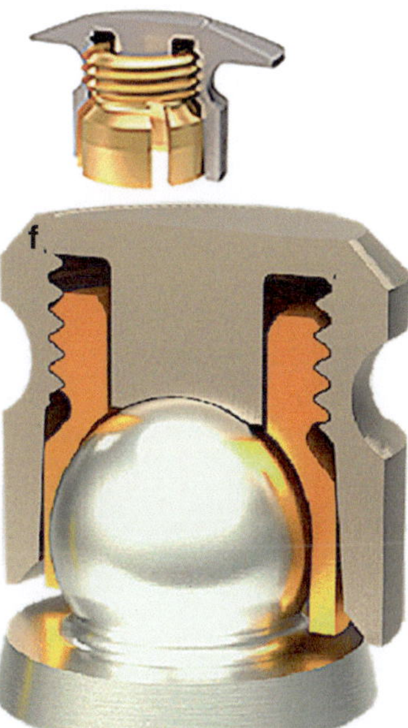

Fig. 3.35 (continued)

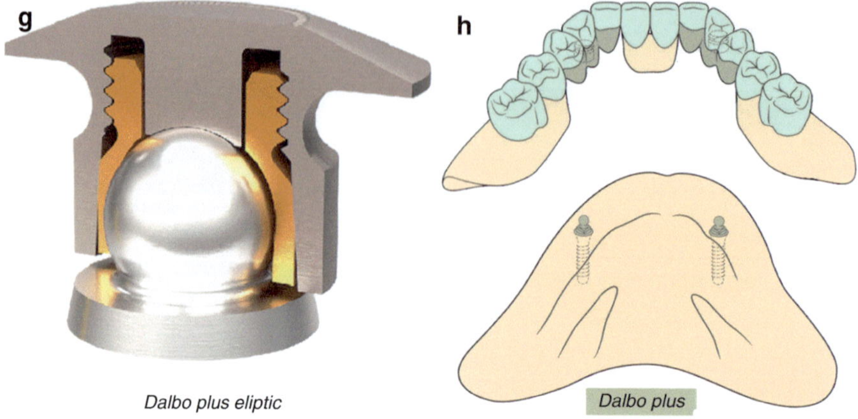

Fig. 3.35 (continued)

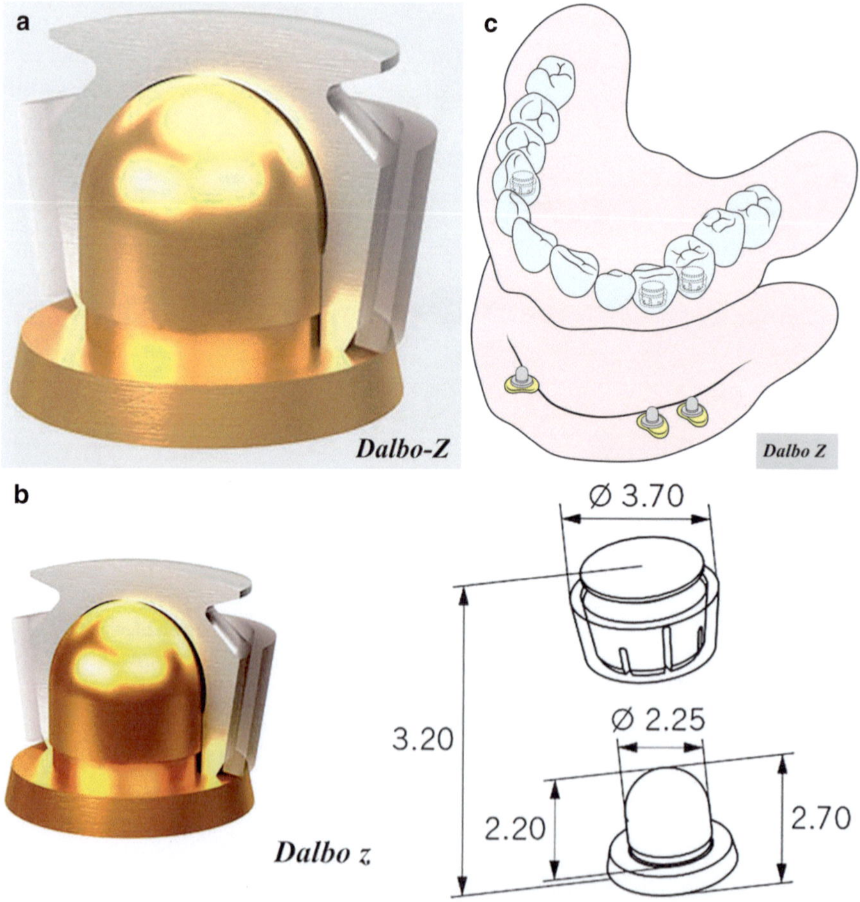

Fig. 3.36 (**a**) The Dalbo z attachment male and female part, (**b**) schematic view, and (**c**) schematic prosthetic view

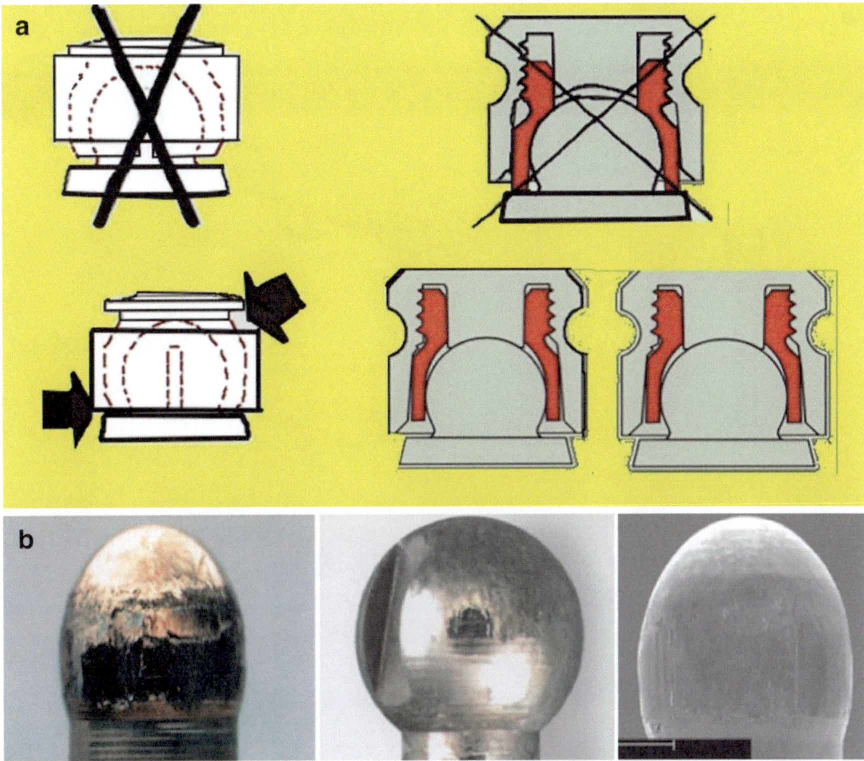

Fig. 3.37 (**a**) Position of the attachment and housing and (**b**) some spherical attachments wear male parts due to plastic female overload

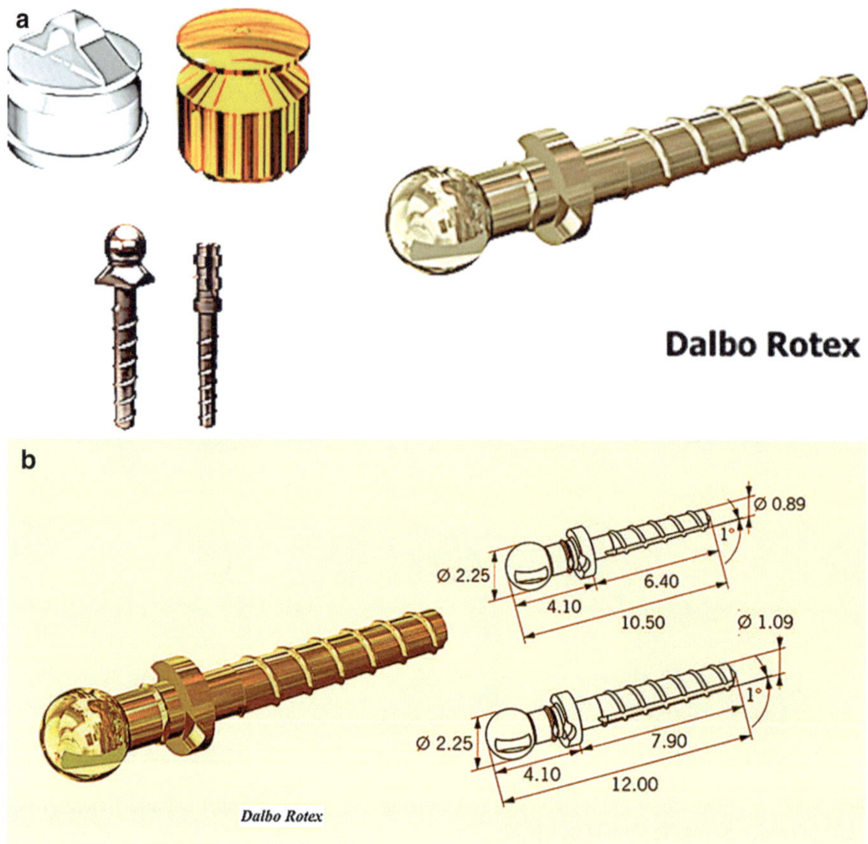

Fig. 3.38 (**a**) The Dalbo Rotex attachment and (**b**) schematic view

placed in the acrylic base (during either laboratory procedures or direct applications). The metal O-ring attachment system is functionally classified as an excellent resilient attachment for overdentures. It does not transfer forces to the root and only serves as a retention device. Additionally, the O-ring system is regarded as the superior attachment because it acts passively on the remaining abutment teeth. This attachment system was chosen because of its low profile and the resilience offered by the rubber retainer. Additionally, it offers sufficient retention, is simple to insert and remove, and is comfortable for the patient.

3.3.6.1 Indications
When resilience and improved oral hygiene are desired for overdentures or partial dentures. The height of the cuff should be at or above the level of the surrounding soft tissue.

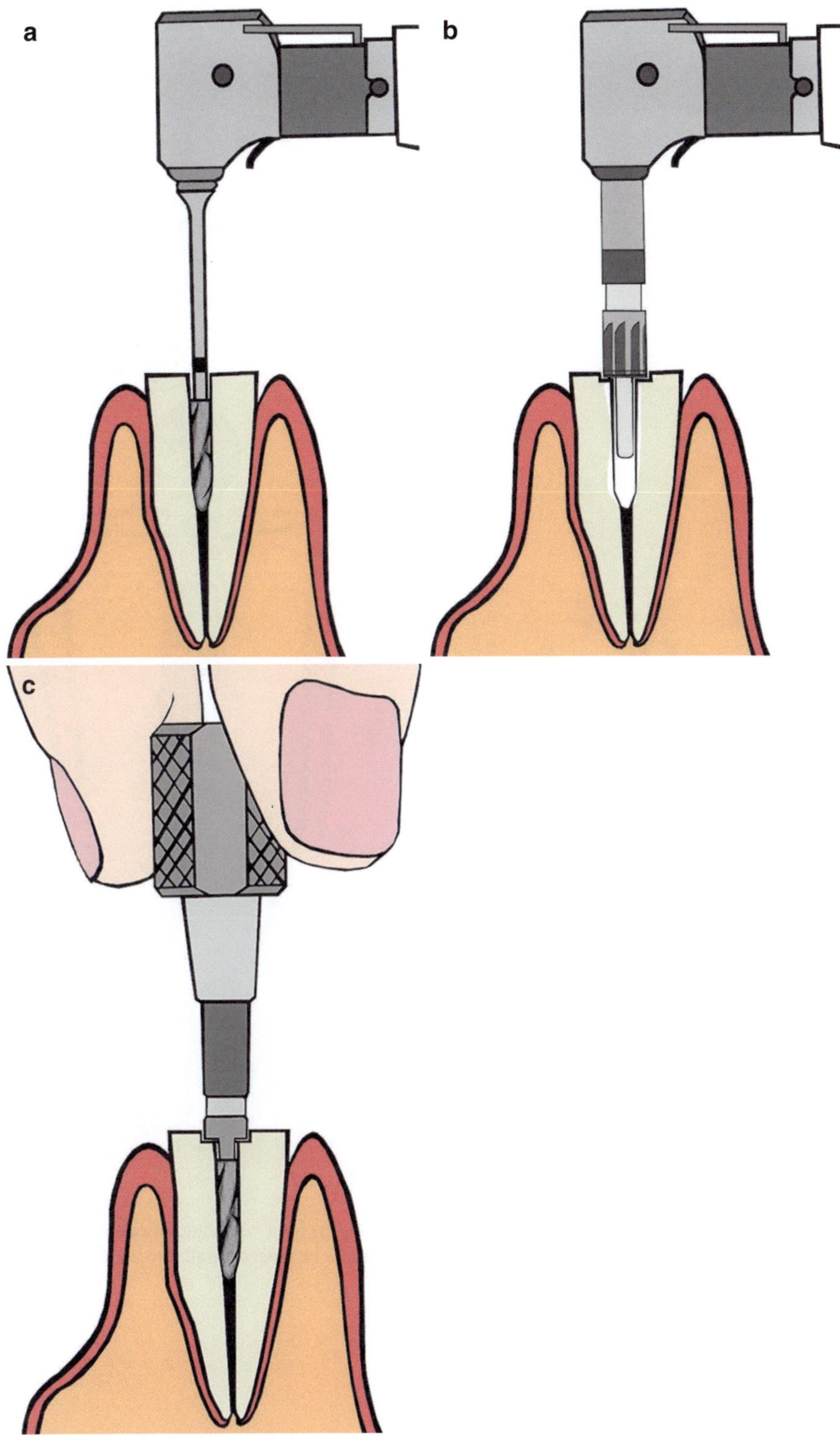

Fig. 3.39 (**a–c**) Preparation of the root for the placement of the Dalbo Rotex attachment

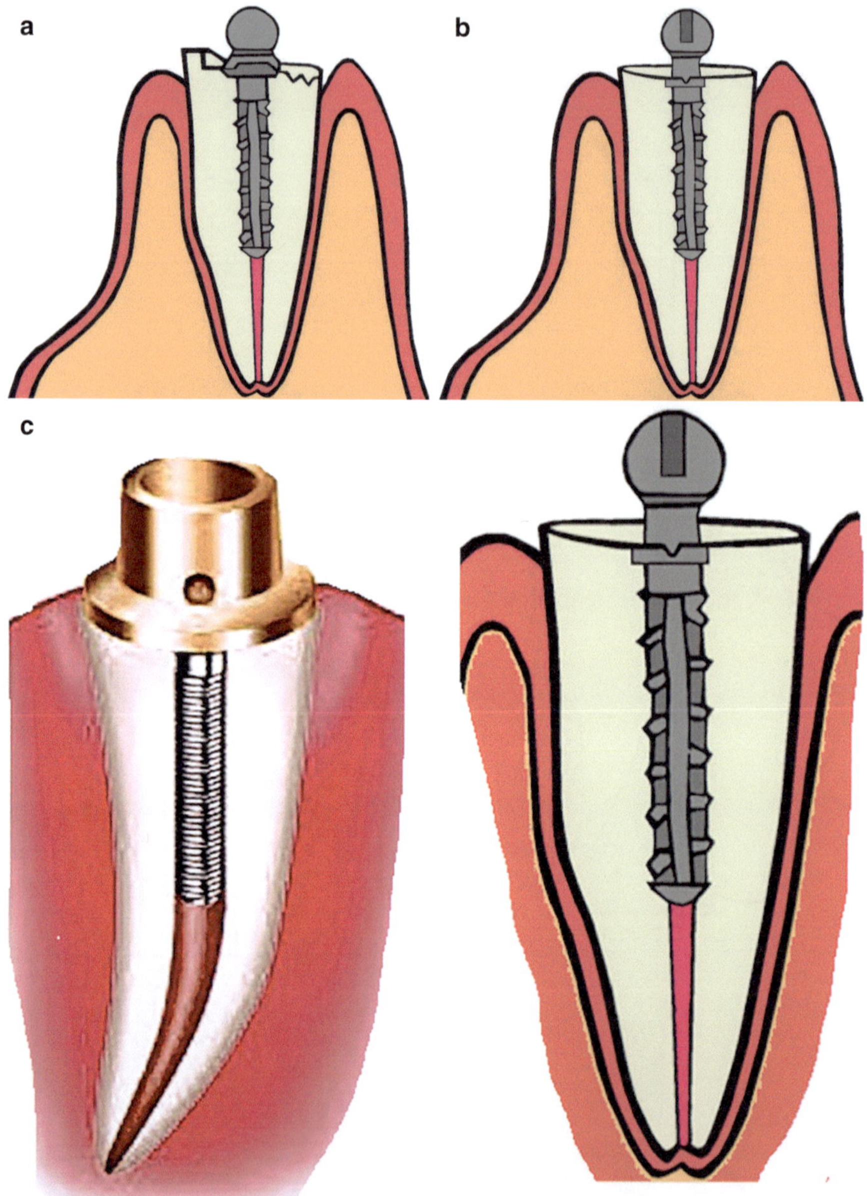

Fig. 3.40 (**a**) Placement of the Dalbo Rotex attachment, (**b**) after cementation occlusal surface should be smoothed and polished, and (**c**) attachment should be placed parallel to the long axis of the tooth

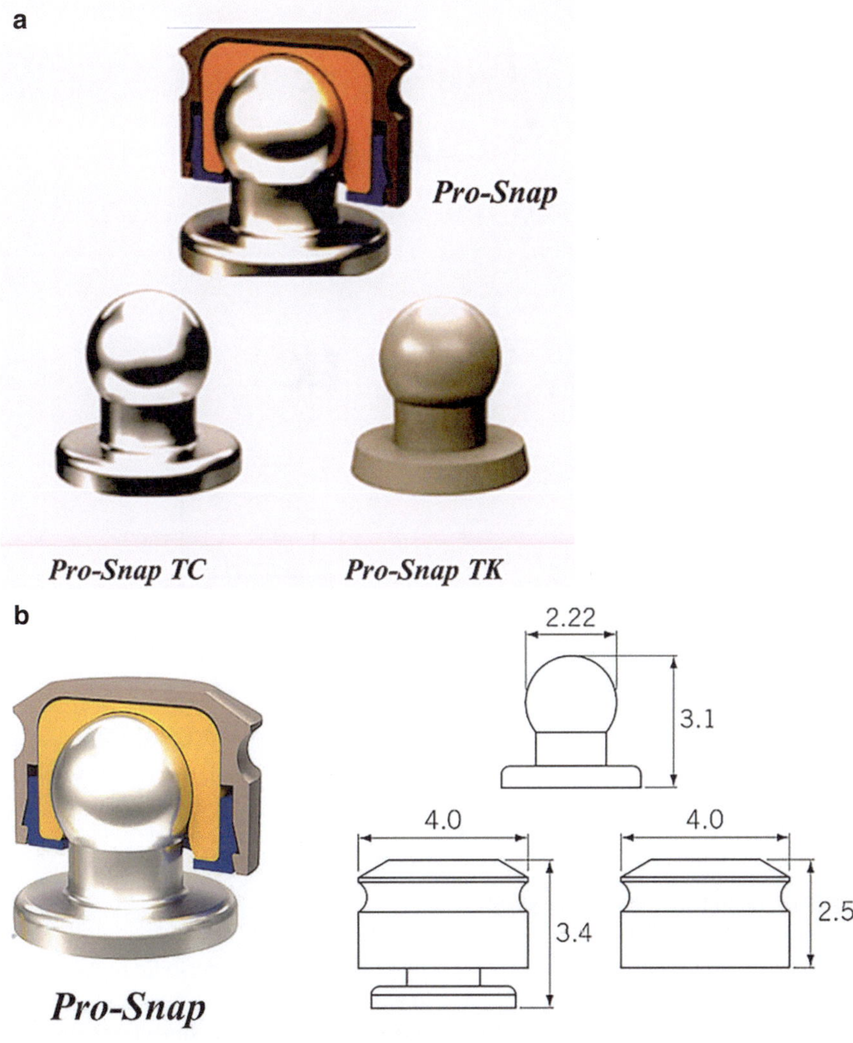

Fig. 3.41 (**a, b**) Pro-Snap attachment system

3.3.6.2 Contraindications

As with the other stud attachments, they should run parallel to one another. It should not be used when teeth are convergent or divergent by more than 10°, when teeth are less than 6.5 mm apart (center to center), or when there is less than 7 mm of space coronal to the teeth. Parallelism is believed to be the chain's weakest link, and non-parallel O-ring abutments may cause fractures at the neck level of the abutments. In addition, a lack of parallelism may lead to attachment wear during insertion and removal movements.

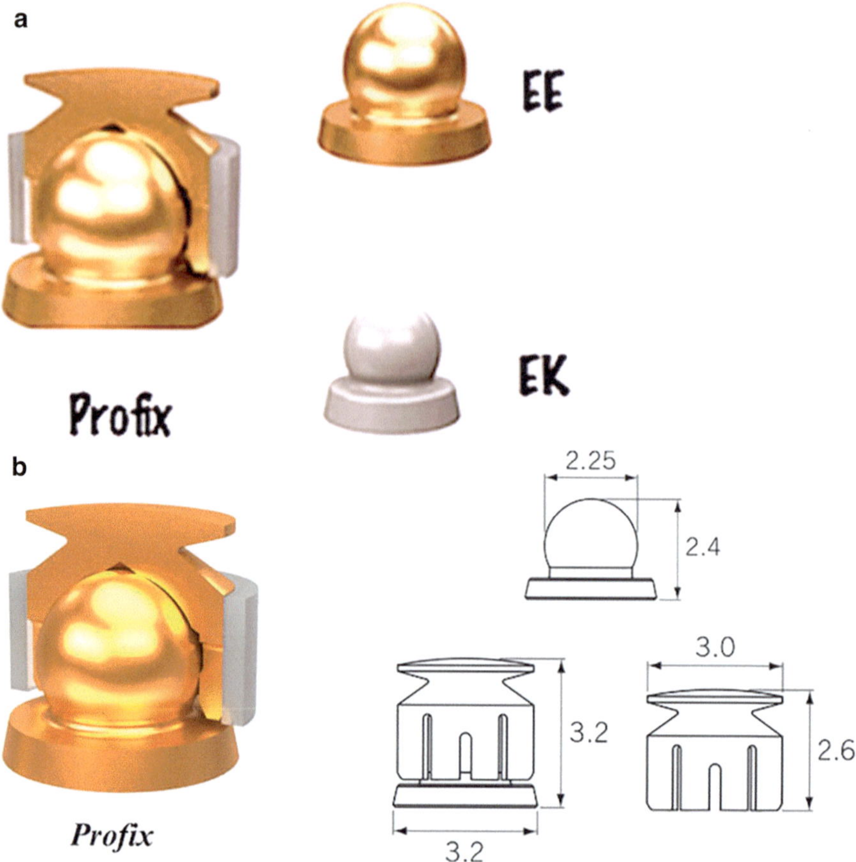

Fig. 3.42 (**a, b**) Profix attachment system

The gradual loss of retention is caused by O-ring wear and periodic replacement is needed. Additionally, this type of attachment is influenced by stress and environmental factors (friction, heat, and water absorption). O-ring attachment perpendicular to the occlusal plane was sufficiently retentive over the first year, and stud inclinations affected the retentive capacity of the O-ring.

The energy absorbed by the attachment is the amount of load necessary to stretch the plastic O-ring component in order to fit at the retentive undercut of the Ti portion of the ball abutment. As the O-ring is stretched and removed from the metal ball, its original shape is restored. If the deformation is elastic, no retention loss is anticipated. In the event of permanent deformation, an imperfect fit results in a loss of retention.

Preci Ball Attachment

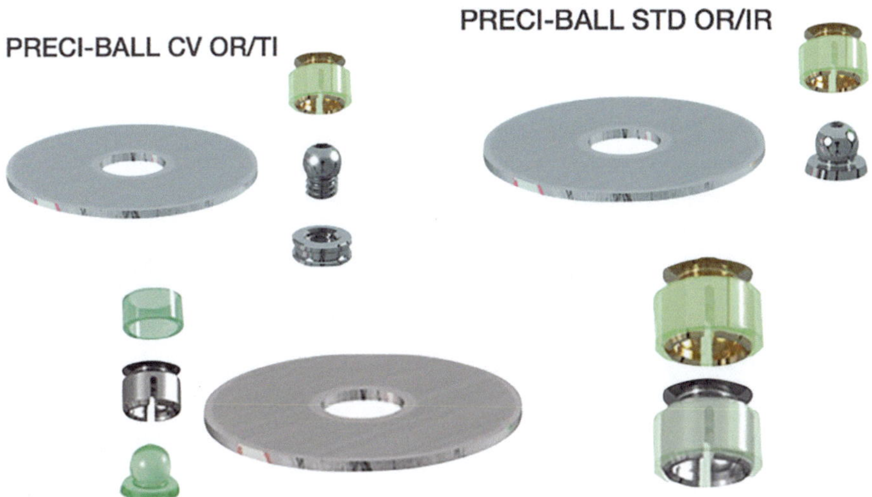

Fig. 3.43 Preci Ball attachment systems

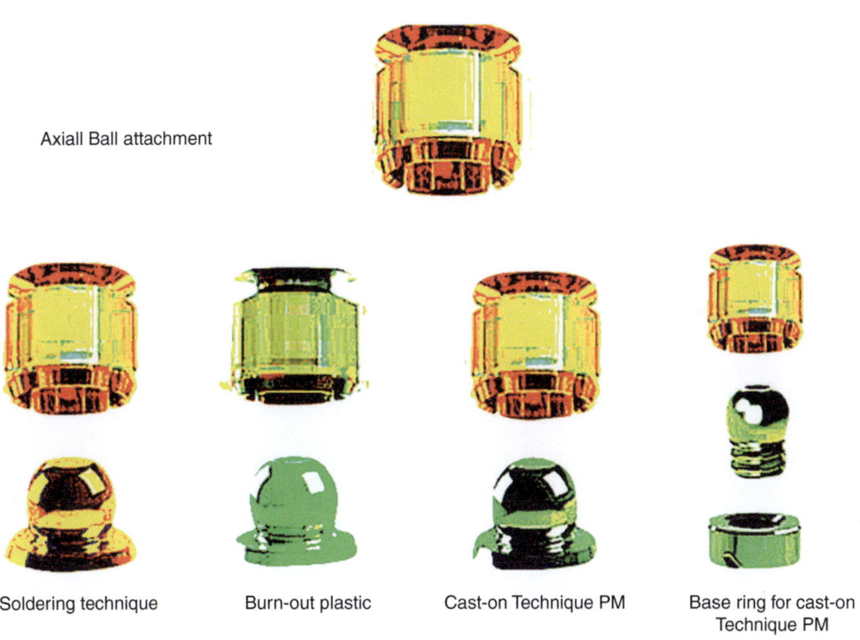

Fig. 3.44 Different types of production of ball attachment systems

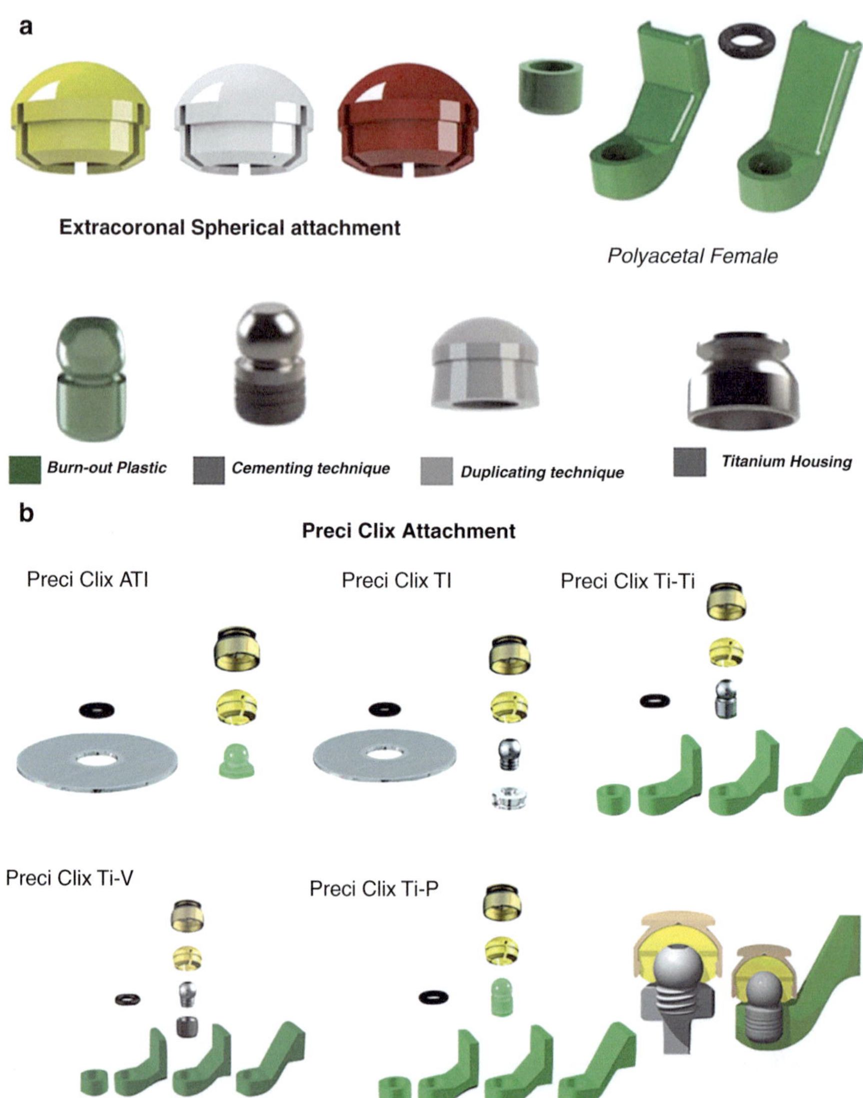

Fig. 3.45 (**a**) Extracoronal spherical attachment and (**b**, **c**) Preci Clix attachment system

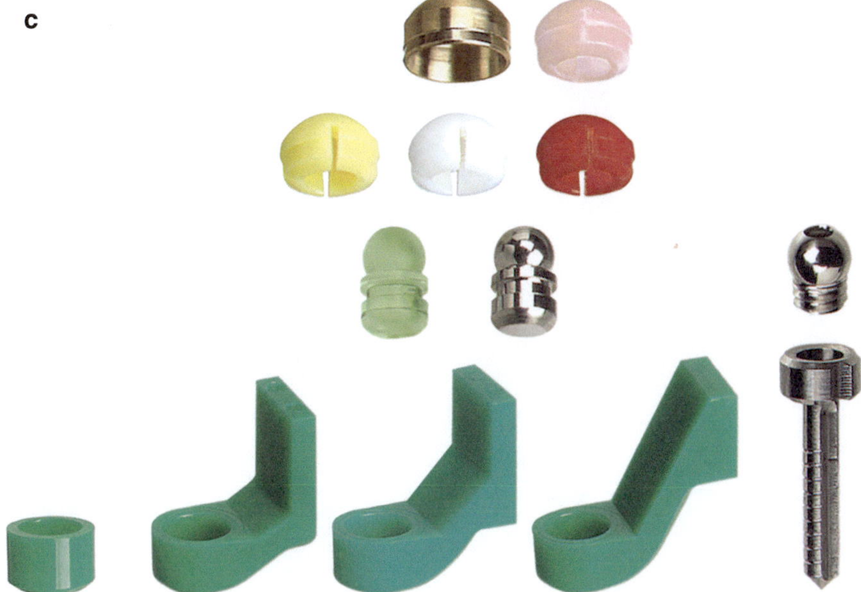

Fig. 3.45 (continued)

3.3.7 Dalbo (Dalla Bona) Attachment

Dalbo attachments are the most popular type of ball-and-socket overdenture attachment and allow for up to 15° of divergence. This attachment utilized detachable, rigid, or elastic attachment prosthetics on implants and root caps (Picture 3.10; Figs. 3.29, 3.30, 3.31, 3.32, 3.33, 3.34, 3.35, 3.36, 3.37, 3.38, 3.39, and 3.40). There are three types, which are named rigid, resilient, and stress-breaker. These are the cylindrical attachments. Attachments from Dalbo feature a cylindrical male component with a round head and ensure a secure connection between the two components. The male portion of the Dalbo cylindrical attachment is soldered to the tooth, and the housing is soldered to the base. The retention is achieved by inserting the flexible attachment rods of the female component into the undercut area on the male component's head. Males are composed of a gold alloy (Elitor), whereas females are comprised of OSV.

Resilient Dalbo is known as a spherical attachment due to his resilience. The male sphere portion permits minimal vertical and rotational motion. Male and female spheres are both made of a gold alloy (Elitor). A PVC ring encircles the

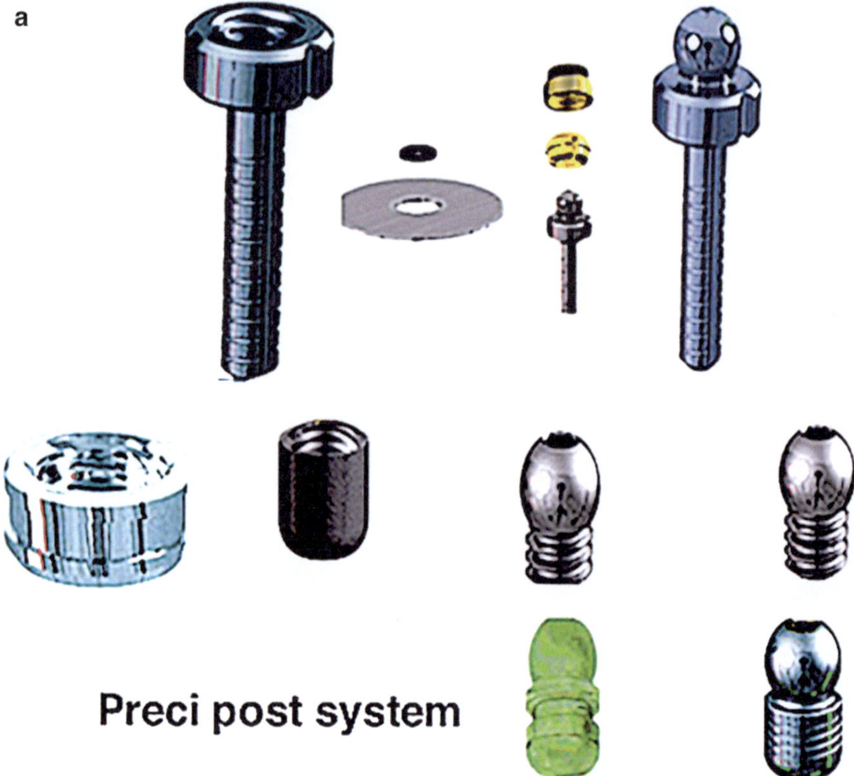

Fig. 3.46 (**a–c**) Preci Clix post attachment

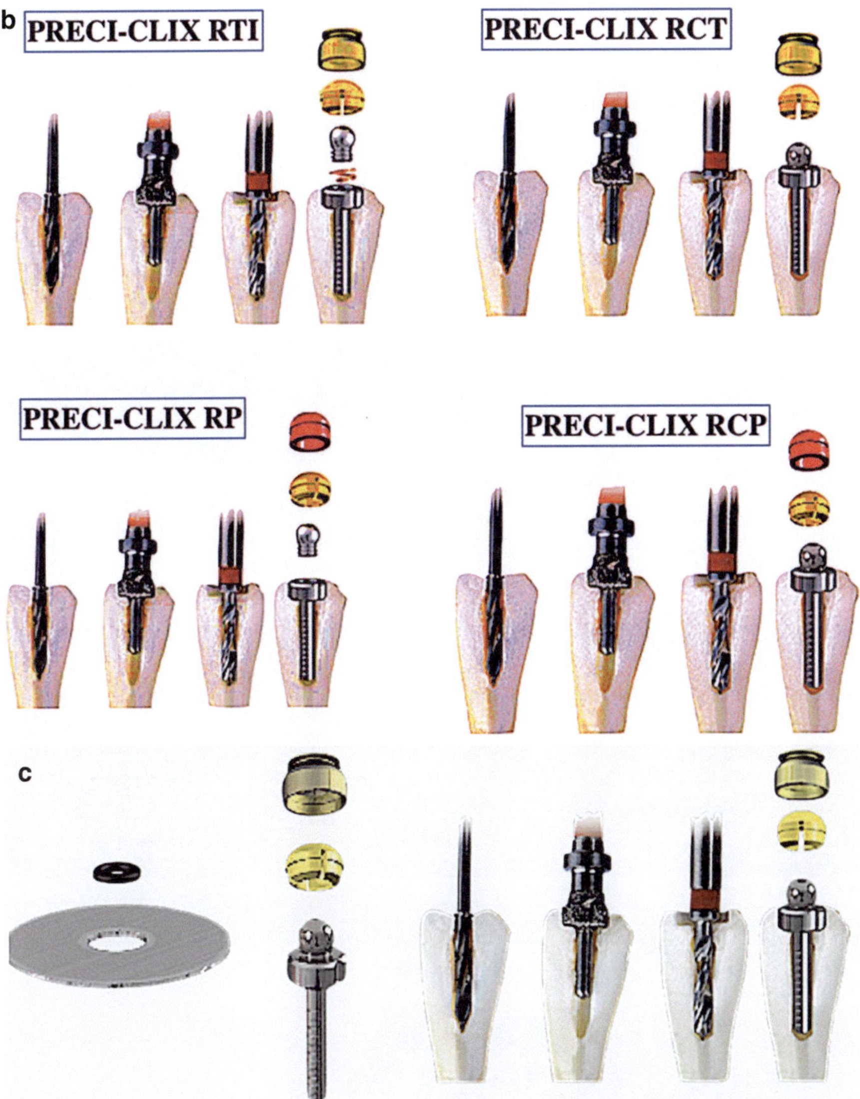

Fig. 3.46 (continued)

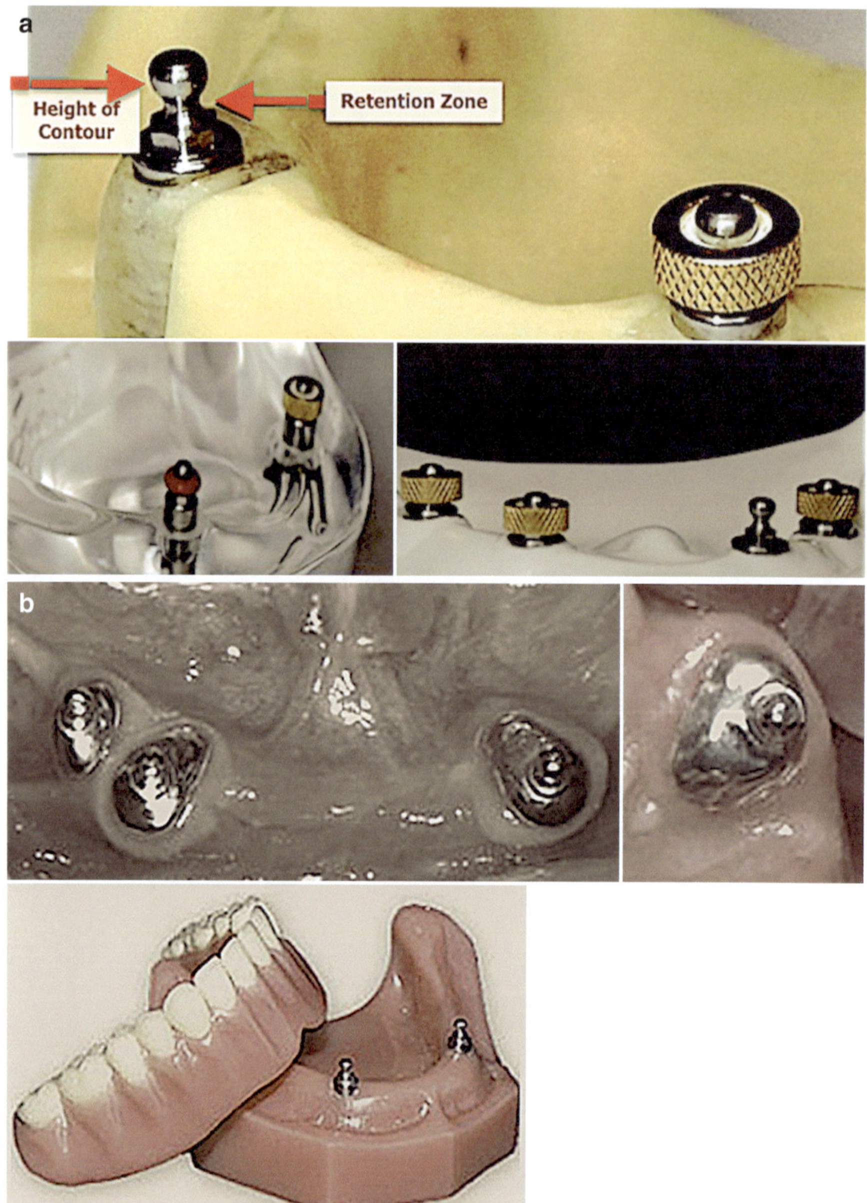

Picture 3.9 (**a**, **b**) O-Ring resilient ball attachment

female to protect adjustment slots from acrylic, and a removable spacer provides vertical and universal hinge movement.

The stress-breaker type resembles a resilient nature. The longer female component is equipped with a helical spring that regulates vertical movement. This system

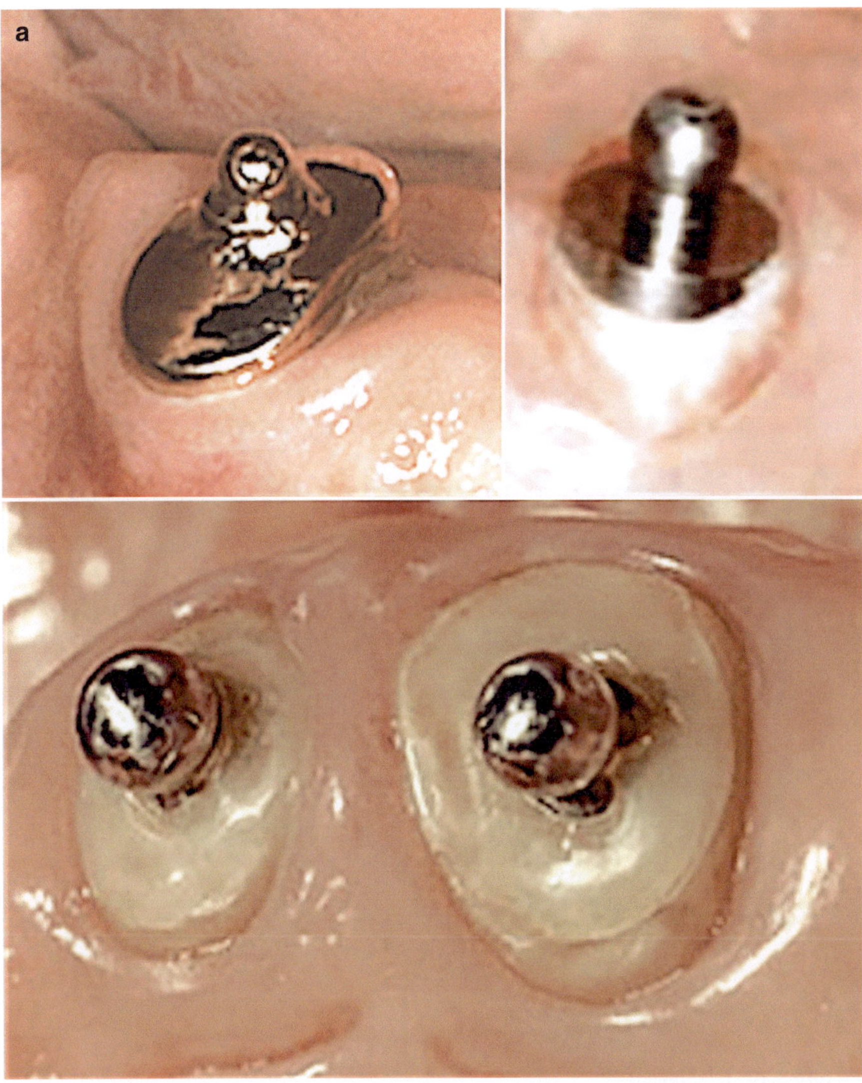

Picture 3.10 Dalbo ball attachment: (**a**) cast on or direct placement and (**b, c**) direct placement of Dalbo attachment

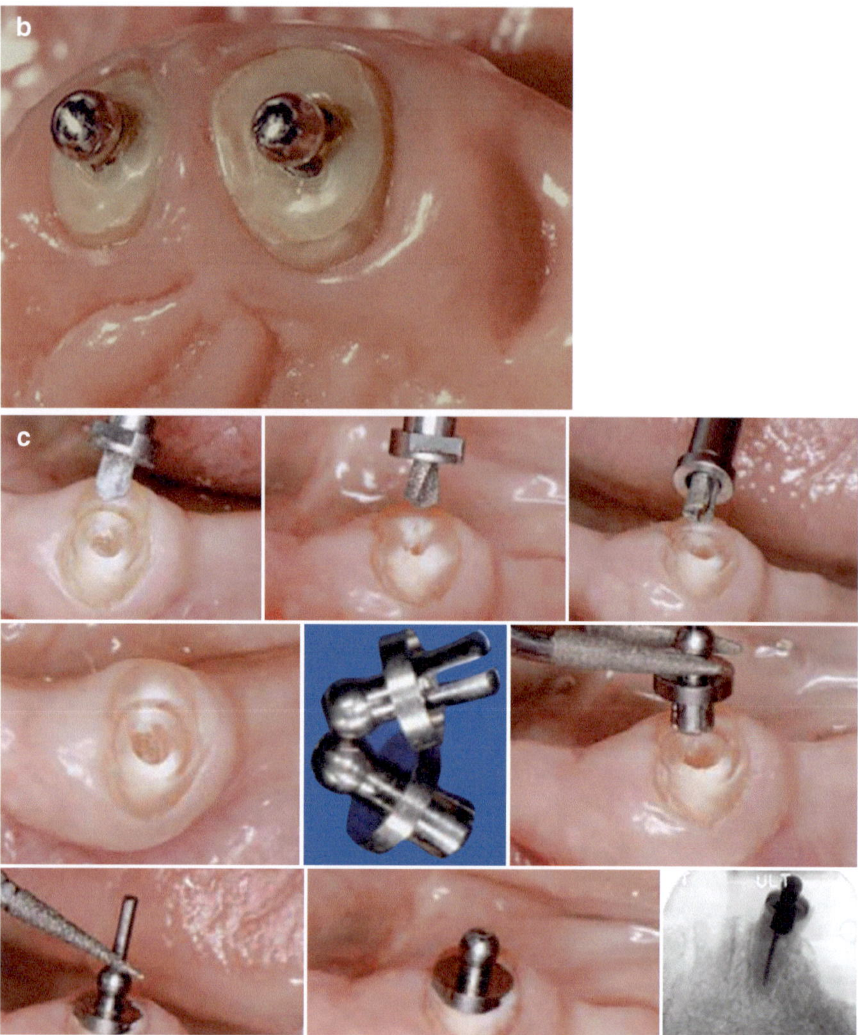

Picture 3.10 (continued)

also permits rotational motions. According to the manufacturer's instructions, these special attachments should be positioned by embedding them in the acrylic base of the denture without soldering the female part to the metal substructure.

3.3.7.1 Advantages

1. The compact spherical shape is exceptionally durable and reliable.
2. The particular precious metal lamellar design ensures reliable and durable functioning.

3. This system is simple to use in the clinic and laboratory and requires minimal maintenance.
4. Universal application: The components of the system have been optimized for the applicable application. A minimal amount of space is required for their incorporation into the denture. There is a male part with a spherical base designed for laser welding.
5. All female components of this system are compatible with the spherical male components of other manufacturers and spherical ball attachments (x 2.25 mm) (Figs. 3.29, 3.30, 3.31, and 3.32).

The Dalbo system minimizes the effects of wear and tear in comparison to other systems. Every female part has flexible precious metal lamellae (Figs. 3.31, 3.32, and 3.35). Lamellae are used to screw into the housing and are made from a yellow precious metal alloy with ideal mechanical properties for long-term function. When inserting the denture, the flexible lamellae open and slide over the spherical male component without causing damage. Additionally, these unique lamellae prevent the accumulation of abrasive plaque and toothpaste. The spacer made of tin that comes with this attachment provides vertical resilience. Generally, the spacers replace the female parts during resin polymerization in the dental laboratory or directly in the patient's mouth after the root canal caps have been cemented. Additionally, the spacers provide superior protection for the male parts during polishing.

There are reportedly more than two million masticatory movements per year, and not all modern materials or attachment designs can withstand this enormous load without sustaining damage. After 50,000 fitting and withdrawal cycles, it was demonstrated that the Dalbo attachment showed almost no signs of wear. The 2:100 N eccentric end loading was used to simulate the loading experienced during functional masticatory movements.

3.3.7.2 Different Types of Dalbo Attachments

Dalbo-Classic attachments are elliptics (Figs. 3.31, 3.32, and 3.33)
These ball attachments are the most space-efficient. It has male and female spherical components that can be combined to provide the optimal solution for a wide variety of applications. The male part's ball allows for a degree of flexibility when placing this attachment. The height of the female part is just 2.2 mm. The activatable, flexible lamellae ensure strong denture retention. The elliptic design differs from the "normal" classic version in that the plastic retention is solid and elliptically shaped, but the height remains the same. The elliptic version enhances retention in denture acrylic and is recommended for use with implants. This version is recommended for direct insertion in the mouth, or when an extra-firm gripping force of the female mold in the denture body is desired.

Dalbo-B attachment (Fig. 3.34)

Over four decades, the ball attachment has maintained its original form. The female component has a height of 3.1 mm and is made entirely of precious metal (elector) with ideal mechanical properties for a durable and secure function. There is a spherical male part base for laser welding. This component can also be conventionally soldered. The activatable, flexible lamellae ensure a strong denture retention.

Dalbo-Plus fundamental and elliptic attachments (Fig. 3.35)

The male component is made of valor for casting. It can only be cast on or soldered to the root cap. Cast-on saves time and eliminates the need for joining materials. Elitor's laser-weldable, definite matrix was developed specifically for this technology. The design of the base plate beneath the ball makes laser welding of this male component to the root caps safe and comfortable. The elliptic version enhances retention in denture acrylic and is recommended for use with implants.

For the replacement of older restorations and those with ball attachments from other manufacturers, it is advised to use the special Dalbo-Plus and Dalbo-Plus elliptic female parts. Enhance existing restorations with Dalbo-Plus female parts. Existing older restorations with worn spherical attachments, regardless of manufacturer, can be improved rapidly.

Dalbo-Z attachment

Dalbo-Z is a cylindrical and rigid attachment for precision work. Adjustable frictional retention is present. Male and female parts (E) are fabricated from elitor. Male components are welded to the root cap, while female components are polymerized in denture acrylic (Fig. 3.36).

Enhancing the proper position of the attachment and housing is fundamental to the effectiveness of the attachment (Fig. 3.37a). Titanium female component with threaded precious metal lamellae is inserted for superior retention force that can be adjusted instantly and permanently with a screw. The lamellar retention insert is the actual holding element in the system. Using the screwdriver or activator to screw the lamellae retention insert into the housing closes the four lamellae and properly adjusts the unit. The range of retentive forces is between 200 and 1200 g.

Some spherical attachments with plastic female parts or plastic inserts may exhibit excessive wear of the male part due to the deposition of substances on the plastic. The Damage is caused by a plastic female component and irreparable damage to the plastic male component due to the accumulation of elements in the plastic are the main disadvantages (Fig. 3.37b). Plaque tends to accumulate on plastic inserts and can be very abrasive. Each female component of the Dalbo attachment has flexible lamellae made of precious metal, so male components experience minimal wear.

Dalbo-Rotex Connection

Root post-copings (RPCs) are indicated when teeth have extensive loss of hard coronal tissues. Dentists can apply prefabricated root screws with a ball attachment in the form of Dalbo-Rotex as a simple and cost-effective alternative. The low profile of Dalbo-Rotex allows it to reduce the crown-to-root ratio. It is rotationally and vertically resilient (Class V function), has a minimum vertical height of 3.5 mm, and permits a 15° root divergence.

The male component is composed of titanium alloy, self-tapping, has a pressure relief groove, and possesses a slight conical root thread to permit direct and immediate engagement of the roots in the retention of the denture. These characteristics permit nearly tension-free root canal attachment incorporation. This technique eliminates the need to cast a root cap and attach a ball attachment. The female component is available in both plastic (Galak) and a precious metal alloy (Elitor®). Female plastic components are appropriate for short-term restorations, while female metal components are adjustable and recommended for long-term restorations (Figs. 3.38, 3.39, and 3.40).

3.3.7.3 Contraindications

- If an adequate fit in root canal preparation is not possible in the case of a root canal that is extensive, the tooth must be extracted.
- In the case of extremely fragile and thin-walled roots.
- Periodontitis, severe gum disease, poor oral hygiene, dental caries, and a narrow inter-occlusal space are all indicators of poor oral health.
- If the long-term prognosis for the teeth to be treated is favorable. Otherwise, there are no restrictions on indications after successful endodontic treatment based on current scientific knowledge.

After 7 years, indirect manufacturing of RPCs had a success rate of 85%. Carious lesions, vertical root fractures, loss of retention, and endodontic pathologies accounted for the majority of complications and failures.

3.3.8 Pro-Snap/Profix Attachment for Ball

These are additional resilience ball attachments (Figs. 3.41 and 3.42). Additionally, they are used as rigid attachments. The Pro-Snap is the cast-on stud attachment for overdentures on root caps (Fig. 3.41a, b). For Pro-Snap male parts, Novostil (high-fusing precious dental alloys can be incorporated directly into the wax up and cast-on) and burn-out plastic should be utilized. By choosing one of the color-coded, interchangeable plastic retention elements, the retention force can be easily adjusted and created. The Snap housing is composed of a titanium alloy (Ti-6Al-4V), a retention element, and a retention ring.

The Profix is also an adjustable press fastener attachment of the stud variety for overdentures. Ancrofil (a light yellow, palladium-free precious metal alloy) and burn-out plastic are available for the male part. Burnt plastic is utilized for cost-effective solutions. The eight-lamellar female portion facilitates activation (Fig. 3.42a, b).

3.3.9 Preci Ball/Preci Clix Attachment (Figs. 3.43, 3.44, 3.45, and 3.46; Pictures 3.11, 3.12, 3.13, 3.14, 3.15, 3.16, 3.17, and 3.18)

3.3.9.1 The Preci Ball System for Attachment

This attachment can be a prefabricated or casted to stud that requires minimal inter-arch distance. The Preci Ball is a durable (360° rotation) stud attachment (Figs. 3.43 and 3.44). It is an easy-to-use system with multiple options for protecting the supporting teeth and retainer overdentures. The spherical male attachment is available in a prefabricated Orax alloy for soldering, a burnout plastic pattern for direct casting, and a threaded male for soldering or direct casting. With a ball diameter of 2.25 mm, the Preci Ball is compatible with the majority of implant systems. The female is offered in both prefabricated alloy and threaded form. There is also an optional, replaceable threaded female. Orax, titanax, and irax should be used to create female and male parts. The Preci Ball features a simple insertion and removal path, an adjustable female, and patient-friendly hygienic maintenance. These characteristics enable the dental professional to adapt the attachment to the patient's needs. The Preci Ball system and Preci Clix system are totally interchangeable.

3.3.9.2 Attachment Choices

1. Insert the male component into the post-coping by soldering. The soldering procedure combines low-cost precision and technique precision.
2. Casting precious alloys on the male component, or include the base ring and make the male component replaceable—the recommended method for combining accuracy and practicality.
3. Cast from a durable dental alloy, which is the most economical solution (Fig. 3.12a).

3.3.9.3 Preci-Ball Attachment Types

Precise-Ball CV

Titanium male is removable with a high-fusing base ring for direct casting with precious alloys and gold female for acrylic fixation.

Preci-Ball OR/OR

The gold female for acrylic resin retention and the gold male (height: 3.5 mm) for soldering to the post-coping (options 1 and 3).

Preci-Ball PC

Option three necessitates a titanium female for acrylic fixation and a burn-out plastic male for casting with post-copying (height: 3.5 mm).

Preci-Ball OR/IR

(Suitable options 2) Gold female for acrylic fixation and high-fusing male for direct casting with precious alloys (height: 3.5 mm) (Fig. 3.43).

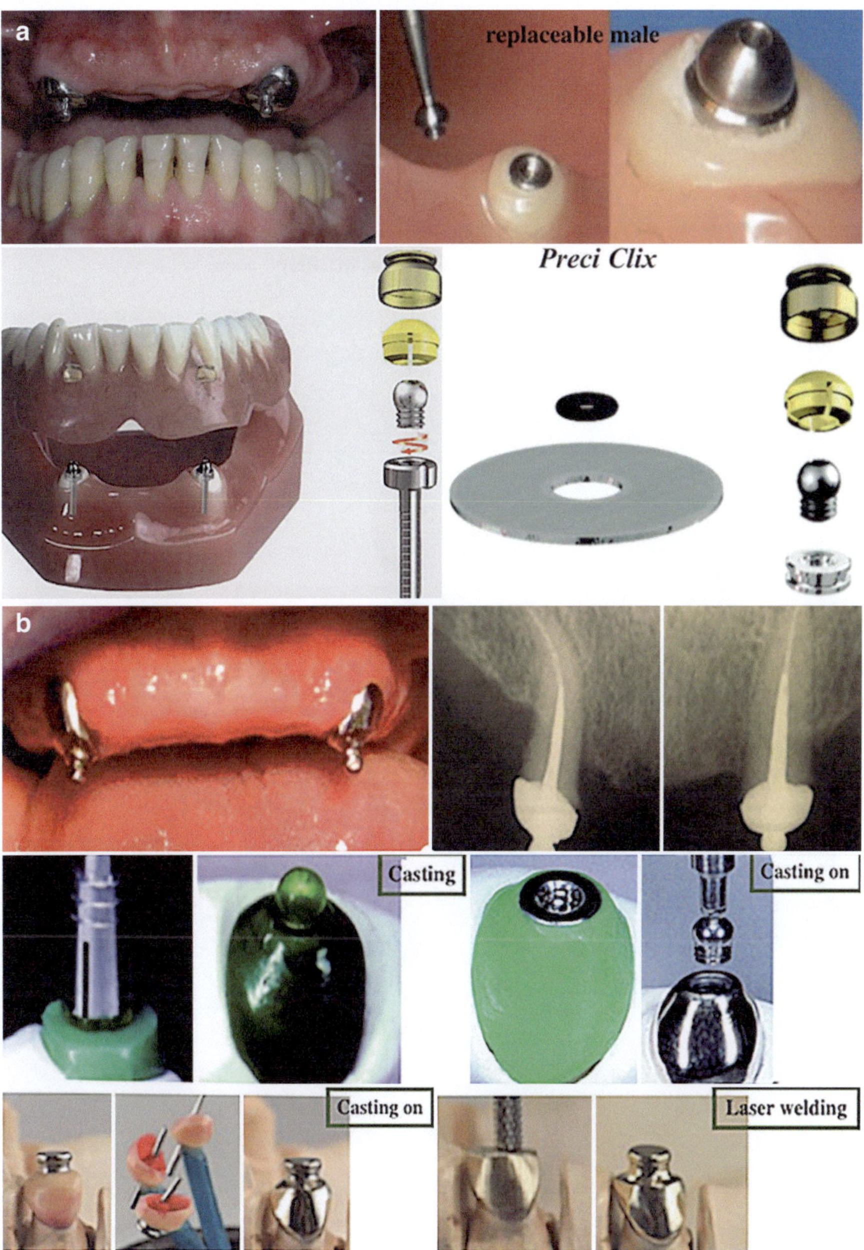

Picture 3.11 (**a**) Preci Clix attachment on cast coping and directly on root; (**b**) extraradicular attachment can be used to cast, solder, or laser weld the threaded base ring into either a coping or ball; (**c, d**) Preci Ball and Preci Clix male plastic attachment cast in hard dental alloy

c

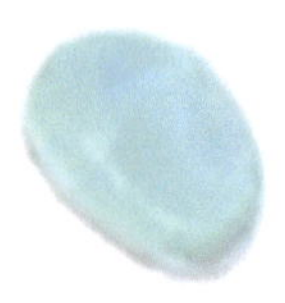
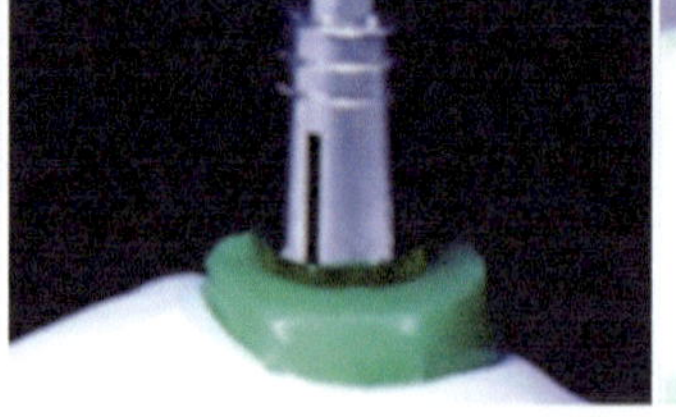
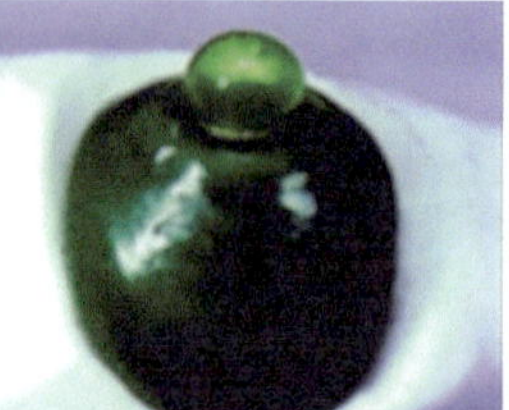

Cast in hard dental alloy

Preci-Ball attachment

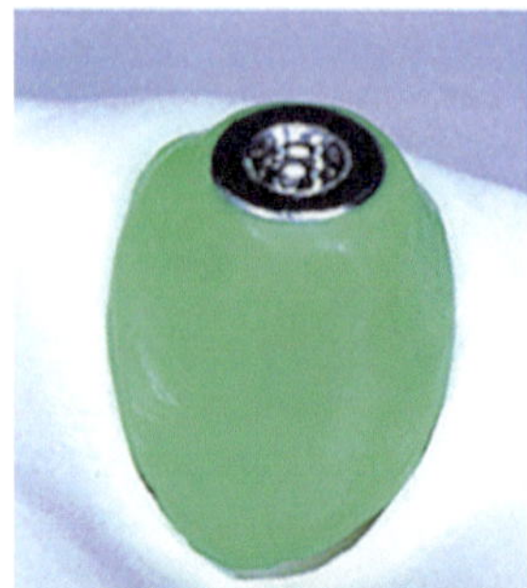
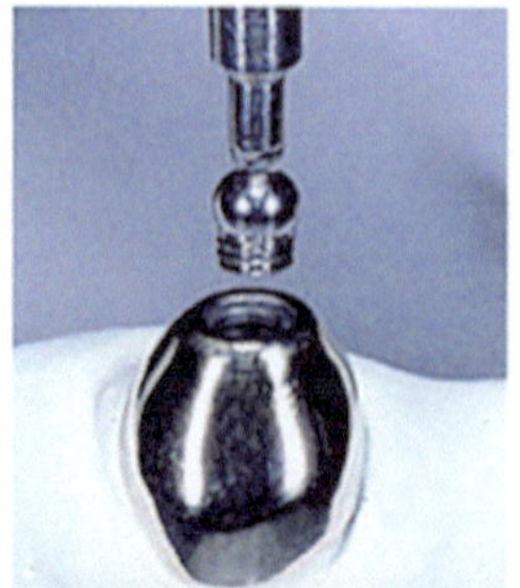
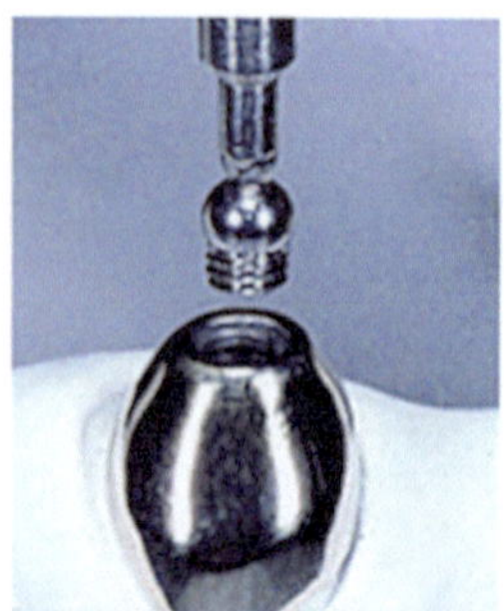

Cast on the male part with the base ring and have the male repleaceable

d

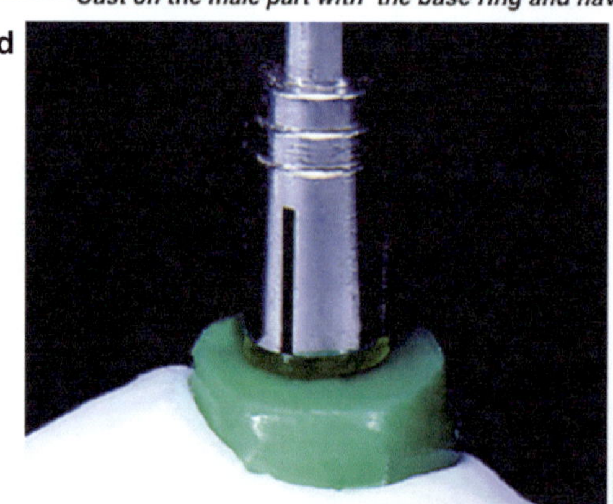
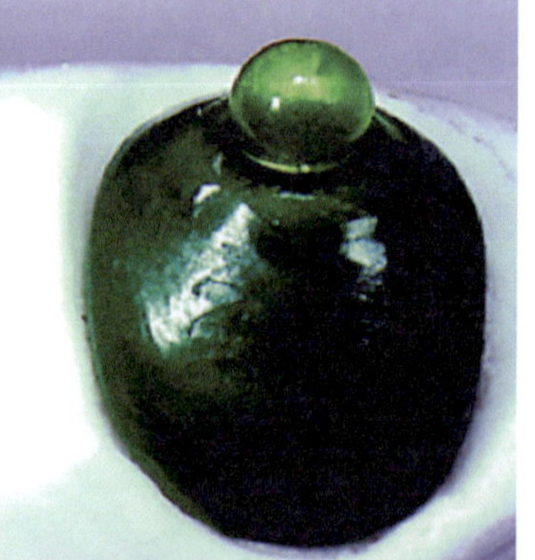

Cast in hard metal alloy

Preci Clix attachment

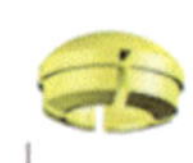
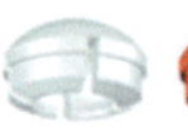
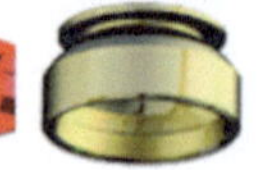
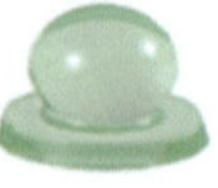
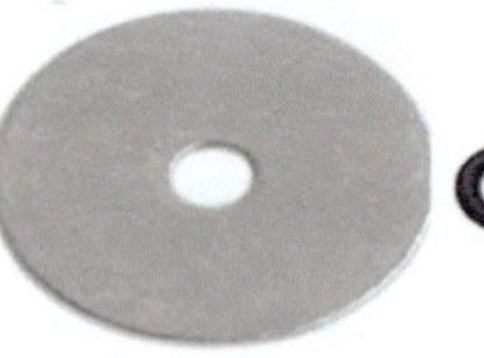

Picture 3.11 (continued)

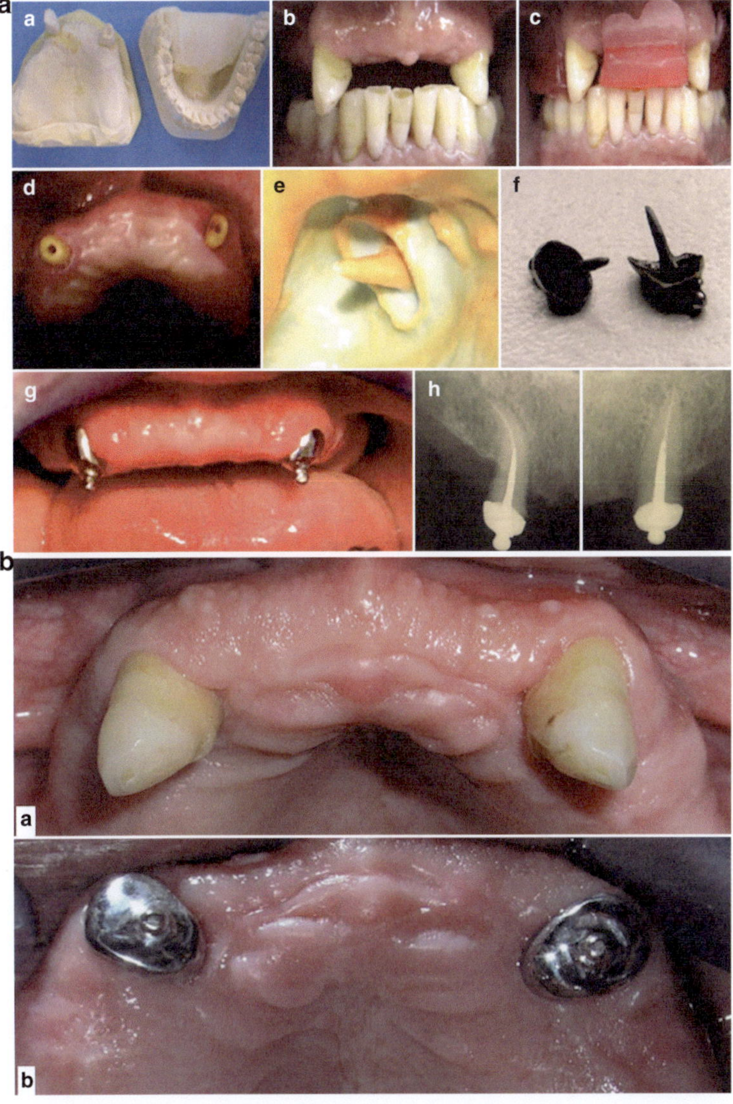

Picture 3.12 (**a**) Extraradicular indirect attachments steps with casting with non-precious alloys using Preci Clix attachment, *a* Diagnostic cast: *b* canine teeth intraoral view; *c* determination of VDO; *d* tooth preparation; *e* impression of coping; *f* attachment cast with post and coping using hard metal alloy; *g* attachment with coping in situ; and *h* radiographic view. (**b**) Intraoral appearance of attachment with coping, *a* Before treatment; *b* After treatment. (**c**) Attachment/coping assembly And metal infrastructure on the model. (**d**) Tooth arrangement done as complete dentures and controlled with an adaptation of attachment/coping assembly. Direct placement of female part in the mouth: (**e**) finished denture controlled in the mouth; (**f**) the yellow female is inserted into the metal housing and the large tinfoil space maintainer used and then the rubber space maintainer placed over the male; (**g**) the low viscous self-cure resin is applied to the inside of denture; (**h**) denture put in the mouth; (**i**) inside and outside appearance of a denture (yellow retention insert placed in the denture; and (**j**) an overdenture in situ, (**k**) Denture seen in the mouth extraoral appearance

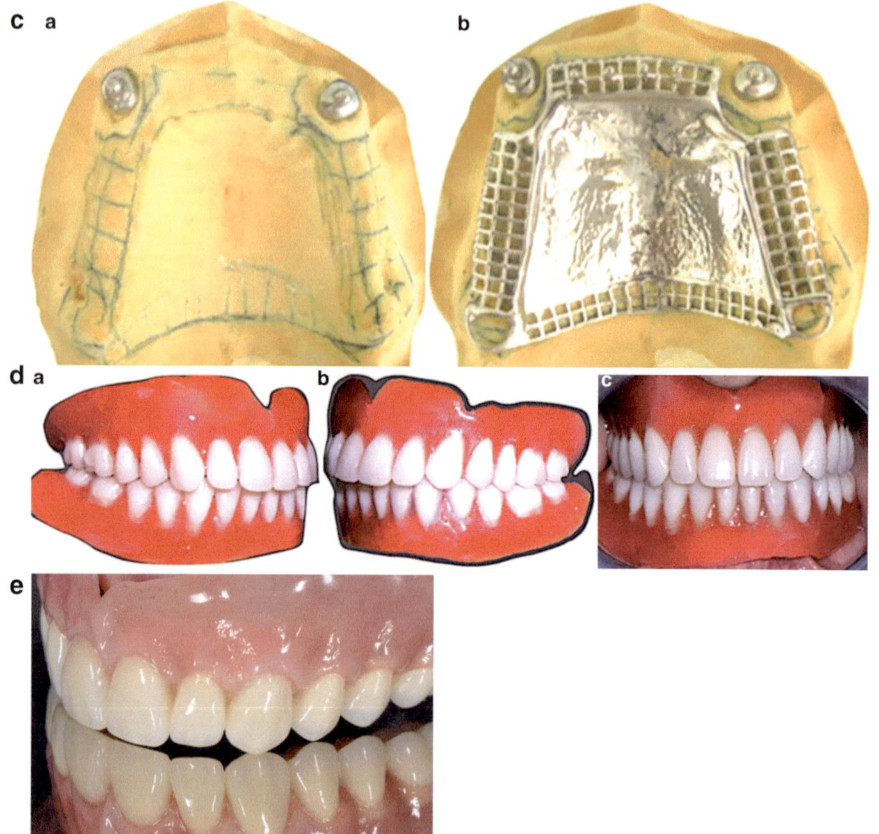

Picture 3.12 (continued)

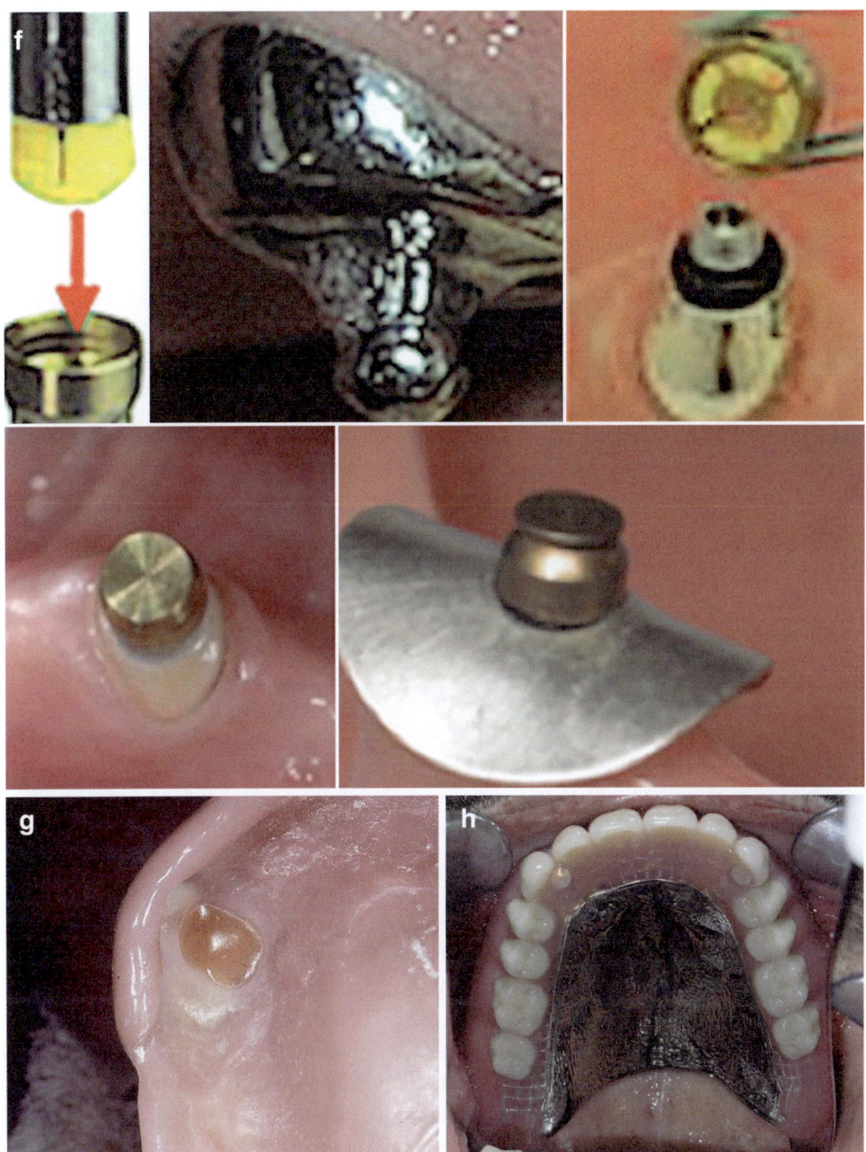

Picture 3.12 (continued)

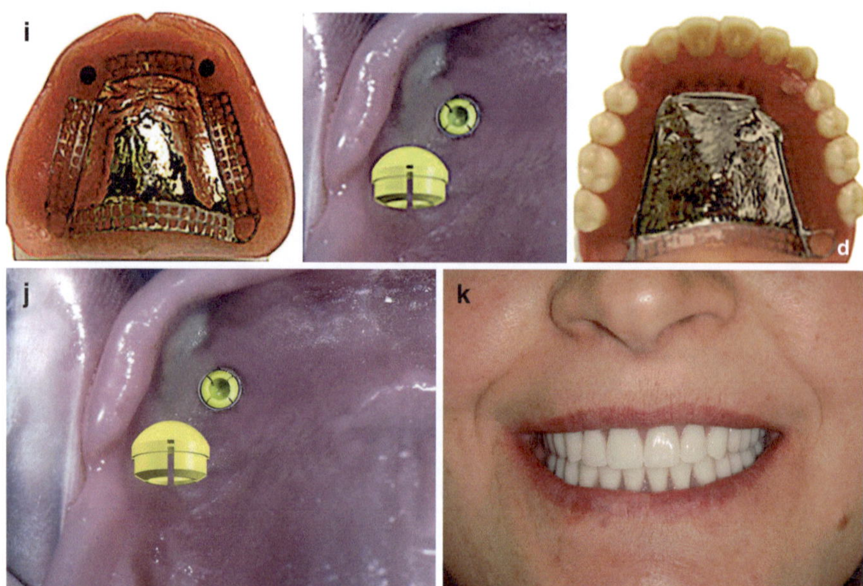

Picture 3.12 (continued)

3.3.9.4 Preci Clix Connection System

It can be used for the roots and implants which retain overdentures, crowns for removable partial dentures, and the tops of bars for implant- or root-supported bridges; all previous retention balls engaged the height of the contour of the sphere. This small area, or "band of retention," may result in attachment wear and replacement of the female unit.

The Preci Clix design enables the female to engage all around the ball, resulting in a larger retention area. In addition to having a retention rate significantly higher than other spherical systems, the clip provides the patient with the reassurance of an audible click. The female component is made of titanium that has been anodized in gold for polymerization into the acrylic resin. This female body part resembles the Hader clips. The sectional cuts of the females allow them to flex over the height of the contour and engage the undercuts of the sphere. A unique female component design surrounds the male component to increase retention. This design necessitates less component corrosion, maintenance, and replacement of female parts. The replaceable plastic female has three retention levels: yellow (2.5 lbs., 1130 g) is standard retention, white (1.7 lbs., 770 g) is reduced retention, and orange (3.3 lbs., 1440 g) is increased retention.

If the attachments are not parallel, the female can be paralleled without compromising retention or stability. Non-parallel females have a steep insertion and removal path, resulting in increased wear on the attachment, and non-parallel females prevent the denture from rotating. Parallel females have an accessible insertion and removal path, which reduces attachment wear. This attachment also permits free

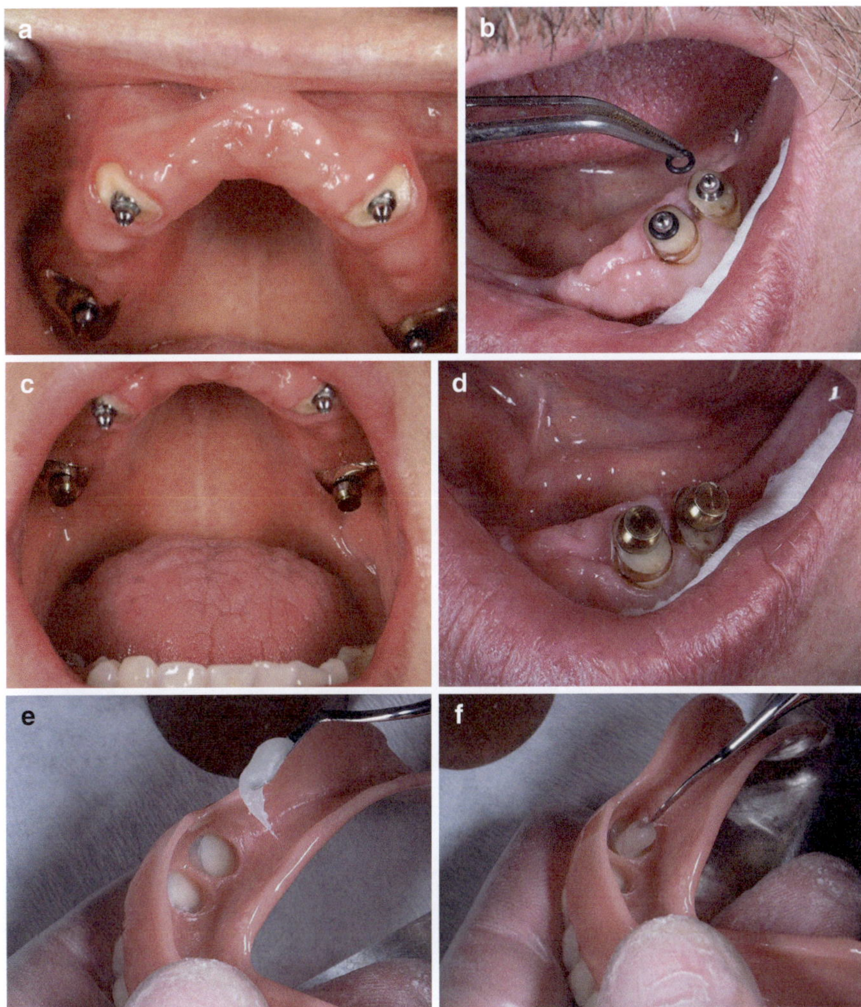

Picture 3.13 (**a**) Preci Clix attachment; (**b**) the Preci Clix attachment is used both directly on the tooth and the cast coping in the same mouth; (**c–e**) placement of black rubber and female attachment part on the male part directly; and (**f, g**) self-cure resin is applied to the inside of the denture and the denture is put in the mouth; (**h**) Intaglio surface of denture

rotation of the denture. Thirty degrees is approximately the maximum divergence at which clix females can still engage the sphere's undercut (Fig. 3.45).

3.3.9.5 Preci Clix Attachment Types

Attachments for Preci Clix CV and Preci Clix TI have interchangeable male and female components. There is a titanium male with a high-fusing base ring for cast-on precious alloy technique. It may be utilized to cast, solder, or laser weld the threaded base ring into a coping or bar. This attachment housing has dimensions of

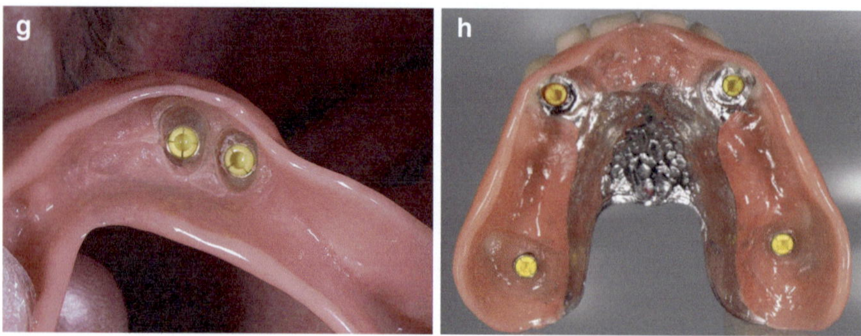

Picture 3.13 (continued)

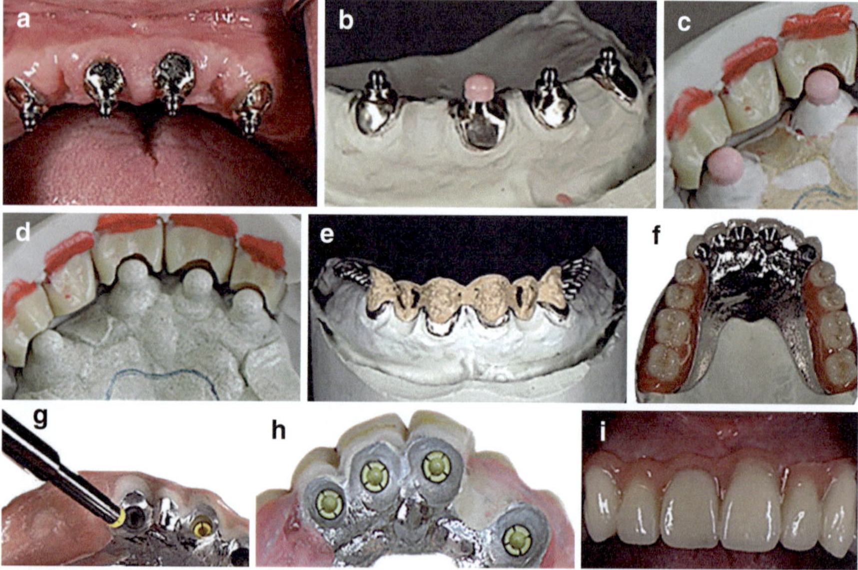

Picture 3.14 (**a**) Casting coping controlled in the mouth, (**b**) İmpressin is taken and cast model obtained, (**c**) pink processing insert placed on the coping, (**d**) duplicate model obtained and teeth arangement controlled for suitability placed on the coping, (**e**) Framework casted as one unit with second part and applied opaquer, (**f**) Finished dentures, (**g**, **h**) yellow retention is inserted placed in the denture, (**i**) Denture placed on the mouth

2.65 mm in height, 4.00 mm in diameter, 2.25 mm in sphere diameter, and 0.9 mm in internal hex. The base ring measures 1.30 mm in height and 3.40 mm in width. The female housing is for acrylic resin incorporation.

The Preci Clix ATI attachment has a male made of plastic for integration into post-copings or bars. The total required vertical space is 4 mm. This attachment housing has a height of 2.65 mm, a diameter of 4.00 mm, and a sphere with a height

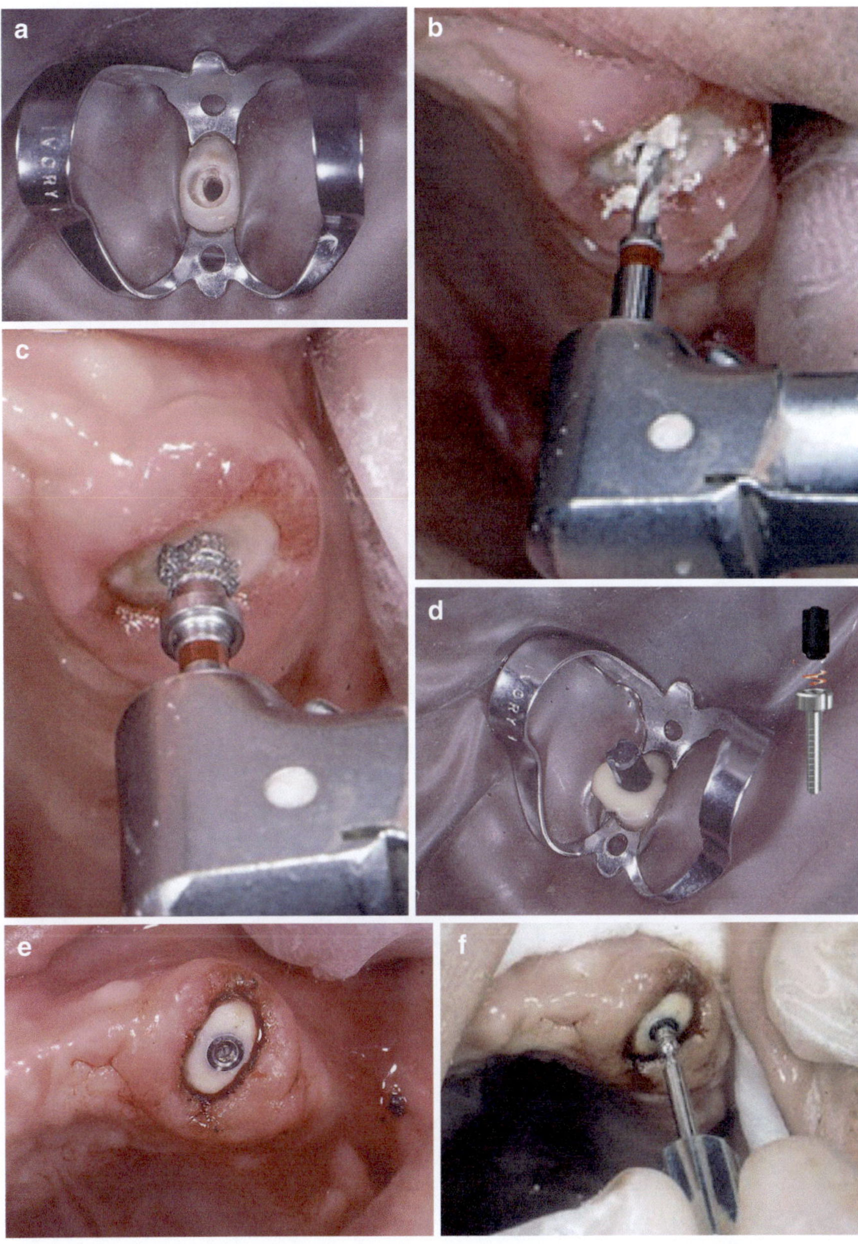

Picture 3.15 (**a**) Direct placement Preci Clix attachment; (**b, c**) the root canal prepared with the penetration bur and use the diamond bur to make the base of the Preci Clix post; (**d, e**) using the RE H2 seating and impression tool as a handle, the Preci Clix post placed into the canal and cemented; (**f**) the male part screwed into the post in the mouth

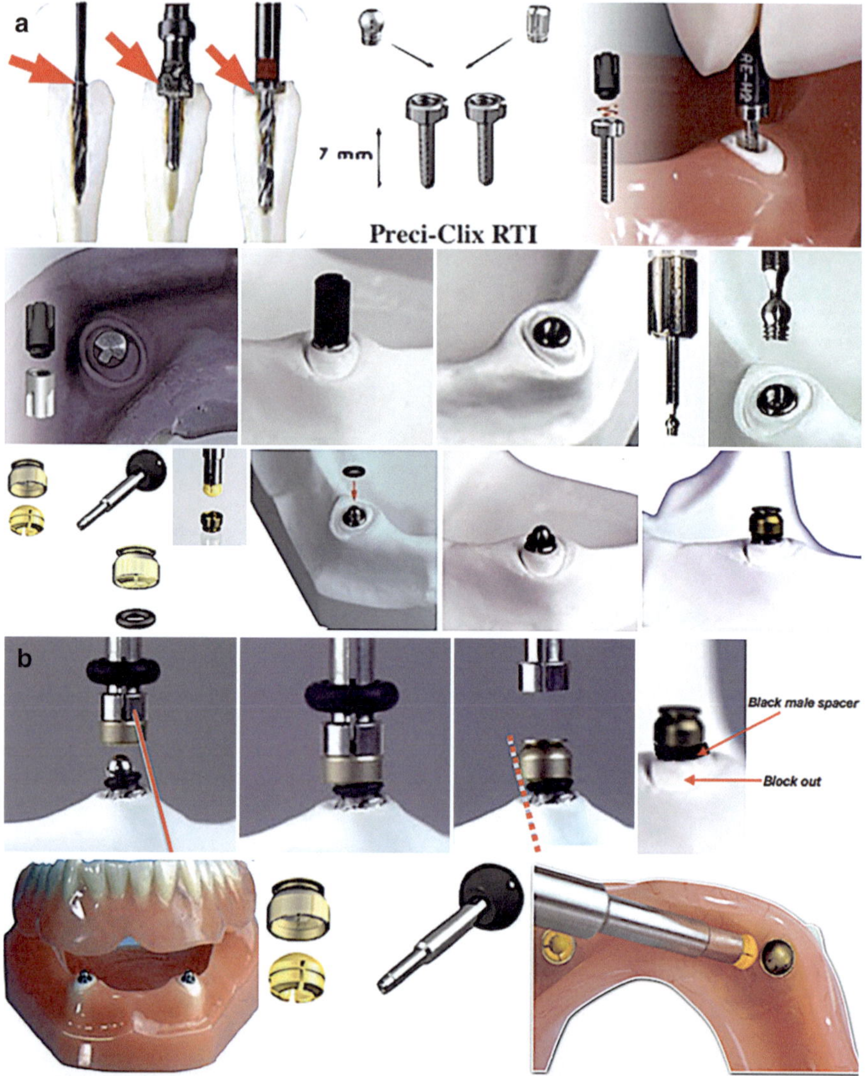

Picture 3.16 (**a, b**) Laboratory processing of the female attachments for direct placement of the Preci Clix attachment (**c**) Direct placement Preci Clix post attachment

of 2.40 mm and a diameter of 2.25 mm. The female housing is for acrylic resin incorporation.

Preci Clix Ti-Ti attachments also feature plastic patterns that can be cast in any dental alloy; the titanium male is then bonded to the attachment using Ceka Site. It also provides clinicians with the convenience of direct casting with a smooth, accurate ball. This attachment housing has a height of 2.65 mm, a diameter of 4.00 mm, a sphere with a diameter of 2.25 mm, an internal diameter of 2.35 mm, and an external hex diameter of 3.40 mm.

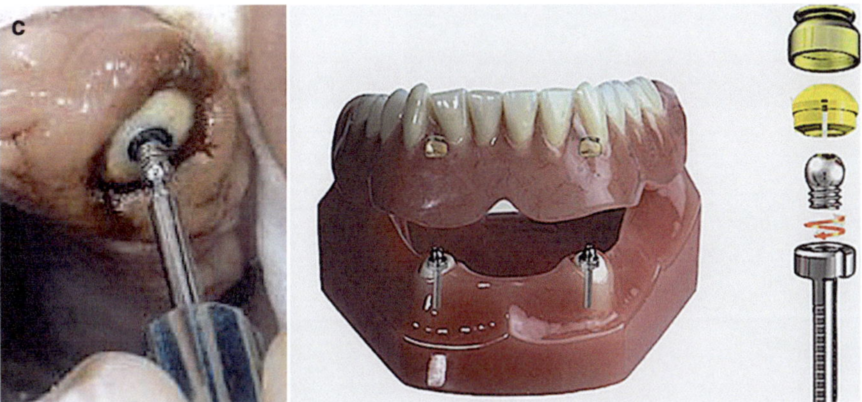

Picture 3.16 (continued)

3.3.9.6 Utilizing the Preci Clix Accessory (Pictures 3.12, 3.13, 3.14, and 3.15)

The Preci Post system is used to prepare the tooth for a post and coping or just a cast coping.

To prepare the final impression model, wax coping is utilized. Post-coping waxing should be kept to a minimum. The castable sphere is coated with the wax. The occlusal surface must be perpendicular to the insertion path at a 90° angle. Casting is performed after the attachment metal alloy has been selected. After try-in procedures, the coping is placed in situ, and a second impression is taken with silicon impression materials using an individual tray. A wax framework is prepared and then cast with precious or nonprecious metal alloys following the pouring of the casting. Then test it in structure with coping, and based on the polymerization process, place it in the denture (Picture 3.12a–e).

3.3.9.7 Acrylic Processing of the Housing

The female connector plugs into the metal housing. The large tinfoil spacer was used for post-copying relief, and then the rubber spacer was placed over the male. The female component was mounted on top of the male. The denture is modified in order to accommodate the female component. Drill a "vent" or small channel in the lingual side of the prosthesis to allow excess acrylic to escape. On the male side, not the female side, the spacers were placed. The low-viscosity self-curing resin is applied to the denture's interior, and the denture is then placed in the mouth. After approximately 5 min of insertion, the denture is extracted (Picture 3.12f–k).

Additionally, the Preci Clix attachment system is used for placement directly on the root. In this system, replaceable male parts are utilized. It should not be forgotten that clinicians should utilize the widest possible spacer. The large tin spacer is placed over the ball, and the flexible tin spacer is shaped around the ball and gingival area to prevent the acrylic from coming into contact with the cast coping. The Clix female is seated in the metal housing, and the black rubber spacer is bonded intraorally to the denture using chairside acrylic materials (Picture 3.13a–h).

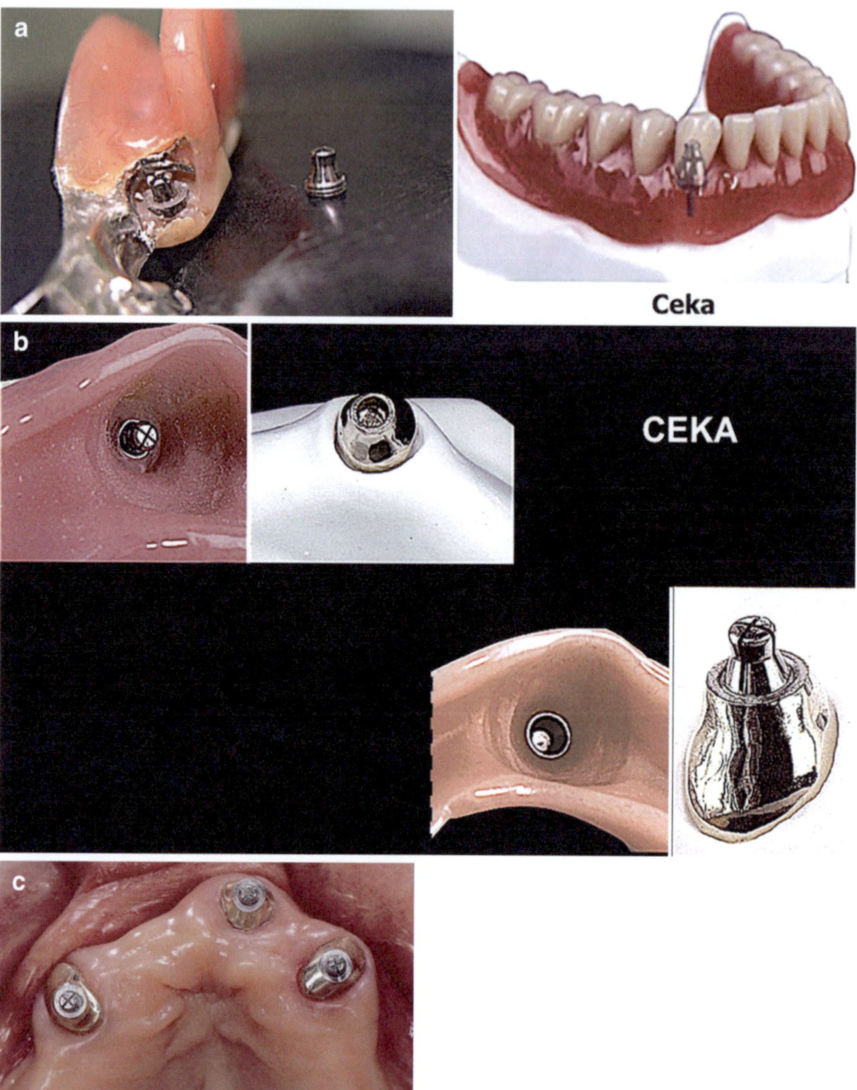

Picture 3.17 (**a**) Ceka attachment, (**b**) Ceka male placed on post coping (Ceka axial classic) (**c**) Ceka attachment on the post coping is shown in the mouth (**d**) Ceka axial classic attachment (**e**) Wax coping with base ring cast together and replaceable male part is placed on coping (**f**) IRAX base ring casting with wax coping (base ring placed with a survivor) and after casting PALLAX base ring for soldering (**g**) **CEKA SOL** use for soldering

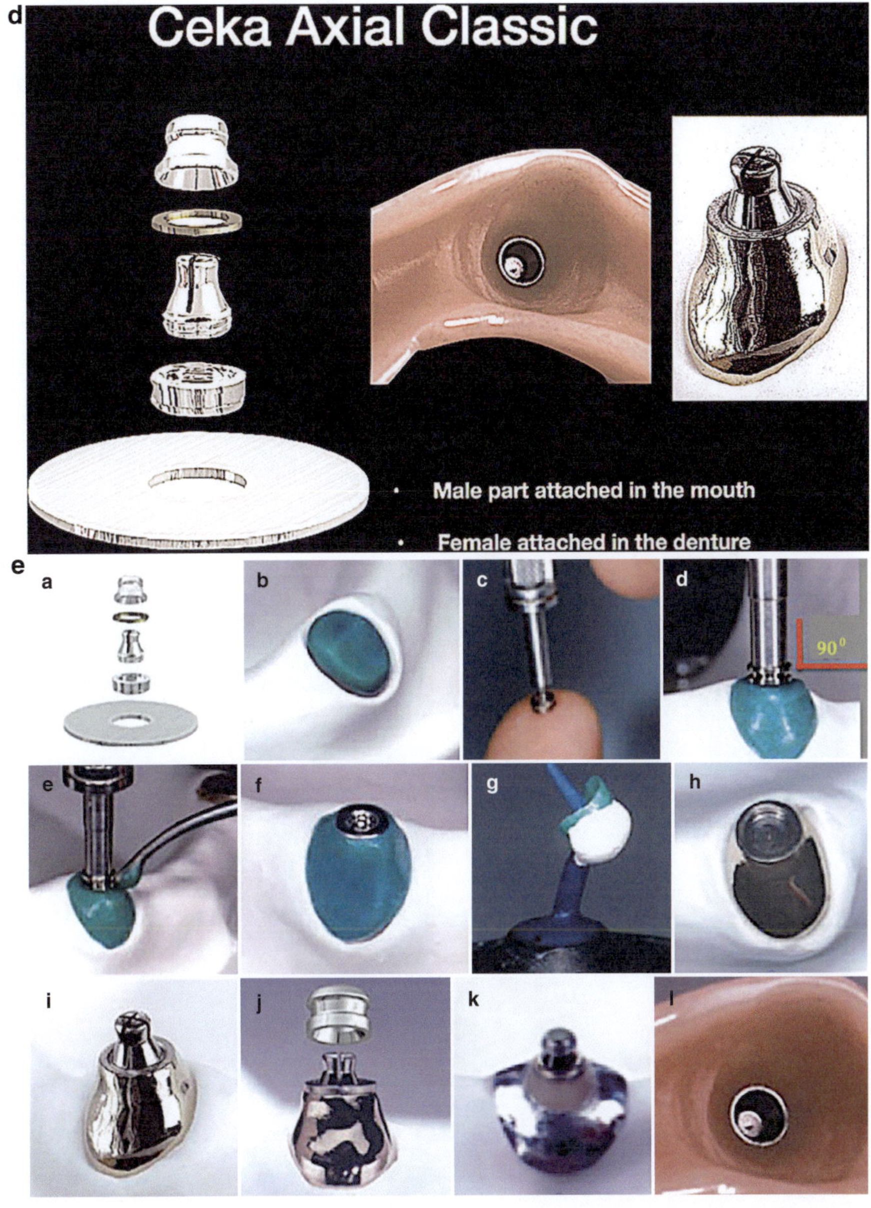

Picture 3.17 (continued)

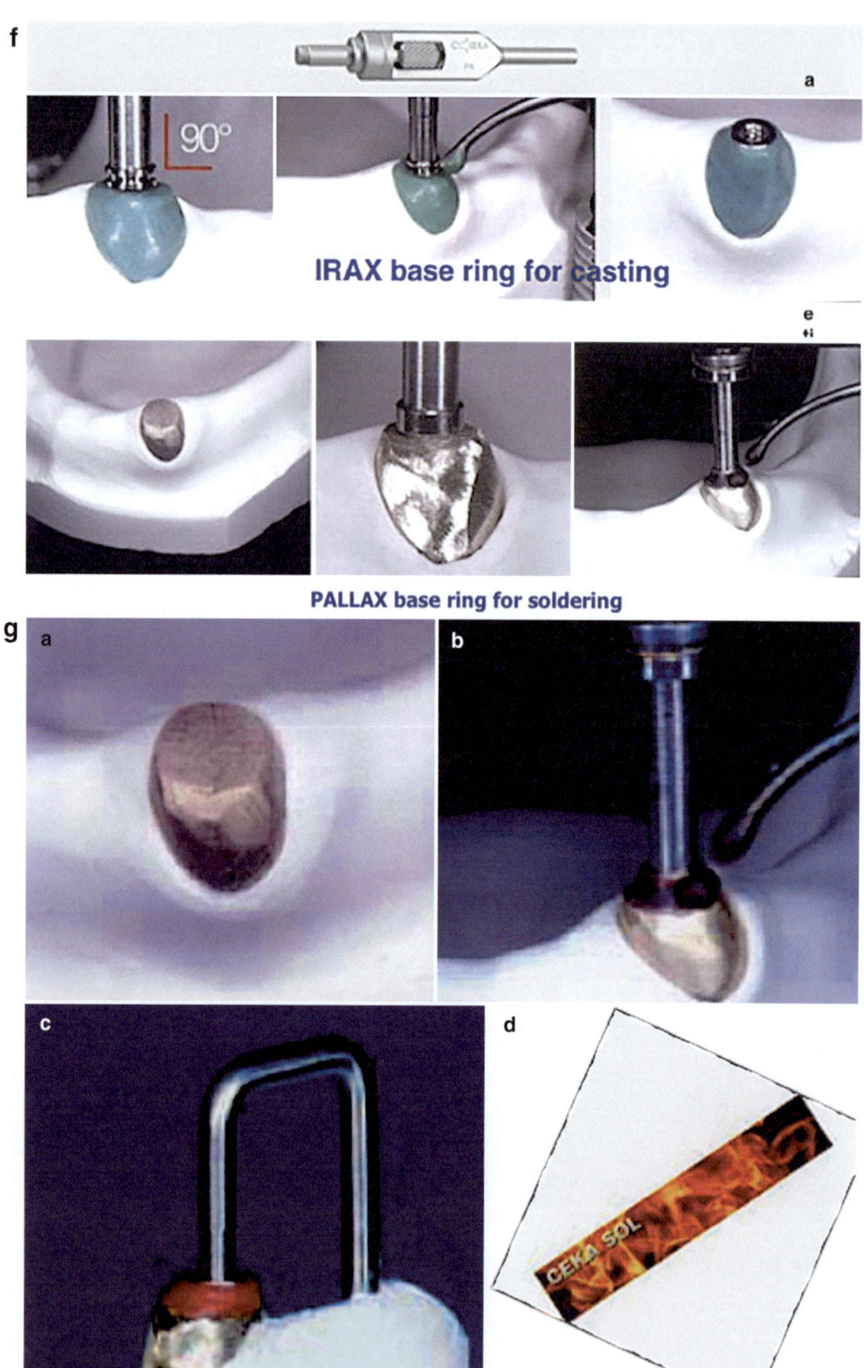

Picture 3.17 (continued)

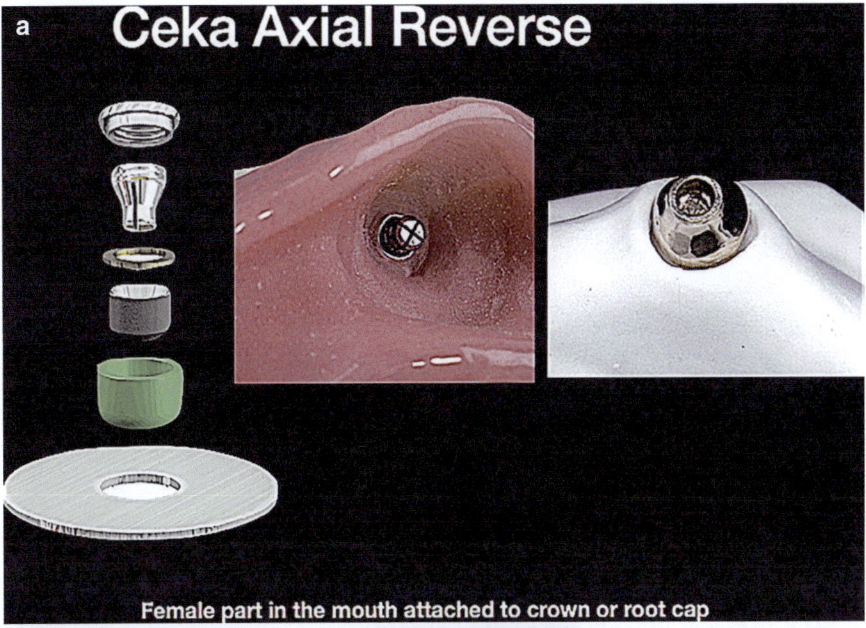

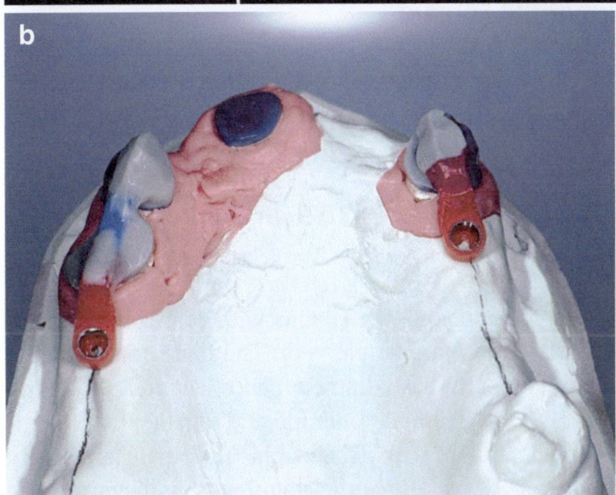

Picture 3.18 (**a**) Ceka axial reverse, (**b**) Ceka attachment placed distally with wax crown male placed on the denture, (**c**) Procedure Caka axial reverse on the coping and the denture

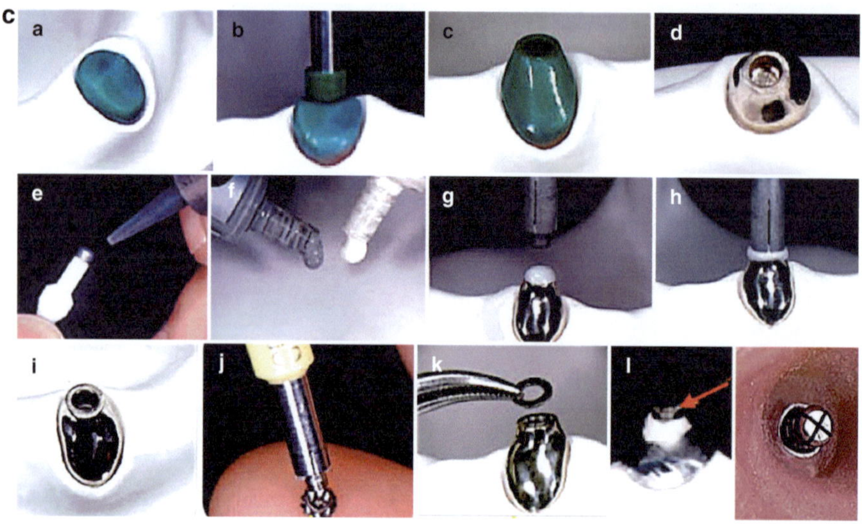

Picture 3.18 (continued)

3.3.9.8 Indirect Placement of the Female

On the male, the duplicating dummy was placed. Then, the model was replicated. Complete the cast frame without damaging the retentive ledge in the female's cavity. Insert the yellow female using the insertion tool into the frame (Picture 3.14).

3.3.10 Accurate Postal System (Figs. 3.38, 3.39, and 3.40, Pictures 3.15 and 3.16)

Clinicians place precise posts (a cementable post in Titanax with a threaded base for the male or a cementable post in Titanax) in a single visit. The male component is composed of metal copings, and its length, base diameter, and diameter are 7 mm, 3.4 mm, and 1.35 mm, respectively. Both the male titanium and female plastic components are easily replaceable. The titanium male and plastic female are easily replaceable and offer a solution for a few remaining abutments with inadequate strength. The attachment clicks into place audibly to ensure patient safety.

Preci Clix RTI has a cementable titanium post with a removable male in Titanax (white, Ti-Al-V) and a Titanax (white, Ti-Al-V) housing with a replaceable plastic female in three retention levels.

Free movement: 10°

It consists of a cementable titanium post and a removable titanium male. The titanium post should be place direct over the denture by using glass ionomer cement to secure the post. The ball is inserted directly into the post. The female housing is for acrylic resin incorporation (Figs. 3.16a, b and 3.46b).

The Preci Clix RCT system is an overdenture with a titanium ball and post for direct placement. It has a titanium cementable post with a titanium male (Fig. 3.46b).

Preci Clix RP is equipped with interchangeable plastic females and a duplicating dummy for cast metal partial frames. Figure 3.46b depicts a titanium post that is cementable with a removable titanium male.

Preci Clix RCP is equipped with interchangeable plastic females and a duplicating dummy for cast metal partial frames. It consists of a titanium cementable post and a titanium male (Fig. 3.46b).

The dentist has the option of incorporating the male into the remaining root and the female into the denture in office or having the laboratory process the female into the overdenture (Picture 3.16a–c). With the penetration bur, the root canal is prepared, and the diamond bur is used to create the base of the Preci Clix post. The reamer is used to prepare the post's diameter. When utilizing the burs, move slowly and avoid horizontal forces. The impression tool is threaded into the Preci Clix post. Using the RE H2 seating and impression instrument as a handle, the Preci Clix post is positioned and cemented within the canal. Before cementation, the Preci Clix post should be sandblasted, and the post and root surface should be coated with bonding composite to improve retention. Following the polymerization of the composite, polish the root surface with a fine sandpaper disk. Fluoride application should be recommended to prevent secondary caries. The ball was secured to the mouth post with a screw.

3.3.10.1   Laboratory Treatment of the Female Attachments

Utilizing impression tools, a mark is made on the stone post. In the impression, the impression tools will create an index. Unthread the impression tool from the post and thread it into the analog model before placing the impression and pouring the master model. Using the screwdriver, thread the male (Preci Clix ball attachment) into the analog. The spacer is positioned over the male. The black rubber spacer is placed over the large tin spacer as a maintainer. Using an insertion tool, the Preci Clix female is inserted into the Clix housing, and then the entire female unit is placed on the clip ball on the model. Eliminate any undercuts. The female Clix is processed into the denture. The large metal and rubber spacers have been eliminated (Picture 3.16b).

3.3.10.2   Direct Insertion of a Female Denture

The tiny black spacer is positioned over the ball and accommodates the entire female (housing and plastic insert). Then, the Preci Clix female (yellow, white, and orange retention rates) was placed in the female house. This enables the denture to be loosened so that the Clix housings can be inserted. There should be no initial contact between the denture and the house. A low-viscosity self-curing acrylic resin is mixed and placed in the area of the denture that has been relieved, and the denture is then seated by applying finger pressure only to the attachment area. It is crucial that the patient does not achieve complete occlusion and displace soft tissue in the saddle region. Because when patients bite, the denture cannot rotate anteriorly to posteriorly, displacing the attachments. According to the acrylic resin manufacturer, the denture is placed in the mouth for approximately 6 min. Along with the tin and black rubber spacers, any excess resin is eliminated. The finishing and polishing steps were then completed. To adjust retention, the female can be easily changed in the metal housing. Patients must be instructed on how to insert and remove their dentures.

3.3.11 Ceka Attachment

The Ceka attachment is composed of a soldering base with a removable male stud that is conical in shape, has a rounded top with an increased diameter for retention, and is vertically divided into four sections. These four sections are adaptable and emphasize small housing for female. The activation of these sleeves achieves retention (Pictures 3.17 and 3.18; Figs. 3.47, 3.48, 3.49, and 3.50).

3.3.11.1 Principles of the System

The Ceka attachment was created 35 years ago as an aesthetically pleasing alternative to the conventional clasp and offers perfect retention. The basic concept is straightforward: a spring pin that precisely fits into a conical female. The denture is correctly seated once the spring pin "clicks" into the female. Today, each Ceka attachment adheres to the same straightforward principle. This design offers dental technicians numerous advantages during laboratory procedures. The system has three primary goals, two of which are pursued daily by dental technicians: simplicity and efficiency. In addition to facilitating maintenance, repair, and precision, Ceka enables the dentist to communicate with the patient regarding the ease of insertion or removal.

The female component is made from titanium alloy. Utilizing a processing spacer permits the attachment of vertical and horizontal movements. During processing, the male intercorperation was maintained by utilizing duplicate processing pieces. Before screwing male threads into female threads, Ceka-Bond cement should be applied to the male threads following processing, finishing, and polishing. Therefore, improve the protection against the male spring pin unthreading during a function. Nevertheless, the male spring pin can be removed at any time with the special tool (Pictures 3.19, 3.20, and 3.21).

3.3.11.2 Advantages

- This attachment allows for both flexible and rigid retention.
- It has greater longevity.
- Its parts are interchangeable.

3.3.11.3 Disadvantages

- This attachment requires a complex torque-producing intraoral adjustment.
- Rigid attachments can produce excessive torque on the teeth.

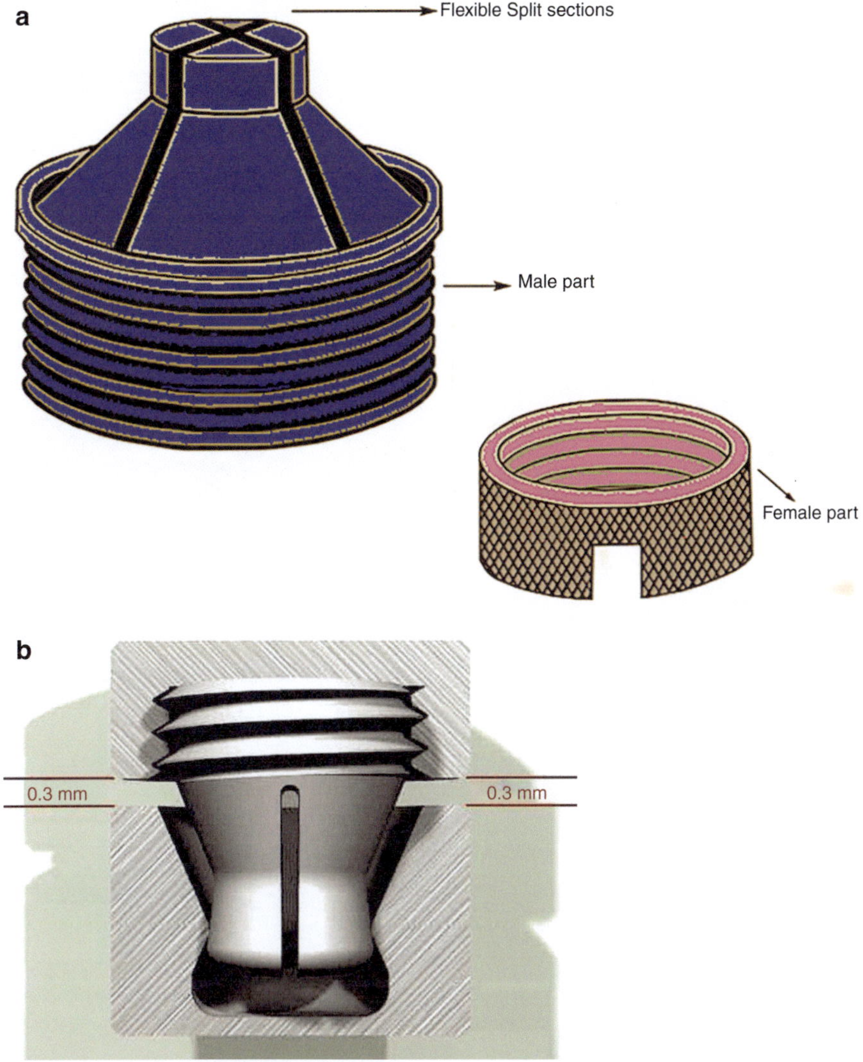

Fig. 3.47 (**a**) Male and female part of Ceka attachment and (**b**) male part of Ceka attachment

Fig. 3.48 Mechanism of Ceka attachment

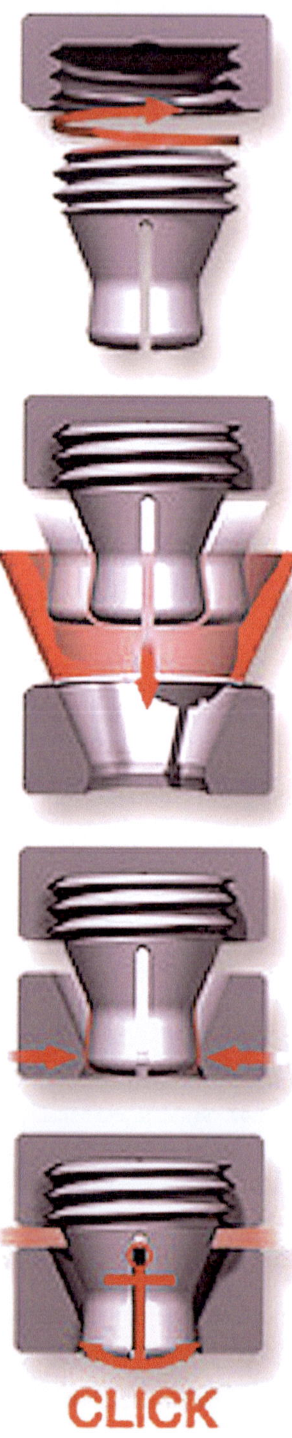

Stability and retention are crucial criteria for the planning of an overdenture. As a means of increasing patient comfort, clinicians may further modify retention in each case. The attachment has 830 g of retentive force, which can be increased at the patient's request. This retention is well above Lehmann and Arnin's recommended minimum of 400 g per attachment. The Ceka Axial attachments, which are available in both M3 (standard) and M2 (smaller) sizes, are favored by numerous dental professionals because they provide the desired stability and spring pin for proper retention. The threaded base diameter is either 2 mm (M2 size) or 3 mm (M3 size). Clinicians should choose the larger M3 size when there is sufficient space, as it is stronger and easier to work with, and the smaller M2 size when there is limited space to maintain proper anatomical contours and space. The M2 attachment is the smallest attachment system that is fully adjustable. The compact size allows for use in "deep bite" situations where space is limited. The space requirements for the Revax (M2) are 3.8 mm in height, 3.4 mm in diameter, and 4.8 mm in height for the attachment, acrylic resin, and teeth.

The adjustable spring pin attachment can be used as a conventional stud (with cast copings) or as an intraradicular connector overdenture on roots and implants (Fig. 3.50).

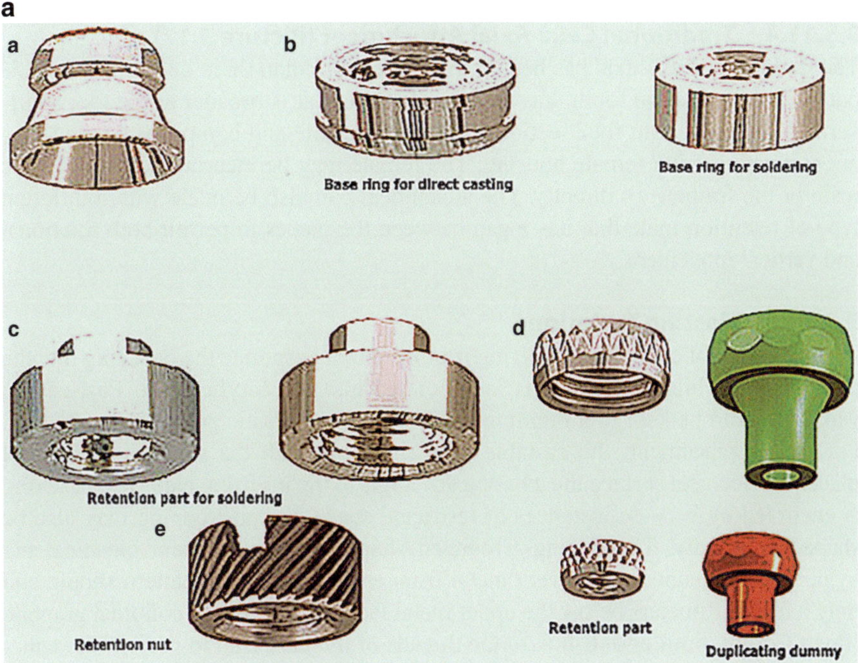

Fig. 3.49 (a) Part of Ceka attachment. (b) *a* Ceka Revax Spring pin (removable resilient spring pin); *b* axial Ceka matrix (female for retention in acrylic resin, for soldering, or direct casting. IRAX alloy); *c* base ring (base ring for direct casting with precious and palladium-based alloys. IRAX alloy); and *d* base ring for soldering (PALLAX alloy)

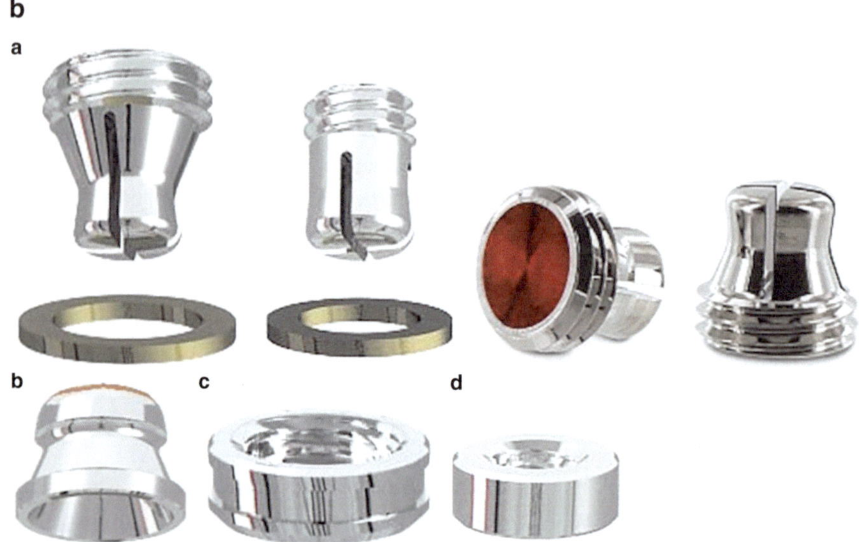

Fig. 3.49 (continued)

3.3.11.4 Traditional Ceka Axial Attachment (Picture 3.17)

The traditional Ceka axis has been utilized for more than three decades. The male part is attached to the tooth, has a rounded shape that is broader at the top, and is vertically divided into four sections. They are flexible and compressible, and they are compatible with female housing. The female may be incorporated into acrylic resin or the framework directly. The attachment can also be made with a different type of retention male that has a gap between the pieces to permit both rotational and vertical movement.

3.3.11.5 Casting Technique

The technique of cast-on or soldering is utilized to incorporate the base ring into the post-coping, while the female is incorporated into the acrylic resin. Post-coping waxing should be kept to a minimum. It should use a plastic post that can be cast. For proper placement, the castable base ring on which the paralleling mandrel places the occlusal surface must be at a 90° angle to the insertion path. The base ring is encircled by wax. In instances of restricted space, the post-coping may also be shaped concavely. The copings' rounded shape facilitates patient cleaning and hygiene maintenance. To prevent metal from entering, the wax pattern should end only a few millimeters below the upper metal ledge. Apply liquid colloidal graphite (Preat Corporation) or anti-flux to the threads of the base ring to prevent the adhesion of any cast metal. Before investing, graphite should be allowed to dry out. A two-step investment process is advised. After 30 min of initial investment setting, the casting and finishing processes are completed (precious alloys are preferred only). Utilize the small space maintainer and the large space maintainer to assemble the attachment. Protect the attachment's inner surface with silicone, and then process the denture.

3.3.11.6   Soldering Technique

Additionally, the attachment can be soldered to a post-coping (made of precious or non-precious alloys). In these processes, either the H4 (M3 size) or RE H4 (M2 size) soldering accessories and CEKA Sol may be utilized. In the laboratory or by the dentist, the precision female is embedded in the acrylic resin. The benefit of this system is decreasing the risk of food impaction in the attachment.

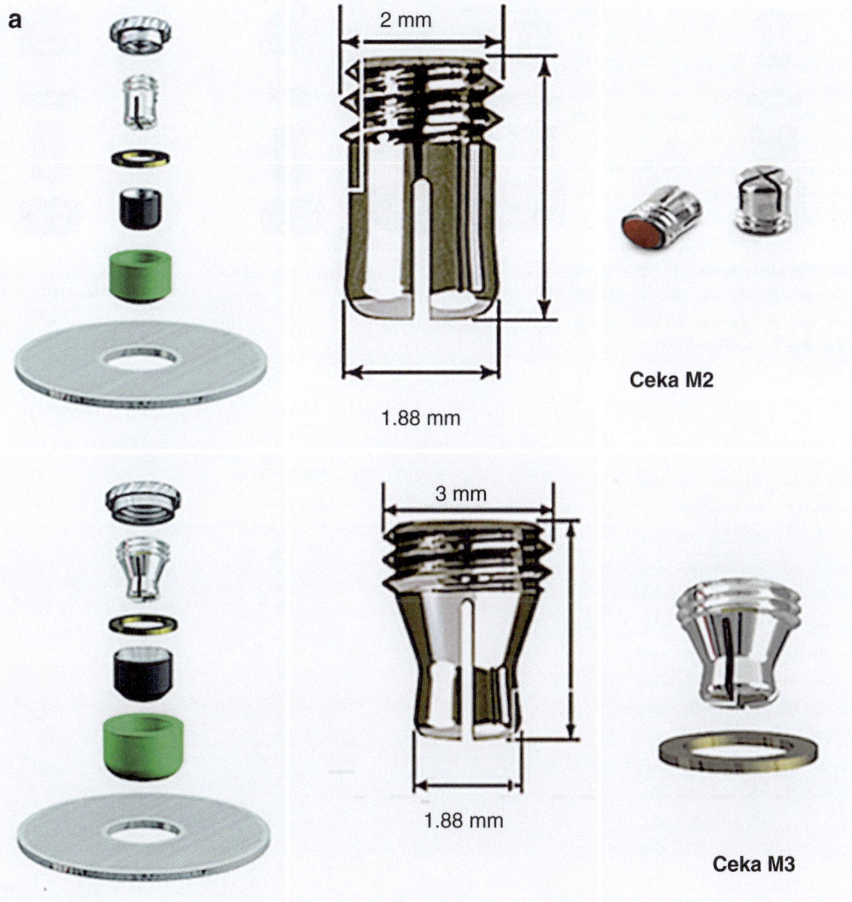

Fig. 3.50 (**a–c**) Ceka M2 and M3 attachment

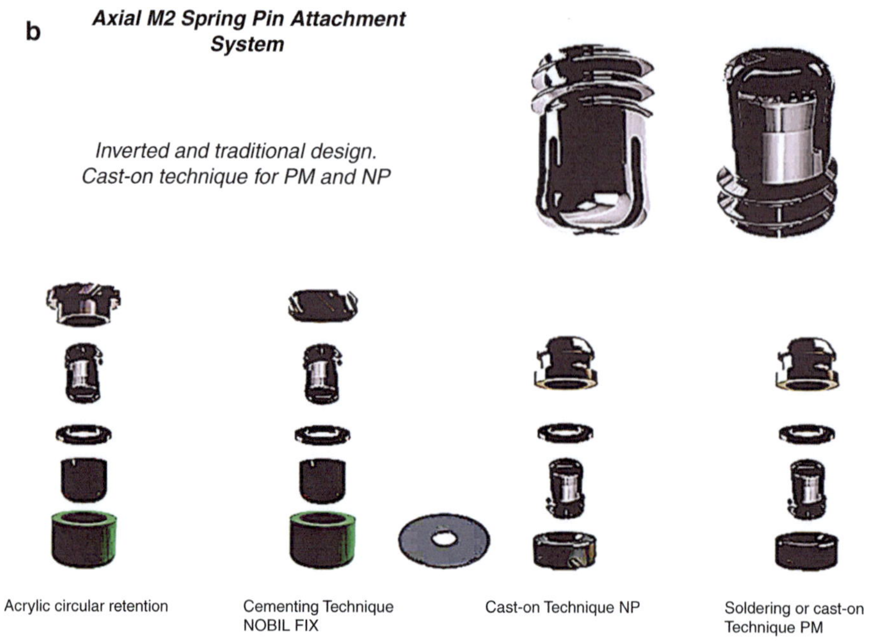

Fig. 3.50 (continued)

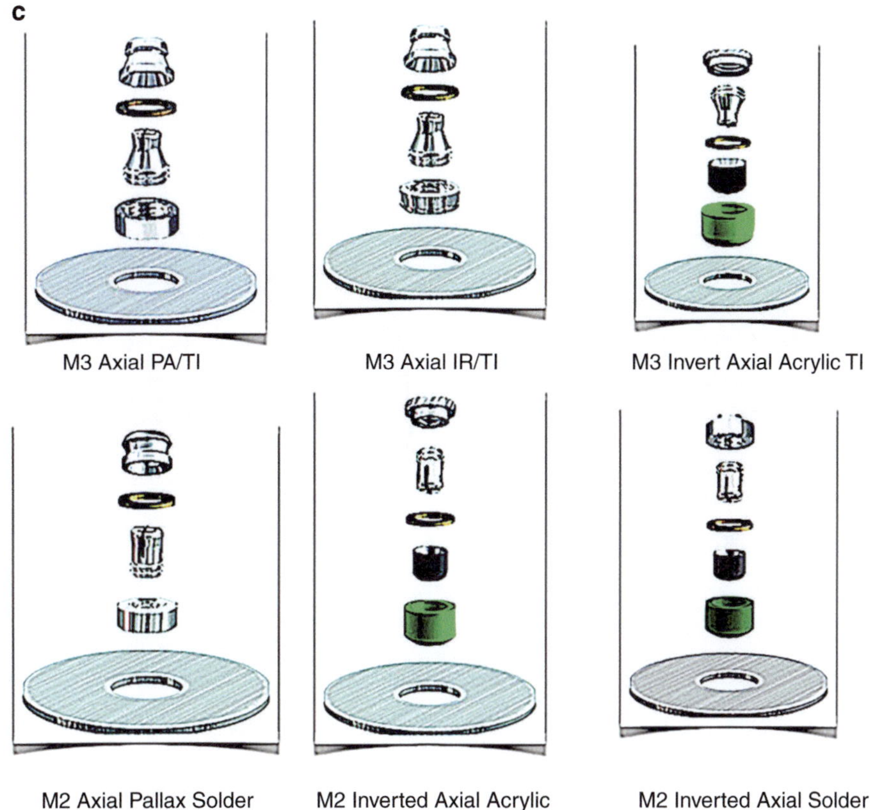

Fig. 3.50 (continued)

3.3.11.7   Inverted Ceka Axial Attachment

The bonding technique incorporates female attachment into the post-coping technique. The male is inserted into the acrylic resin of the removable denture, which enables simple maintenance and oral comfort (Fig. 3.18). Any dental alloy, precious or nonprecious, may be used to cast the post-coping. After determining the path of insertion and incorporating the plastic pattern with the paralleling mandrel before investing and casting procedures, the plastic pattern is incorporated with the paralleling mandrel. Place the titanium female on the parallel mandrel and sandblast it with coarse aluminum oxide. The titanium female is bonded to the Ceka Site in the post-coping. Attached to the female component are the spring pin, retention part, and space maintainer. If a resilient structure is necessary, the tinfoil is modified to maintain a space above the post-coping.

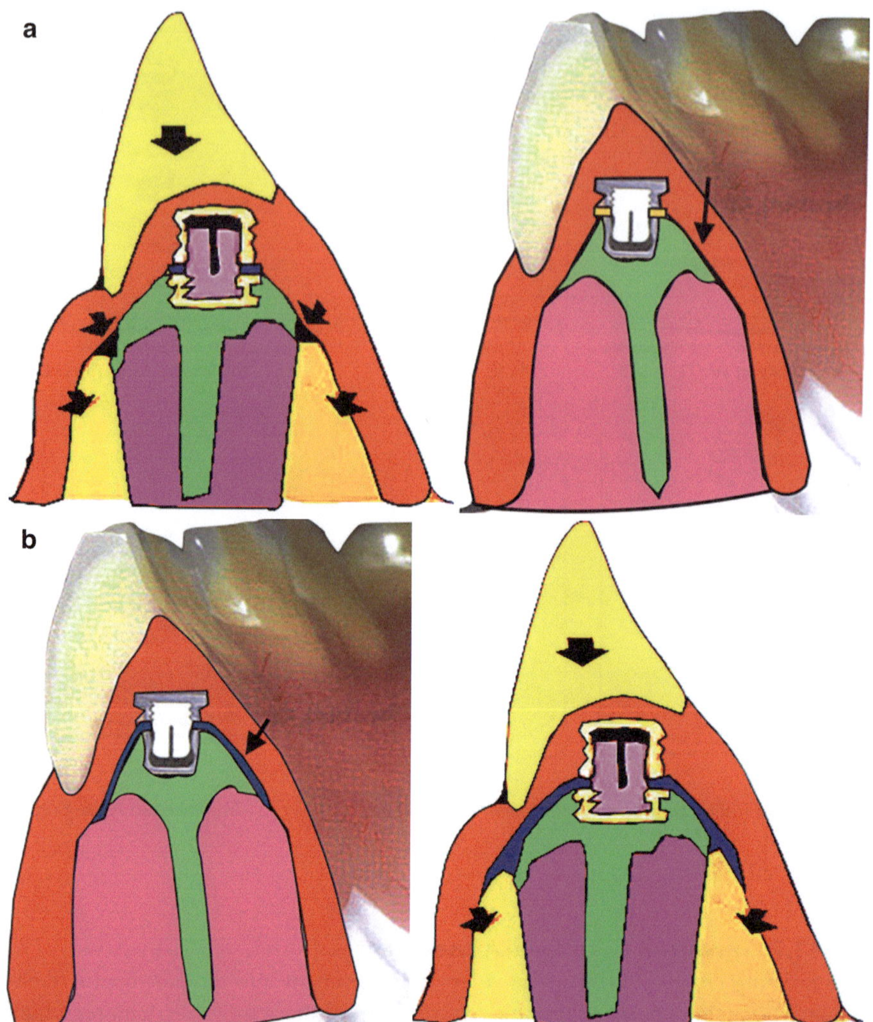

Picture 3.19 (**a**) An overdenture fabricates with the thin spacer; this eliminates all movement of the denture. (**b**, **c**) An overdenture fabricates with a large spacer, the large spacer creates free space between the denture and the post and attachment to allow this free movement

The denture is then polymerized and space maintainers are eliminated. The utilization of spacers is an important aspect of overdenture treatment. If an overdenture is fabricated without a large spacer, the denture's mobility is restricted since the attachment is a rigid system. In this circumstance, the base of the denture is in direct contact with the post and attachment. The forces are transmitted directly to the post and attachment. Using a large spacer allows the denture to move; it is now a resilient (tissue-bearing) attachment. During this procedure, a large spacer is used to create a gap between the denture and its attachment in order to permit free movement and

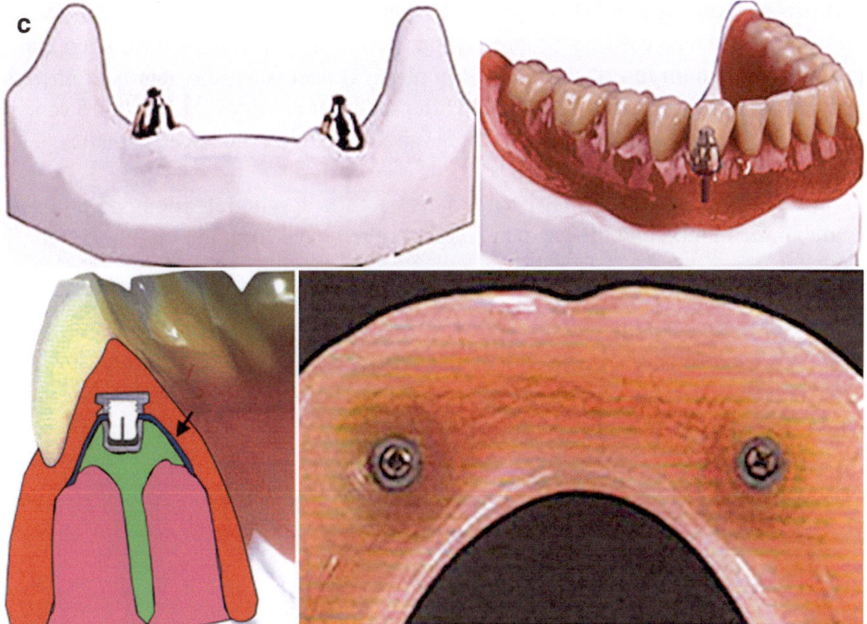

Picture 3.19 (continued)

transmit forces to the supporting soft tissue. The greater the height of the space, the greater the force distribution and the lesser the force transmitted to the abutment (Figs. 3.19 and 3.20).

3.3.11.8 Types of Ceka Connection (Fig. 3.50)

M3 Type
M3: 691 PA/TI Axial
Pallax base ring for soldering to the bar or post-coping. Titanax female for retention in male position acrylic resin on the post-coping or bar.

M3: 693 Axial IR/TI
Irax base rings are utilized for direct casting with precious metals and alloys containing palladium, or for soldering to the post-coping. Female Titanax is used to retain acrylic resin. On the post's coping or bar, there are males. The direct cast is simple.

M3 Invert Axial Acrylic TI
For bonding, a female Titanax is used in the casting with Ceka Site. The titanax retention component is used to hold the acrylic resin in place. With an alloy, a cast (coping or bar) can be produced. After all other steps have been completed, the titanium inserts are bonded in place.

M3 Invert Axial Spacer TI

Alloys can produce castings (coping or bar). After all other steps have been completed, the titanium inserts are bonded in place. If necessary, the abutment crowns and female attachment can be modified after try-in. It provides the option to veneer the metal frame of a removable partial denture directly for enhanced esthetics.

In clinical procedures, it is simple to connect the acrylic retention cap to a cast frame in the mouth, and the cap can be quickly removed from the mouth.

M2 Type
M2 Axial Pallax Solder

A Pallax base ring is used to solder the post-coping or bar to the post. Female Titanax is used to retain the acrylic resin. The male component is placed on the post-coping or bar to increase the stability of the denture.

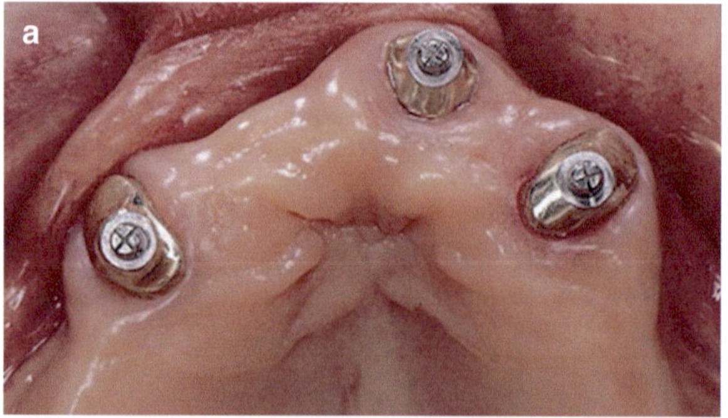

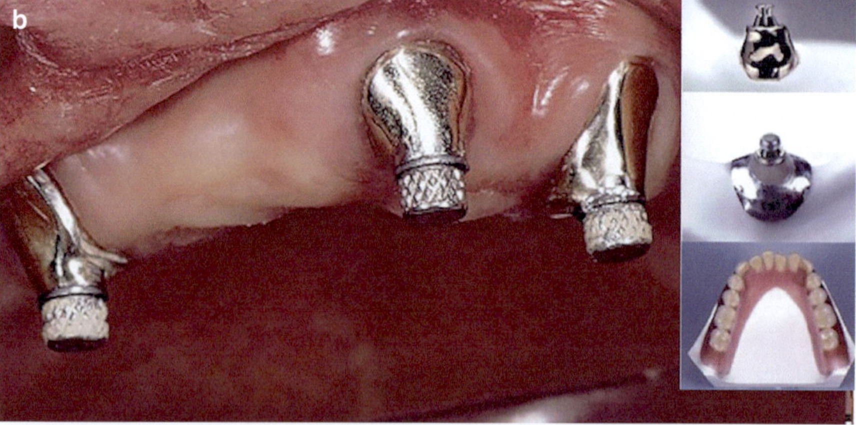

Picture 3.20 (**a–e**) Direct placement of CEKA female to the denture: (**a**) Ceka male attachment is placed on coping in the mouth; (**b**) metal housing is placed on the male in the mouth; (**c**) CEKA SITE bonding material; (**d**) bonding material placed in the inside of denture is relieved for female area; and (**e**) female part of Ceka attachment in the denture

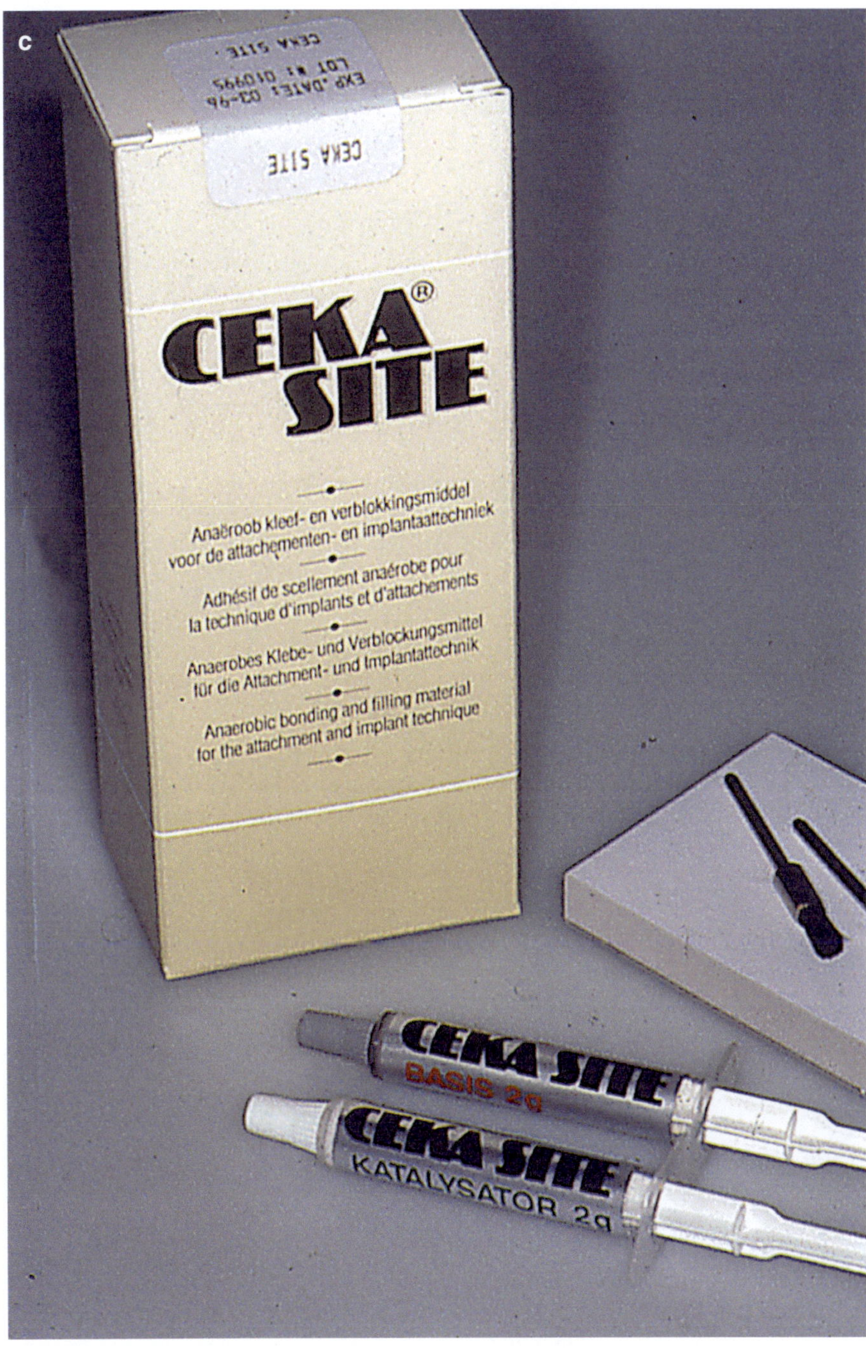

Picture 3.20   (continued)

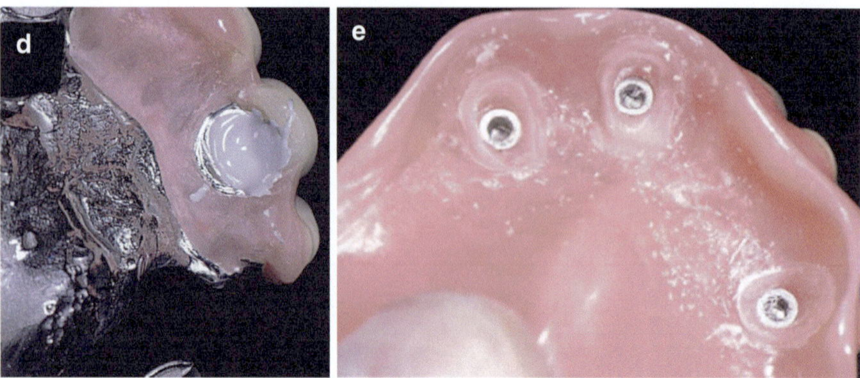

Picture 3.20 (continued)

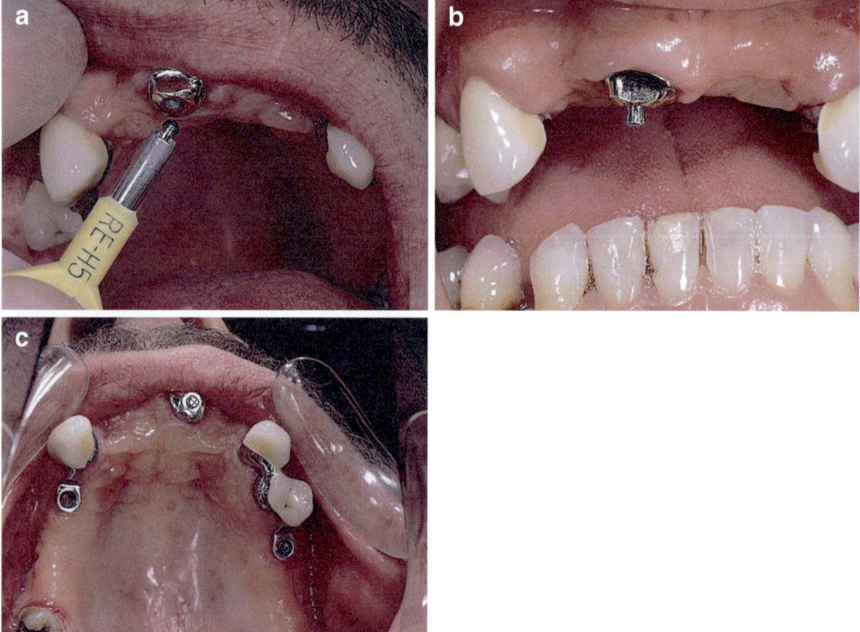

Picture 3.21 Female part is processed in the acrylic model using indirect methods: (**a**) male part is placed on the coping in the mouth; (**b, c**) male part in situ; (**d**) male part in the model; and (**e**) female attachment is placed in the finished denture

M2 Inverted Axially Inverted Acrylic

For bonding, a female Titanax is used in the casting with Ceka Site. The Titanax retention component is used to hold the acrylic resin in place. An alloy may be used to create a casting (coping or bar). There are no miscasting or devesting errors. The

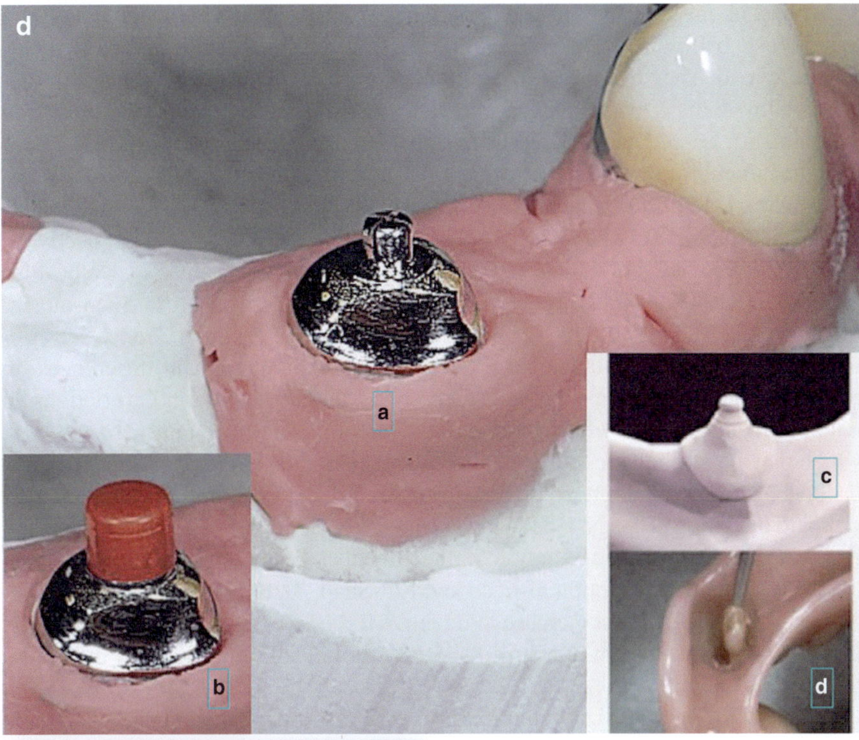

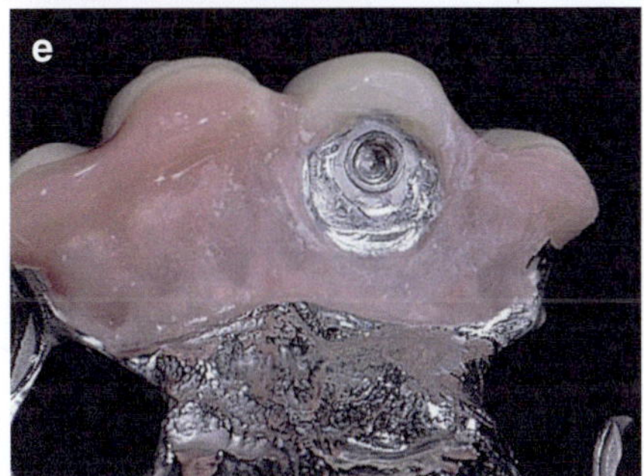

Picture 3.21 (continued)

titanium female is bonded into place after all other procedures have been completed. If necessary, the abutment crowns and female attachment can be modified after try-in.

Solder M2 Inverted Axial

Alloys may be used to produce castings (coping or bar). There are no miscasting or devesting errors. The precise titanium female is inserted in and bonded after all other procedures have been completed. The abutment crowns and female attachment can be modified after the try-in if necessary.

Wolf et al. investigated the retention, wear, inserting, and separating cycles of a commercial ball attachment when a unilateral denture was subjected to a 100 N eccentric load. They examined five ball attachments [Dalbo-Plus elliptic with precious alloy ball (Cendres & Metaux), Dalbo-Plus elliptic with titanium ball (Straumann), Ecco (Unor), Tima (Unor), and Pro-Snap (Metalor)] as well as a ball-like attachment locator (Zest Attachments). The retention values of Dalbo-Plus precious alloy, Dalbo-Plus titanium, Ecco, Locator, Tima, and Pro-Snap attachments were 9.350 N, 9.850 N, 8.300 N, 13.950 N, 11.300 N, and 8.150 N, respectively, after 10,000 cycles. Following 50,000 cycles, the retention values of Dalbo-Plus precious alloy, Dalbo-Plus titanium, Ecco, Locator, Tima, and Pro-Snap attachments were 2.100 N, 10.400 N, 0.950 N, 2.000 N, 1.150 N, and 3734 N, respectively. The different attachment systems exhibited significant differences in retention, but within some groups, there were initially substantial variations in retention. Some attachments exhibited initial retention values of approximately 3 N, which may be attributable to the manufacturing tolerance of the retention elements. Dalbo-Plus elliptic ball attachment with titanium balls exhibited the smallest first standard deviation of 1.6 N and the lowest retention of 9.875 N. Except for Ecco and Pro-Snap attachments, the retention of attachments initially increased with increasing cycles, with the exception of Ecco and Pro-Snap. At 1000 cycles, the Ecco system exhibited the smallest increase in retentive forces. For specific test samples, the Locator and Tima system attachments revealed clinically questionable maximum values of 38 N and 45 N.

In contrast, the median retention force of Pro-Snap attachments gradually decreased from 8150 N at the start to 3734 N at the end. The increase in retention is accompanied by a rise in the roughness of the retentive parts, particularly the equators of the balls. This increased wear led to an increase in joining and separating forces as well as an increase in wear. Due to this material loss, a long-term decrease in retention caused the majority of specimens to be lost.

In contrast, retentive plastic inserts or frictional attachments with activating lamellae demonstrated less abrasion and superior retention performance. However, the tested ball attachments with retentive plastic inserts did not confirm the benefit of plastic inserts for ball attachments in the present study. A combination of a titanium-based alloy for the ball and a precious gold-based alloy for the flexible metal lamellae of the matrix seems preferable.

3.3.12 Attachment to the OT Equator/Sphere

This attachment was originally constructed in accordance with the OT CAP standard (Rhein 83, Bologna, Italy) (Figs. 3.51 and 3.52; Picture 3.22, 3.23, and 3.24).

3.3.12.1   Single Castable Spheres

In addition to the spherical inner surface of the elastic cap, the design of the sphere with a flat head permits vertical movement during mastication. Rhein83 female caps are made from a special nylon material that remains stable and functional in the oral cavity for extended periods. The available clinical data indicates that stability can be achieved with minimal wear. All types of alloys can be used to cast these attachments, but it is essential to use a metal with a high Vickers hardness to prevent wear. Furthermore, the hardness of titanium single spheres and tin for welding or bonding is 1600 v (Fig. 3.22a).

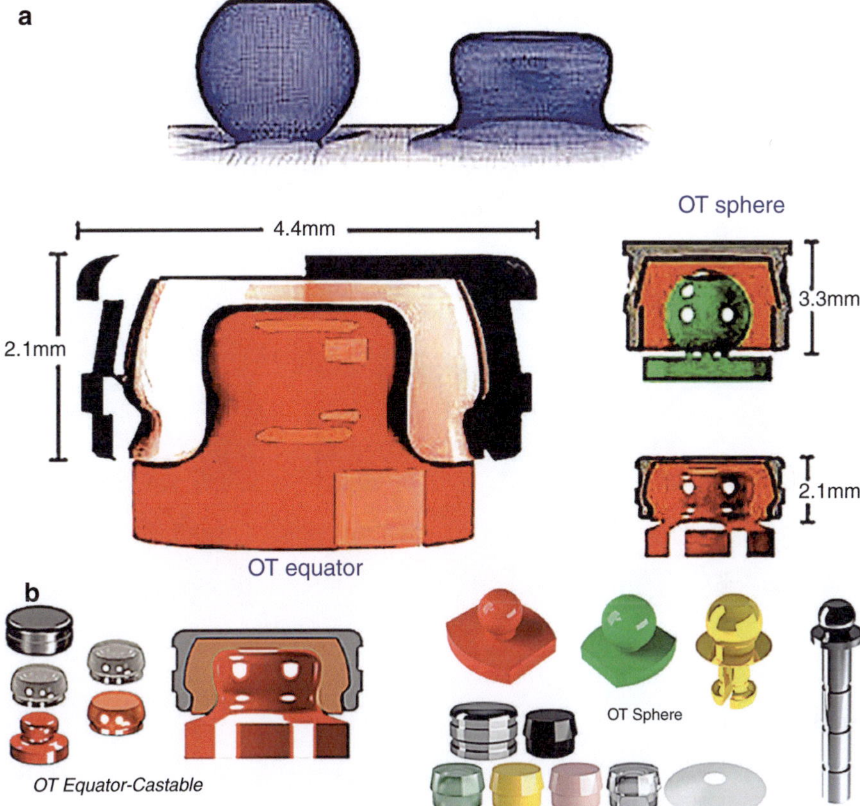

Fig. 3.51 (**a**, **b**) The OT Equator and Sphere attachment. (**c**, **d**) The design of the sphere with a flat head of the elastic cap permits vertical movement during mastication. (**e**) The OT Sphere attachment assembly. (**f**) Different types of caps for OT attachment

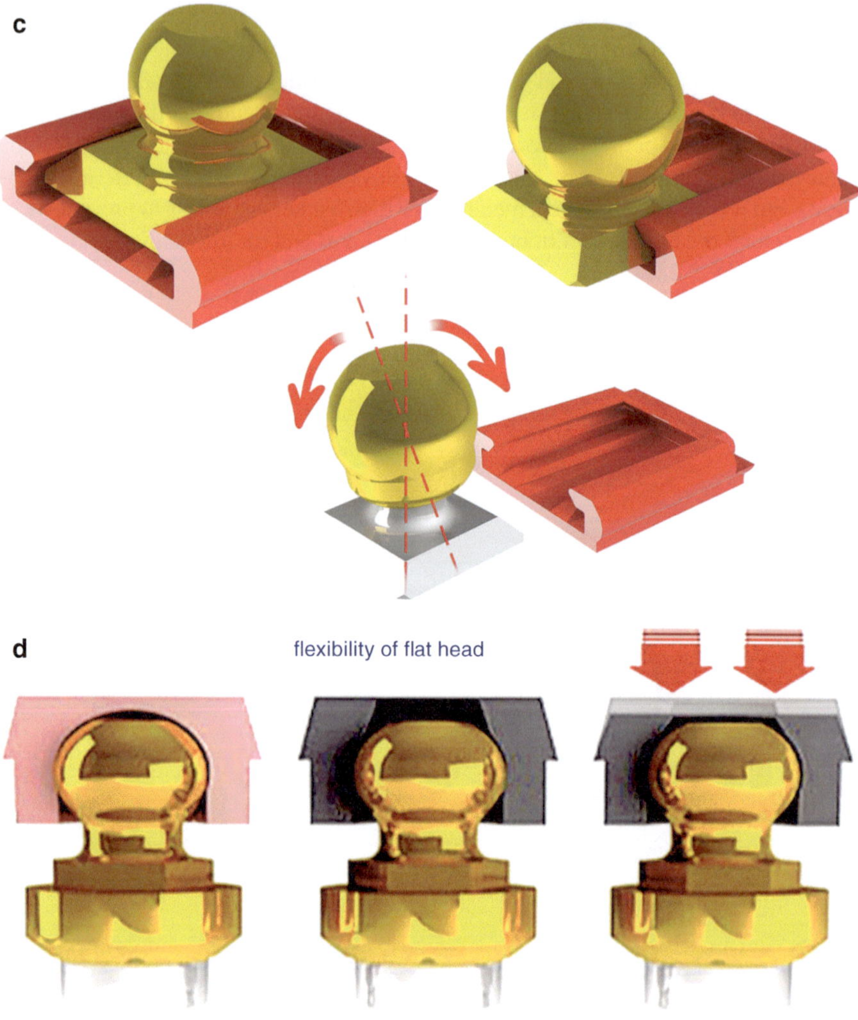

Fig. 3.51 (continued)

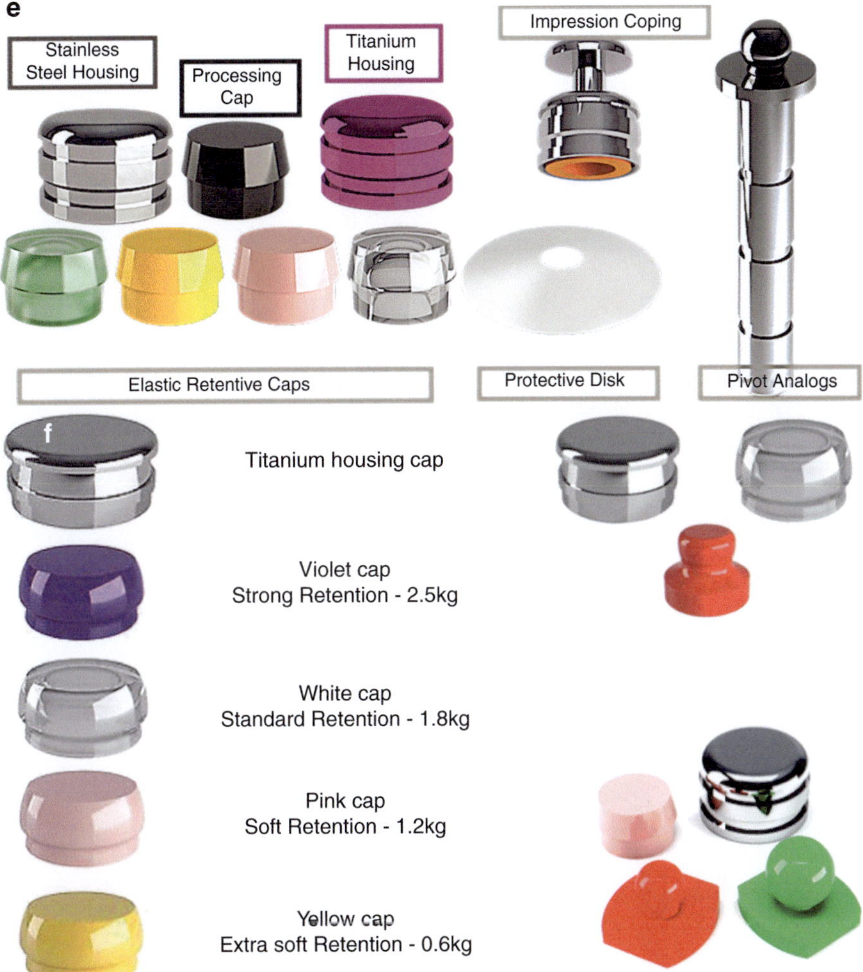

Fig. 3.51 (continued)

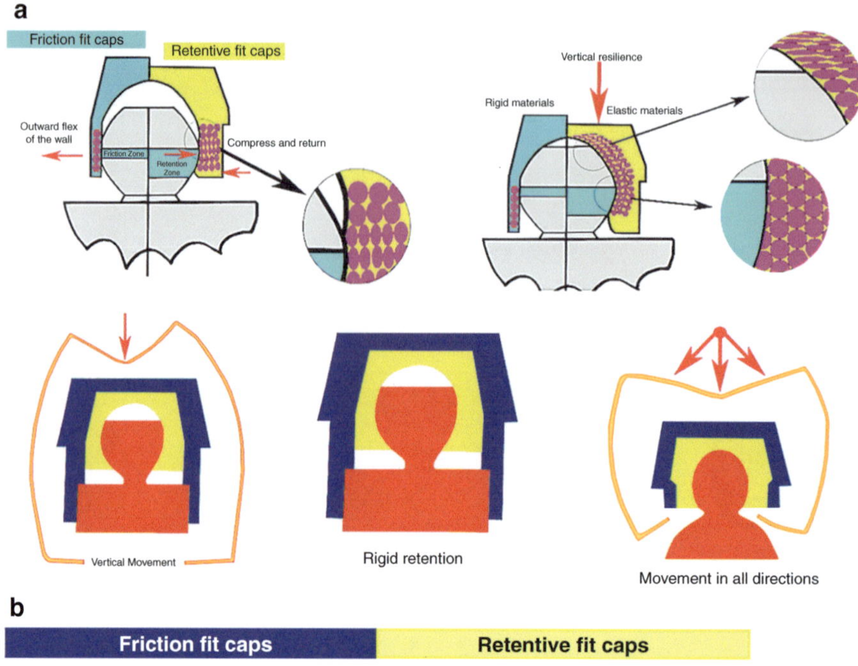

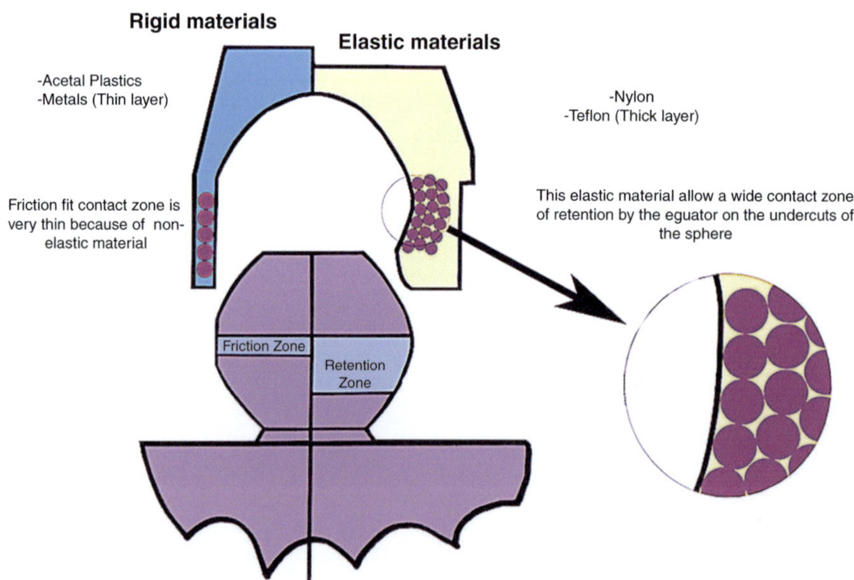

Fig. 3.52 (**a–d**) Comparison of friction fit and retentive fit caps (rigid vs. elastic materials): Characteristics and retentive functionality

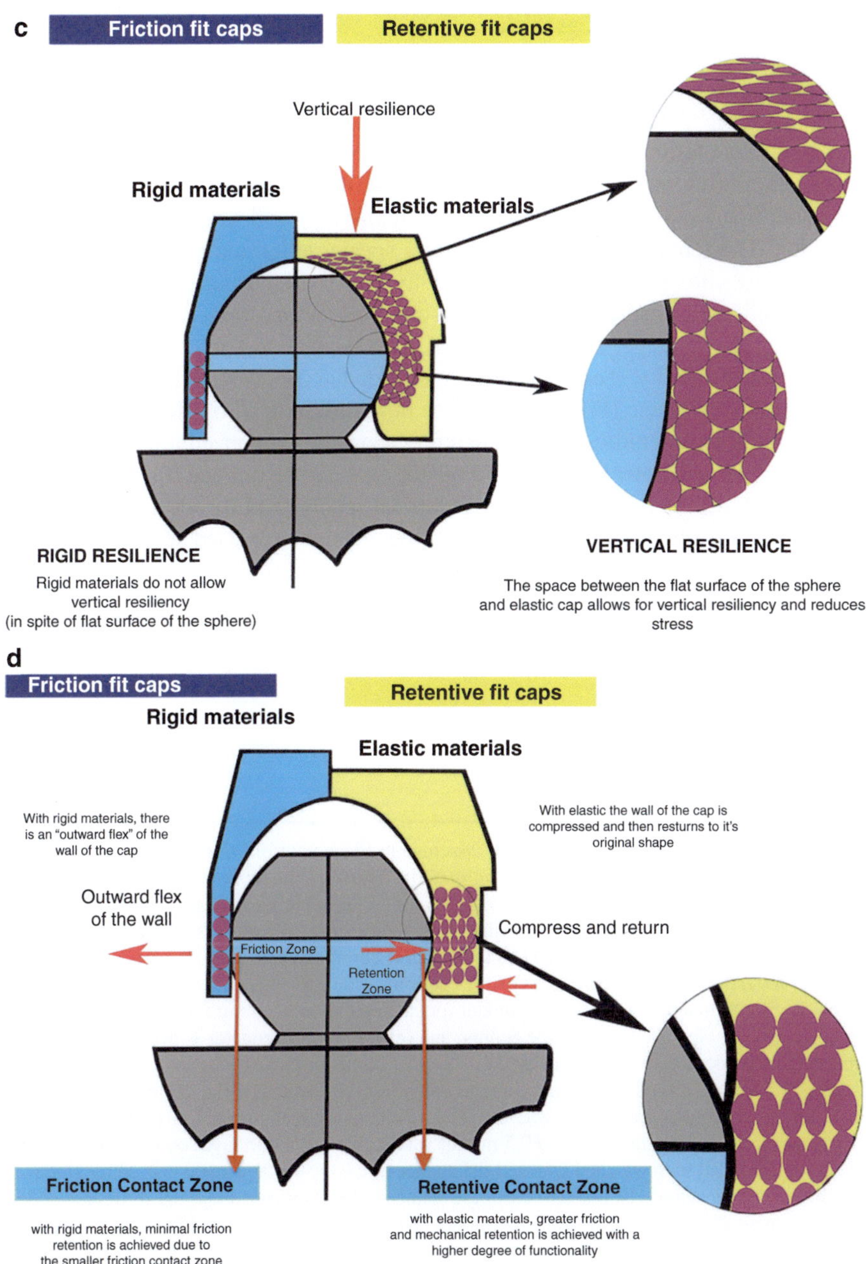

Fig. 3.52 (continued)

3.3.12.2 OT Equator Castable

The significant change is the elimination of the head and neck of the sphere, with only the central portion, known as the OT Equator single attachment, remaining unchanged (Fig. 3.51a, b; Pictures 3.22 and 3.23). In addition to the spherical inner surface of the elastic cap, the design of the sphere with a flat head permits vertical movement during mastication (Fig. 3.51c, d). With overdentures, resiliency can be regulated using a variety of retentive caps with varying degrees of elasticity and retention. The female caps are made from a special nylon material that is durable and continues to function in the oral cavity for extended periods. Standard and micro-sized extra-resilient caps will absorb masticatory forces without causing implant or root damage. The new stainless steel housing design offers reduced size and increased stability; it can be directly embedded in the resin, welded to the frame, or bonded to the frame (Fig. 3.51e, f). The new version is also offered in titanium. If the clinical case requires resilient denture bearings, the conventional OT cap can be utilized. On the other hand, nylon Equator caps can be utilized if retentive activity is desired. If the denture requires additional retention in this system, OT cap is used. Standard retentive caps and metal housings can be used to cover any OT

Picture 3.22 (**a**) OT Sphere and Equator attachment. Placement of OT Equator Castable using the indirect technique. (**b**) *a* The separating material brush on the stone model for the prepared areas to receive the castable posts; *b* it should be longer castable posts in the room channels for easy removal and reline with castable resin, for higher accuracy; *c* the castable post placed and using resin materials margins finished and then resin is cured, the post cut to the required length at the root; and *d* the OT equator is placed on the occlusal surface by using a surveyor and the waxing technique is continued. (**c**) *a* Final cast model for casting OT attachment; *b* the waxing of coping and placing castable attachment on the coping; and (**c**) OT castable equator with coping. (**d**) Build up the framework directly on master model: *a, b* after cementing of attachment/coping assembly, impression coping placed on the attachment and impression taken; *c* the OT analog placed in impression; and *d* the plaster model with the OT equator analog seen in position. (**e**) *a* The stainless steel housing placed on the analog; *b* 0.5 mm of wax applied as a thin layer on the model, all the undercuts are filled with wax and attached the connectors; *c* the castable resin is used for connecting the parts. Care should be taken to cover the stainless steel housing; and *d* the sprues are added to the framework and removed from the model. The stainless steel housing should not remain inside. After careful investigation, the framework invested and cast choice of alloy. (**f**) The last controlled wax framework with silicone index. (**g**) *a* After casting the metal framework, the framework verified the position on the model and controlled; *b* the composite resin materials used to bond the stainless steel housing to the frame and controlled the metal frame with the stainless steel housing in place and then any excess materials cleaned off the inside of metal framework; *c* the stainless steel housing cemented into the framework; and *d* using conventional methods, acrylic prosthesis finished on a metal frame. After processing, the black caps are replaced with pink caps

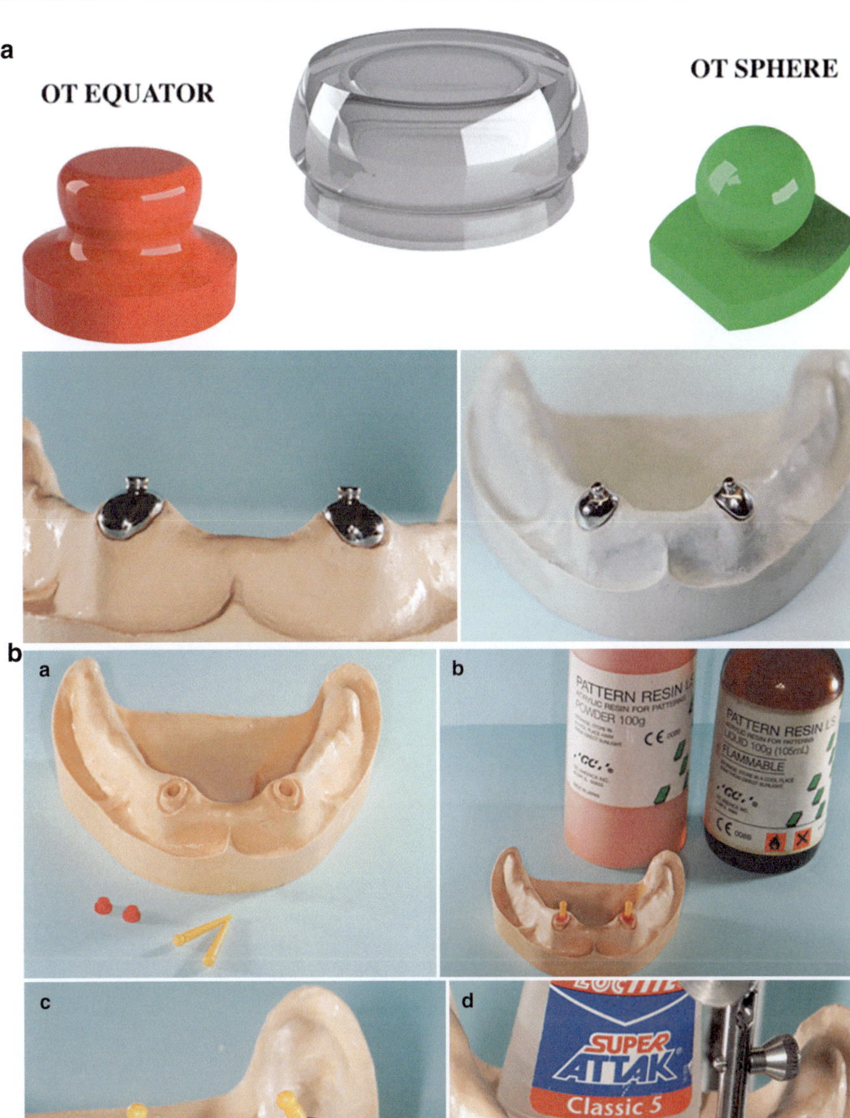

OT EQUATOR
OT SPHERE
a
b
a
b
c
d
PATTERN RESIN
POWDER 100g
PATTERN RESIN LS
LIQUID 100g (105mL)
FLAMMABLE
SUPER
ATTAK
Classic 5

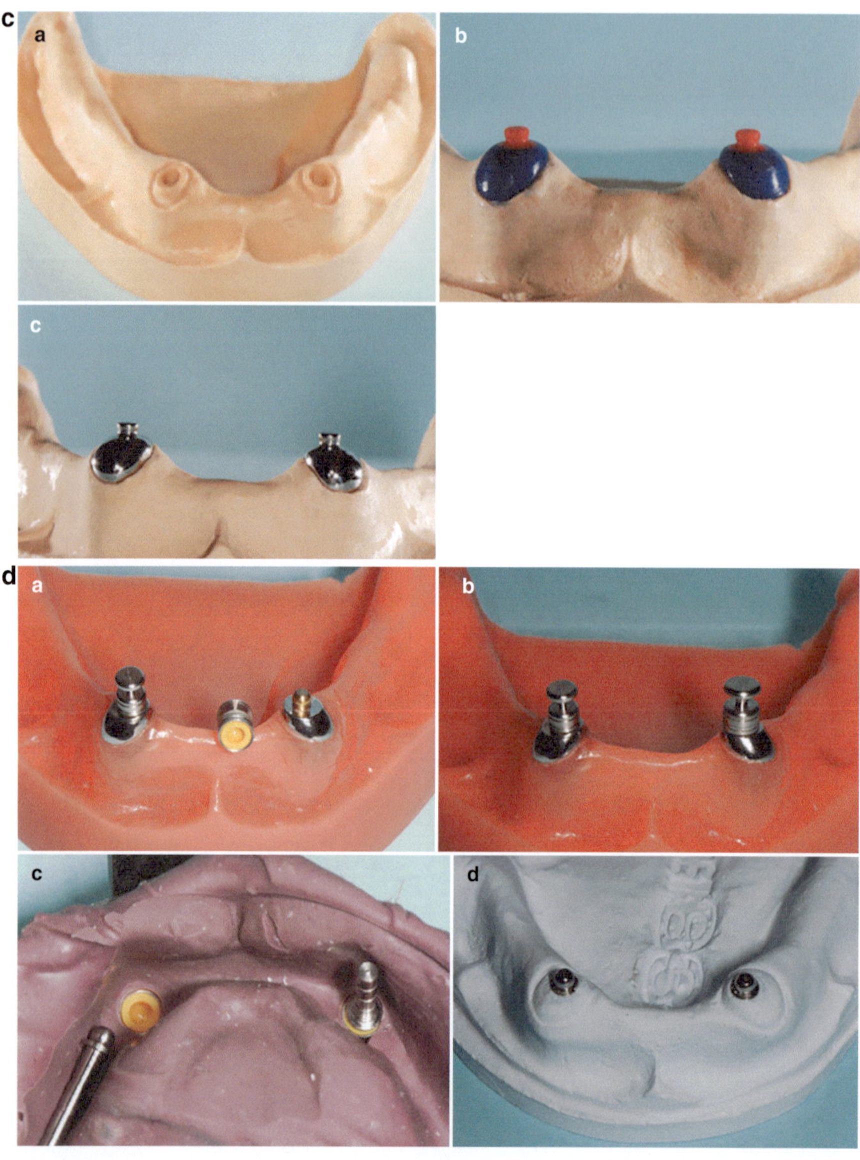

Picture 3.22

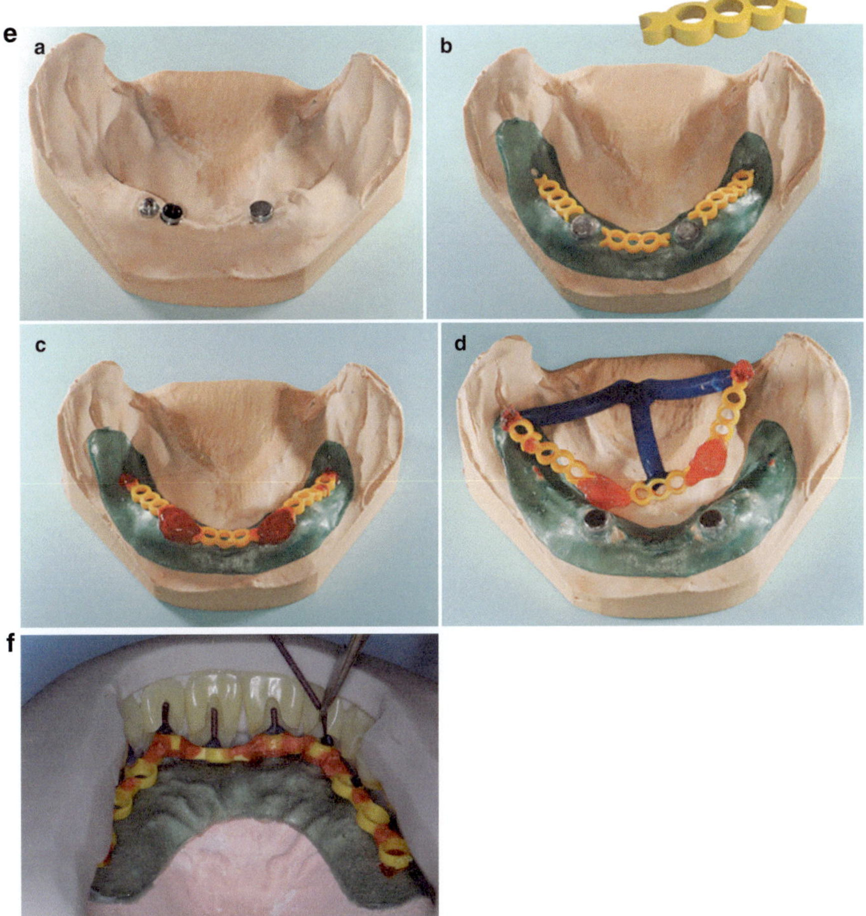

Picture 3.22 (continued)

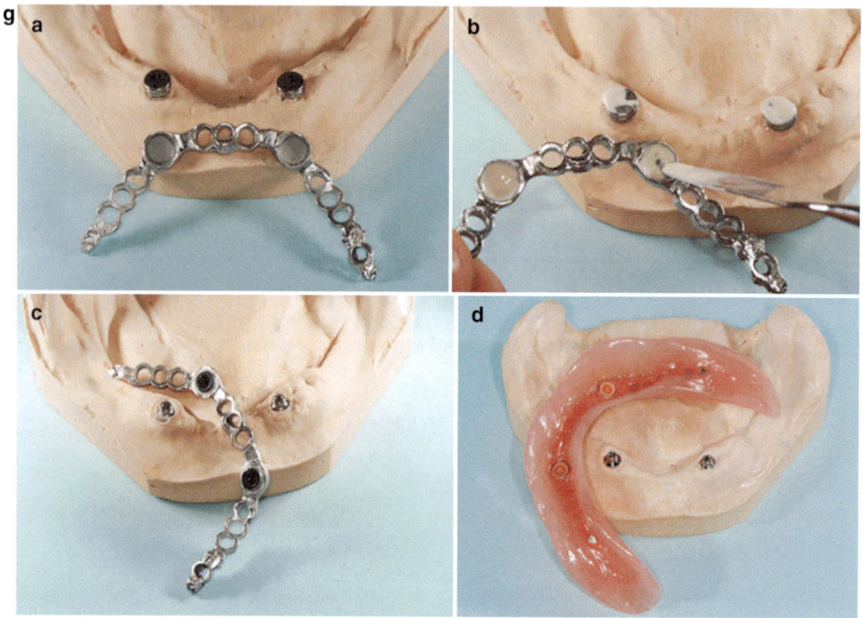

Picture 3.22 (continued)

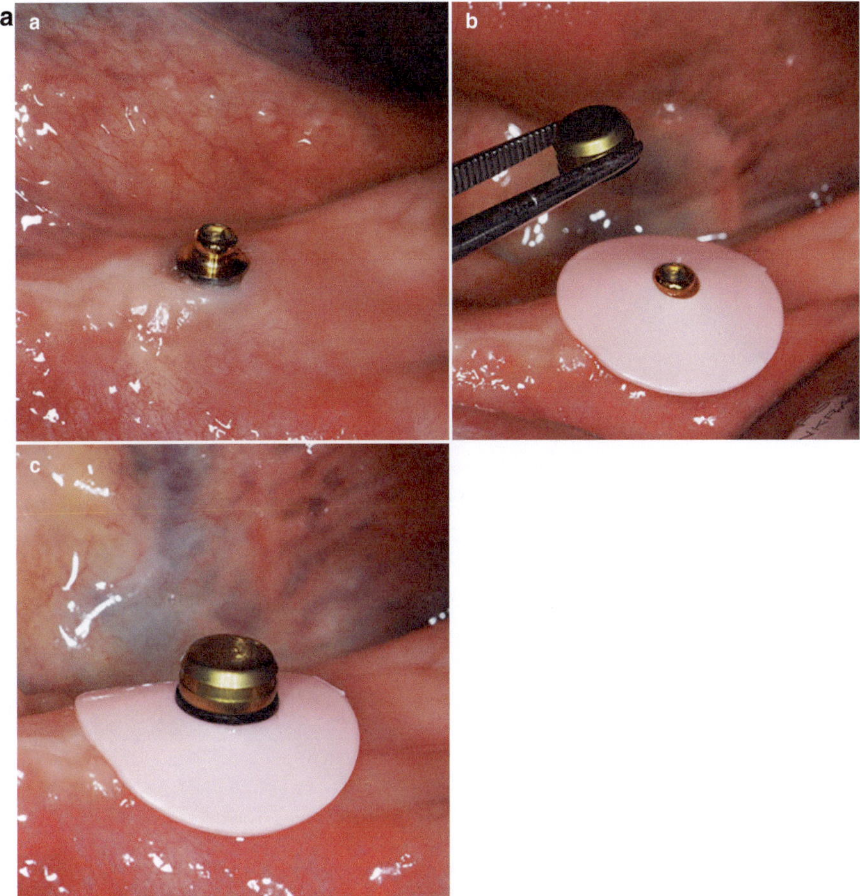

Picture 3.23 (**a**) Chairside procedure for Smartbox positioning: *a* the OT equator attachment in situ; *b* the protective disk placed over the OT equator; and *c* the Smartbox with the black cap placed securely on the attachment (fully engage black cap securely onto the OT equator and verify the positioning of the prosthesis before bonding the stainless steel housing). (**b**) *a* On the prosthesis, the space in the corresponding house is filled with a self-curing resin and denture insert into the patient's mouth. Once the resin has cured, the protective disk is removed; *b* the excess resin is removed carefully and polished for passive connection; *c* the Smartbox is removed with a cap extractor tool and verify that the positions of the attachments are correct; and *d* the cap insertion tool places the OT Equator female caps for desired retention

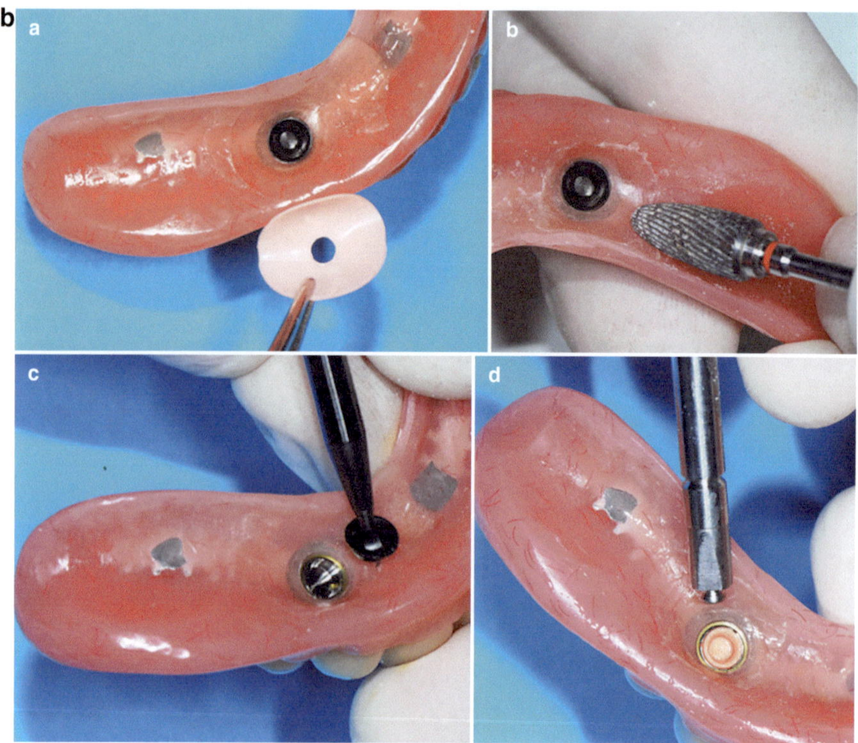

Picture 3.23 (continued)

Equator Profile sphere. The denture will be retained in the same manner; however, the connection will be made more rigid. Only the attachment's dimensions will be altered. The Titan cap is an elastic nylon cap with an internal titanium ring that has an oblique cut around its circumference. It can pass through the sphere without causing any friction, leaving the perimeter smooth for an extended period. In this cap system, after adjustment, the titanium ring maintains constant compression and retention over time, despite nylon wear, because it is encased between the titanium and the housing (Fig. 3.52a–d).

3.3.12.3   OT Equator Castable Attachment with Metal Coping (Indirect Technique for Overdenture)

Following tooth preparation and root canal impression, a castable plastic post and a stone model are obtained. Then, separating material was brushed onto the stone model's areas that had been prepared to receive castable posts. The castable post is installed, and the edges are finished with resin. The resin is cured, and the root of the post is cut to the required length. Using a surveyor, the OT equator is placed on the occlusal surface, and the waxing technique is continued. It is also essential to center the attachment relative to the post's long axis. When the finishing-controlled OT equator reaches its final position, the cast pole and the OT equator reach their final position. For optimal results, cast an alloy with a Vickers hardness of at least 220 (Picture 3.22b, c). After a controlled model and fit, the tooth is cemented with glass ionomer or another cement attachment or coping assembly. The impression cap is placed on the OT equator attachment for the final impression. After taking the final impression with PVS impression materials for metal framework fabrication, impression analogs were inserted into the impression copings, and the model was then poured (Picture 3.22d).

3.3.12.4   Building Up the Framework Directly on Master Cast

On the plaster model, a stainless steel housing with a black processing cap was placed. The model was then coated with a thin layer of wax, all undercuts were filled with wax, and the connectors were attached. The components are then joined with castable resin, and the sprues are added to the framework and removed from the model. After a thorough examination of the framework's invested and cast alloy selection (Picture 3.22e), the stainless-steel housing must be retained.

Later, the casted framework with base metal alloys validated the position of the model and governed the composite resin materials used to bond the stainless-steel housing to the framework.

After the centric relation and vertical dimension of occlusion are provided and the teeth are arranged, the denture is completed on the metal frame. Following processing, selected retentive caps are substituted for black caps (Fig. 3.22f).

3.3.12.5   Direct Placement of the Caps in the Clinic (For Implants)

After the attachment assembly for the cast cement coping was installed, the protective disk was placed over the OT equator. The housing and cap of stainless steel were then screwed onto the attachment. For accurate placement of the cap, the interior of the denture should be reshaped using a metal bur. The positioning of the denture should then be confirmed prior to bonding the housing made of stainless steel. This relief area was then filled with self-curing resin, and the denture was placed in the patient's mouth. After the resin has hardened, the denture is removed from the mouth and the protective disk is eliminated. The denture is meticulously trimmed of excess resin, and a black processing cap is removed. Then, using a cap insertion tool, OT Equator female caps for the desired retention were inserted into the housing (Picture 3.23a, b).

3.3.12.6　Direct Placement of Denture Crowns in the Clinic (For Root Coping and Attachment Assembly)

The protective disk is placed on top of the metal-cast spheres. The housing and cap of stainless steel were then screwed onto the attachment. For accurate placement of the cap, the interior of the denture should be reshaped using a metal bur. Remove the disc and trim the excess material around the housing once the resin has hardened. Completed prosthesis is delivered to the patient.

3.3.13　Attachment of Pivots for Direct Placement

The pivot Flex line of titanium posts (RHEIN 83) was designed as a cost-effective alternative for "in-root" supported overdentures (Fig. 3.53a–h).

There are three types of pivot attachments used for direct placement on roots (Fig. 3.53, Pictures 3.24, 3.25, 3.26, 3.27, and 3.28).

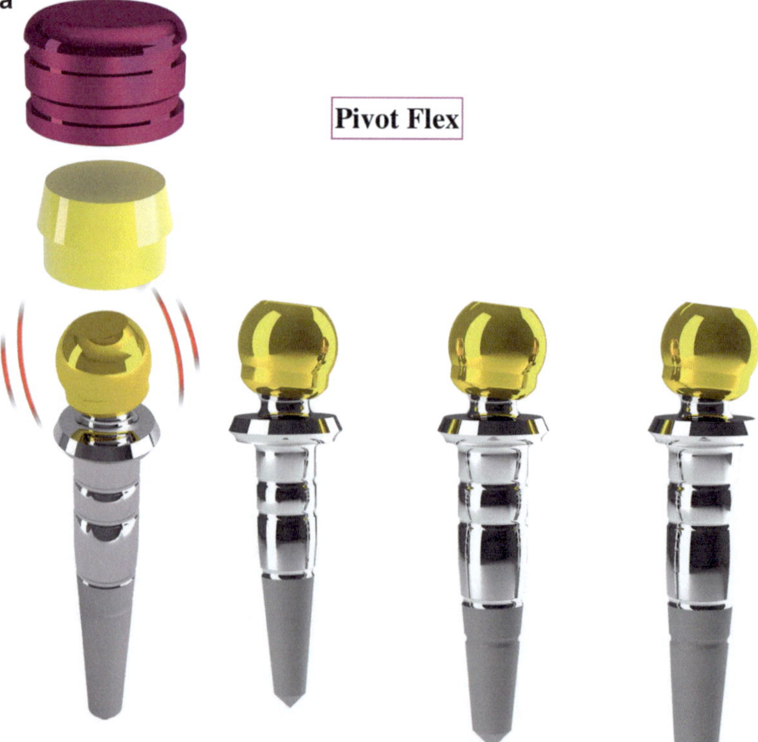

Fig. 3.53 (**a**) The Pivot Flex. (**b**) The Pivot block. (**c**) The OT Equator Pivot. (**d, e**) The *OT Equator Smartbox* housing; it's possible to correct divergency up to 50°. (**f**) Notches were drilled on the post surface for a permanent solution. (**g**) Directional cap with a different angle. (**h**) The Pivot OT Equator correct divergency up to 50°

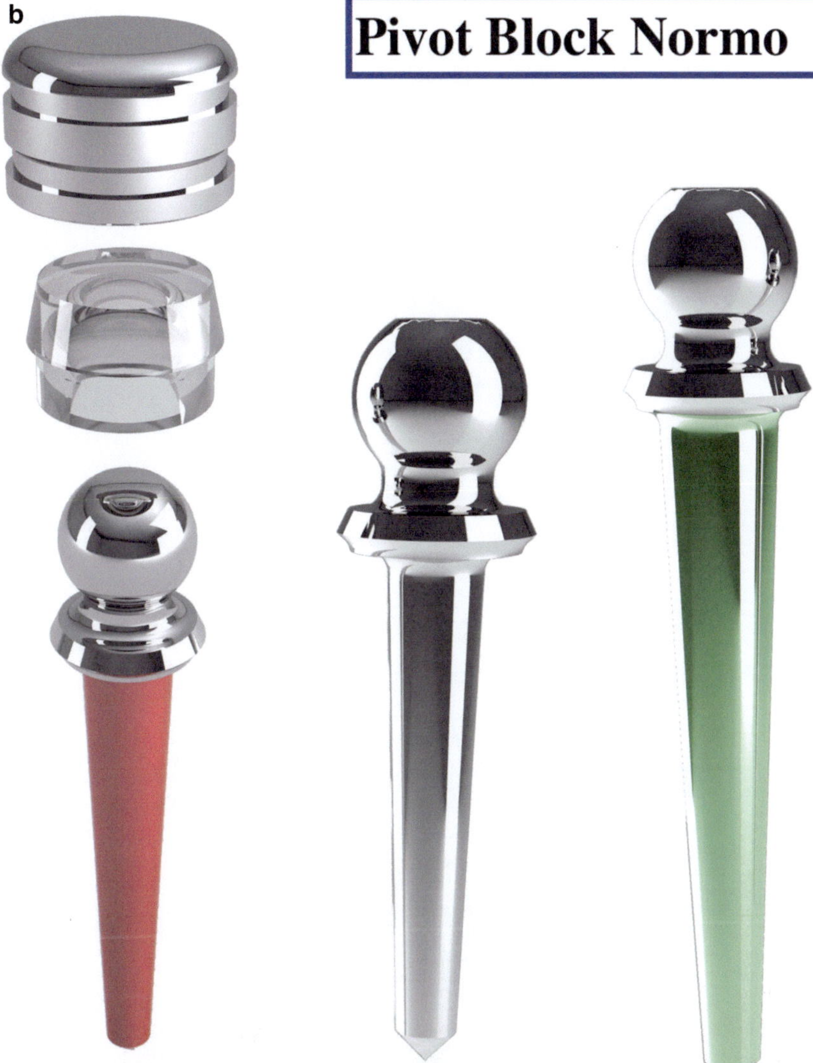

Fig. 3.53   (continued)

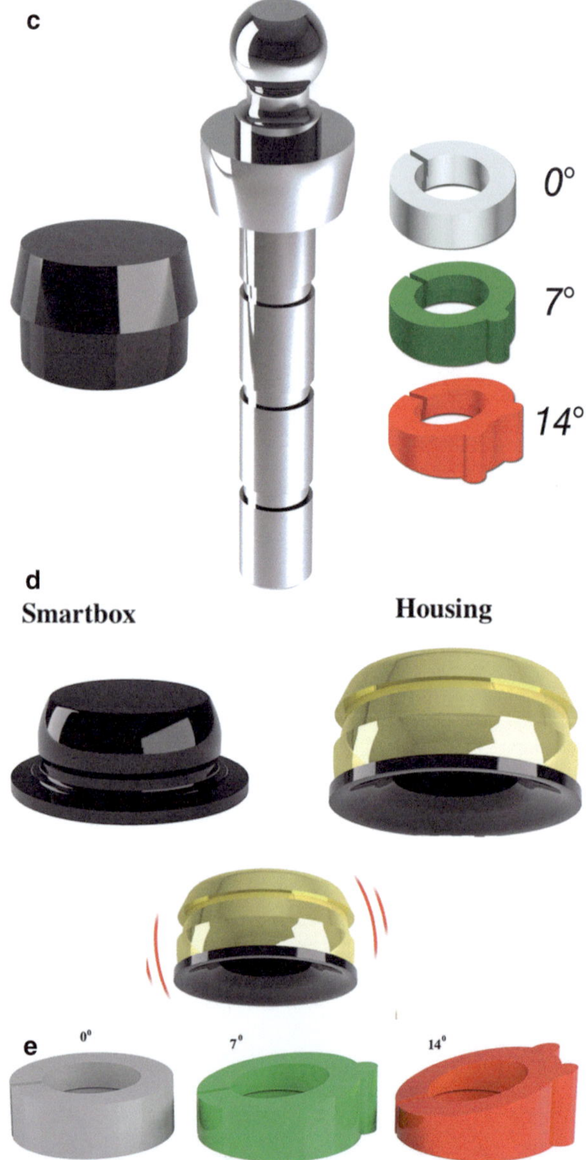

Fig. 3.53 (continued)

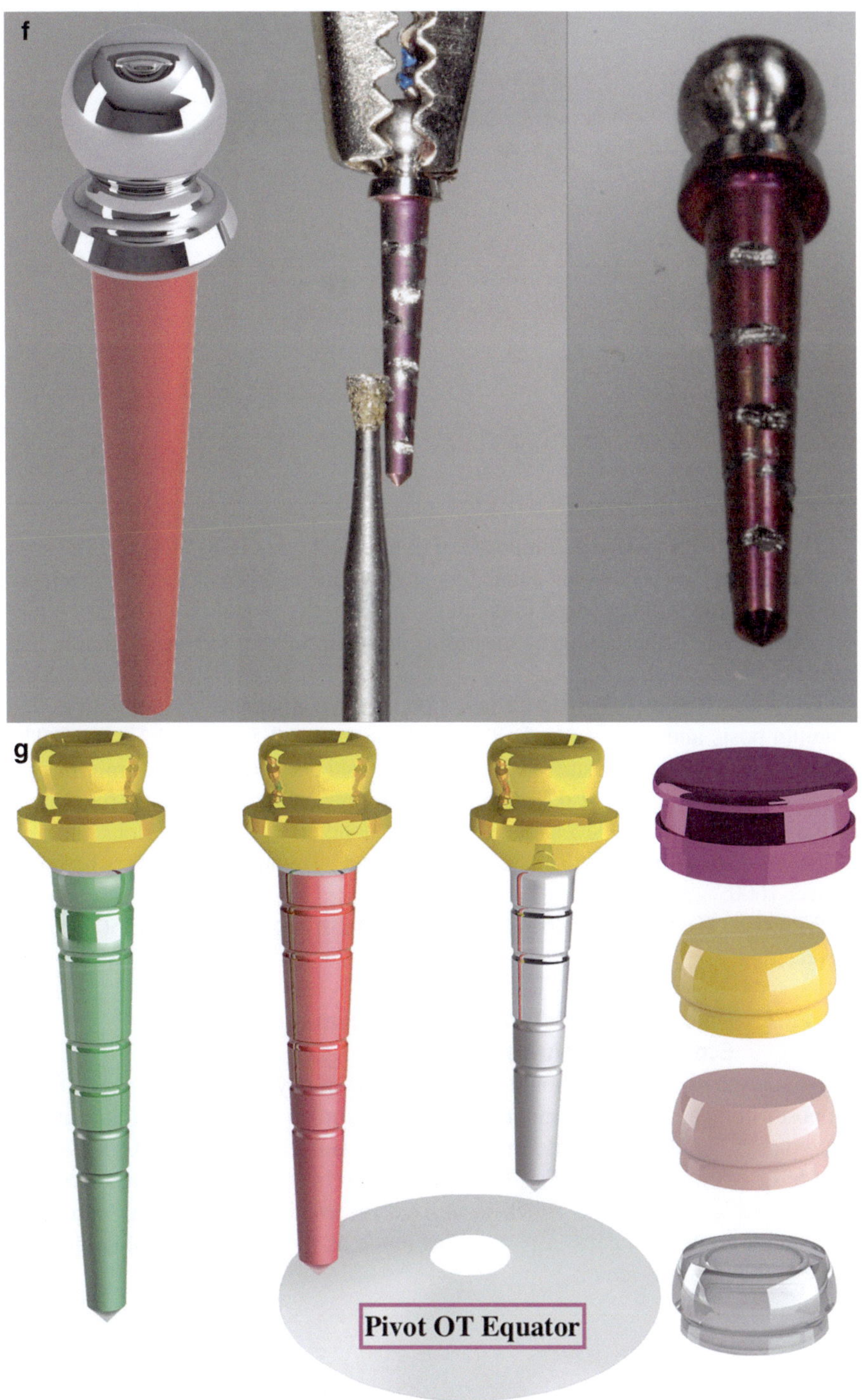

Fig. 3.53 (continued)

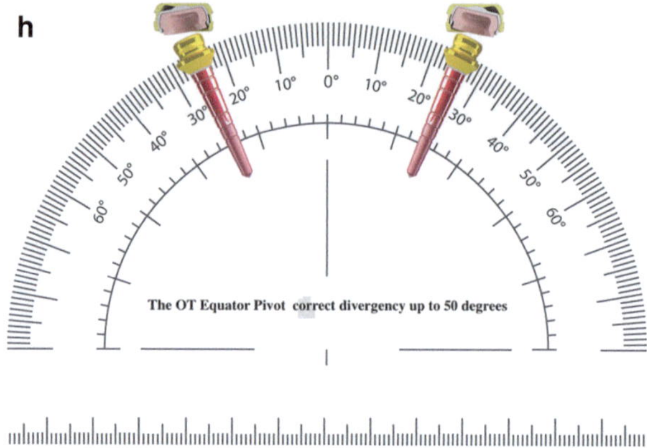

Fig. 3.53 (continued)

The Pivot Flex sphere is composed of titanium and tin (1600 Vickers). The self-aligning pivot Flex post with a 2 mm diameter rotating ball is indicated for divergent roots. When the posts are used in conjunction with directional rings to align retentive caps prior to the curing of the resin, insertion of the denture is simple and painless.

The Pivot Block (PB) sphere is a temporary or permanent solution with milled titanium posts and a stationary ball (with diameters of 2.5 mm and 1.8 mm). The elastic caps of Rhein83 ensure optimal retention and performance while minimizing wear. There are five tiers of retentive caps, including extra-resilient caps for vulnerable root situations. The levels of retention are denoted by caps of various hues.

The OT **Equator Pivot** is made of Titanium and Tin and has a Vickers hardness of over 1600.

With the OT *Equator Smart Box* housing, the divergence of up to 50° can be corrected.

3.3.13.1 Pivot Block: For Temporary or Permanent Economical Solutions

As a temporary fix, the PB should be cemented with oxyphosphate cement. Due to the post's conical shape and smooth surface, it is simple to remove. Before cementing, notches should be cut into the post and the surface should be roughened for long-term solutions (Fig. 3.25). There are five levels of different colored retentive caps available. A Flex and Block is utilized on titanium posts for aligning and attaching the retention caps in parallel (as much as possible) on a mobile denture while in the patient's mouth.

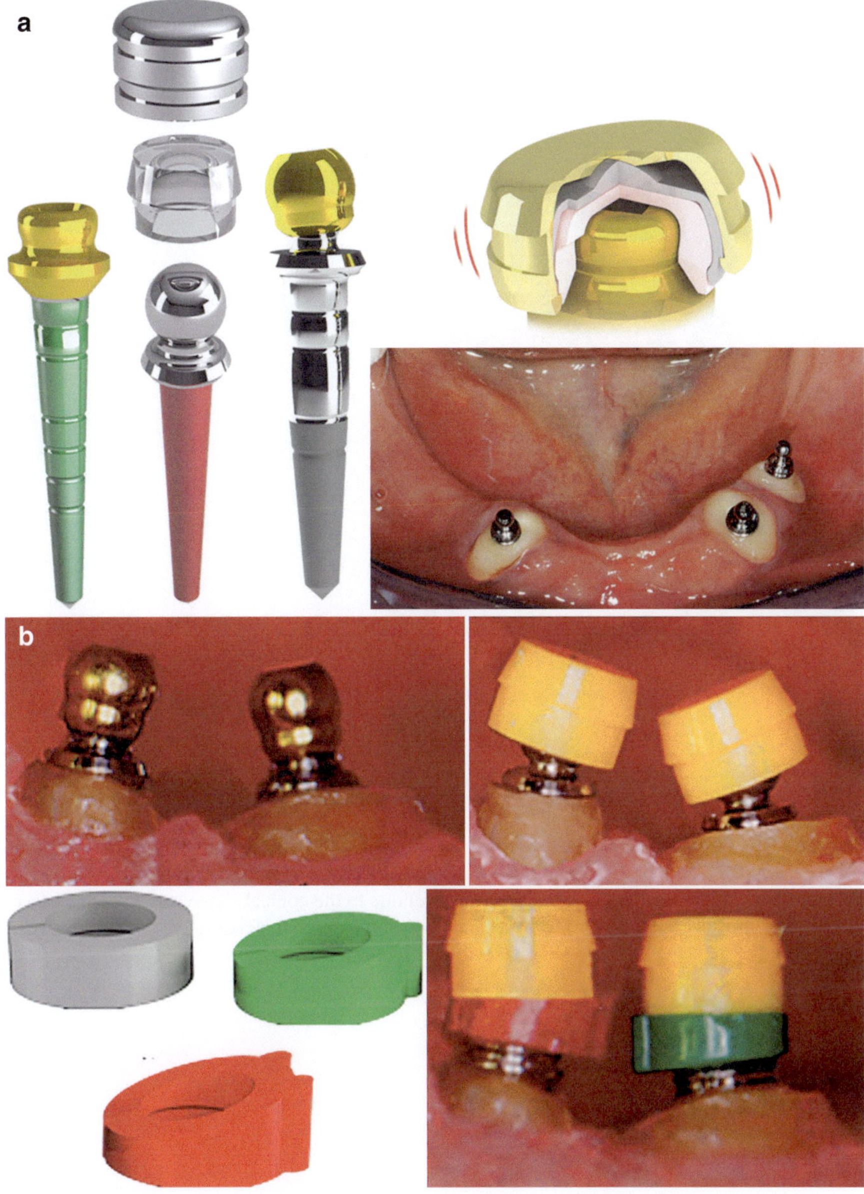

Picture 3.24 (**a**, **b**) The Pivot flex application: (**a**) the Pivot Flex posts placed in divergent roots and (**b**) nylon caps placed without directional roots. In these positions, the caps are not supported in the same horizontal plane. When Nylon caps are placed with directional rings. Caps are now supported in the same horizontal plane

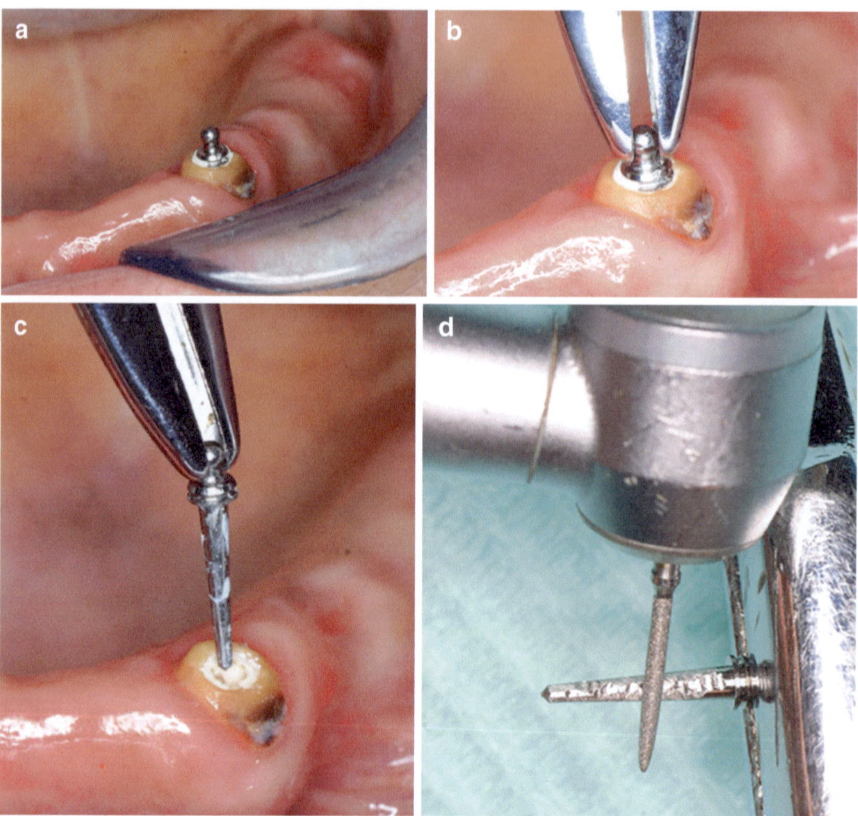

Picture 3.25 (**a–d**) The application of Pivot Block: (**a**) the Pivot Block cemented with polyphosphate cement for a temporary solution; (**b**) to remove the post from the root, grasp the sphere with the pliers and rotate carefully in both directions; (**c**) due to the conical shape and smooth surface, the post is removed easily; and (**d**) for permanent solutions, create notches in the post and roughen the surface before cementation

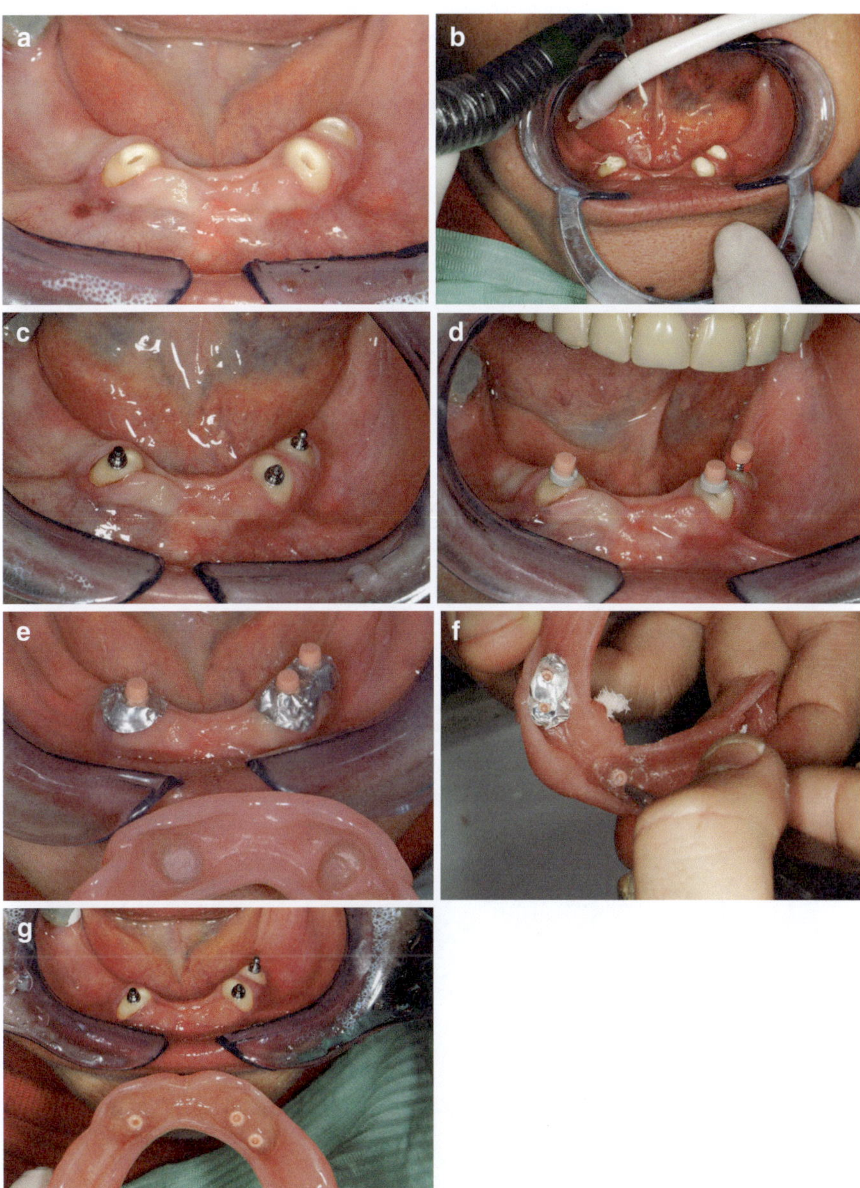

Picture 3.26 (a–e) Pivot Block used for permanent cost-effective solutions: (**a**) the roots were prepared by the mucosal level and adjusted the radicular cavity by using a Mooser Bur with the proper dimensions; (**b**) the radicular cavities filled up with proper composite cement than the spherical titanium pivots insert to the root cavities; (**c**) cemented micro block pivot in position, retentive notches were applied to support the permanents fixation; (**d**) the directional rings are placed in position between the roots and retentive caps; (**d**) The directional rings are placed in position between the roots and retentive caps, (**e**) The protective disk is placed between the directional rings and the retentive caps. (**f**) The self-curing resin was placed in the hole for the cap and then placed in the prosthesis in the patient's mouth. vhen the resin will be hard enough remove the protective disk and clean up any excess resin (**g**) Finished Denture

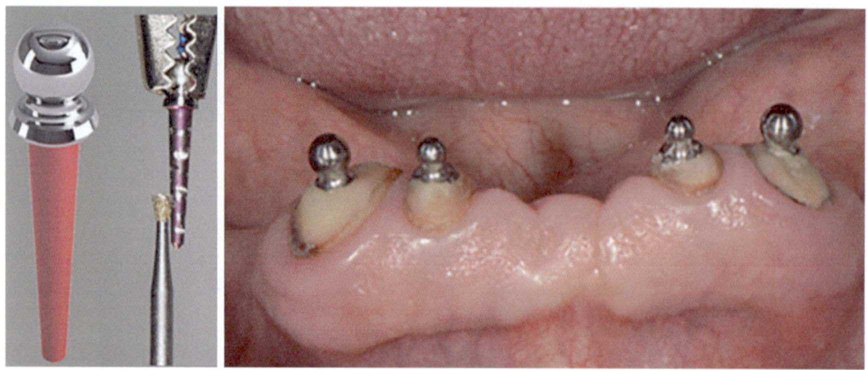

Picture 3.27 The cases with Pivot Block used for permanent cost-effective solutions

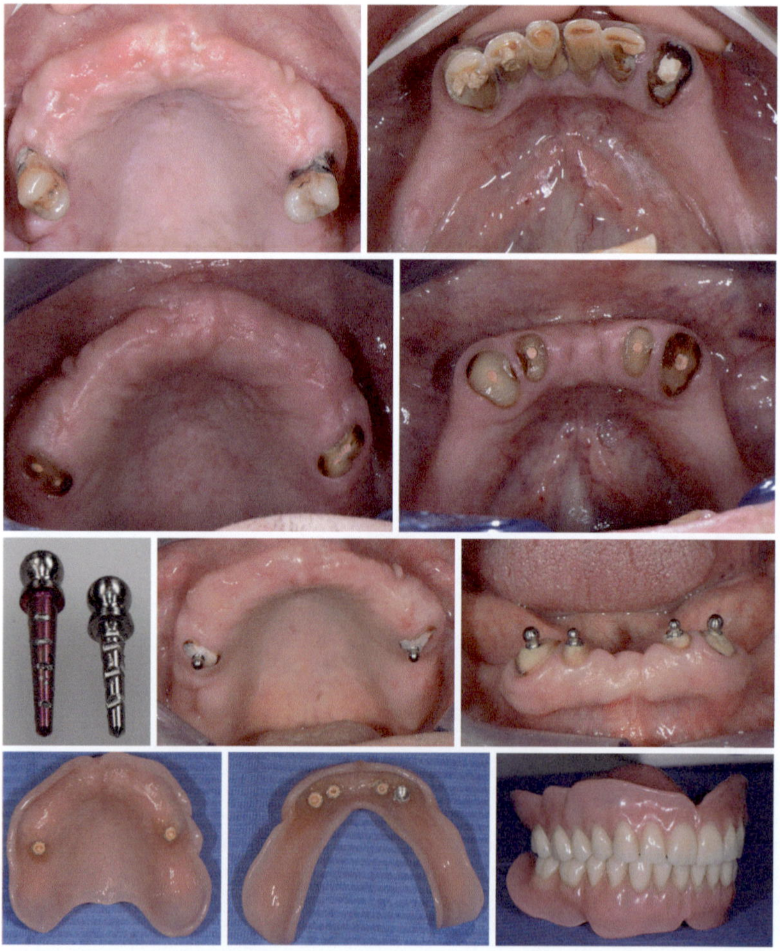

Picture 3.28 The cases with Pivot Block used for permanent cost-effective solutions

3.3.13.2 Permanent Economical Solutions

The PB should be utilized after taking impressions and determining a more comfortable vertical size for the patient. Using a properly sized Mooser bur, I adjusted the radicular cavity after preparing the root to the mucosal level. After filling the root canal cavities with the proper composite cement, spherical titanium pivots were inserted. On the conical surface of the PB, retention notches should be recommended for cementing the PB. The PB is then inserted into the root canal to increase retention in the canal after cementation, and the denture is completed in the laboratory using conventional techniques involving traditional steps. PB attachments were utilized to regain the correct vertical dimension and the lost maxillary relationships by taking advantage of the root retention (Pictures 3.26, 3.27, and 3.28).

At the time of denture delivery, all preceding steps are reviewed, and any necessary adjustments are made. For the placement of the denture's female portion, the directional rings are positioned between the roots and retentive caps, and the protective disks are inserted between the directional rings and the retentive caps. The self-curing resin was used to fill the denture and prepare it for the placement cap before it was placed in the patient's mouth. When the resin has hardened sufficiently, remove the protective disk and remove excess resin. The restoration was then completed and polished (Fig. 3.26). Pictures 3.27 and 3.28 illustrate the direct attachment placement with PB.

3.3.13.3 Directional Rings: For Fixed and Rotating Spheres

When the attachment is placed directly in the divergent root in order to correct the divergence, directional rings with angles of 0°, 7°, and 14° are utilized. After placing the pivot flex post on divergent root directional rings placed at the desired angle on the post, nylon caps are inserted on the directional rings (Fig. 3.53e).

When nylon caps are affixed to posts without directional rings, they are not supported in the same horizontal plane. If the nylon caps are attached to the post by means of directional rings, they can be supported in the same horizontal plane (Picture 3.24b).

3.3.14 Flexi-Post Direct System

Flexi-Post and Flexi-Flange have achieved clinical success for many years (EDS Company). Through the incorporation of the patented split shank, insertion stresses are absorbed by the post (rather than the root) during placement. Flexi-Post consistently offers maximum retention with minimal stress (Fig. 3.54).

The head of the Flexi-Post is highly compatible with Ti-Core and other composites, glass ionomers, and amalgam. The vertical and horizontal grooves prevent the core material from rotating.

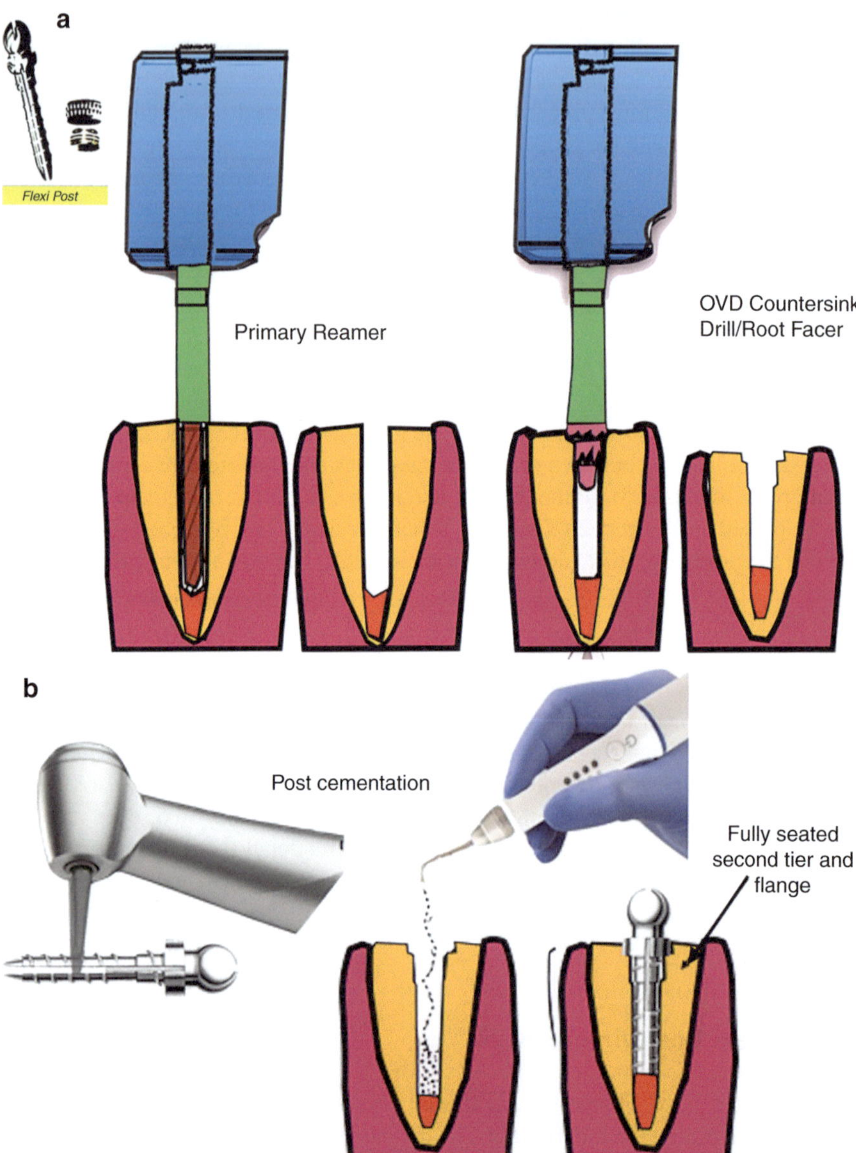

Fig. 3.54 (**a–c**) Flexipost placement with direct (non-coping) technique

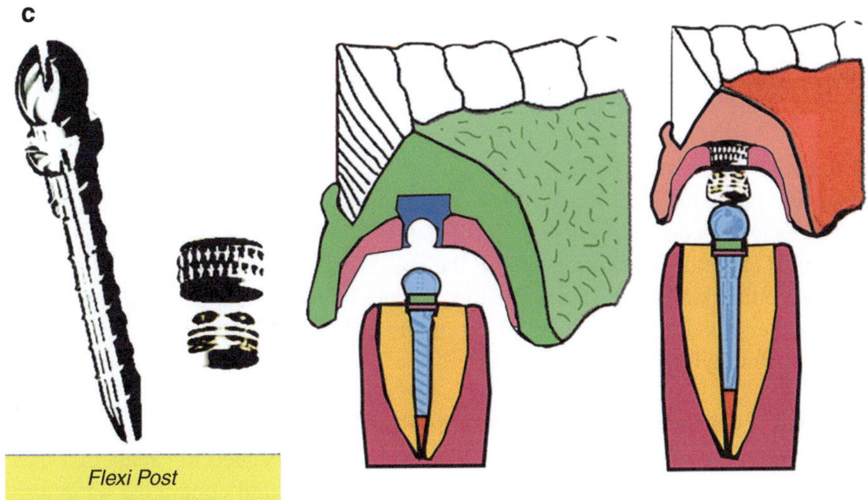

Fig. 3.54 (continued)

3.3.14.1 The Flexi-Post Access Post Overdenture of EDS

Access Post is the most advantageous passive overdenture position offered by EDS. The patent-protected design of the thick-walled, hollow tube and the undercuts of the head and shank provide strength, retention, and stability, as well as the assurance of repeatability.

The attachment can be placed without lab assistance, allowing for the chairside fabrication of a simple, inexpensive overdenture.

Based on a patented split-shank post, the ball-and-socket attachment provides all the advantages of the Flexi-Post for maximum retention of full and partial dentures. The system is compatible with the patented EZ-Change keeper and cap inserts system, enabling "quick and easy" replacement of nylon caps. The attachment can be placed without lab assistance, making EZ-Change chairside overdentures simple and affordable. When worn, the cap insert can be quickly removed from the permanent metal keeper and replaced in mere seconds. Countersinking the post into the tooth prevents the high apical stress typical of other passive posts under function.

3.3.14.2 Direct/Non-coping Technique

After using the primary reamer, the countersink drill is utilized to simultaneously cut two preparations. It prepares the seat for the second tier and the location for the post's flange. The drill's smooth extension is merely a guide to facilitate parallelism between the primary post-hole, second tier, and flange. The post must always be filled with the maximum capacity. Deepen the countersink or root-facing surface sufficiently to create a complete 360° preparation within the root to ensure that the hole is completely seated. There is no risk associated with over-countersinking the post. If, on the other hand, the dentist does not completely seat the post, the retention and stability of EDS's Access Post Overdenture are compromised, increasing the tendency to the post loosening or cracking under function. To achieve complete seating in post-hole preparations, it is necessary to reduce the length of the post's shank. The dentist must remove sufficient apical post length to permit complete seating of the second tier and flange of the post.

3.3.14.3 Post Insertion

As a test, insert the EDS Access Post Overdenture post. The flange and second tier must always be completely seated. If the flange is not seated within the preparation, the apical end must be shortened until the post is completely seated.

The countersinking drill lacks a stop. If there is insufficient occlusal space, you can countersink deeper into the root to provide additional clearance for the overdenture post and nylon cap.

3.3.14.4 Cementing the EDS Access Post Overdenture

- The use of composite cement should only be recommended in canals that have been etched or grooved and in which all traces of eugenol-containing temporary cement or root canal paste have been eliminated.
- Because of its fragility, glass ionomer cement shouldn't be used.

The second tier and flange are completely seated in the preparation and cement; remove the post and cement it with the clinicians' preferred cement. Extra care must be taken to ensure that the flange is fully seated. Prior to concluding the procedure, the excess cement must be removed (Fig. 3.54a–c and 3.55).

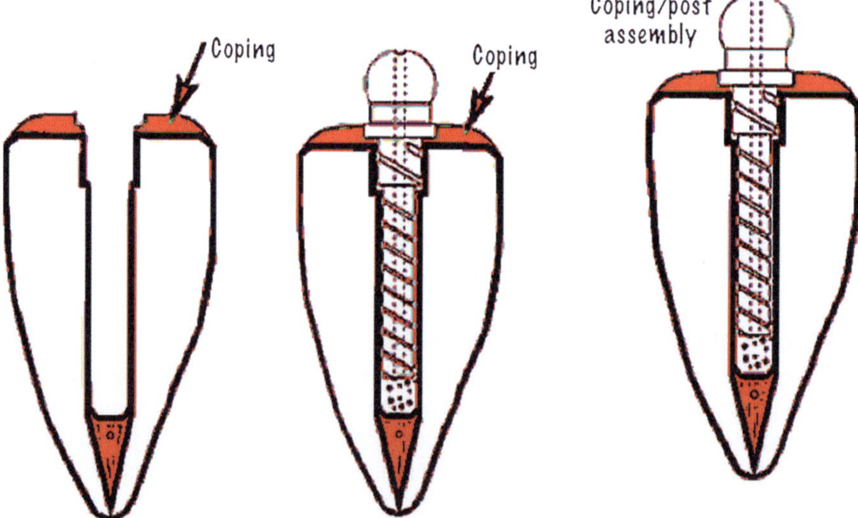

Fig. 3.55 Flexipost placement with coping

3.3.14.5   Indirect/Coping Strategy

In the coronal post-hole preparation, the second drill is used after the primary reamer to create the second-tier preparation. The drill's smooth extension is merely a guide to facilitate parallelism between the primary post space and the second phase.

In order to place the coping using the indirect coping technique, 0.25 mm of space is required between the post's flange and the coronal tooth structure. To create a 0.25 mm space, the post must be completely seated and, if necessary, its apex must be shortened. When full seating is complete, remove the post and install the *corresponding-sized brass transfer stud* so that there is a 0.25 mm gap between the flange and the coronal tooth structure for placement of the coping. After seating the brass transfer stud of the corresponding size, take an impression of the brass transfer stud. Remove the impression from the root canal using the transfer stud. Send the impression and the transfer stud made of brass to the laboratory. In the lab, the coping is then waxed and cast. For cementing the EDS Access Post Overdenture, either etched or grooved root canals should be filled with resin cement. Temporary cement or root canal pastes containing eugenol should be removed first. Due to its fragility, glass ionomer cement should be avoided. The coping can then be cemented. Following the installation of the coping, the EDS Access Post Overdenture is cemented in place (while the cement is still wet). When the flange is fully seated within the coping, insertion is complete. Finally, the female cap (or optional EZ-Change attachment) can be placed into the overdenture (Fig. 3.54d).

3.3.14.6   Incorporation of the Attachment Cap

After attaching the overdenture attachment, the dentist has two options:

1. *At the chairside*, the dentist can use a direct one-visit technique (Fig. 3.56a, b).
2. *Alternatively, the laboratory* may attach the attachment cap to the denture (Fig. 3.56c, d).
1. *Chairside Technique*: The attachment cap is placed on the post and scored with a scoring paste using the chairside technique. The denture is then positioned over the ridge and extracted. The marking ensures that the clinicians can remove the acrylic from the denture. Repeat this procedure until the denture fits passively over the crown. The portion of the denture that has been relieved is then filled with cold-cure acrylic, which is placed over the ridge and allowed to set. The rubber band must encompass the height and contour of the post's head. If not, there is a chance that the cold-cured acrylic will harden under the head, making it difficult to remove the denture. The self-curing acrylic is placed in the denture's relieving area. When the acrylic is polymerized, the denture is removed, and the rubber band is lifted off the post and discarded.

The rubber band around the base of the overdenture attachment should not be damaged until after the attachment cap has been incorporated into the denture. If this occurs, the acrylic material may lock into the undercut of the ball, preventing the denture from being removed from the mouth. When seated on the post's ball, the

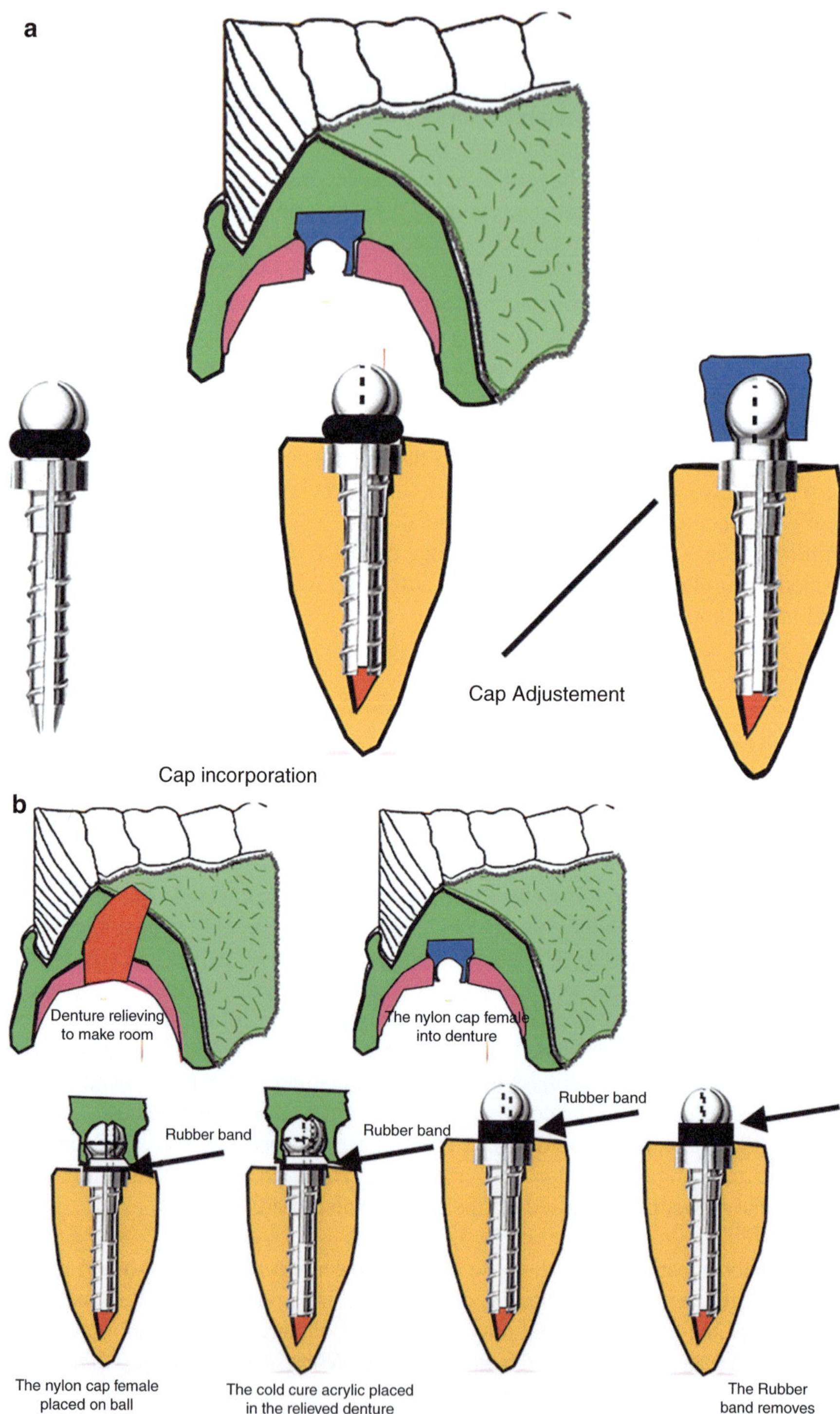

Fig. 3.56 (**a–d**) Incorporation of the attachment cap

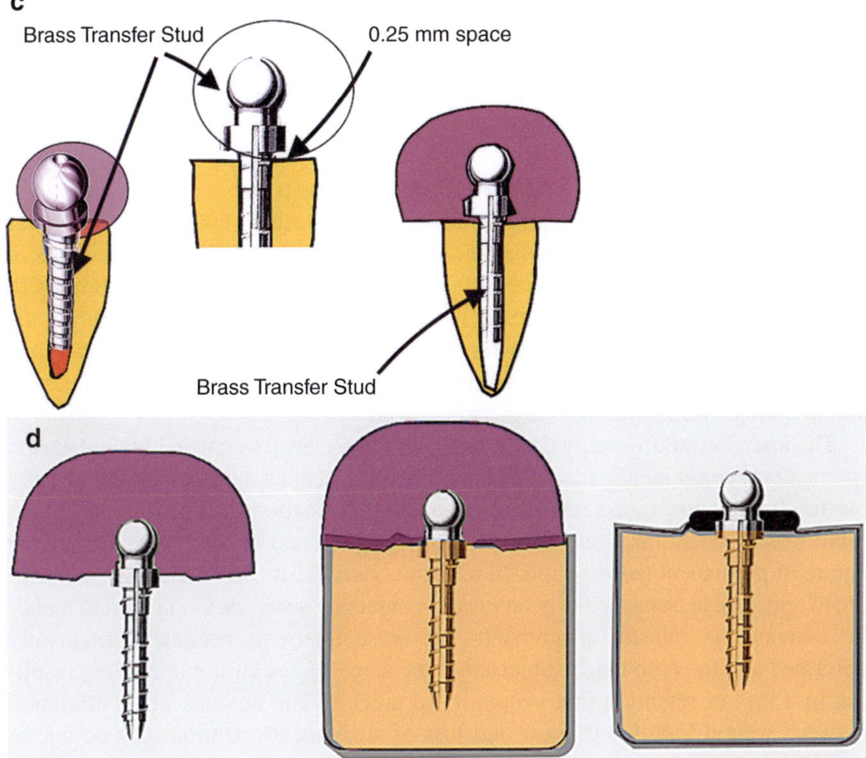

Fig. 3.56 (continued)

attachment cap should always maintain a small distance from the root. If this is not the case, the attachment cap cannot rotate on the ball. A small amount of nylon is removed from the cap's lip, if necessary, to create this space.

3.3.14.7 Laboratory Technique

The rubber band is adhered to by the EDS Access Post Overdenture attachment and then removed by it. Make an impression and send it along with the attachment cap and brass transfer stud to the laboratory for adaptation.

In the laboratory, a stone cast is created by inserting the transfer stud into the impression. The laboratory incorporates polymerized acrylic into the denture cap. The denture is returned to the clinician with the crown already attached.

3.3.15 Sphero Post Direct System

The Sphero Flex Post system is a rotating ball attachment for endodontic posts that corrects up to 15° of misalignment in any plane. This self-paralleling system's benefits include the flexibility (resilience) that protects weak abutments, the biocompatibility of titanium, the simplicity of conventional techniques, and the small size of the sphere (2.5 mm). Additionally, no potential debris can enter the female, which eliminates potential insertion issues. The female can be seated in a denture or cast into a frame. The available lengths for the posts are 6.75 mm, 8.40 mm, and 9.75 mm. The precision 2° reamer guarantees accuracy. This system is also compatible with cast copings (Fig. 3.57).

3.3.15.1 Kit for Concave Sphere Reconstruction

It is widely accepted that attachments will gradually lose their holding power over time. The deterioration of attachment components has been attributed to this loss of retention. Even though the mechanisms of wear are poorly understood, the loss of retention may be attributable to the deformation mechanisms that occur during the insertion and removal of attachment components. Chung et al. correlated a low strain with matrix dislodgment and matrix configuration attachment with a snap action during overdenture insertion and removal.

The insertion strain energy can be separated into elastic (recoverable) and plastic (permanent) components. Ideally, the strain on the contact surfaces should be fully elastic. It is demonstrated that if a permanent deformation occurs, there will be a rapid loss of retention. Loss of retention may be related to the energy-dependent nature of permanent deformation. In addition, viscoelastic creep may also contribute to retention loss, particularly on plastic-contacting surfaces. Compared to metallic components, plastic attachments are more likely to become permanently deformed and to creep when subjected to the same forces during operation, resulting in a loss of retention that occurs more quickly. The absence of a correlation between weight loss due to wear and loss of attachment retention may be due to plastic deformation and creep.

As with most other mechanisms, dental attachments are subject to wear. When stud attachments become worn, new reconstruction kits are utilized to restore them. Rhein83 manufactures spheres for replacing worn ball attachments, restoring and stabilizing the denture in a single visit. Over the worn ball, reconstructive spheres are bonded, restoring the attachment to its original size.

The titanium sphero reconstruction kit is designed to allow the rebuilding of worn spheres in the mouth using concave titanium spheres to achieve long-term retention and stability for the patient. This kit can also be used to increase the diameter of a small sphere in the mouth or to convert an O-ring attachment to a ball attachment. When the ball attachments exhibit excessive wear, concave reconstructive spheres (CRS) are the best long-term restoration option. The CRS restore the worn male to its original diameter of 1.8 mm, 2.2 mm, or 2.5 mm, and is manufactured with a titanium nitride coating and a Vickers hardness rating of over 1600. The chairside procedure for using reconstructive spheres is quick, straightforward, and a cost-effective alternative to replacing the old restorations.

3.3.15.2 Application

The concave sphere is placed within the plastic instrument. It is placed over the deteriorated sphere in the mouth. If the concave sphere does not fit passively, a diamond or carbide cylindrical bur is used to slightly reduce the diameter. When

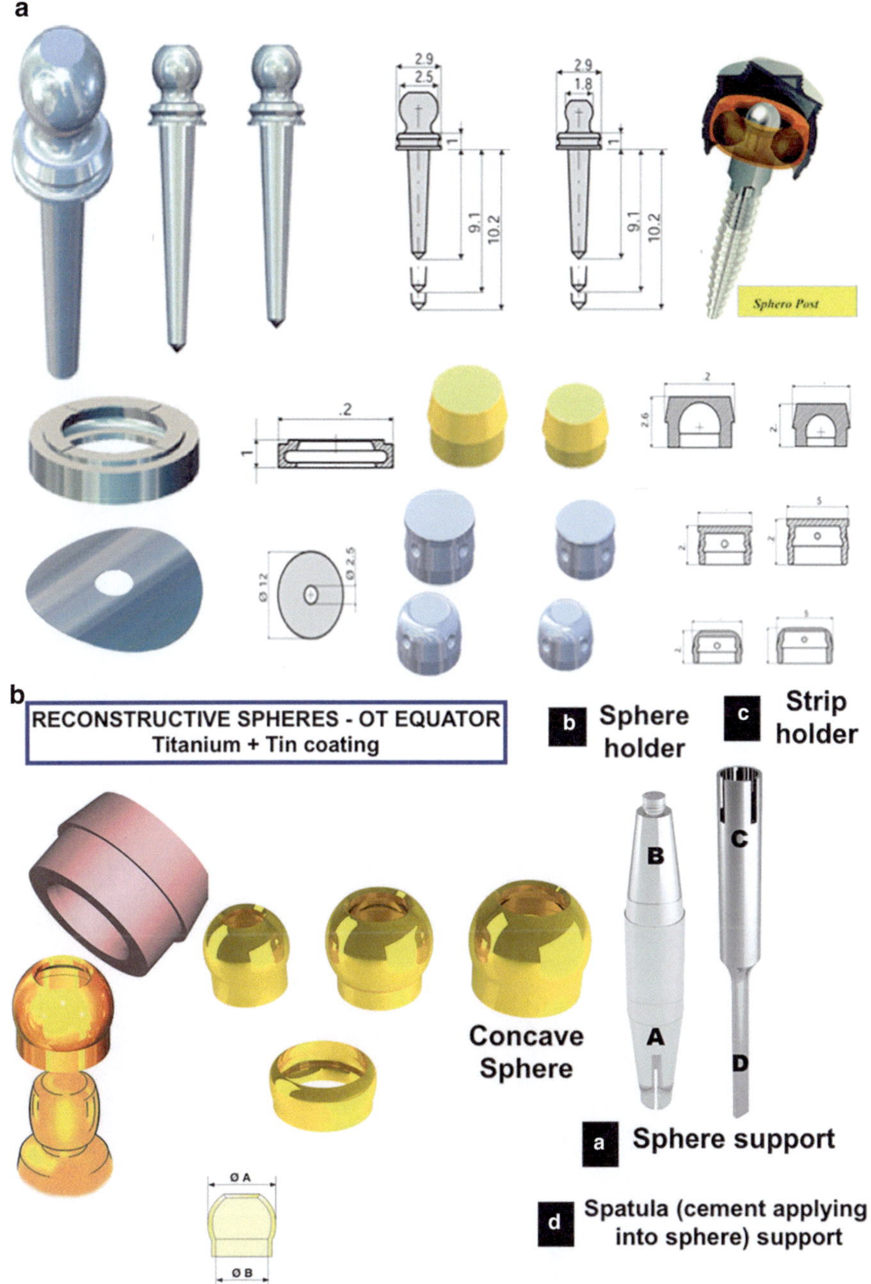

Fig. 3.57 (**a**) The Sphero Flex Post system. (**b**) Concave Sphere reconstruction kit

necessary, the process is repeated and the fit is rechecked. The position of the concave sphere on the worn sphere was evaluated, and the two components were cleaned. The additional surface can be eliminated by using the tool's reverse side. After a diamond strip has been inserted into the notches, the instrument is manually rotated over the sphere. For the "metal to metal" bond, a small amount of self-curing resin is inserted into the sphere. The resin is cured after the concave sphere is positioned over the worn sphere. After the resin has hardened, the excess resin must be removed. The cap can be repositioned if maintenance is required (Fig. 3.58, Picture 3.29).

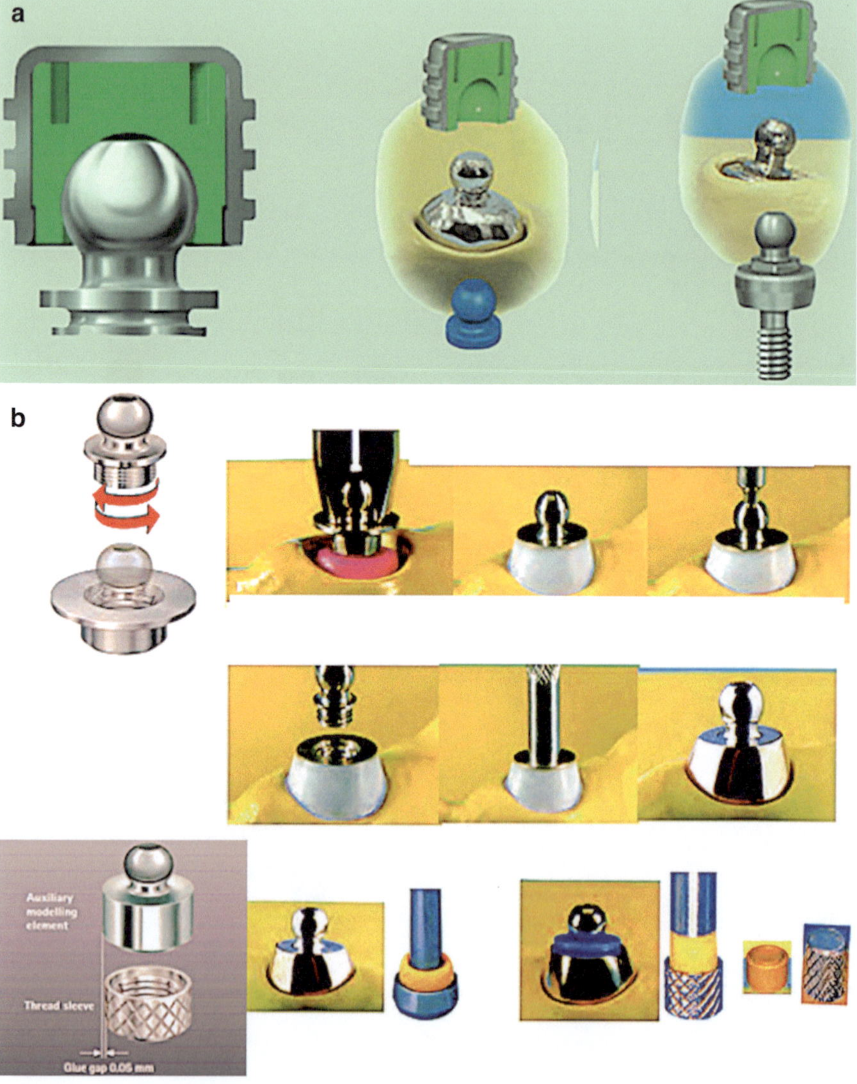

Fig. 3.58 (**a, b**) Vario-Kugel-Snap VKS-OS exchangeable stud

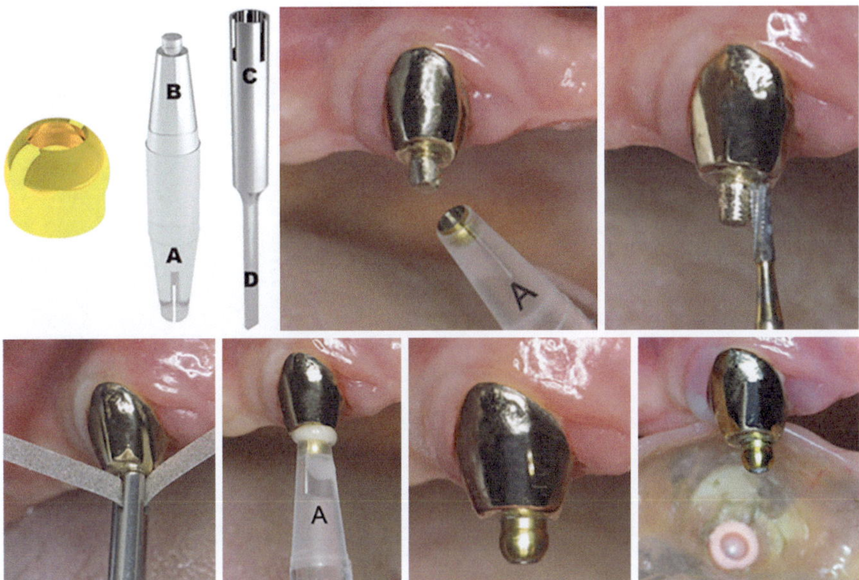

Picture 3.29   The Sphero Flex Post system

3.3.16 Vario-Kugel-Snap VKS-OC Exchangeable Stud (VKS-OC Attachment System)

These attachments are beneficial for cases with restricted diameters. Due to the interchangeable titanium stud, it is safe, accurate, and biocompatible. Using the paralleling mandrel, the stud-head screw is only slightly screwed into the threaded sleeve and held to the waxed root cap. To model the determined insertion path, the attachment matrix is adhered to the wax. The screwdriver was used to remove the stud-head screw from the threaded sleeve by turning it counterclockwise. Before purchasing the model, the stud-head screw must be substituted with a fixation screw. The cast is sandblasted, and the fixing screw is unscrewed. Using titanium polishing paste, the stud head screw is turned in and polished after the root cap has been polished (Fig. 3.58).

3.3.17 Stern ERA Attachment

The Sterngold dental attachment was created for the first time in 1921. They have produced precision attachments longer than any other organization. It produced attachments for removable partial dentures, overdentures, and segmented bridges, making it the most popular American manufacturer of attachments. They created the patent-protected Stern ERA, one of the most popular resilient semi-precision attachments available today. Class IV function occurs universal hinge with vertical

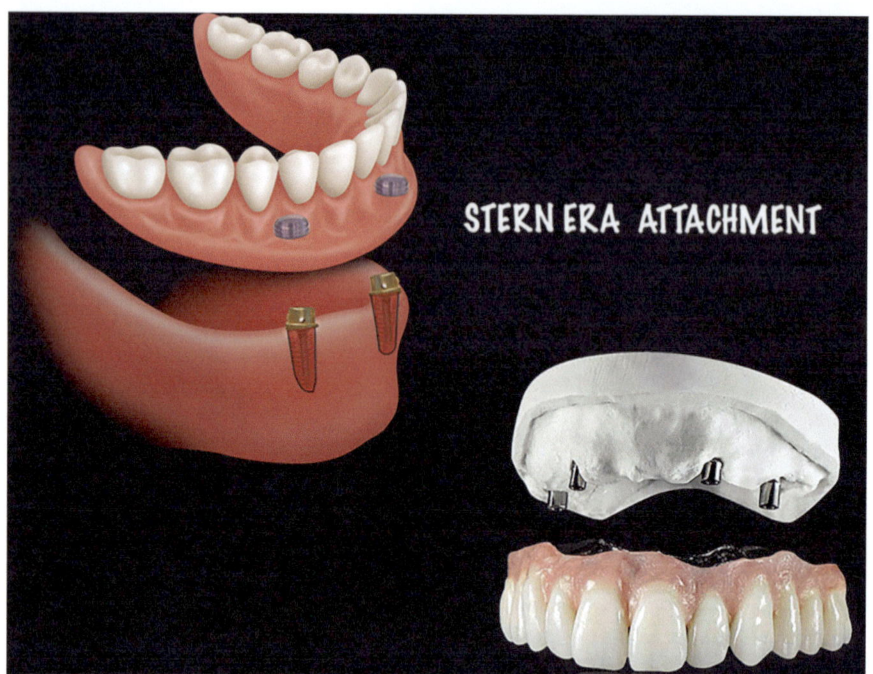

Picture 3.30 Stern-ERA attachment

motion (Picture 3.30; Figs. 3.59, 3.60, 3.61, and 3.62). Because the Stern ERA attachment can be placed at the point of occlusal force application within the root, it has a minimal crown-to-root ratio.

The ERA Female Overdenture Attachment is a plastic pattern that is incorporated into the wax pattern for a post and root-cap coping. It is composed of a hard alloy. The female component has two distinct designs (standard size and mini) that are compatible with the same male component. The Micro ERA attachment is 20% smaller than the standard type (0.5 mm less in length and nearly 1 mm in width) with no reduction in retention or durability. Additionally, it requires only 3.0 mm of vertical space, although more is preferable.

It features a nylon male, a plastic pattern female, or a stainless-steel female with titanium nitride coating, a black fabrication male with an integrated spacer, and six color-coded males for six retention levels (from lightest to strongest: white, orange, blue, gray, yellow, and red). The final males are white and orange. Males that are blue and gray are oversized. The male component features two distinct designs. The standard design has a vertical resilience of 0.4 mm and requires 0.5 mm less vertical distance than the alternative design. The Stern ERA male can be replaced without the use of auto-polymerizing acrylic and can be directly attached to processed denture acrylic or an ERA metal jacket. Additionally, an optional ERA overdenture metal jacket is preloaded with a black fabrication male and holds the attachment male in the denture base.

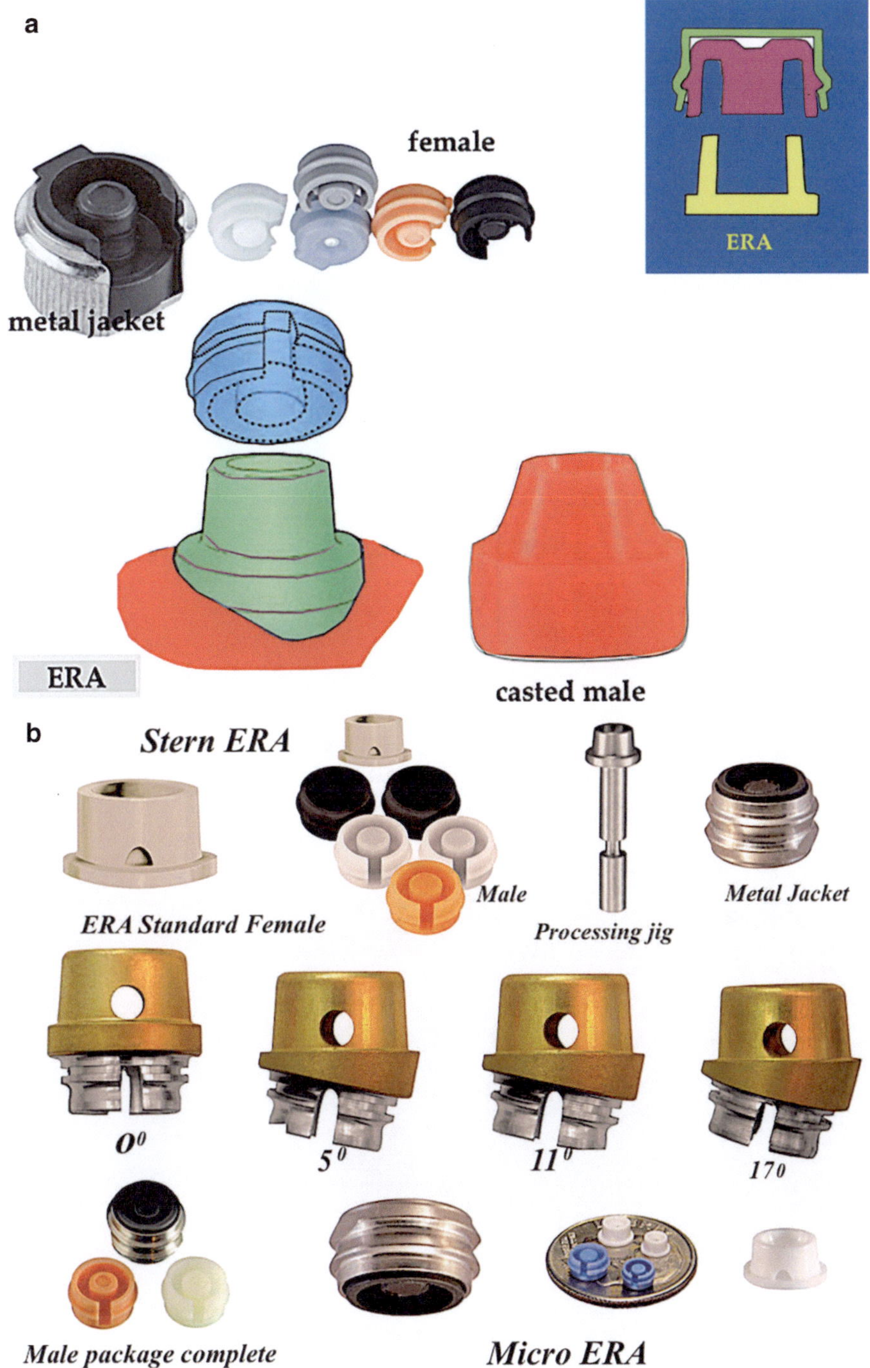

Fig. 3.59 (**a**, **b**) The Stern ERA and micro ERA attachment

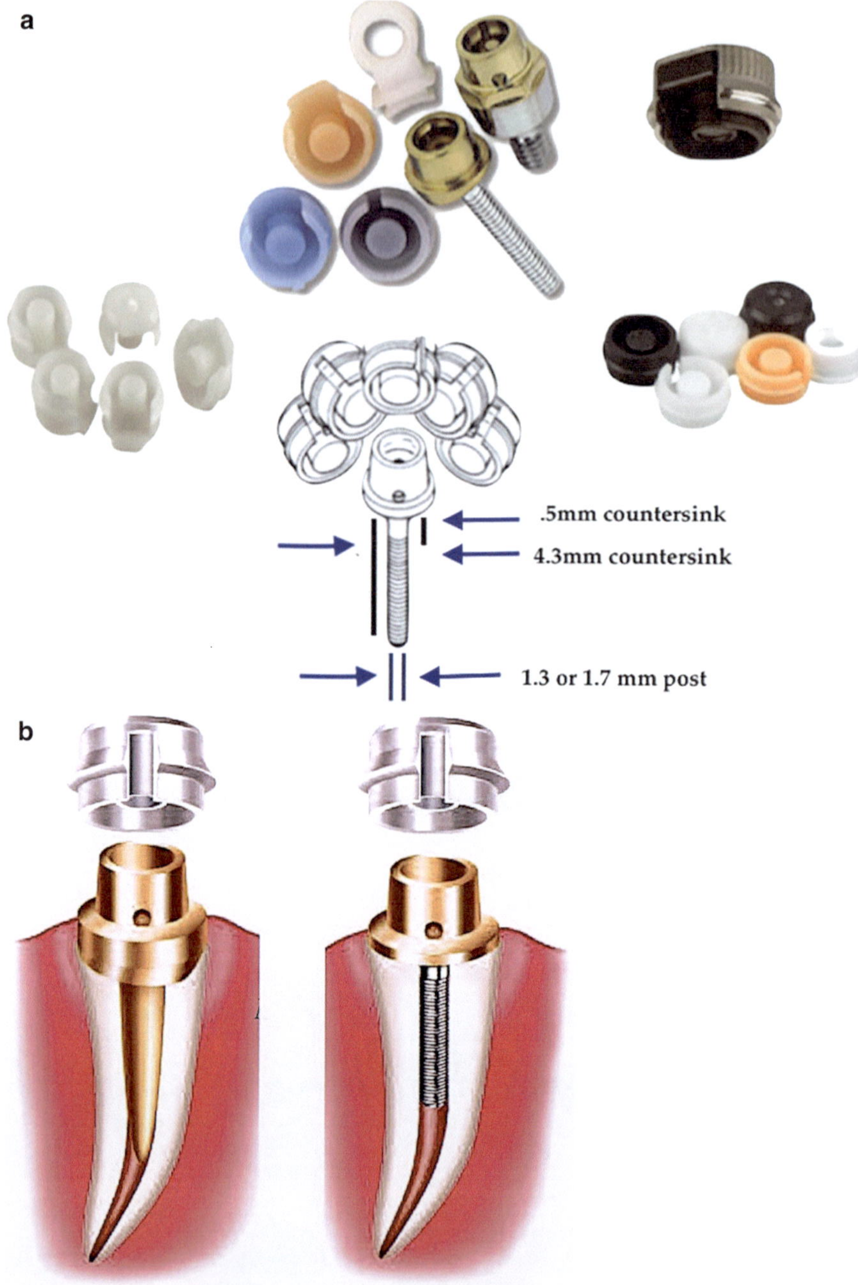

Fig. 3.60 (**a**, **b**) The Stern ERA direct root attachment

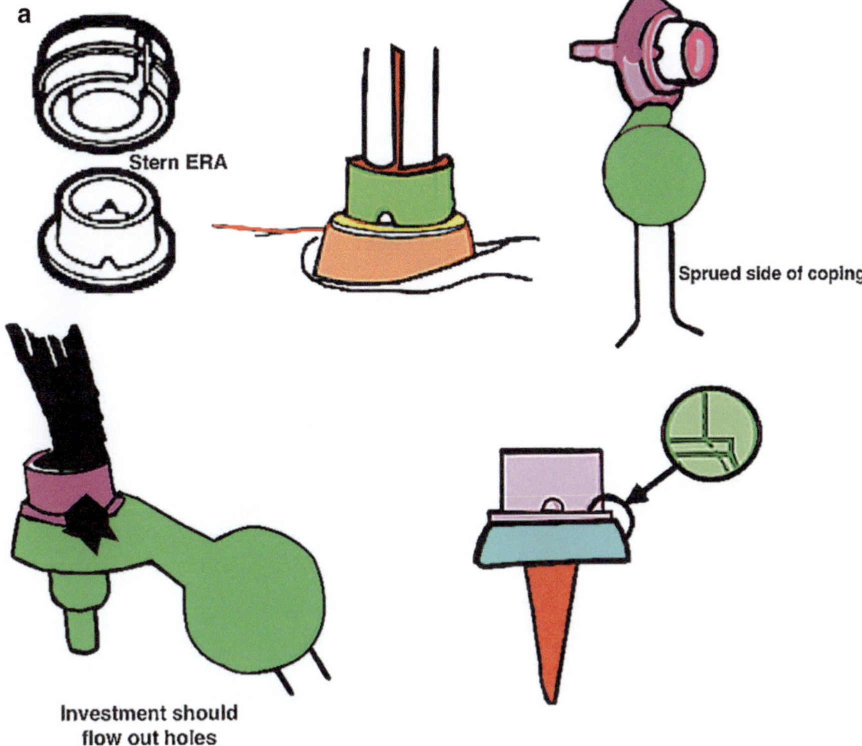

Fig. 3.61 (**a–d**) Steps for cast on ERA attachments

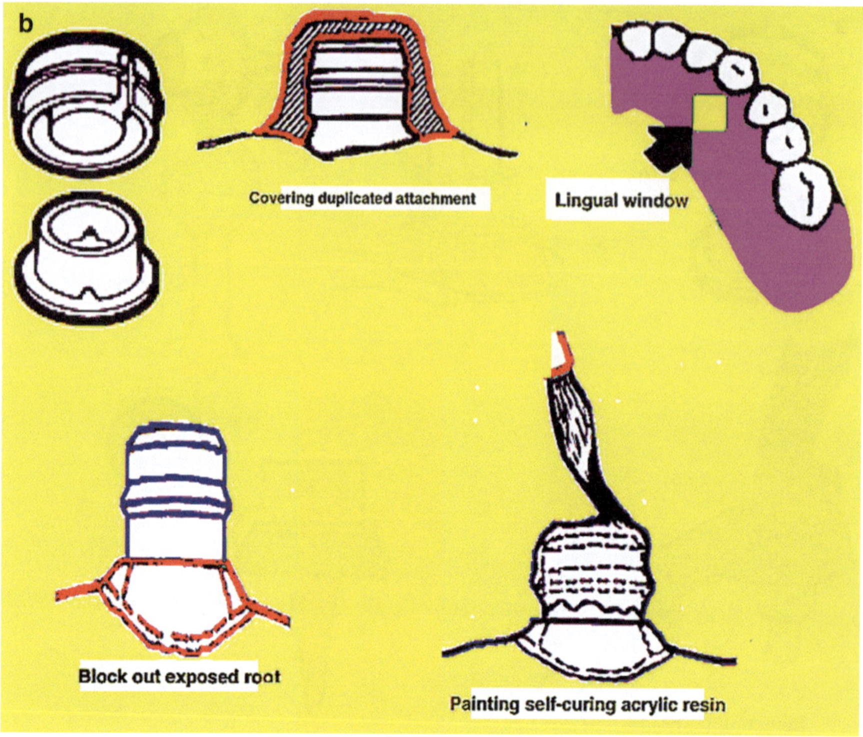

Fig. 3.61 (continued)

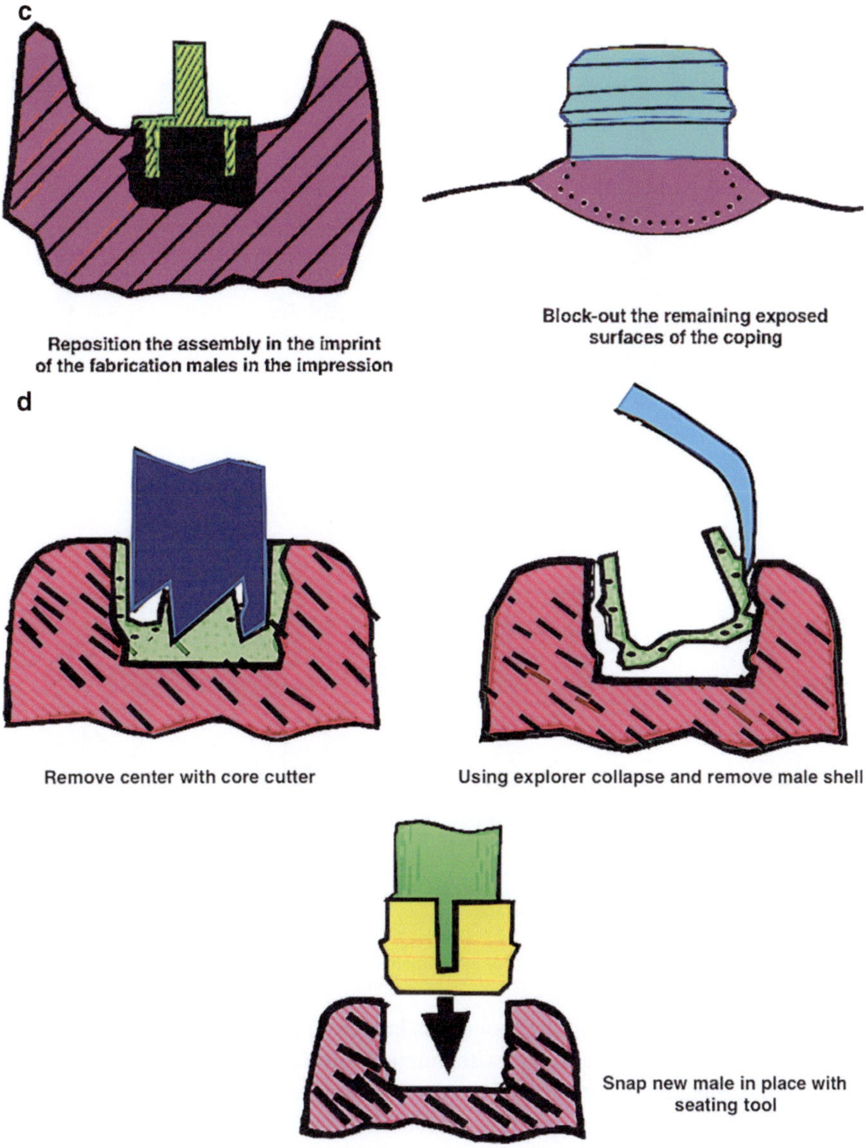

c

**Reposition the assembly in the imprint
of the fabrication males in the impression**

**Block-out the remaining exposed
surfaces of the coping**

d

Remove center with core cutter

Using explorer collapse and remove male shell

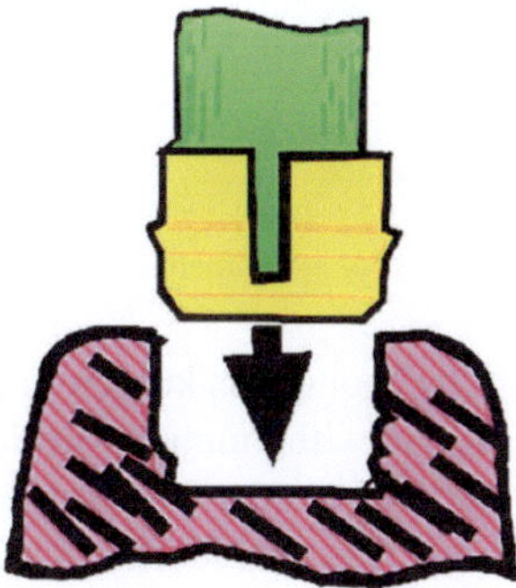

Snap new male in place with
seating tool

Fig. 3.61 (continued)

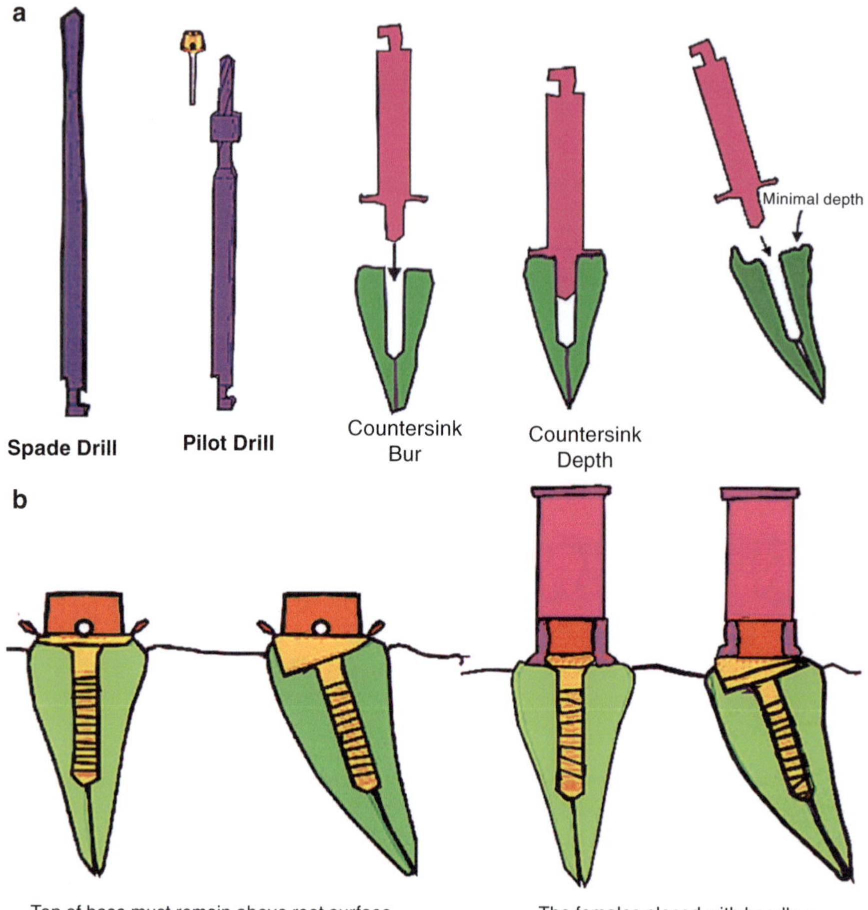

Fig. 3.62 (**a**, **b**) Steps for direct ERA root attachment

The female component of the root cap is known as coping. In comparison to the female component's stainless steel with titanium nitride coating, the mechanism for varying the amount of retention between the various nylon male components becomes increasingly oversized. This procedure increases the surface area, tightens the fit, and enhances retention.

The manufacturer suggests casting plastic components using alloys with a minimum Vickers hardness of 200 and an ultimate tensile strength of at least 85,000 psi. For yellow gold castings, Pegasus ceramic alloy and Sterngold 100 crown and bridge alloy are suitable options.

Additionally, the Stern ERA is placed directly on the endodontically treated root (Fig. 3.60). It includes two different post diameters and four different post angles: 0 (straight), 5, 11, and 17 (3 mm or 1.7 mm, both 9.0 mm long). It applies the least amount of lateral load compared to other attachments, making it preferable when bone loss exceeds 50%. The stainless-steel females are available in two post diameters and four post angles to meet the needs of the majority of patients and are cemented into a root that has been specially prepared to receive them. The attachment functions normally when positioned 7° out of parallel with the insertion path of the case. All ERA direct placement females are titanium nitride coated. The intraradicular connection of the attachment components decreases the root's occlusal stress. The male is polymerized in the denture using acrylic resin, while the female is directly bonded to the root structure (Figs. 3.59 and 3.60).

3.3.17.1 Instructions for Fabrication

The Pattern of Female Plastic
The root-cap copings are constructed from wax. The occlusal surface should be as low and as flat as possible. The female plastic pattern is placed on the mandrel while the female is held against the shoulder of the mandrel, the thumbscrew is tightened to secure the female, and the base of the plastic female is glued to the coping. This surface must remain clean and uncontaminated by the wax. The patterns are sprues for affixing the sprues away from the attachment base to the copings, and the sprues patterns are invested. The capital should flow through the relief openings near the female pattern's base. Then, casting is produced using a hard alloy in accordance with the manufacturer's instructions. Keep in mind, when finishing and polishing the attachment females, that the interior dimension should not require additional refinement.

Notably, the base and coping may be rounded from the external surface of the female ring to the coping's edge. The master model's copings must be seated, and the fabrication males must be snapped into the females. After blocking out the model, a duplicate impression is made. Then, the refractory model is constructed, the framework surrounding the ERA male representations is waxed and cast, and the framework is completed. With this option, the males are snapped into the overdenture framework's custom metal housing (Fig. 3.61).

Positioning of the Males

Throughout the Laboratory
The black fabrication males are snapped into the females on the master model, and both the copings and attachments are wrapped in a sheet of foil or wax. The model is then duplicated for processing, and wax is used to create the denture. Over each abutment, the wax-up will contain recesses. After approval, proceed with normal denture processing. Following the completion of the procedure, the denture and cast copings are delivered.

At Chairside
The parapet is cemented. For each coping, a lingual window is carved into the denture using a round bur. Then, an artificial black male is inserted into each female. After blocking out the remaining surfaces of the copings, the self-curing acrylic is

added and cured; it will not come into contact with the copings. This small space between the copings and acrylic will allow the ERA attachments to function with resilience. The overdenture is seated to avoid contact with the copings, black fabrication males, and the ERA metal jacket. If it touches, a round bur is used to remove the remaining acrylic. The self-curing denture repair resin is applied on top of and all around the black fabrication males. It is preferable to ensure that the external retentive portion of each male's cylindrical housing is completely coated with resin. In addition, the prepared surfaces of the overdenture are filled with acrylic resin prior to placement in the mouth. As the acrylic cures, the denture should be passively seated on the tissue. After removing the denture, the gaps should be filled with acrylic resin. If no missing parts are discovered, finishing and polishing are carried out. Before delivering the overdraft, white fabricators can now replace the black fabricators (Fig. 3.61b).

Laboratory Assignment of Males

There are two ways to complete the model for laboratory processing of male fabrications:

1. Using attachment coping strategies.
2. Using the processing jigs rather than the copings.
1. *Using attachment coping strategies*: With the copings in place, the black fabrication male is inserted into each female and an impression is made. A passive impression of the tissue is required to obtain an accurate stone cast from which the denture can be fabricated. If the copings and fabrication males were not removed with the impression, they should be carefully positioned within the impression. The master dies are repositioned on the copings. Then, a stone mold is cast.
2. *Using the processing jigs in place of the copings*: The black fabrication male is inserted into each female, and an impression with copings in place is created. During the impression procedure, the edentulous tissue should be subjected to pressure. A mucostatic impression of the tissue is required for the creation of an accurate stone cast. After separating the black fabrication males from the females on the copings, the processing jigs are broken. After assembly, the males resemble the impression, and a stone cast is produced.

The try-in dentures, which have already been modeled in wax, are then prepared for the flasking procedure. The black fabrication males must be properly seated, and the under-cut areas surrounding it must be carefully blocked off so that the acrylic resin does not touch the copings. This small space between the copings and acrylic will allow the ERA attachment to function with resilience. After polymerization and finishing procedures, the intraoral fit of the denture must be evaluated. If there is no problem, the black fabrication males are replaced with the final white fabrication males. This method allows for both vertical elasticity and hinges. If black men are not altered, the dentures will lack resilience.

If the denture lacks adequate retention in the mouth, the clinician can easily replace the white males with more retentive alternatives (Fig. 3.61b, c).

Altering the ERA for Males

The core cutter is mounted on a straight handpiece to cut the male part's core at low RPM with a brief cutting cycle and an in-and-out motion. After a one-second pushing motion, it should be determined whether the core has been extracted. During this procedure, the core should be ejected by sliding a thin blade along the side slot of the core cutter. Using a blade or instrument resembling an explorer, collapse the remaining ring into the void created by the removal of the core, lift it out, and position a new male on the seating tool. The tool containing the new male is inserted into the acrylic and pushed firmly until it is securely in place (Fig. 3.61d).

Era Direct Attachment

Location of Direct ERA Females

The final tooth reduction should be 1 mm above the gingiva. The particular spade drill is used to remove the gutta-percha, and the plastic depth reference ring is set to a depth slightly greater than the length of the female post on the pilot drill. When different roots are chosen, the occlusal root surfaces must be prepared in the same plane, perpendicular to the proposed insertion path.

The root canal has been prepared using the pilot drill. In general, the alignment of this initial preparation will follow the canal's direction. On non-parallel roots, the divergence of the female attachments will be corrected by employing angled female components.

The countersink bur is utilized to prepare the root surface to a depth equal to the countersink bur's collar thickness. The depth of the countersink will vary on roots where the root surface plane is not approximately 90° from the axis of the canal preparation. At the highest point, the countersink depth should be minimal, just imprinting the collar of the countersink bur. Remember that the top surface of the female base must always remain above the root surface for the nylon male to snap in without obstruction.

Due to countersinking, a portion of the original Pilot Drill canal preparation will be lost. Re-establish the full depth of the canal preparation to the initial setting of the depth reference ring on the pilot drill. The individual inserts the females with handles into the completed preparations and visually verifies the parallel alignment of the female eyelets. If the alignment can be improved, select the most suitable female from the 5, 11, and 17 angles and rotate it in preparation to determine the placement that provides the best visual parallelism among the females.

Cement the Direct ERA females in place with composite cement, ERA Lock Cement, or an alternative material that is suitable. Follow the procedures for surgical or laboratory placement of the males when incorporating the nylon males into the device (Fig. 3.62a, b).

3.3.18 Determine Root Attachment Position

In clinical situations where healthy tooth roots can be prepared for the placement of attachments to retain an overdenture, the Locator Root Attachment demonstrates exceptional adaptability. It is intended for use with overdentures or partial dentures retained in whole or in part by mandibular or maxillary endodontically treated roots. The unique dual retention innovation gives the Locator attachment a larger retention surface area than other attachments have ever had. A combination of inner and outer retention guarantees the most durable performance (Pictures 3.31 and 3.32; Figs. 3.63, 3.64, 3.65, 3.66, 3.67, 3.68, and 3.69).

The self-aligning feature of the Locator attachment (LOCATOR and LOCATOR R-Tx are registered trademarks of Zest Attachments, LLC) enables a patient to seat their overdenture comfortably without the need for precise alignment of the attachment components. The new LOCATOR R-TxTM is utilized for implant dentures in particular. Multiple layers of titanium carbon nitride and titanium nitride provide a harder, more abrasion-resistant surface for the abutment's exterior. It is over 30% harder, more than 25% more resistant to wear, and has a surface roughness reduction of nearly 65% compared to ZEST, the industry-leading titanium nitride coating. Increased strength is accompanied by an aesthetically pleasing gingival tone that is distinct enough to provide the patient with adequate visibility.

The Locator attachment is an extraradicular design comprised of a straight post, two angles (10° and 20°) to accommodate divergent roots, and a special cast-to version. The retentive nylon male retains full contact with the female socket, while the metal denture cap has complete rotational movement over the male. The three retentive males allow clinicians to select regular, heavy, or extra-heavy retention based on the needs of the patient. In addition, the design of the pivoting male locator allows for a resilient connection between the denture and the locator without compromising retention. Locator standard and extended range males permit a more durable denture connection and safeguard males during insertion. Dual retention and a pivoting action that accommodates up to 20° of divergence between two implants are standard for males. Males with extended range can tolerate up to 40° of total divergence between two implants.

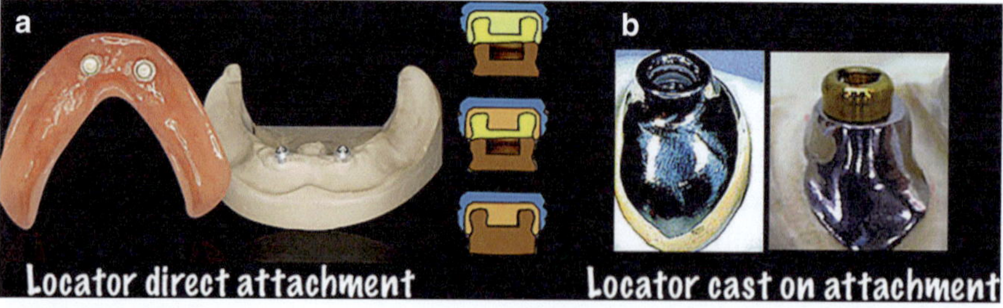

Picture 3.31 (a) The Locator attachment and (b) Locator direct attachment and cast on attachment

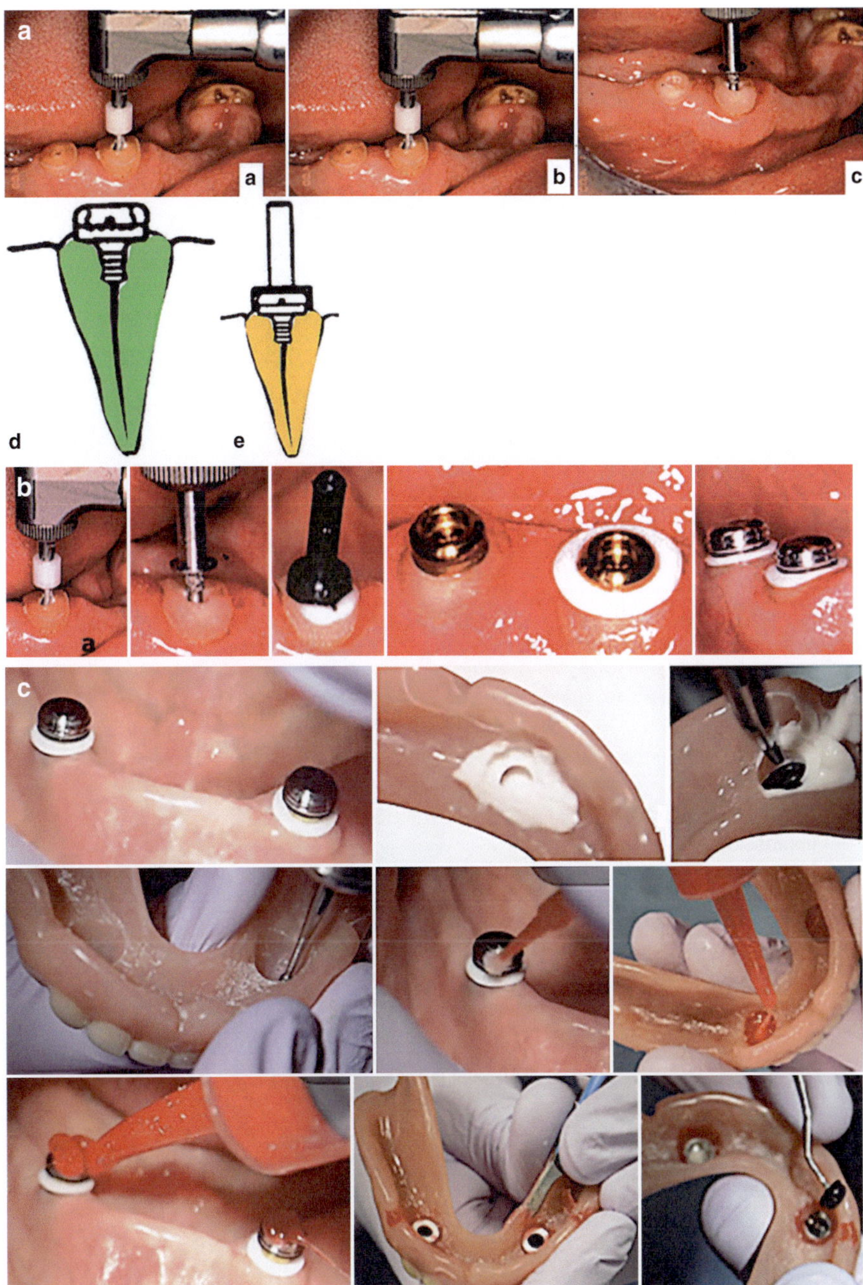

Picture 3.32 (**a**, **b**) The steps for the direct placement of Located root attachment; (**c**, **d**) the steps for Locator male direct placement by a dentist; (**e**, **f**) the steps for Locator male placement by the laboratory; and (**g**) Locator male attachment in the mouth and female in the denture

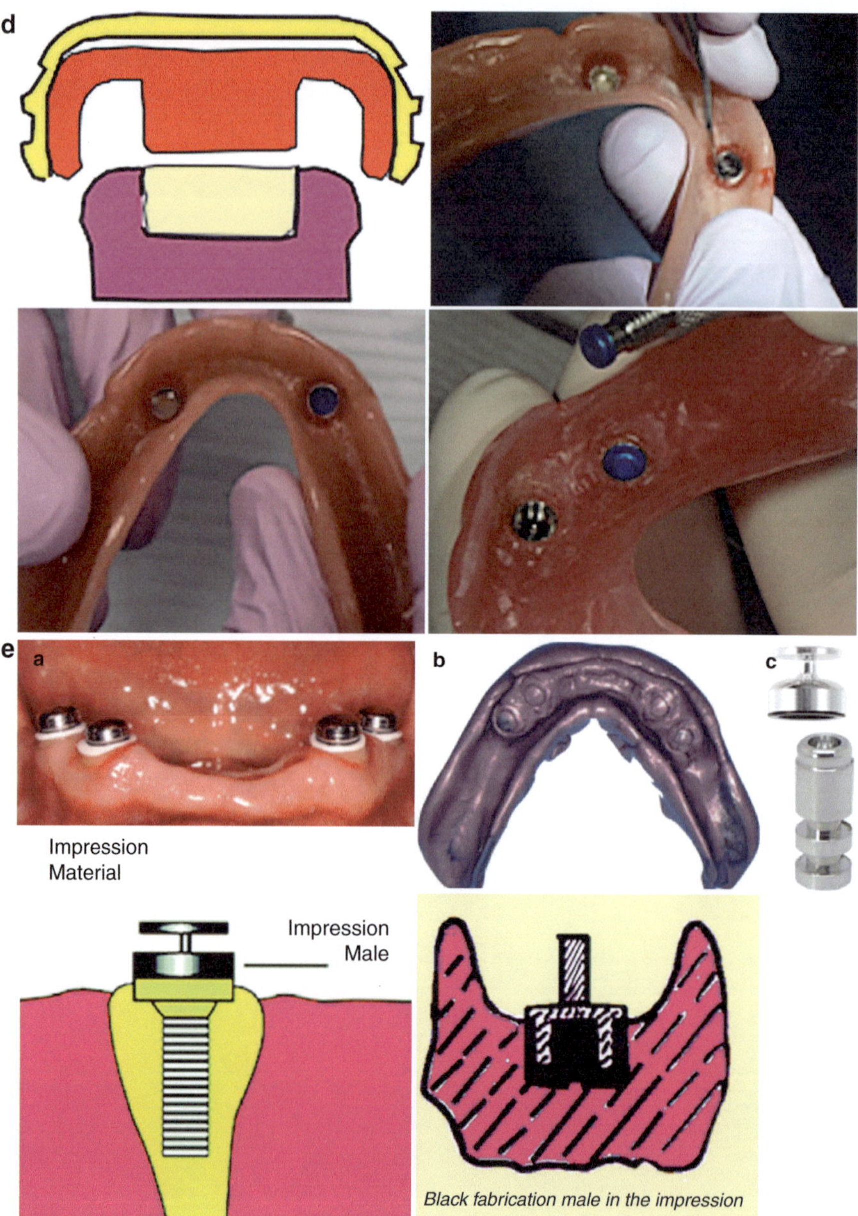

Picture 3.32 (continued)

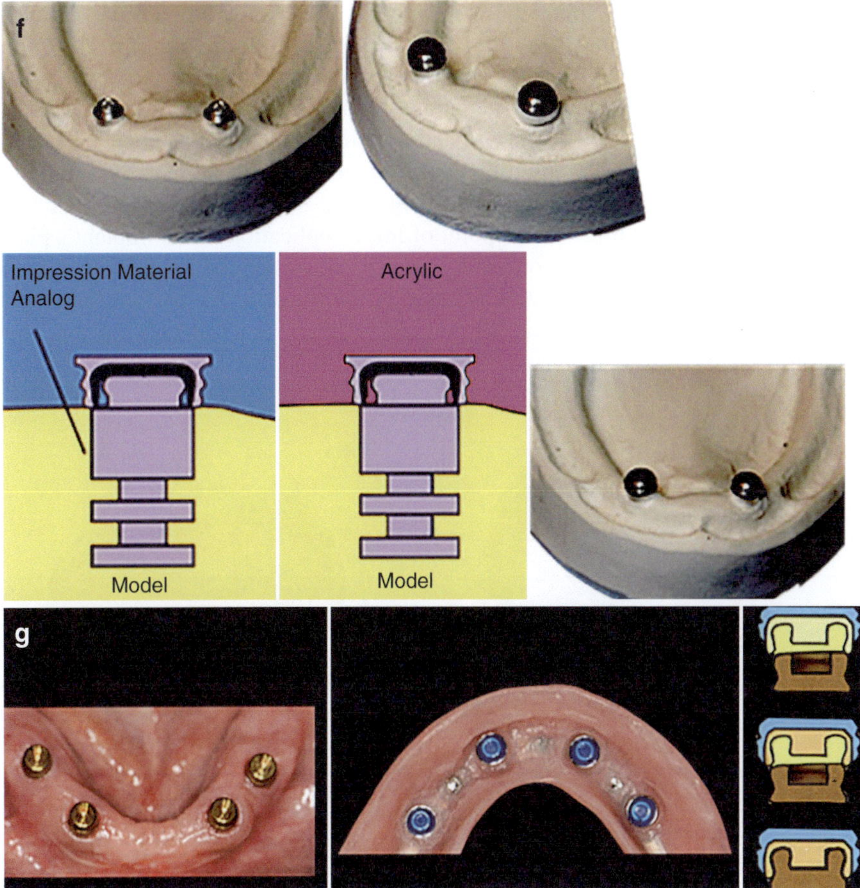

Picture 3.32 (continued)

The Nylon Retention Insert pivots within the denture attachment housing during insertion/removal, resulting in a resilient system that has allowed patients to seat their overdenture without damaging the components, even when implants/roots diverge or converge. Eliminating the need for pre-angled abutments, the denture attachment housing can now pivot up to 30° over the seated LOCATOR R-Tx Nylon Retention Inserts to treat a maximum of 60° convergence or divergence between implants. In vitro durability tests revealed that 60,000 insertion-removal cycles occurred without incident.

For implant dentures, the minimum vertical space required for the Locator attachment is only 8.5 mm from the osseous level to the superior surface of the acrylic resin (as 1.8 mm from the osseous level to the shoulder of the implant, 1.5 mm for the shortest abutment including the bevel, 3.2 mm for the attachment and processing matrix, and 2 mm of acrylic resin above the attachment), and the minimum horizontal space required is 9.0. Depending on the implant system, the transmucosal height of the abutment can range from 1 to 4 mm, 1 to 5 mm, or 1 to 6 mm. Due to the proximity of the point of force application to the implant's platform, optimal biomechanical conditions are achieved when the implant's height is chosen precisely. Consequently, it is essential to measure the maximum height between the implant platform and the mucosal edge and to allow only 1.5 to 2 mm of protrusion.

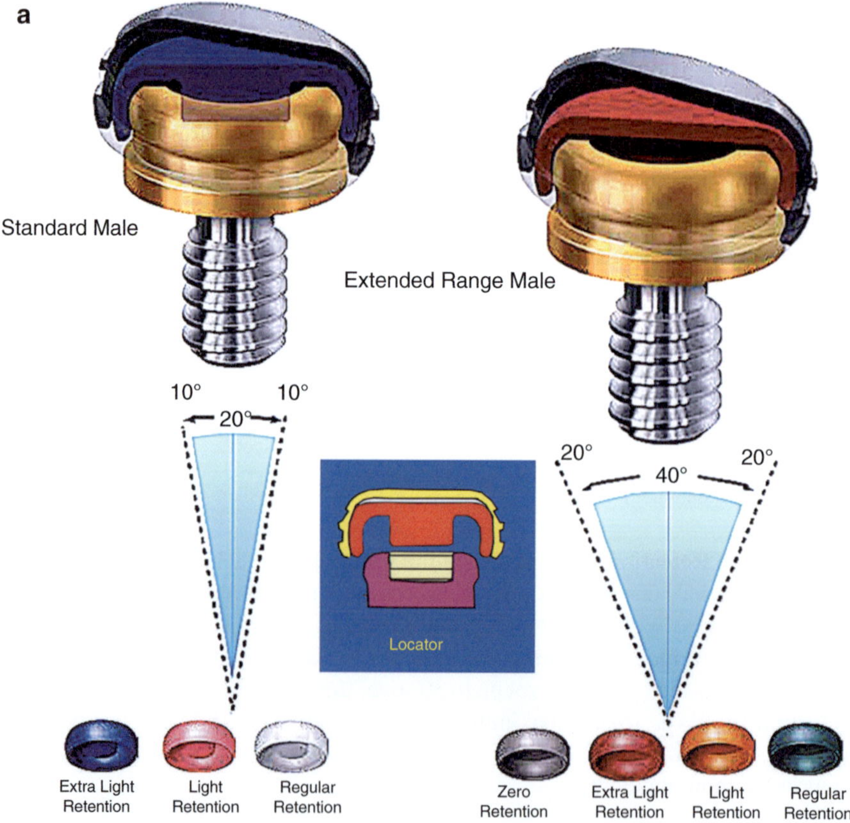

Fig. 3.63 (**a**) The Locator attachment, (**b**) types of Locator attachment insert, and (**c**) Locator female attachment type

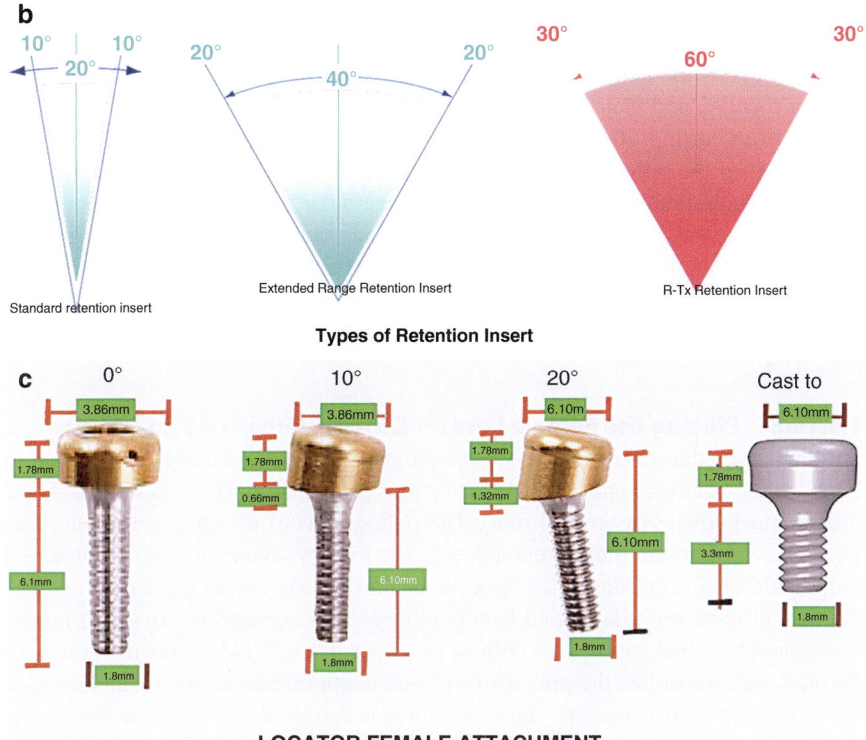

Fig. 3.63 (continued)

3.3.18.1   Cast-to-Coping Location Attachment

Following endodontic therapy, the root is finished by removing the desired amount of gutta-percha using a standard clinical procedure. The final reduction should position the root surface 1 mm above the gingiva and be finished with a beveled shoulder or chamfered margin. Holding the cast-to-locator abutment (LRA) next to the pilot drill and setting the plastic depth reference ring on the pilot drill to a depth that slightly exceeds the cast-to-coping thread length are two methods for determining the cast-to-coping thread length. The size of the canal was determined using a pilot drill that stopped at the depth ring. In general, the alignment of this initial preparation will conform to the canal. On a non-parallel root, the divergence can be corrected with a 10° or 20° angled LRA. Complete the site preparation with a dental burst of choice to ensure that the cast gold coping will encompass the LRA. Place the plastic parallel post with the attached LF in parallel with other LOCATOR attachments using a surveyor. The arch and the prepared roots have been imprinted in as much detail as possible, and the master cast is currently pouring and preparing the dies. Using a surveyor, position the parallel port with the LRA attached in position and parallel to other abutments. Directly wax the LF into the die. The wax should be built up to the bottom corner of the female base, leaving the majority of the base's outer surface above the coping level (*wax must surround the entire area of the 3 mm stainless steel post to provide mechanical retention of the locator inside the casting*). If this is not possible, please fabricate the coping with a 4.5-in. top, level or parallel, and then consider incorporating laser weld or drill and tap locator females after casting. Remove the parallel post and leave the stainless steel attachment open for the inflow of investment material. Then spruing is a combination of the investing and burnout processes (only precious or semi-precious alloys should be used for casting root copings; base metal alloys should not be used). The coping was cast per the manufacturer's specifications. After completing and polishing the coping, the LOCATOR Processing Male (LPM) was inserted into each LF, checked for a proper fit, and then cemented intra-orally onto the prepared tooth root (Fig. 3.64).

3.3.18.2   Placing the Female Locator Directly (Figs. 3.65 and 3.66)

The teeth are reduced to 1 mm above the gingiva, and the root width is measured to establish the available space for a locator root implantation (the width of the root surface must equal or exceed 4 mm). The radiographs of the abutment tooth roots are used to determine the correct angle of the locator abutment's post. Following endodontic treatment, the dentist removes the desired amount of gutta-percha using standard clinical procedures and then completes root contouring. The final reduction should be 1 mm supragingival from the root surface. Hold the abutment next to the pilot drill and adjust the pilot drill's plastic depth reference ring to the length of the screw thread. If necessary, the screw threads can be shortened. The size of the canal is determined by the pilot drill stopping at the depth ring. In general, the alignment of this initial preparation will conform to the canal. On a non-parallel root, the divergence can be corrected with a 10° or 20° angled locator abutment, utilizing the spot-face diamond bur to a depth where a full 360° recessed seat appears first on the occlusal surface of the root. When preparing a countersink for a divergent root, the countersink depth will vary across the surface. Create the smallest recess possible on the flat surface of the specimen. Create the smallest recess possible on the side of the preparation that is shallow. If a portion of the original depth from the pilot drill

Fig. 3.64 Steps for cast on Locator root attachment (LRA) placement. (**a**) Reduce the teeth and measure the root width to determine the space available for an LRA (at least 4 mm width); (**b**) the final reduction should place the root surface 1 mm supragingival; and (**c**) the waxing limit should be at least 1 mm above the gingival level. (**d**) *a* Finish the contouring of the root; *b* using a pilot drill with the plastic depth reference ring determines the cast-to coping thread length; *c* size the canal using the pilot drill stopping at the depth ring; and *d* complete the preparation of the site with dental burs. (**e**) *a, b* impression of the arch and the prepared roots are taken *c* Master cast obtained and attachment placed using mandrel, *d* Using a surveyor, place the parallel post with the cast-to LRA attached in position, wax coping and then coping casted with LRA attachment. (**f**) Snap a denture cap with a black processing male onto each LRA and proceed with the fabrication of the denture

a
Min. 4 mm
b
4 mm
1 mm
c
wax limit
Locator attachment and depth reference ring
wax limit

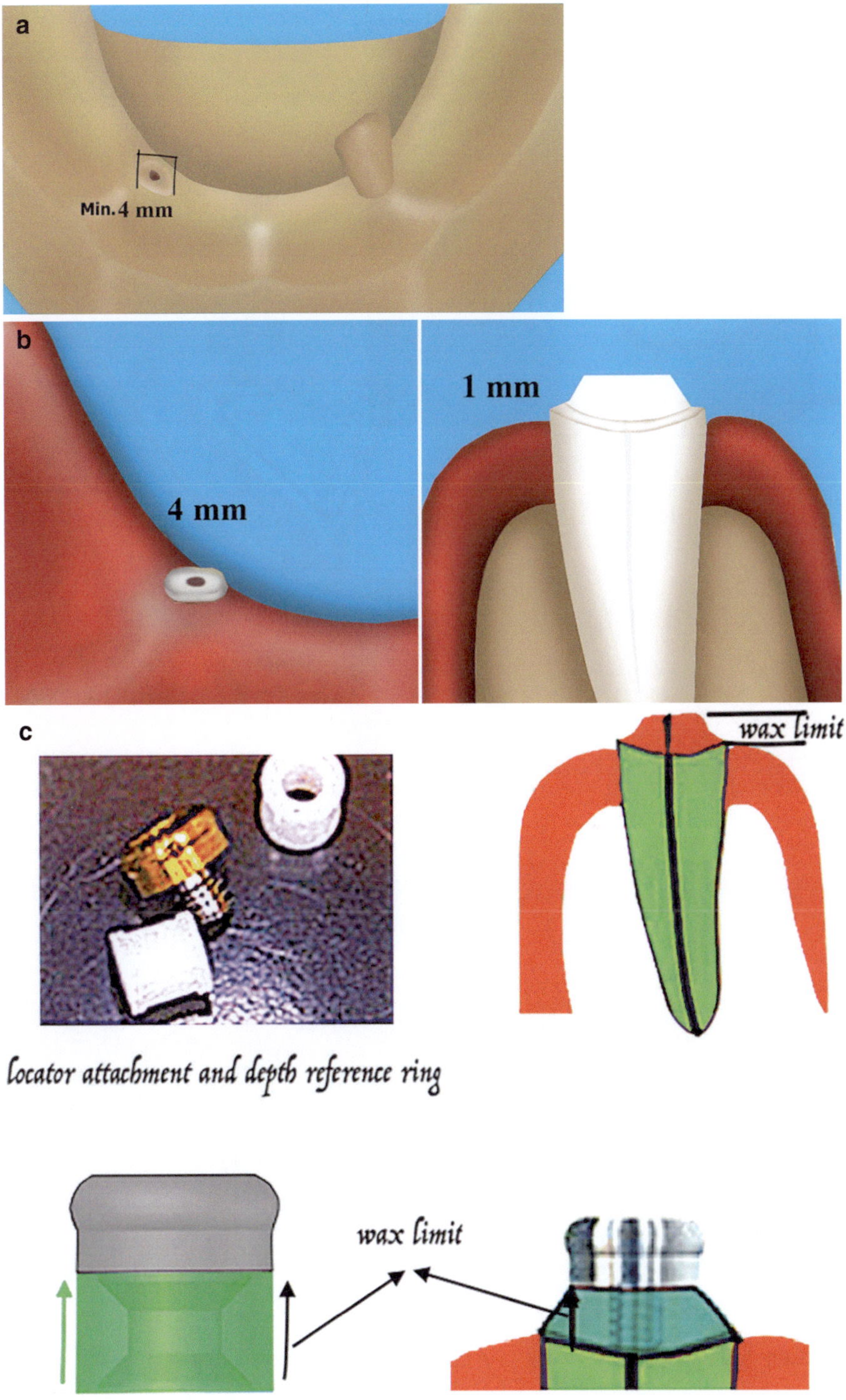

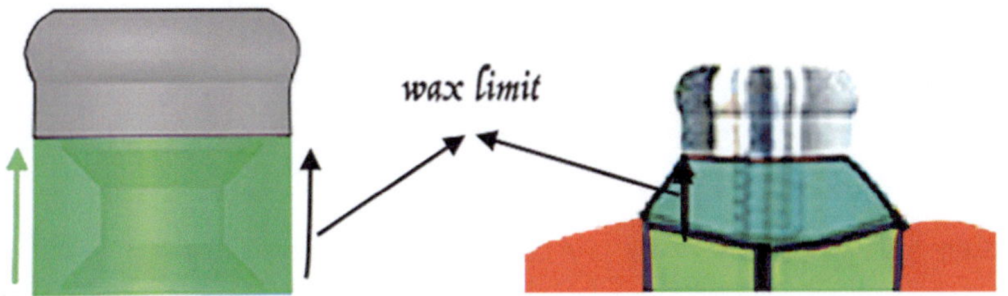

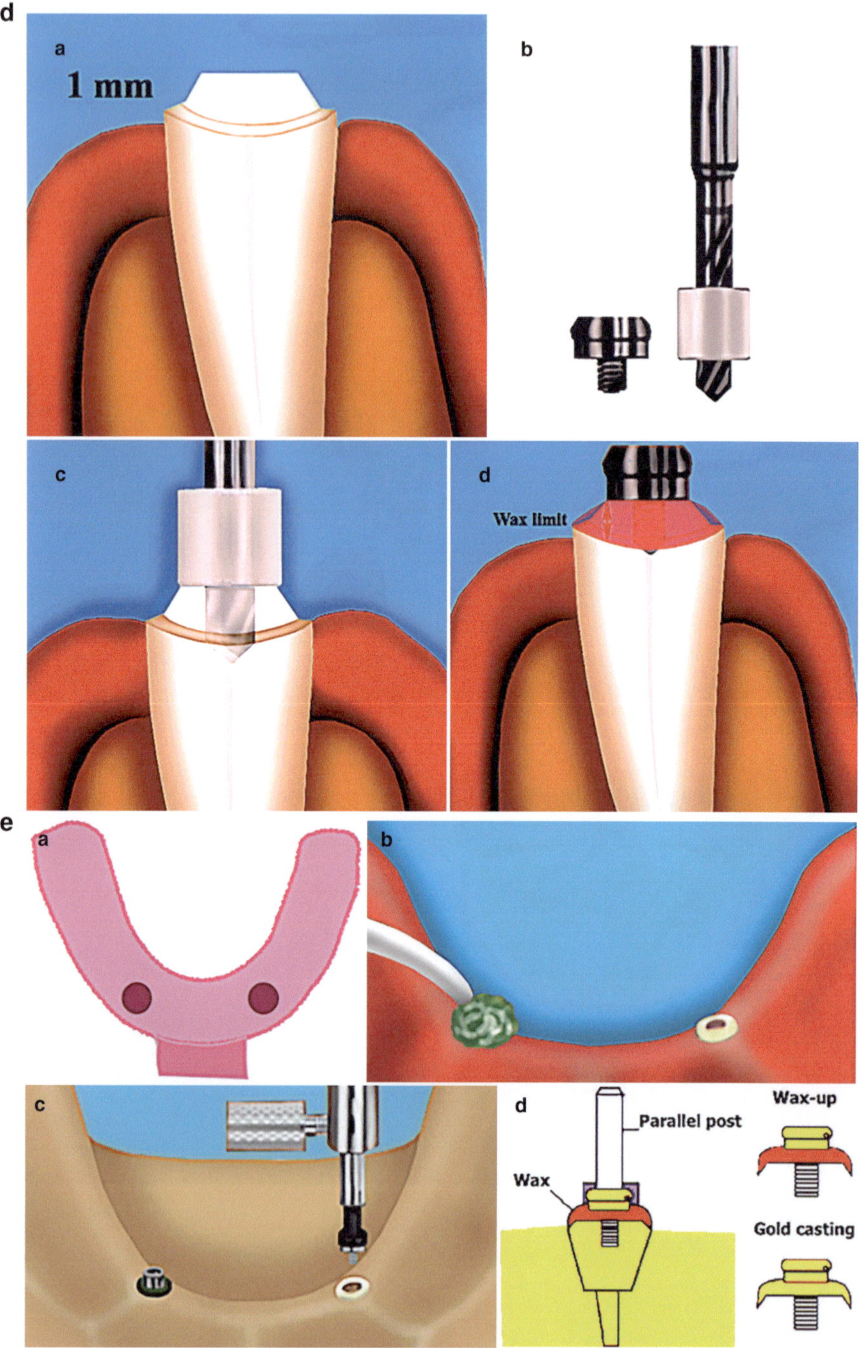

Fig. 3.64 (continued)

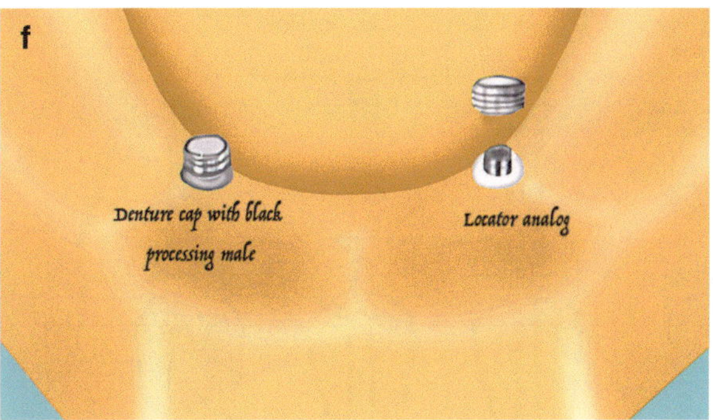

Fig. 3.64 (continued)

canal preparation is lost due to countersinking, reestablish the full depth of the canal preparation with the pilot drill using the original depth reference setting.

The placement of a locator parallel post on a 0° locator root abutment serves as a handle and verifies the proper fit and parallel alignment of multiple abutments. If the alignment of any of the abutments can be improved for a draw, choose the most appropriate angled Locator root abutment (10° or 20°) and test it in the preparation to determine the optimal parallelism. Position root abutment cement using the recommended dental cement. After the cement round has hardened, polish the root surface from the metal flange to the tissue. To protect the abutment during polishing, the parallel post should be placed on it. Utilize a dental cement of your choosing to affix the LRA in place. Permit the cement to harden before polishing the root surface of the tissue. The parallel post can be used to shield the LRA during polishing (Fig. 3.67).

3.3.18.3 Locator Male: Placement Made Directly by a Dentist

Chairside Technique

The advantage of the chairside technique is that the attachment can be made passively using bite force, ensuring that the denture is fully seated on the underlying tissues. This technique is more difficult, but it allows attachments to be added to an existing denture.

The rings are blocking undercuts to prevent the flow of acrylic material. To avoid "locking into" additional undercut areas, care should be taken to block off any additional undercut areas. The root contouring and cementing of the locator females (LF) have been completed. The white block-out spacer (WS) is placed over the head of every female that has been cemented. The spacer is used to cover the remaining exposed surfaces of the root so that the self-curing acrylic does not come into contact with the root after it has been applied and cured. Using the undercut bur to cut an undercut around the circumference of the recesses for mechanical retention, the space created between the root and denture base will permit the complete, resilient

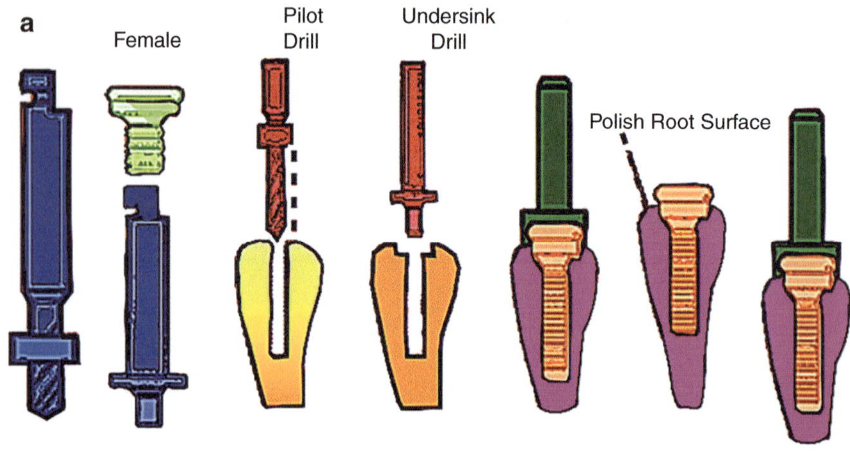

Placement of Locator root attachment

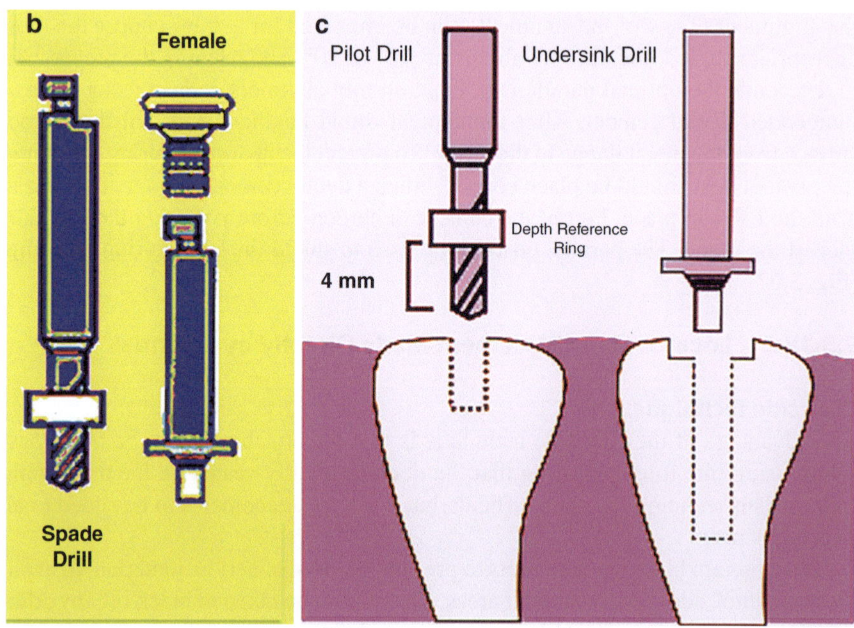

Fig. 3.65 (**a**) Steps for direct placement of Locator root attachment (LRA); (**b**) the spade drill; (**c**) the pilot drill with depth reference ring and Undersink drill; and (**d**) Locator parallel post places 0° LRA, e 0° and angled LRA

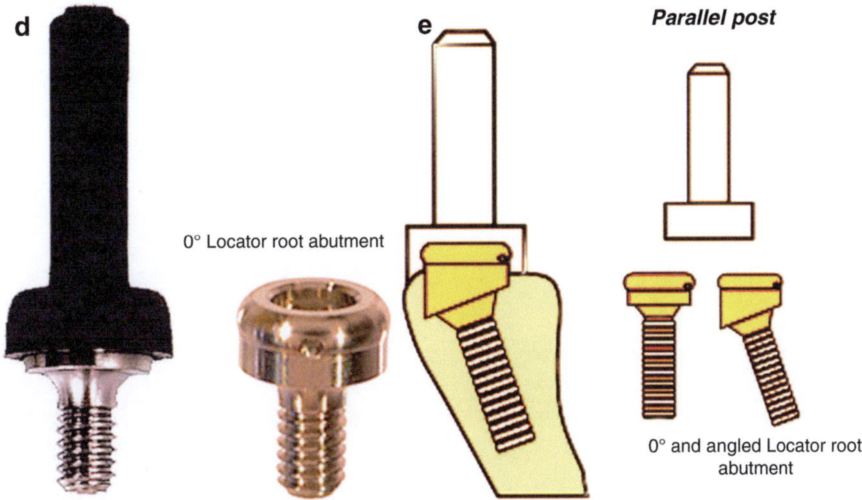

Fig. 3.65 (continued)

function of the pivoting metal denture cap over the locator male (LM). Use a vent burst with lingual and palatal vent windows in the overdenture to visualize full seating and vent excess material.

The LOCATOR Black Processing Cap Male (BPCM) was inserted into each cemented female while the WS was left beneath it. During the processing procedure, the BPCM will maintain the overdenture at the upper limit of its vertical resiliency. A small amount of fit checker paste was applied to the intaglio surface of the overdenture, and the denture was positioned over the denture cap in the mouth. This procedure will identify the pressure areas in the overdenture where space must be created for the crowns. Remove the burr from the areas that are marked to indicate where to stop drilling for the denture cap.

Each cap is surrounded by a small amount of chairside processing material. Place chairside processing material in the overdenture's recesses and seat it over the caps and onto the tissue. The patient should request a light occlusion and hold it while the chairside processing material polymerizes, after which the overdenture should be disengaged from the abutments and removed from the mouth. The denture cap is processed securely into the overdenture. The voids are filled with a flowable material that is then light-cured within 30 s. Use a bur to remove excess acrylic and polish the denture base prior to switching to the final male, the LM Removal Tool is for removing the BPCM and the metal denture cap. Insert the new tip into the cap/male assembly and push it directly into the base of the nylon male. Invert the instrument so that the sharp edge of the tip will grab the male and extract it from the

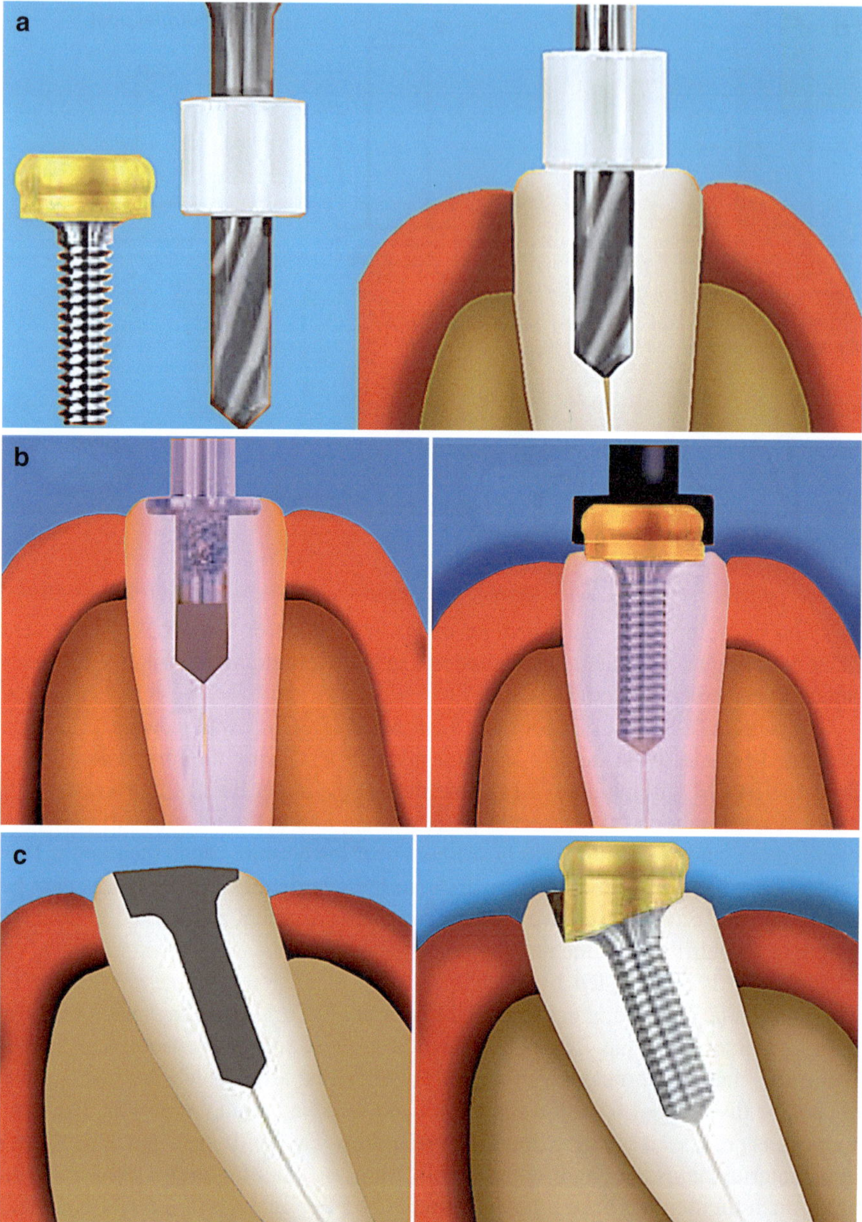

Fig. 3.66 (**a**) Hold the abutment next to the pilot drill and set the plastic depth reference ring on the pilot drill to the length of the screw thread; (**b**) spotface the root surface; (**c**) when making a countersink preparation into a divergent root, the depth of the countersink will vary across the surface; (**d**) place a 0° or angled (10° or 20°) LRA into each of the prepared roots and verify the proper fit; and (**e**) cement LRA in place with appropriate dental cement

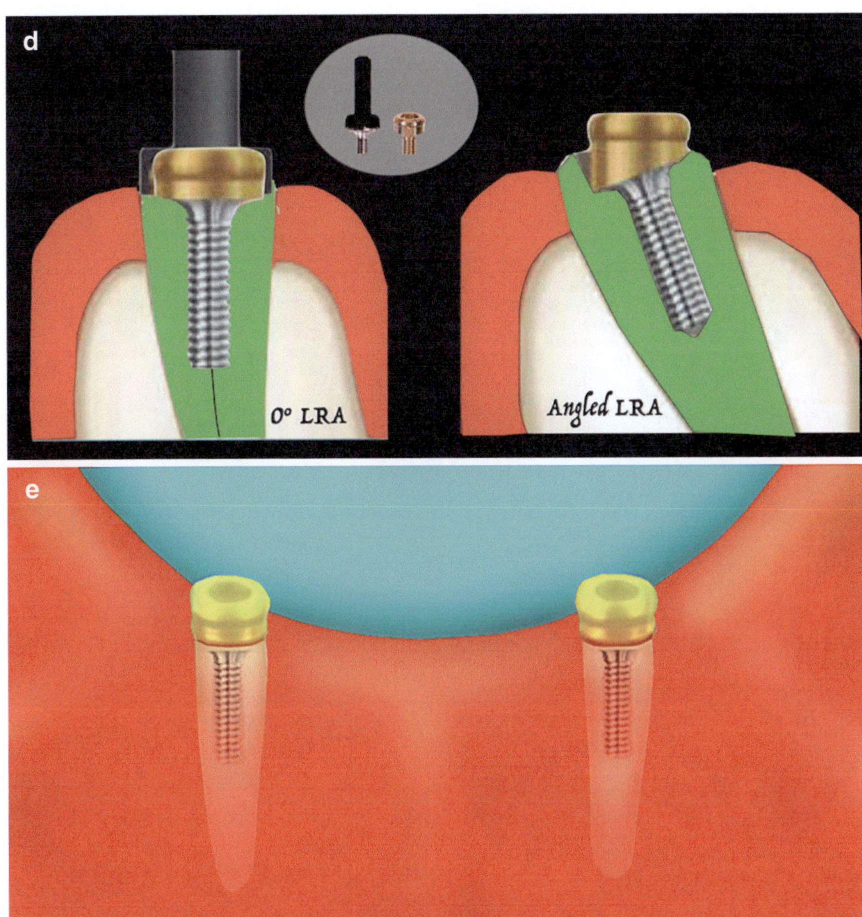

Fig. 3.66 (continued)

cap. Throw away the nylon male by pointing the tool away from you and rethreading the Male Removal Tool onto the Core Tool in a clockwise direction. This will trigger the removal pin and detach the nylon male from the tip. The LM Seating Tool is utilized to push a LOCATOR Replacement Male firmly into an empty metal denture cap. The replacement male must be firmly secured in place, flush with the cap's rim (Fig. 3.67).

Laboratory Operations

Incorporating laboratory attachment reduces technique sensitivity, but does not account for the level of compression necessary to ensure complete tissue seating. It is recommended that laboratory curing of attachments be performed in the base

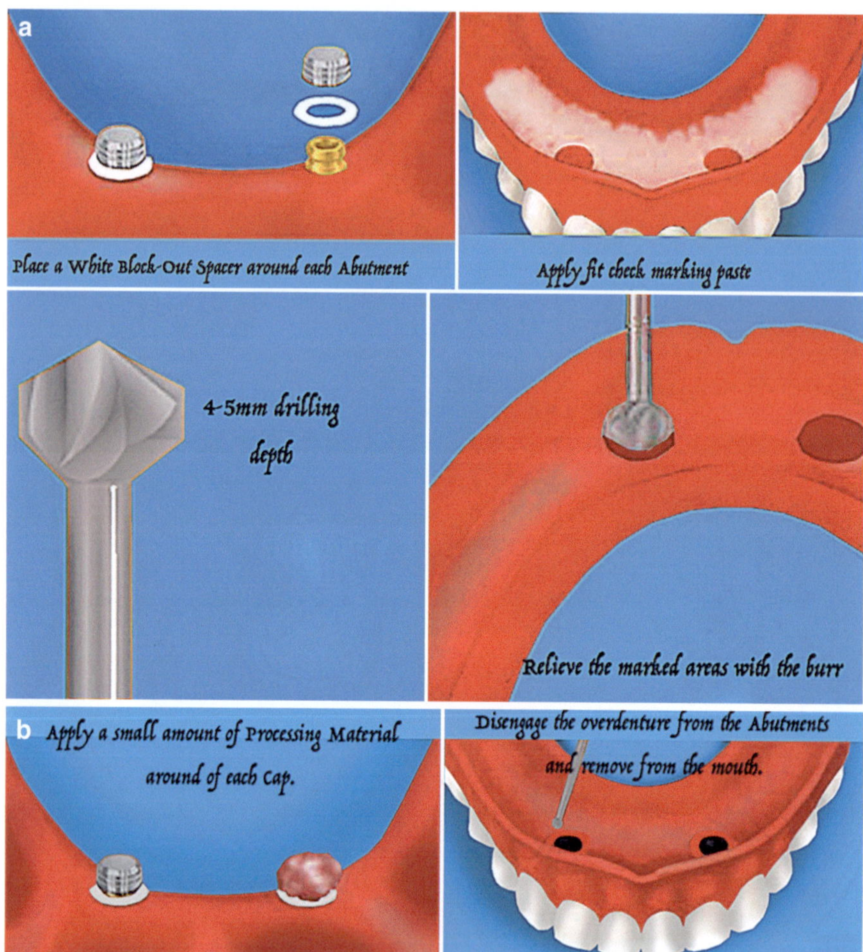

Fig. 3.67 (**a–f**) Processing Locator denture caps into the overdenture direct technique

plate prior to processing the denture at the wax rim try-in or the set-up appointment in order to evaluate full seating on the tissues and minimize distortion caused by curing the bulk of acrylic during processing. This procedure will permit the attachment position to be monitored and adjusted prior to the scheduled delivery date. The most important concerns are preventing acrylic from flowing into any undercuts, preventing the denture from being removed, and ensuring that the denture can fully seat on the tissues without interference from the attachments. After cementing the LF and finalizing the root contouring, BPCM is inserted into each cemented female. During the processing procedure, the built-in spacer of the BPCM will maintain the overdenture at its maximum vertical resilience. A lightweight impression material was used to avoid compressing soft tissue. Once the impression is removed, the

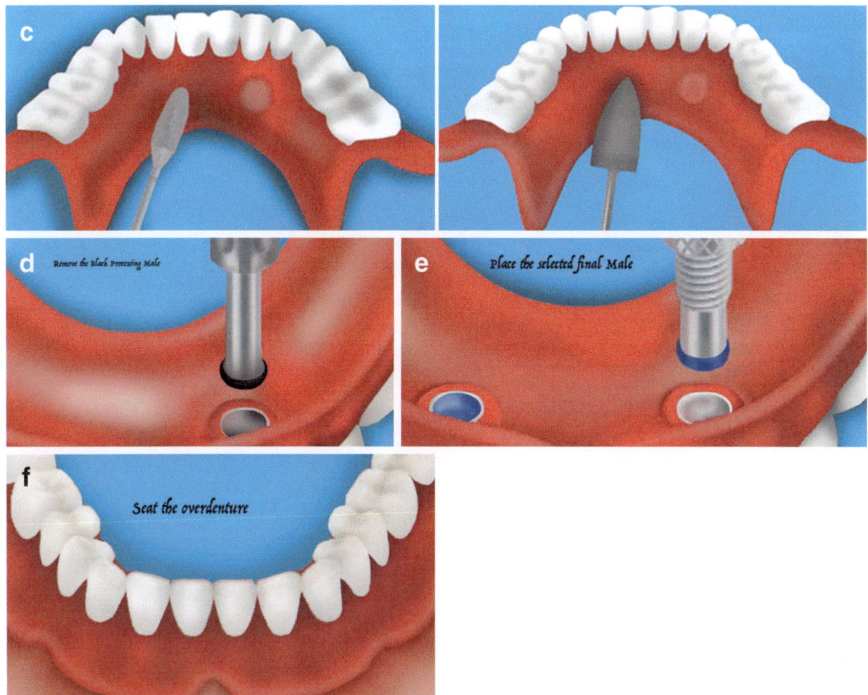

Fig. 3.67 (continued)

BPCM will remain in the cemented females. BPCM is from an LF female and it should be snapped securely into an LF analog before sending it to the lab.

The following are laboratory procedures:

The master mold should be cast. The LF analog becomes a component of the master cast upon separation, replicating the position of the cemented LF in the oral cavity. Place a BPCM into each LF analog in the master cast before waxing and processing the appliance. BPCM was eliminated after tooth arrangement and processing technique. The WS is placed over each LF analog's head. The spacer is used to cover the root's remaining exposed surfaces, preventing the processed acrylic from coming into contact with the root. The space created between the root and denture base will permit the metal denture cap to perform its full, resilient function over the LM. The BPCM was reintroduced into each LF analog, with the WS remaining below it. During the processing procedure, the BPCM will maintain the overdenture at the upper limit of its vertical resiliency. Finish processing and dispose of the white spacer. Polishing the denture base prior to switching to the final male will prevent damage to the final male. Remove BPCM from the metal cap of the denture. The replacement male was then inserted into the empty denture cap (Fig. 3.68).

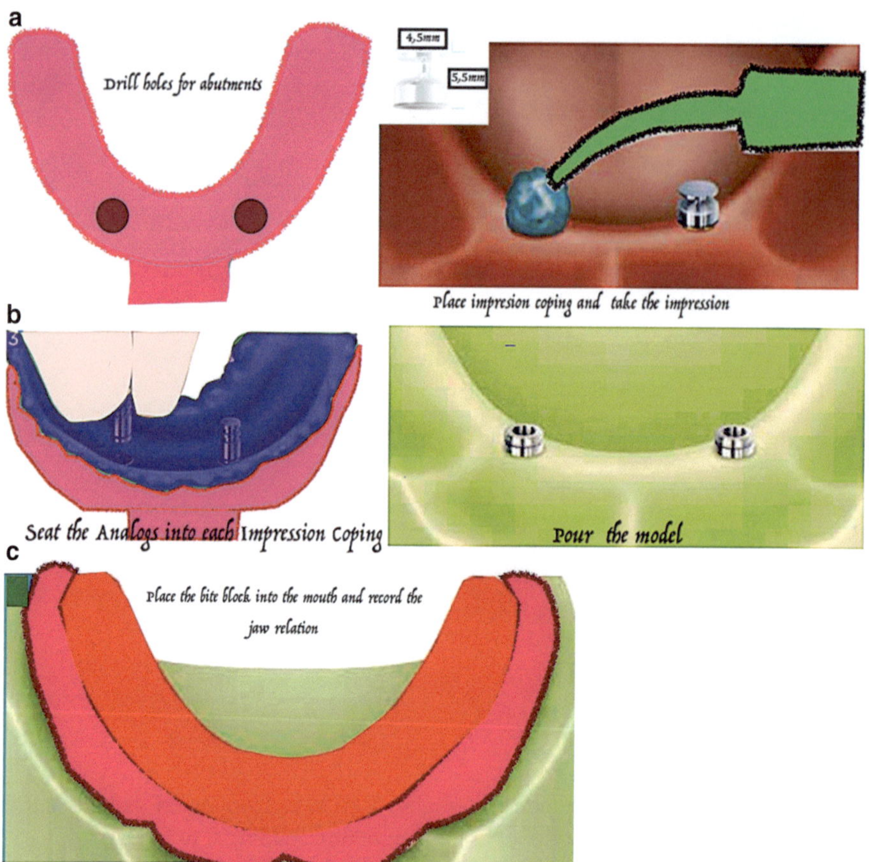

Fig. 3.68 (**a–d**) Processing Locator denture caps into the overdenture laboratory technique and (**e**) different types of attachment (Locator, ERA, and OP attachment)

To ensure the full seating of the final denture without interference from attachments or housings, housings were placed. Prepare the final denture for incorporation into the housings.

- "Vent Holes" are placed in the area of the accessories to allow excess material to escape and prevent the tissues from becoming completely seated.
- Looking through the patient at the black processing males that are tacked in place with acrylic while maintaining a moderate biting force in the centric position. Vacancies surrounding the housings are filled in extraordinarily, and black processing males are replaced with final retentive inserts (available in various amounts of retention).

It is advised that a metal framework or lingual reinforcing bar be used to prevent denture fracture due to inadequate acrylic thickness or excessive occlusal forces.

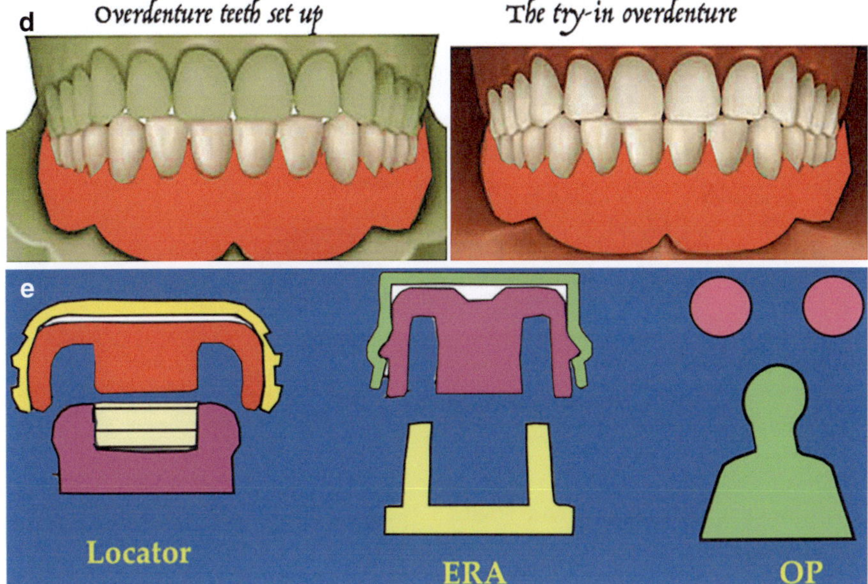

Fig. 3.68 (continued)

The locator attachments appear to function adequately, but a long-term evaluation is lacking. A long-term evaluation may provide the clinician with useful guidelines for selecting the type of attachment system and overdenture design. In terms of retention and stability, Locator attachments outperform Nobel Biocare Ball connectors for implant-supported overdentures. Abi-Nader et al. reported that while simulated mastication resulted in minor modifications to the ball attachment, it reduced the retention of locator attachments to 40% of baseline values with a nonlinear descending curve. The nylon capsules were significantly impacted. Kleis et al. concurred that the self-aligning attachment system required more maintenance than ball attachments. Also, when implant angulations are increased from 0° to 30°, there is a decrease in retentive force, as well as an increase in metal component wear and maintenance.

Rotation of dentures is one of the difficulties associated with ensuring resilient attachments. Especially when food is chewed on the anterior teeth, denture rotation can lead to food particles entering under the dentures and difficulty chewing.

Retrofit-ERA Locator Root Attachments

This attachment is intended for use with overdentures or partial dentures retained in whole or in part by mandibular or maxillary endodontically treated roots.

The LOCATOR® Retrofit for ERA® Root Attachment is intended for use with overdentures or partial dentures retained in whole or in part by endodontically treated mandibular or maxillary roots. The flexible attachment converts worn or damaged standard-sized ERA® attachments into the new Locator attachment for

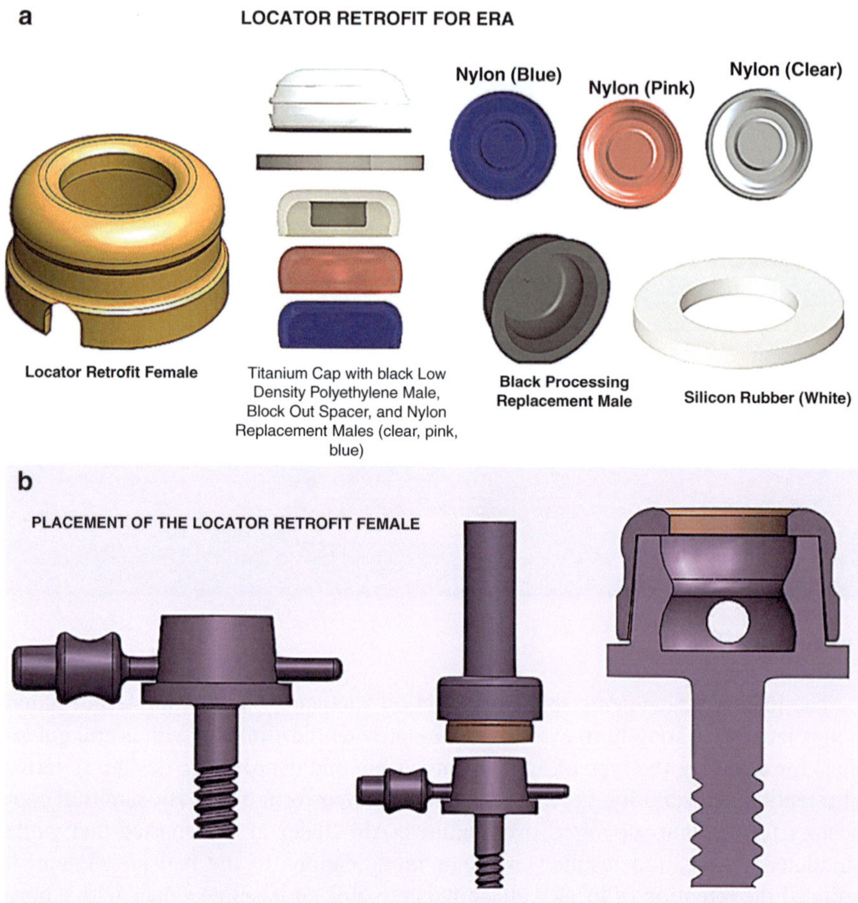

Fig. 3.69 (**a**, **b**) Locator Retrofit ERA attachment

endodontically treated roots. It is designed to retrofit existing worn ERA abutments and is unsuitable for micro-sized ERA attachments or situations where a rigid connection is required.

Placement of the Locator Retrofit Female

The weep hole alignment pin is inserted through the ERA attachment's two weep holes. This allows clinicians to prevent this small part from being dropped and lost, as well as aid in the pin's removal after cementation. The female locator retrofit was placed onto the ERA attachment using a black parallel post to visually verify the proper fit.

Crown cement was utilized to affix the Locator Retrofit Female in place. Apply the adhesive around the perimeter of the ERA attachment. The Locator Retrofit Female's slots must align with the Weep Hole Alignment Pin shaft, which has been inserted into the ERA attachment. The pin is arranged for weep hole alignment. Using the floss, remove it from the assembly before the adhesive has fully hardened. Before removing the parallel post, allow the cement to harden somewhat, as the retention may dislodge the locator. The female bonded locator retrofit should be firmly seated on the ERA's top (Fig. 3.69a, b).

3.3.19 Custom-Made Stud Attachment

Approximately three decades ago, custom-made precision attachments were utilized; today, their fabrication is more prevalent. Prefabricated attachments are more precise, but they are often not preferred due to their cost and various other factors, such as the lack of availability of the exact size, which may result in an improper fit. In addition, the precision of the sophisticated prefabricated attachments, which is essential for achieving a satisfactory function, is lacking in the custom-made attachments. The acceptance level of the patients is comparable to that of expensive attachments, or perhaps it is higher because the attachments are less expensive.

The attachment was less expensive and simpler to manufacture, and it offered adequate retention and stability for the dentures. Nemcovsky et al. (1990) described a straightforward method for fabricating stud overdenture retainers with custom attachment castings and Teflon retention discs. This system enables selective placement of the retention sphere on the root surface and retention regulation by means of the retention sphere's diameter. This technique enables the replacement of Teflon discs at the chairside.

The pattern wax can be used to create attachment patterns, but it is extremely fragile and soft, leading to pattern distortion. It was also time-consuming. Patterns were created using pattern resin, which served its purpose. Less analytical techniques and a straightforward approach are recommended. The choice of attachment was determined by the root's length and diameter. In the case of shorter root lengths, the full-length serrated attachments can be used, whereas the sandblasted attachments were effective for larger-diameter roots. The attachment size for a specific root can be chosen based on its surface texture, length, and width (size) (Fig. 3.70).

3.3.20 Rothermann Attachment

Vertically, the Rothermann is the smallest rigid (Class 1a) or flexible (Class V) overdenture attachment currently available (Figs. 3.71 and 3.72). When space is limited and the teeth are asymmetrical, a Rothermann attachment is the best option. It is made up of a male stud with a solder core for forehand soldering to a coping and a female clip made up of a perforated retention beam with a split C-ring extension. The height of the male portion differs between the resilient and non-resilient attachments, with the resilient attachment measuring 1.7 mm and the non-resilient attachment measuring 1.1 mm. The flexible Rothermann permits both vertical and

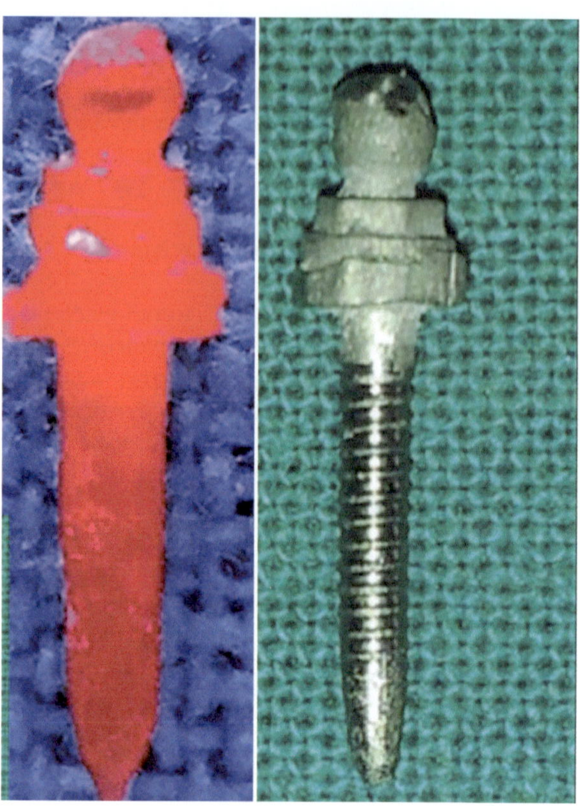

Fig. 3.70 Custom-made attachment

rotational motion. One end of the groove on the male part is deeper than the other. The housing contains a "C"-shaped ring, the ends of which fit in the retaining groove's thickest portion. The gold females can be altered. The flexible Rothermann attachment allows for approximately 5° of divergence. There are two available configurations: the anterior (retention area on the lingual) and the posterior (retention area along the ridge). The Rothermann male in white gold incorporates solder directly; no additional solder is required. Before processing acrylic, the solid male spacer is used to block the male attachment occlusally.

3.3.20.1 Advantages

When multiple coping strategies are employed, parallelism is unnecessary.

It is one of the shortest attachments that are available.

Torque is not required.

By spreading out the retention ring, one can obtain the lowest possible retention.

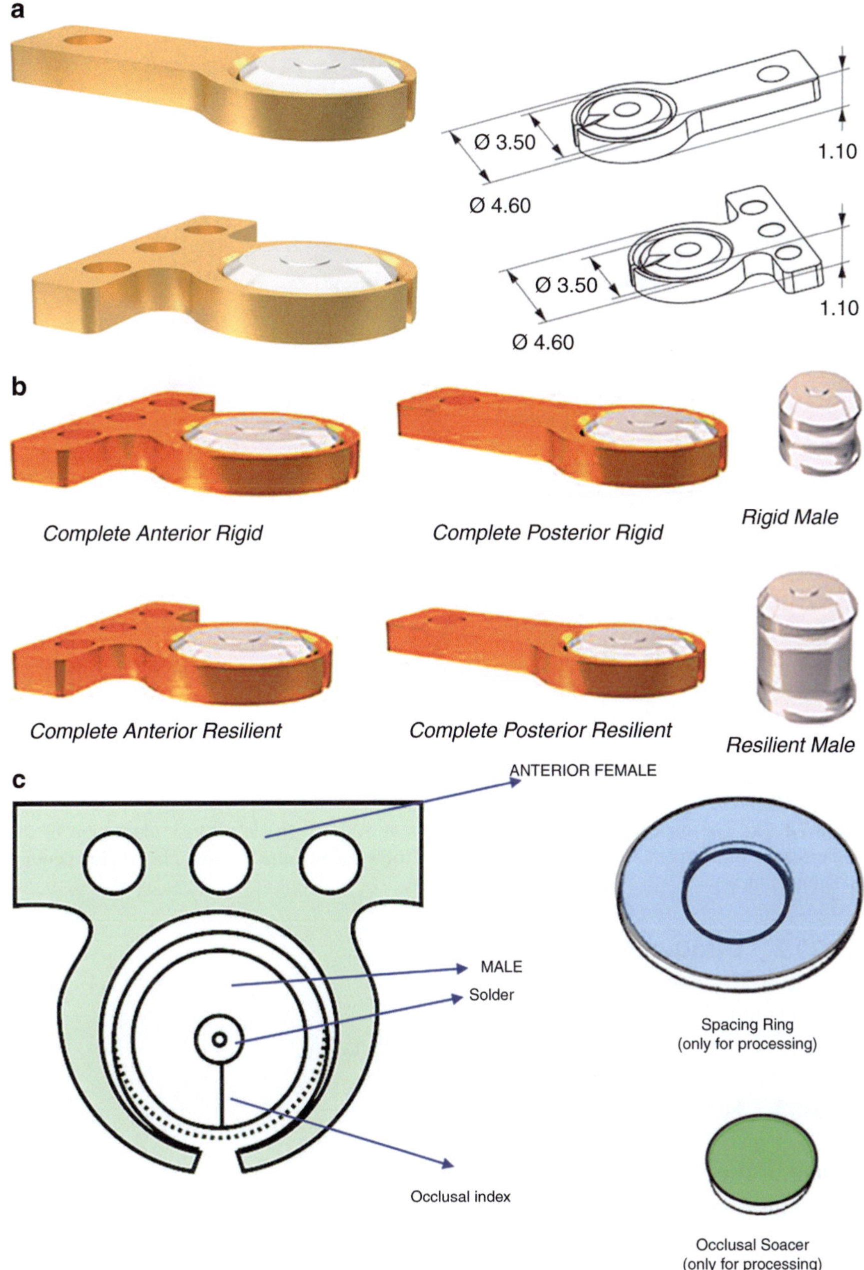

Fig. 3.71 (**a–c**) The Rothermann attachment

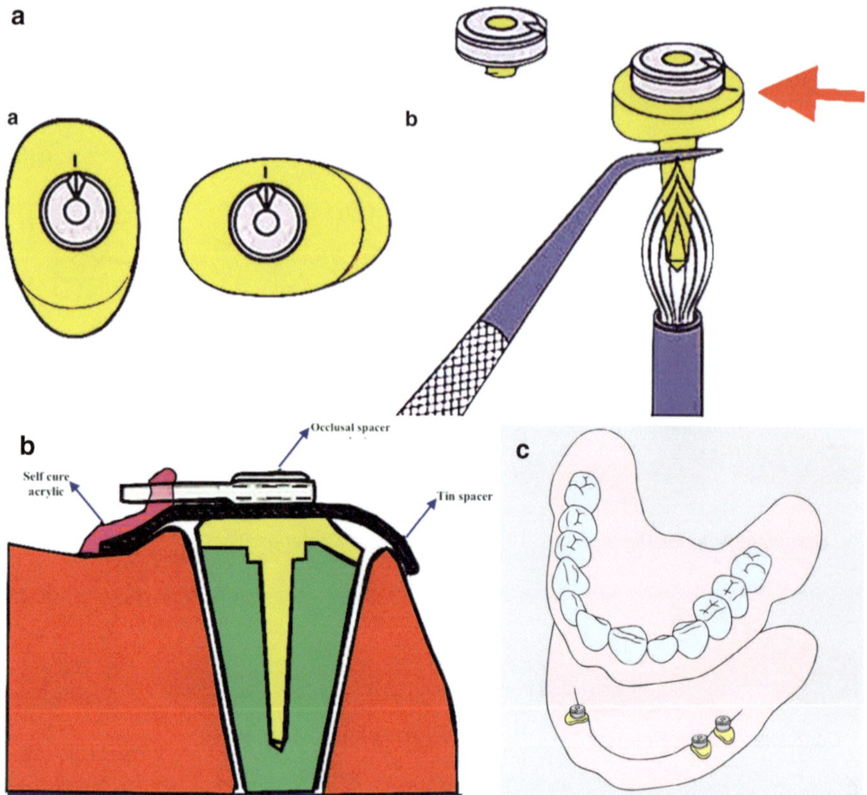

Fig. 3.72 (**a**) The male contains solder that flows at 800 °C, (**b**) laboratory placement of the Rothermann attachment female, and (**c**) the Rothermann attachment placed in denture (Schematic view)

3.3.20.2 Disadvantages

There is no mechanism for "C" ring activation.

Rebasing is challenging.

There is lingual bulk in the attachment's orientation.

3.3.20.3 Fabrication Instructions

Attaching the Male

The occlusal surface of a root coping is manufactured to be flat to accommodate the male. If the resilient Rothermann males are utilized, they should be within 5° of being parallel to the path of insertion of the overdenture. The rigid males of Rothermann must be within 10° of parallel.

The male is situated on the coping with the occlusal index facing upward. The female C-opening clip must align with the male's occlusal index. Therefore, if clinicians use the anterior C-clip, the occlusal index must be positioned facially with the

C-anchor clip's bar on the lingual. If the posterior C-clip is utilized, the occlusal index must be positioned mesiodistally so that the C-anchor clip's bar is along the ridge. The male contains solder that flows at 1470 °F (800 °C). It is unnecessary to pre-drill the coping before soldering (Fig. 3.71a, b). A small amount of flux is applied to the bottom of the male, and, using small tweezers, the coping is removed from the Bunsen burner flame as soon as the solder flows from the male's center.

Laboratory Placement of Female
Using Rothermann processing jigs, females can be processed directly over males or indirectly using jigs. The anchor bar of the anterior C-clip is lingually positioned. The anchor bar of the posterior C-clip is positioned mesiodistally along the ridge (Fig. 3.71c).

Resilient Rothermann Attachment
The cast is fitted with a spacing ring that is placed over the male or jig. The sections are cut from the spacing ring so that they do not overlap when forming the coping's shape. The excess material is trimmed to conform to the coping's final dimensions. For the rigid Rothermann attachment, the spacer is not required. The female is then found on the male. For the resilient Rothermann attachment, the top of the male or processing jig is coated with sticky wax. The occlusal spacer is omitted from the rigid Rothermann. Cover all exposed areas of the male and occlusal spacer (if used) as previously.

3.3.21 Quinlivan Attachment

It is a type of resin stud attachment with a wax-up (wax prepared for casting) post and coping. It is bonded to teeth that have received endodontic therapy. The female component is located within the denture, and retention is provided by an O-ring of rubber within the female component. Among its advantages are its simple and inexpensive construction as well as the simplicity of replacing the O-ring as its retention decreases.

3.3.22 Introfix Attachment

This attachment is a stable cylinder that can be used for overdentures. The long stud has torque-producing potential. Therefore, it is only utilized in a tooth-supported system, or OD, with superior support. It consists of three components: a soldering base, an adjustable male post with a split, and a female housing. The design is straightforward and provides a frictional connection between the two components. The male stud has a longitudinal slit that can be attached for increased or decreased retention. As it is screwed onto the solder base, this is replaceable.

3.4 Intraradicular Stud Attachments

Regarding space requirements, intraradicular attachments have the advantage of requiring no additional metal casting; rather, drilling is made into the root preparation made with the manufacturer-supplied bur (Figs. 3.73, 3.74, 3.75, 3.76, 3.77, and 3.78).

These attachments ensure retention from within the root; the male portion of the attachment is a component of the base plaque and is located in a housing tailored to the root's contours. Intraradicular attachment systems require less vertical space. In addition, forces are transferred to the root along the entire length of the tooth's axis. Although placement is dependent on the root shape, a significant difference in root inclination can affect the path of denture insertion. The male portion of the attachment is embedded within the female portion, which is positioned at the root. The female parts are designed to accommodate the majority of remaining root structures. Even with minimal bone support for the remaining teeth, intraradicular attachment is successful. Simple laboratory and chairside procedures render the system cost-effective.

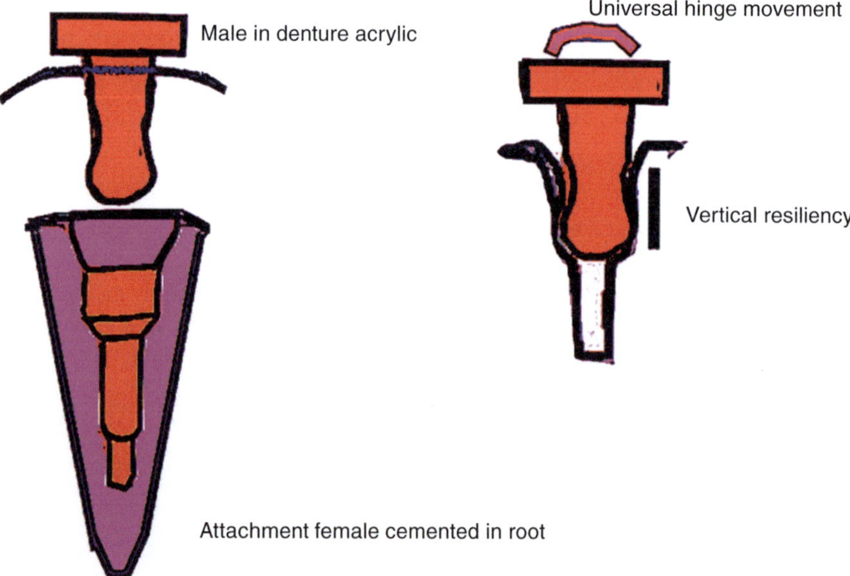

Fig. 3.73 Intraradicular stud attachment schematic view

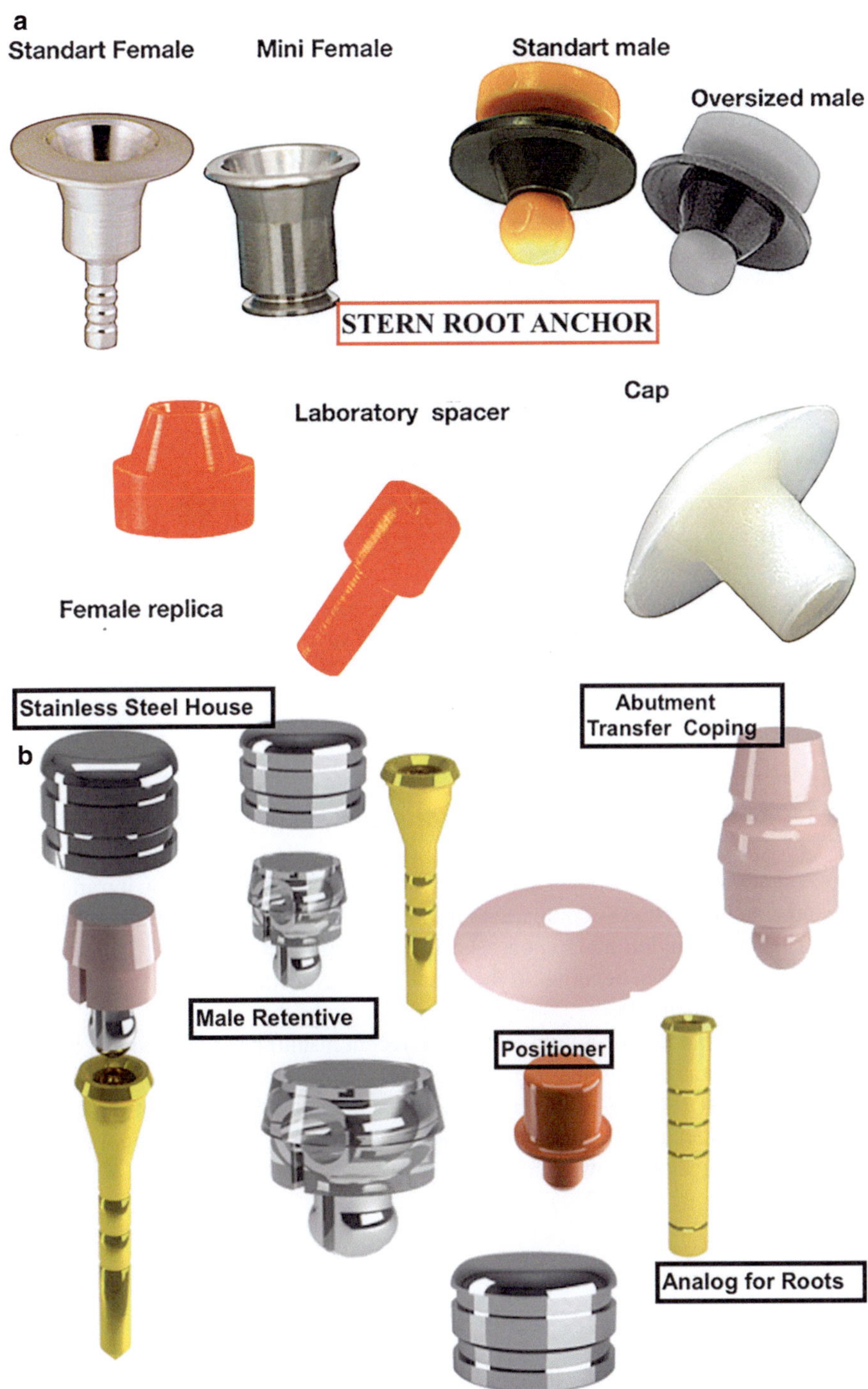

Fig. 3.74 (**a**) The Stern ROOT anchor intraradicular stud attachment and (**b, c**) the OT Reverse 3 direct pivot attachment

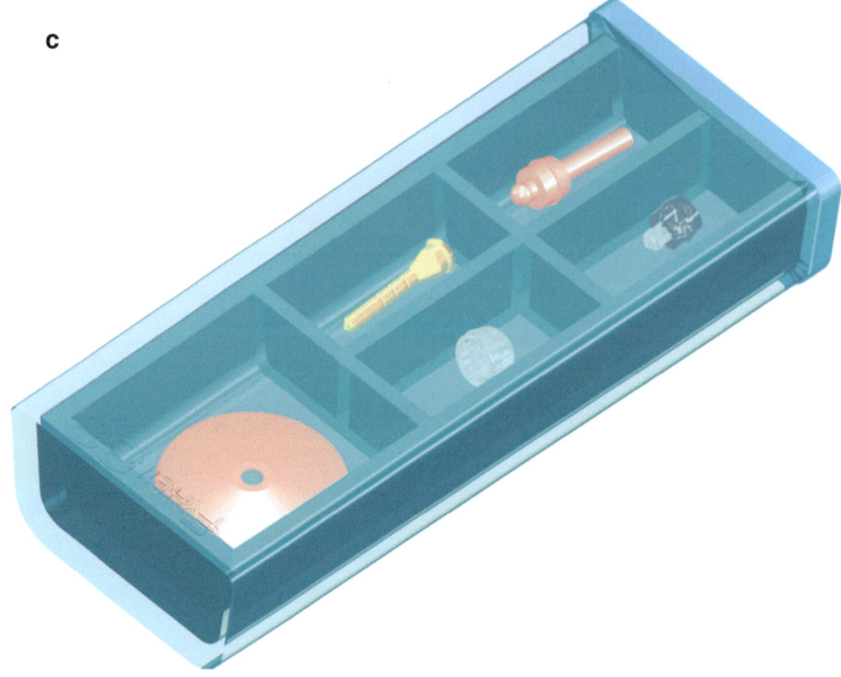

Fig. 3.74 (continued)

3.4.1 Zest Attachment (ZAAG Root Attachment System)

The Zest advanced anchorage generation (ZAAG) attachment is a new intraradicular stud attachment that is comparable to the Zest attachment but not interchangeable. The ZAAG nylon male is encased in a pivoting metal housing. This feature prevents the male from bending. In the metal housing, worn-out males can be easily replaced at the chairside.

The Zest advanced generation is the most recent installment in this line of highly developed intraradicular units. It is suitable for use with all dental appliances that utilize non-vital roots as abutments. The attachment is designed for direct root placement without a cast coping. For bridge alloys that require a cast coping, a precious or semi-precious crown may also be cast-to.

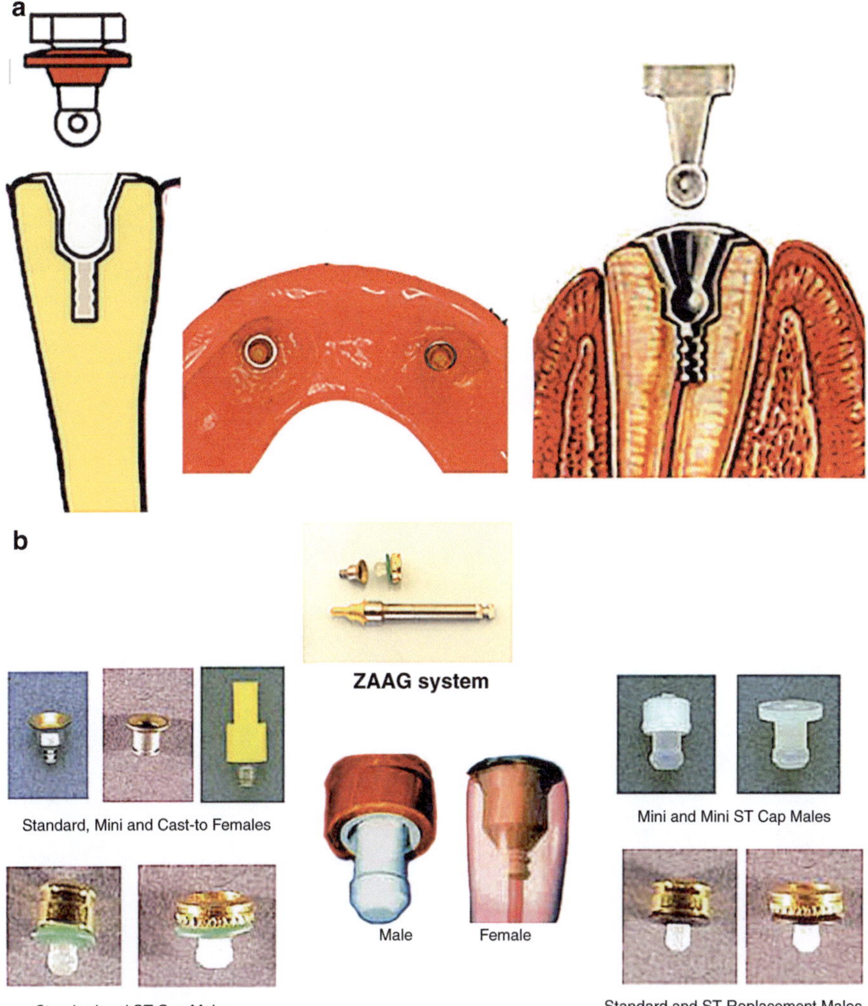

Fig. 3.75 (**a–c**) The ZAAG intraradicular stud attachment system

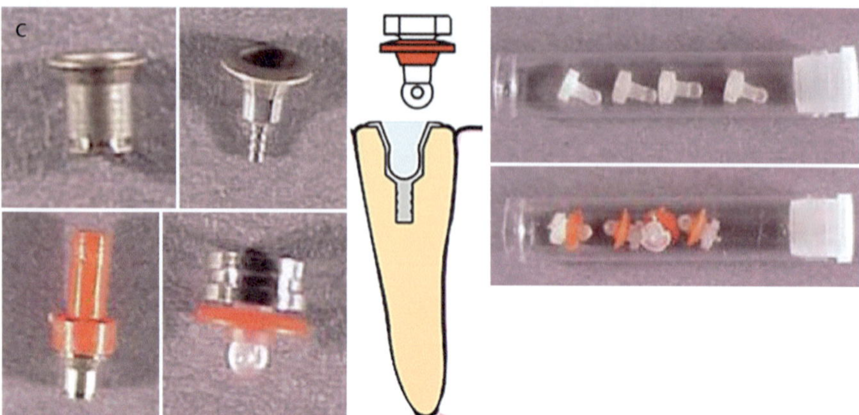

Fig. 3.75 (continued)

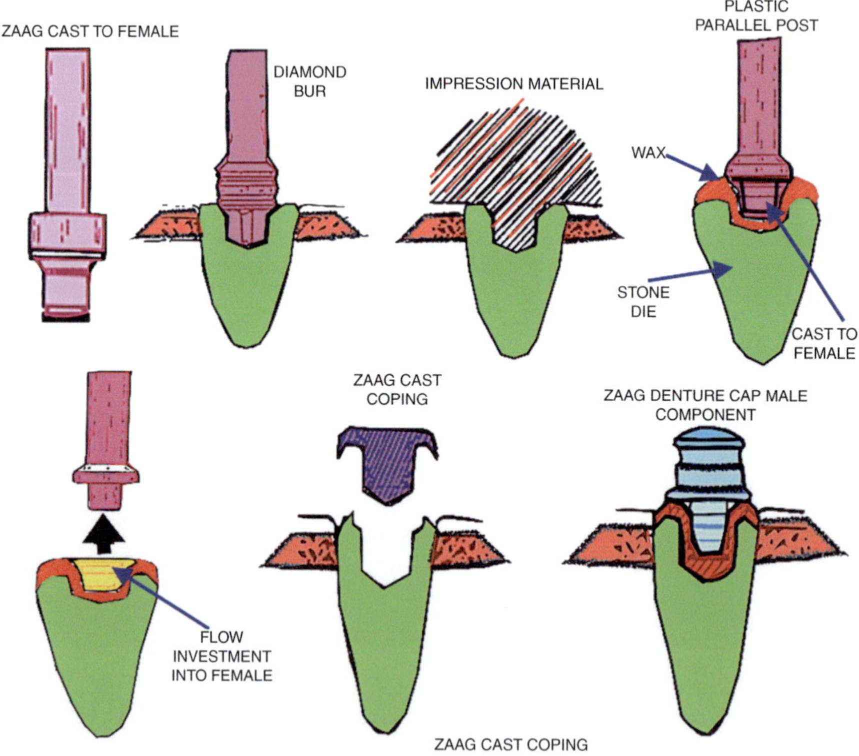

Fig. 3.76 Placement of the ZAAG intraradicular stud attachment with coping

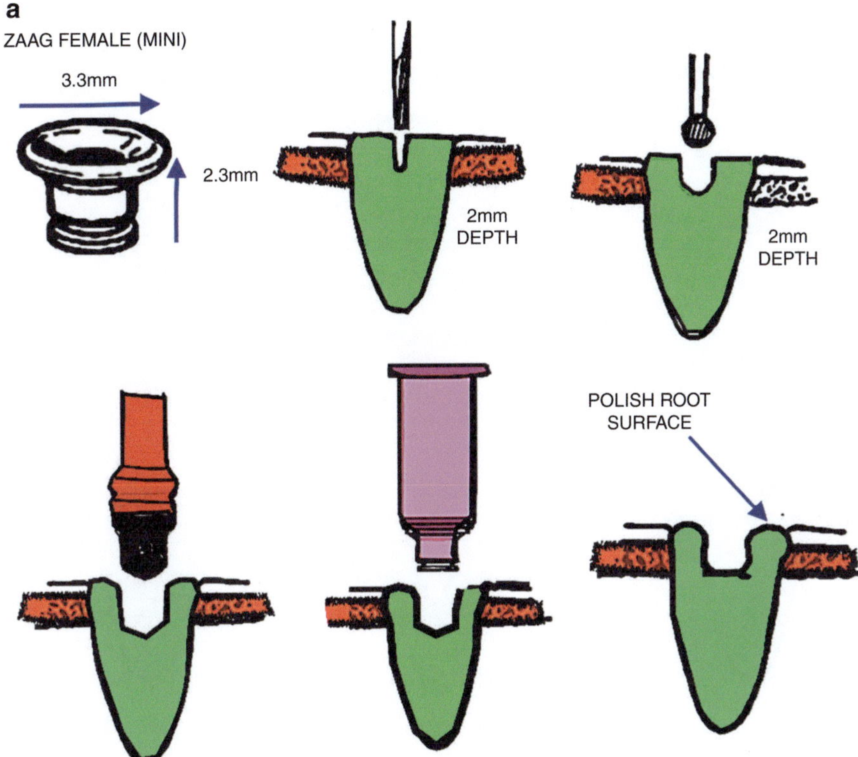

Fig. 3.77 (**a**) Placement of the ZAAG intraradicular stud attachment female (3.3 mm diameter) and (**b**) placement of the ZAAG intraradicular stud attachment female (3.8 mm diameter)

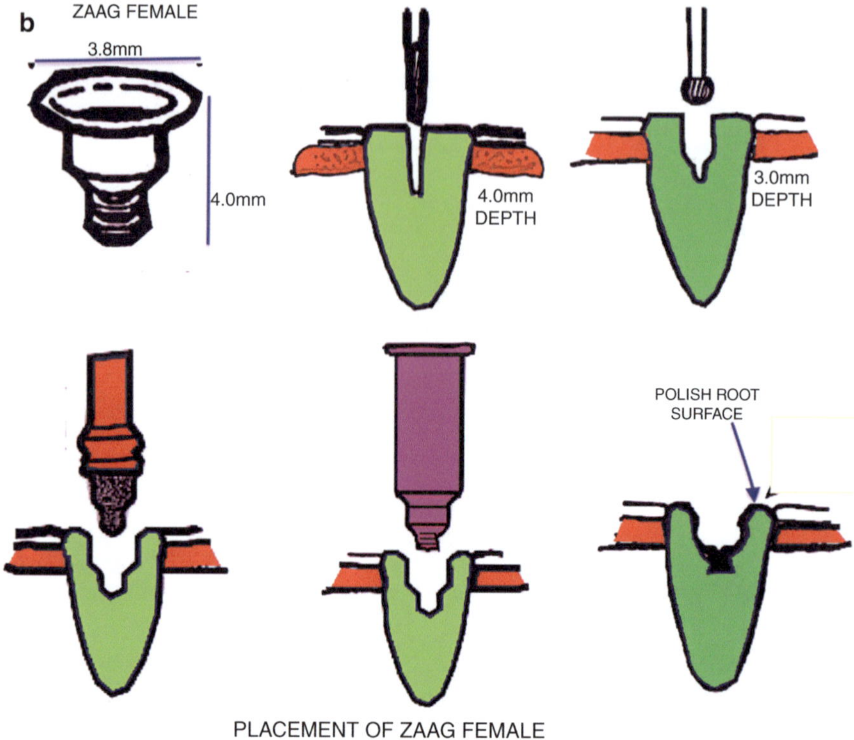

Fig. 3.77 (continued)

The retention of the impression surface of a denture with Zest attachments is derived from the root. Within the root, a post-preparation was made, and the female sleeve was cemented in place. As a chairside procedure, the male portion consists of a nylon post and a ball-head attachment to the overdenture. The post is inserted into the sleeve, and the overdenture is placed on top of it using self-curing resin. It was made up of a metal funnel cemented to the root canal of the endodontically treated tooth and a polyethylene structure extending from the denture base. This design reduces the need for vertical distance and the risk of the denture base weakening. There are two dimensions of Zest attachments, depending on the length and diameter of the root.

The systems' requirements are similar to the Rothermann attachment's vertical distance requirements, but with more straightforward technical specifications. It reduces the cost and eases the mechanical procedure (Fig. 3.75a–c).

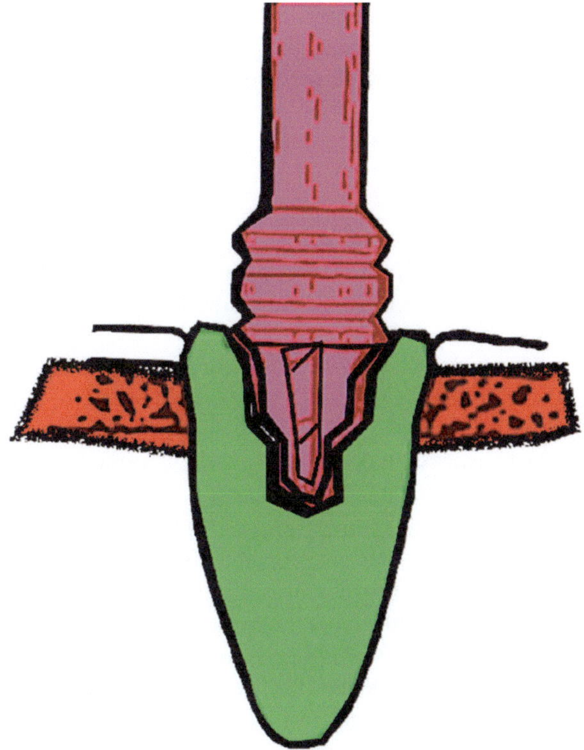

Fig. 3.78 Fabrication technique using the ZAAG One-Step Drill Standard

3.4.1.1 Features

- Subgingival attachment results in the application of forces close to the root's support center.
- A complete wear band on both the nylon male and the metal female extends the life of the attachment.
- The nylon male shaft's large diameter reduces bending and breakage.
- Rapid removal and snap-lock replacement of male dentures without the need to remove acrylic.
- Universal relief from joint stress with vertical resilience.

3.4.1.2 Advantages

- Exceeds any space limitations (when there is a small interocclusal distance).
- Reduces the leverage on the abutment tooth.
- The attachment process is straightforward.
- Due to the flexibility of the nylon, parallelism is not required if more than one tooth is used.
- This precise attachment system can be utilized for root preparation without requiring laboratory work.

3.4.1.3 Disadvantages

- There is technique sensitivity because there is no coping mechanism in place.
- Bendable nylon studs prevent seating (this part twists and prevents placement).
- Frequent recall visits are necessary to correct this.
- Without an overdenture, food particles can accumulate on the female reproductive organ.

3.4.1.4 ZAAG Cast Coping

When a cast gold crown covering and protecting the root surface is desired, a special ZAAG Cast-to-Female (Standard or Mini Size, without Titanium Nitride Coating) is used.

After endodontic treatment has been completed and the tooth structure has been reduced to the gingiva level, a beveled shoulder or chamfer margin is prepared on the tooth.

Drill a hole with the One Step Drill at a slow enough speed (750 RPM) to create a recessed seat on the occlusal surface. The Cast-to Drill is then utilized to create an adequate reduction preparation (and space) for the wax-up and Cast-to Female. The master mold and dies are prepared after an impression is made. Using a surveyor, the plastic paralleling post was positioned with the attached cast-female parallel to the other ZAAG attachment. Directly wax the female cast-to into the die. The stainless steel should be completely encased in wax up to, but not beyond, the plastic Paralleling Post junction. Utilize a hard wax to hold the female securely while removing the paralleling post. Following the manufacturer's instructions, the plastic Paralleling Post was removed, leaving the stainless-steel attachment cavity unobstructed for the flow of investment material. For casting root copings, the manufacturer recommends using only precious or semi-precious alloys. After polishing the coping, insert a male attachment into each Cast-to-Female and ensure that it fits properly. A male (stainless steel cap, nylon male, and centering sleeve) is snapped into each bonded coping for chairside pickup into the denture (Fig. 3.76; Picture 3.33).

3.4.1.5 The Female

After preparing and measuring study casts to determine the space available in the root for the standard size ZAAG Female (the width of the root surface must be equal to or greater than 4.0 mm), endodontic treatment is performed with the coronal surface of the root prepared as low as possible. A pilot hole is drilled to a depth of 4 mm and then enlarged to a depth of 3 mm using a carbide bur. Using the ZAAG Diamond Bur, the surgical stainless-steel female prefabrication was completed (Standard). On the occlusal surface of the root, the diamond bur should be used to a depth where a 360° recessed seat is created.

The ZAAG Parallel Post was used as a handle and tried in the metal female component to ensure proper fit. The metal female component was then cemented in place with composite resin cement or a durable adhesion material, and the root surface from the metal flange to the tissue was rounded off and polished (Fig. 3.77).

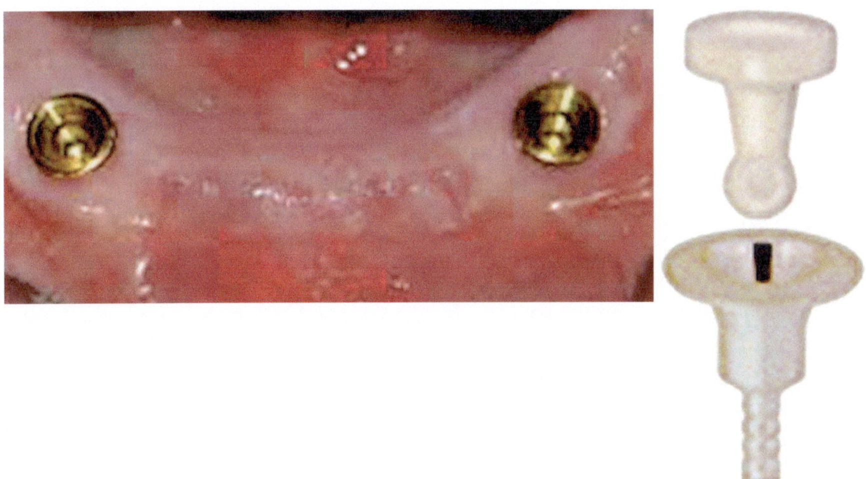

Picture 3.33 The ZAAG intraradicular attachment

3.4.1.6 Standard Fabrication Method Employing the ZAAG One-Step Drill

After reducing the non-vital teeth to the gingival level, drill a hole with the standard drill at a slow enough speed (750 RPM) to create a full 360° recessed seat on the occlusal surface of the dental root (Fig. 3.78).

3.4.1.7 Placement of the Female

After completing the preparation for the prefabricated stainless-steel female surgical instrument, accompanied by the ZAAG Diamond Bur (the diamond bur should be used to a depth where a full 360° recessed seat is created on the occlusal surface of the root), maintain the diamond bur's rotation throughout the entire procedure, including instrument insertion and removal. Utilizing the ZAAG Parallel Post as a handle, test the metal female's compatibility. Cement the female metal component in place with a composite resin cement or other durable adhesion material. After the cement has hardened, the root surface from the metal flange to the tissue should be rounded and polished.

Studies revealed that the ZAAG system provided high retentive forces; however, the increased retention led to greater forces and moments on the abutments. According to reports, the most common prosthetic complication associated with the ZAAG system is the loss of retention over time due to the wear of the male part. Comparing various stud attachments, Petropoulos et al. demonstrated that the Zest Anchor Advanced Generation Intraradicular Attachment System was highly retentive and resistant to dislodging forces. Epstein et al. investigated the difference in retention forces between six prefabricated attachment systems at initial placement and throughout 2000 insertions and removals of the denture. The authors discovered that ZAAG was one of the attachment systems exhibiting the least rate of change.

3.4.2   OT Reverse 3

OT Reverse 3 (OT 3) is a root-supported direct pivot attachment system for full dentures that provides retention and stability. Titanium is embedded within a soft nylon material to create the "split" male portion of the attachment. The female pivots have a distinctive shape designed to accommodate the majority of remaining root structures (Picture 3.34).

3.4.2.1 Placement of the Attachment

The diamond bur prepares the root for the attachment. Cement was applied after the plastic pivot was inserted using the handpiece. After affixing pivots to the root, the male transfer catheter was inserted into the pivot, and a laboratory impression was taken and sent. The technician poured the stone model after placing an analog into the impression (Picture 3.35a–e).

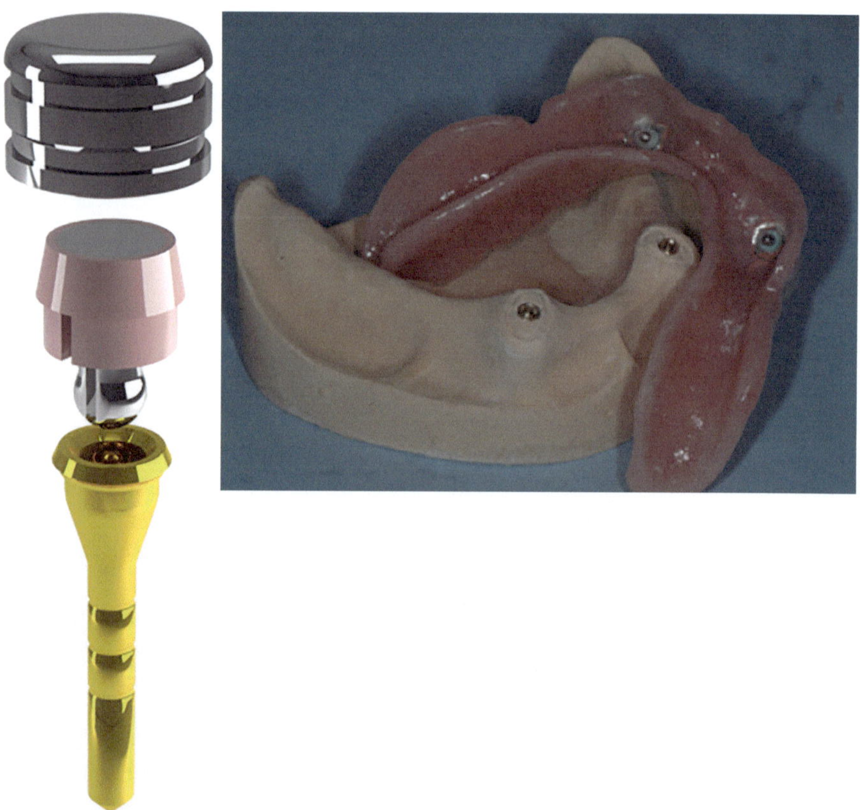

Picture 3.34 The OT Reverse 3 intraradicular attachment

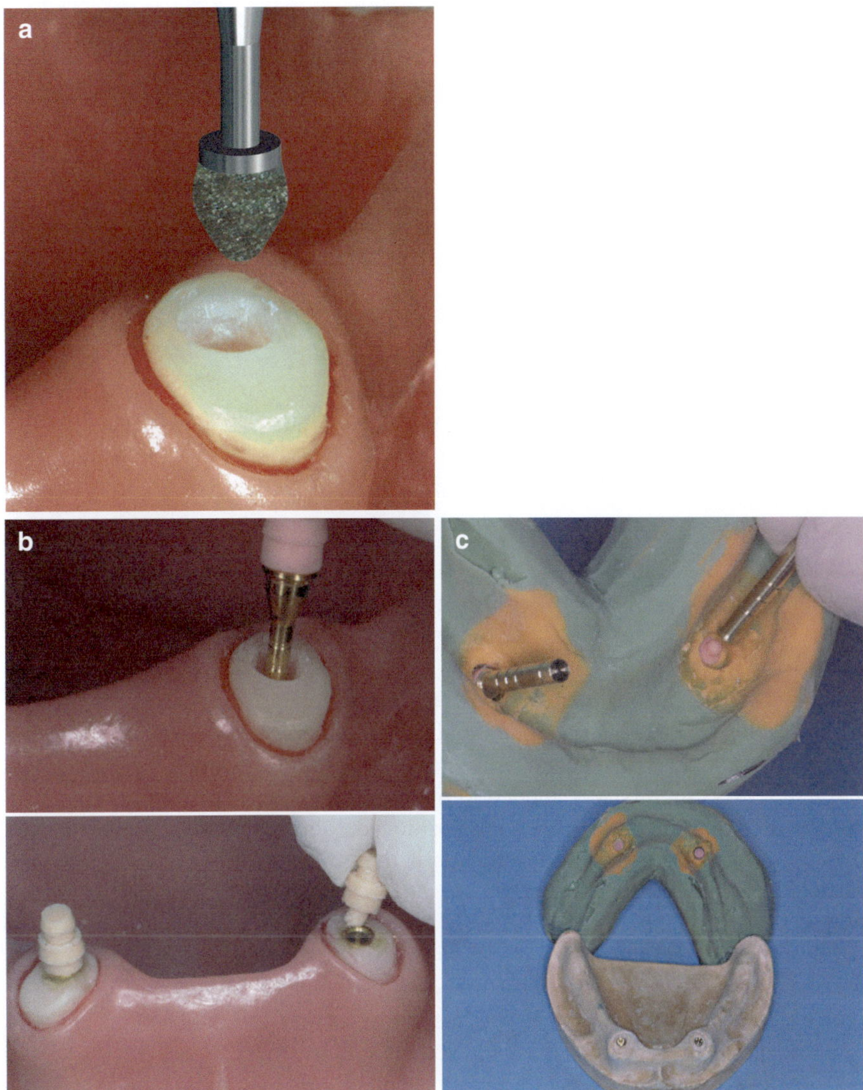

Picture 3.35 (a–e) Direct clinical application steps of the OT Reverse 3 intra-radicular attachment

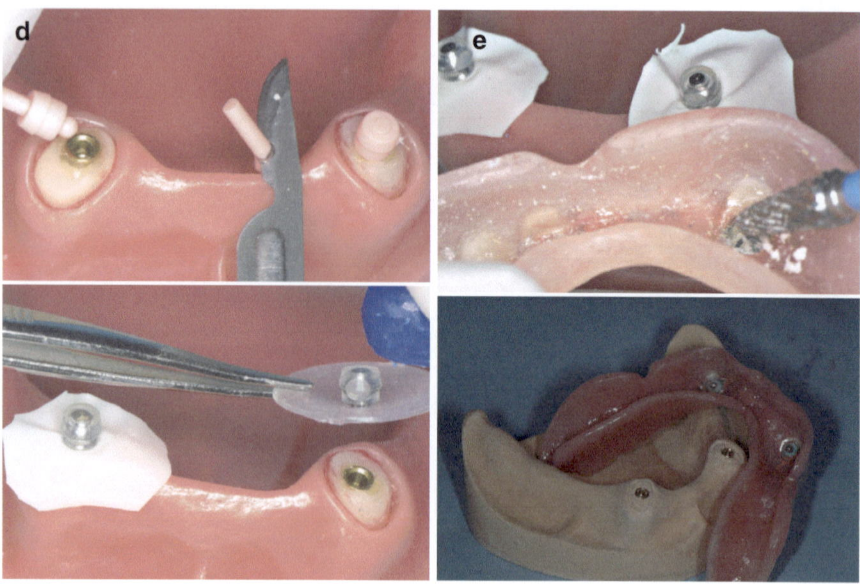

Picture 3.35 (continued)

3.4.2.2 Fabrication of Frame for Direct Roots

After pouring analogs into a stone mold, the denture setup and silicon guide are used to create space for the denture. The positioners were inserted into the analogs, and a thin layer of wax was applied to the gingival ridge. Using the surveyor, the sectioned OT Box housing of choice is positioned, followed by the reinforcement of the castable connectors. Self-curing resin is used to hold all of the parts together. Each tooth is fitted with a wax pin while the silicon mask provides additional support. On the model, the OT Box framework was removed, and any voids were filled with wax. Then, the procedures of investment and casting are executed. After casting, the reinforcement section of the framework is sandblasted, and opaque white or pink paint can be used to conceal the metal framework. The attachments are then inserted into the cast housings, and the denture is delivered.

3.4.2.3 Chairside Procedures

Remove the stem if the clinician decides to use the plastic retentive male. The male retentive plastic must be properly inserted. If the denture is improperly inserted, it may bend and no longer fit into the female housing. The attachment was then submerged in resin that hardens on its own. It is essential to always use the protective disk around the attachment's perimeter. When using OT Box Large, enlarge the space with a carbide bur to reduce male interference. The gaps should be filled with a resin that cures on its own. Insert the denture into the patient's mouth and instruct them to bite down until the resin hardens. Remove the prostheses and shave off any excess resin.

Further Reading

Abi Nader S, De Souzan RF, Fortin D, De Koninck L, Fromentin O, Albuquerque Junior RF. Effect of simulated masticatory loading on the retention of stud attachments for implant overdentures. J Oral Rehabil. 2011;38:157–64.

Alsiyabi AS, Felton DA, Cooper LF. E role of abutment- attachment selection in resolving inadequate interarch distance: a clinical report. J Prosthodont. 2005;14:184–9.

Assemat T, Amzalag G. Overlay dentures with push-button type axial attachment use of isolated roots for retention of overlay dentures. Inf Dent. 1990;72:867–75.

Bassi F. Comparing overdenture therapies with teeth and implant abutments. Int J Prosthodont. 2009;22:527–8.

Bureau GP. Tooth-supported stud retained prosthesis. Dent Update. 2003;30:389–94.

Castleberry DJ. Philosophies and principles of removable partial overdentures. Dent Clin N Am. 1990;34(4):589–92.

Chao YL, Meijer HJ, Van Oort RP, Versteegh PA. The incomprehensible success of the implant stabilized overdenture in the edentulous mandible: a literature review on the transfer of chewing forces to the bone surrounding implants. Eur J Prosthodont Restor Dent. 1995;3:255–61.

Chen L, Xie Q, Feng H, Lin Y, Li J. The masticatory efficiency of mandibular implant-supported overdentures as compared with tooth-supported overdentures and complete dentures. J Oral Implantol. 2002;28:238–43.

Chikunov I, Doan P, Vahidi F. Implant-retained partial overdenture with resilient attachments. J Prosthodont. 2008;17:141–8.

Cohen BI, Pagnillo M, Condos S, Deutsch AS. Comparative study of two precision overdenture attachment designs. J Prosthet Dent. 1996;76:145–52.

Chung K-H. Retention characteristics of attachment systems for implant overdentures. J Prosthodont. 2004;13:221–6.

Dodge CA. Prevention of complete denture problems by use of "Overdenture". J Prosthet Dent. 1973;30:403–6.

Evtimovska E. The change in retentive values of locator attachments and Hader clips over time. J Prosthodont. 2009;18:479–83.

Feine JS, de Grandmont P, Boudrias P, Brien N, LaMarche C, Tache R, et al. Within-subject comparisons of implant-supported mandibular prostheses: choice of prosthesis. J Dent Res. 1994;73:1105–11.

Gamborena JI, Hazelton LR, NaBadalung D, et al. Retention of ERA direct overdenture attachments before and after fatigue loading. Int J Prosthodont. 1997;10:123–30.

Alfred GH, Kundert M, Charles KC. Complete denture and overdenture prosthetics. New York: Thieme Medical Publishers Inc.; 1993.

Gotfredsen K, Holm B. Implant-supported mandibular overdentures retained with a ball or bar attachments: a randomized prospective 5-year. Int J Prosthodont. 2000;13:125–30.

Guttal SS, Tavargeri AK, Nadiger RK, Thakur SL. Use of an implant o-ring attachment for the tooth-supported mandibular overdenture: a clinical report. Eur J Dent. 2011;5:331–6.

Jain DC, Hegde V, Aparna IN, Dhanasekar B. Overdenture with access post system: a clinical report. Indian J Dent Res. 2011;22:359–61.

Krawczykowska H, Panek H. Applying the overdentures in the geriatric patients with residual and reduced dentition. Dent Med Probl. 2004;41:255–61.

Langer Y, Langer A. Root retained overdentures. Part I– Biomechanical and clinical considerations. J Prosthet Dent. 1991;66:784–9.

Majer HJ. E stern ERA attachment. Exacting retention made easy. J Can Dent Assoc. 1992;58:615.

Meijer HJ, Raghoebar GM, can't Hof MA, Geertman ME, van Oort RP. Implant-retained mandibular overdentures compared with complete dentures: a 5-years follow-up of clinical aspects and patient satisfaction. Clin Oral Implants Res. 1999;10:238–44.

Menicucci G, Lorenzetti M, Pera P, Preti G. Mandibular implant-retained overdentures a clinical trial of two attachment systems. Int J Oral Maxillofac Implants. 1998;13:851–6.

Mensor MC. Removable partial overdentures with mechanical (precision) attachments. Dent Clin N Am. 1990;34:669–81.

Mericske-Stern R, Piotti M, Sirtes G. 3-D in vivo force measurements on mandibular implants supporting overdentures. Clin Oral Implants Res. 1996;7:387–96.

Morrow RM, Feldmann EE, Rudd KD, Trovillion HM. Tooth-supported complete dentures. Approach to preventive prosthodontics. J Prosthet Dent. 1969;21:513–22.

Morrow RM. Handbook of Immediate overdentures. St. Louis, MO: Mosby; 1978. p. 48.

Pavlatos J. The root-supported overdenture using the Locator overdenture attachment. General Dent. 2001;50:448–53.

Petropoulos VC, Smith W. Maximum dislodging forces of implant overdenture stud attachments. Int J Oral Maxillofac Implant. 2002;17:526–35.

Preiskel HW. Overdentures made easy: a guide to implant and root supported prostheses. Chicago, IL: Quintessence; 1999. p. 189–232.

Prieskel HW. Precision attachments in prosthodontics over denture and telescopicture prosthesis, vol. 2. Chicago, IL: Quintessence International; 1985.

Quirynen M, Naert I, van Steenberghe D, Dekeyser C, Callens A. Periodontal aspects of osseointegrated fixtures supporting a partial bridge. An up to 6-years retrospective study. J Clin Periodontol. 1992;19:118–26.

Reitz PV, Weine MG, Levin B. An overdenture survey: preliminary report. J Prosthet Dent. 1977;37:246–58.

Rissin L, House JE, Manly RS, Kapur KK. Clinical comparison of the masticatory performance and electromyographic activity of patients with complete dentures, overdentures, and natural teeth. J Prosthet Dent. 1978;39:508–11.

Rodrigues RC, Faria AC, Macedo AP, Sartori IA, de Matros MD, Ribeiro RF. An in vitro study of non-axial forces upon the retention of an O-ring attachment. Clin Oral Implants Res. 2009;20:1314–9.

Rutkunas V, Mizutani H, Takahashi H. Evaluation of stable retentive properties of overdentures attachments. Baltic Dent Maxillofac J. 2005;7:115–20.

Rutkunas V, Mizutani H, Takahashi H. Influence of attachment wear on retention of mandibular overdenture. J Oral Rehabil. 2007;34:41–51.

Rutkunas V, Mizutani A, Takahashi H. Wear simulation effects on overdentures stud attachments. Dent Mater J. 2011;30:845–53.

Sadowsky SJ, Caputo AA. Effect of attachment systems and extension base contact on load transfer with mandibular implant-retained overdentures. J Prosthet Dent. 2000;84:327–33.

Samra RK, Bhide SV, Goyal C, Kaur T. Tooth supported overdenture: a concept overshadowed but not yet forgotten! J Oral Res Rev. 2015;7:16–21.

Schuch C, Pinheiro de Moraes A, Onofre RS, Cenci TP, Boscato N. An alternative method for the fabrication of a root-supported overdenture: a clinical report. J Prosthet Dent. 2013;109:1–4.

Schwartz IS, Morrow RM. Overdentures. Principles and procedures. Dent Clin N Am. 1996;40:169–94.

Shah FK, Gebreel A, Elshokouki A, Habib AA, Porwal A. Comparison of the immediate complete denture, tooth and implant-supported overdenture on vertical dimension and muscle activity. J Adv Prosthodont. 2012;4:61–71.

Sposetti VJ, Gibbs CH, Alderson TH, Jaggers JH, Richmond A, Conlon M, Nickerson DM. Bite force and muscle activity in overdentures wearers before and after attachment placement. J Prosthet Dent. 1986;55:265–73.

Staub SL, Teubner E, Zitzmann NU. Clinical follow-up evaluation of Dalbo®-Rotex® retention elements in private practice. Swiss Dent J. 2018;12:210–6.

Steen RP, White V, Markowitz NR. E use of ball clip attachments with an implant-supported primary-secondary bar overdenture. J Oral Implantol. 2004;30:234–9.

Tallagren A. The continuing reduction of the residual alveolar ridges in complete denture wearers: a mixed-longitudinal study covering 25 years. 1972. J Prosthet Dent. 2003;89:427–35.

Thayer HH, Caputo AA. Occlusal force transmission by overdenture attachments. J Prosthet Dent. 1979;41:266–71.

Thayer HH, Caputo AA. Photoelastic stress analysis of overdenture attachments. J Prosthet Dent. 1980;43:611–7.

Tokuhisa M, Matsushita Y, Koyan K. In vitro study of a mandibular implant overdenture retained with the ball, magnet, or bar attachment: comparison of load transfer and denture stability. Int J Prosthodont. 2003;16:128–34.

Tokuhisa M, Matsushita Y, Koyano K. In vitro study of a mandibular implant overdenture retained with the ball, magnet, or bar attachments: comparison of load transfer and denture stability. Int J Prosthodont. 2003;16:128–34.

Van Kampen F, Cune M, van der Bilt A, Bosman F. Retention and postinsertion maintenance of bar-clip, ball and magnet attachments in mandibular implant overdenture treatment: An in vivo comparison an er three months of function. Clin Oral Implants Res. 2003;14:720–6.

Van Waas MA, Jonkman RE, Kalk W, Van't Hof MA, Plooij J, Van Os JH. Differences two years after tooth extraction in a mandibular bone reduction in patients treated with immediate overdentures or with immediate complete dentures. J Dent Res. 1993;72:1001–4.

Verma R, Joda T, Brägger U, Wittneben JG. A systematic review of the clinical performance of tooth-retained and implant-retained double crown prostheses with a follow-up of =three3 years. J Prosthodont. 2013;22:2–12.

Wolf K, Ludwig K, Hartfil H, Kern M. Analysis of retention and wear of ball attachments. Quintessence Int. 2009;40:405–12.

Wang X, Ohkubo C, Hosoi T, Shimpo H, Kurihara D, Murata T. Retentive forces of 3 types of attachments for root-retained overdentures. Prosthodont Res Pract. 2007;6:104–8.

Williamson RT. Retentive bar overdenture fabrication with preformed castable components. a case report. Quintessence Int. 1994;25:389–94.

Winkler S, Piermatti J, Rothman A, Siamos G. An overview of the O-ring implant overdenture attachment: clinical reports. J Oral Implantol. 2002;28:82–6.

Yadav B, Guttal S. Implant O-ring attachment used for tooth-borne overdenture. Int J Prosthodont Restor Dent. 2013;3:115–8.

Bar Attachments Used in Tooth-Supported Overdentures

4

Yılmaz Umut Aslan

4.1 Bar Attachments

Implant-supported restorations and bar-retained teeth are the most common types of prosthetic treatment. A bar attachment—as compared to a stud attachment such as a Locator, O-Ring, Ball, or Magnet—provides greater denture stability (ideal for a patient with a flat or atrophied residual ridge), splinting of questionable implants, and will readily compensate for divergent implants. This type of attachment is commonly used for overdentures (tooth/implant) if adequate vertical space is available and patients have good oral hygiene. If the patient oral hygiene is poor, the dexterty and ability of practising good hygiene should be improved for an extended bar pontic area.

The secondary advantage of bars is that they splint the abutments together, which protects weak implants and roots and is frequently indicated in the softer bone of the maxilla. As a result of their proximity to the alveolar bone and the rotation point of the tooth, bar attachments reduce the lever force on the teeth (Figs. 4.1, 4.2, 4.3, 4.4, 4.5, 4.6, 4.7, 4.8, and 4.9; Pictures 4.1, 4.2, 4.3, 4.4, 4.5, 4.6, 4.7, and 4.8).

The Advantages of Bar Attachments.

- They are applicable to both teeth- and implant-supported prostheses.
- They can reinforce the support of teeth or implants with splints.
- These connections improve retention and stability.
- They are capable of being affixed to non-parallel teeth or implants.
- They permit the rotation of the denture in place.
- The load is distributed across the teeth, implants, bars, and soft tissues.

Y. U. Aslan (✉)
Faculty of Dentistry, Department of Prosthodontics, Marmara University, Istanbul, Turkey
e-mail: umut.aslan@marmara.edu.tr

© The Author(s), under exclusive license to Springer Nature Switzerland AG 2023
Y. Özkan (ed.), *Treatment Options Before and After Edentulism*,
https://doi.org/10.1007/978-3-031-37582-8_4

Disadvantages of Bar Attachments.

- Clinical and laboratory processes require technical skills.
- There can be some problems during the placement of artificial teeth (aesthetic problems) due to the bulkiness of the bars.
- The bar attachment placed lingually to the crest limits the tongue distance, and if placed labially to the crest causes rotational movement.
- Difficulty in plaque control (maintenance of oral hygiene) is complicated which can lead to problems like mucosal irritation.
- They require sufficient vertical and buccolingual dimensions according to the crest formation.
- The higher cost compares to the stud attachments.
- Frequent retention loss of clips.

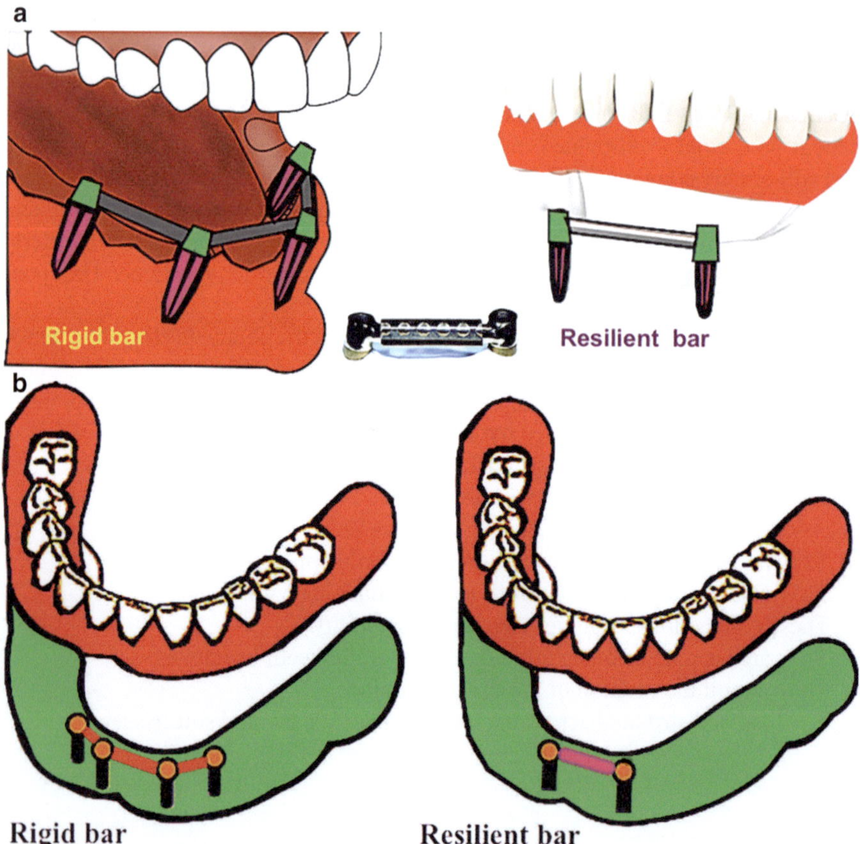

Fig. 4.1 (**a–c**) Rigid and resilient bar attachment used in TSO, (**d**) rigid bar attachment used for splinting the mandibular few and weak supporting teeth

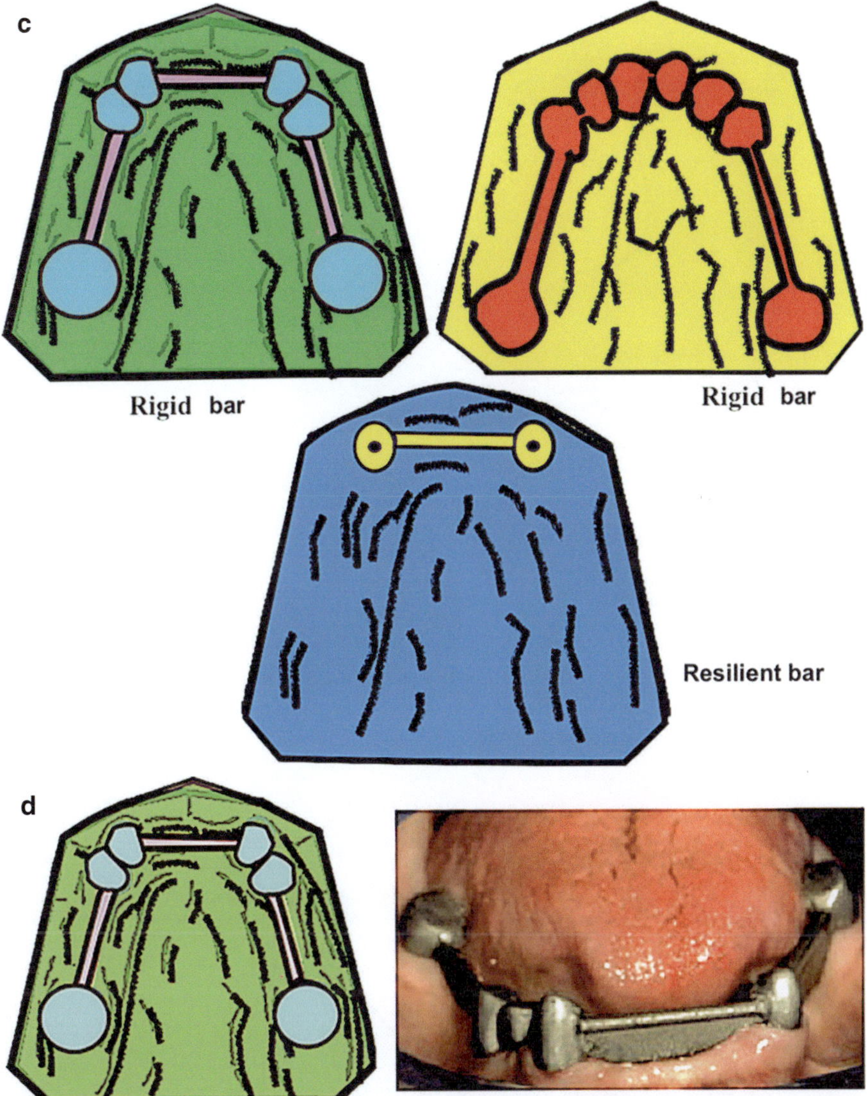

Fig. 4.1 (continued)

A typical bar attachment assembly for tooth-supported overdenture (TSO) consists of a one-piece cast bar that is connected to copings that are cemented to the supporting teeth as direct retainers. Two or more teeth are splinted with a bar, with retention provided by a "clip" or "sleeve" attached to the bar. The bar and clip are the connecting elements between the teeth and the overdenture, where the bar connects and splints the teeth and the clip is located on the denture's fitting surface (Fig. 4.2).

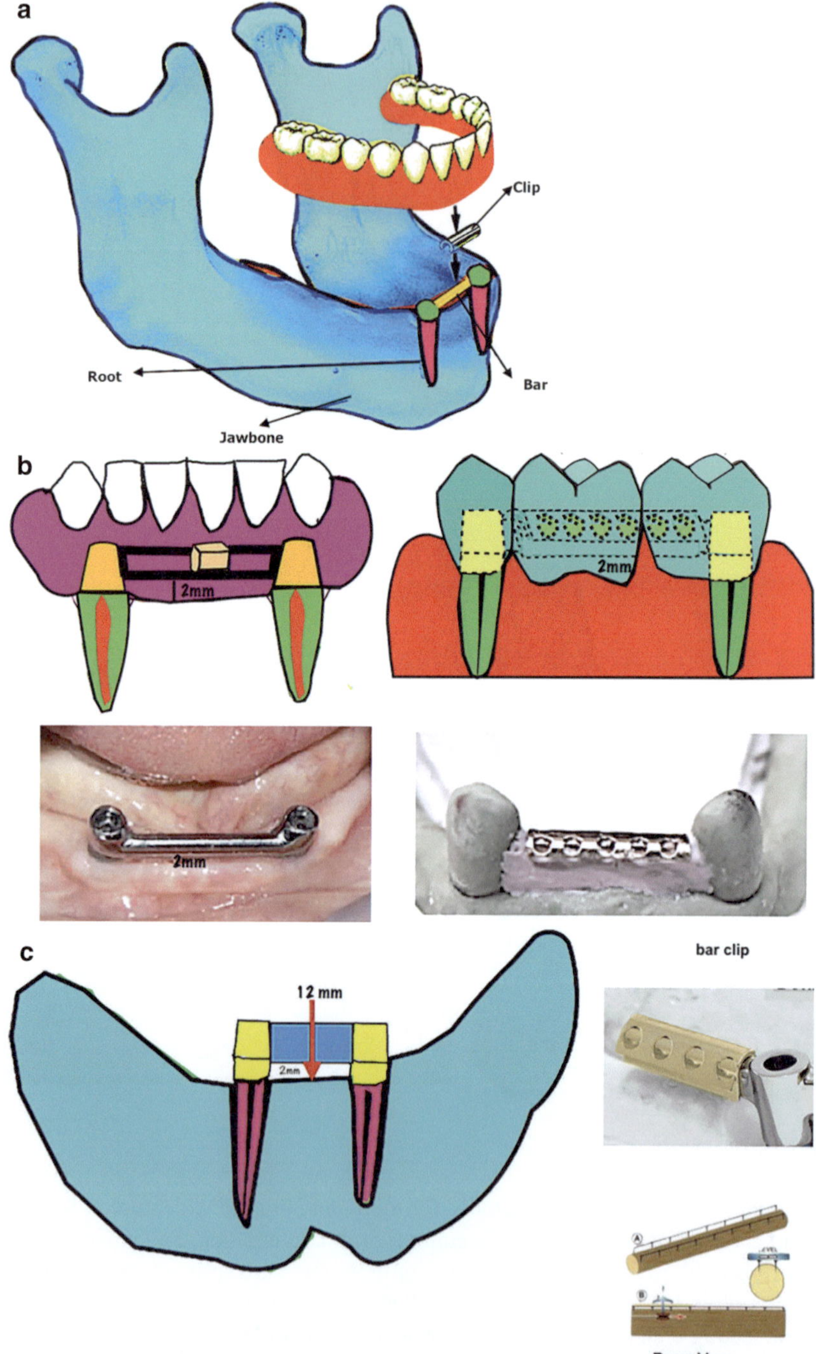

Fig. 4.2 (**a**) The bar assembly is widely used in the TSO, (**b**, **c**) bar attachments generally are combined with the copings on root canal–treated teeth (the most tissue-born available, it allows for both vertical and rotational movement)

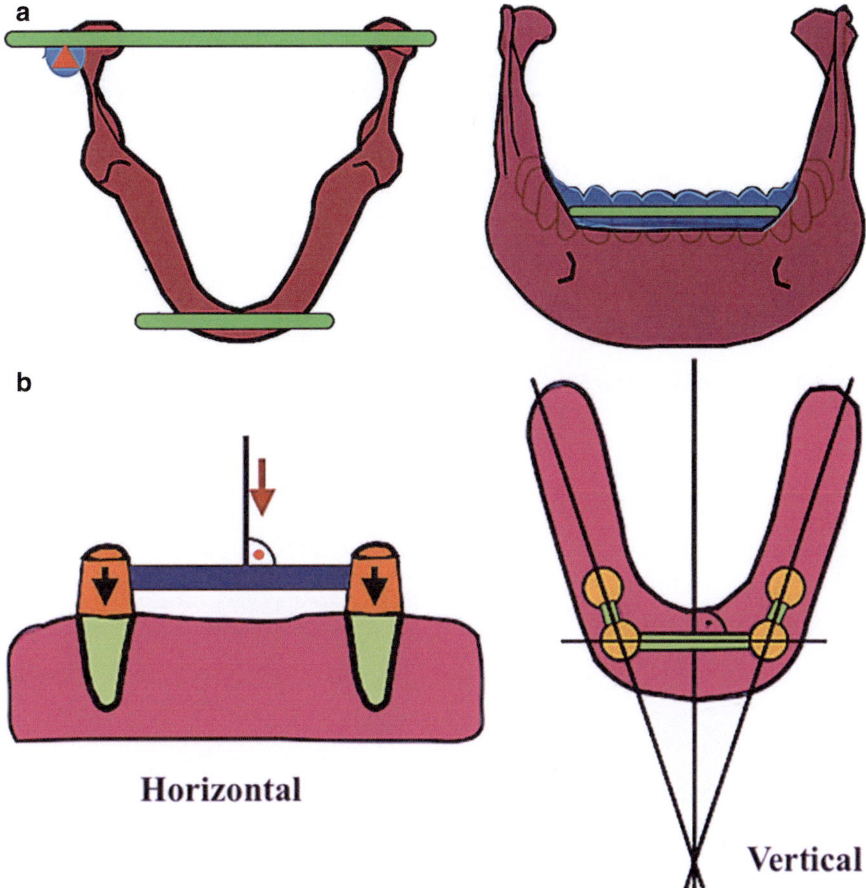

Fig. 4.3 (**a**) The bar should be positioned horizontally to the ideal occlusal plane and the arbitrary hinge axis, (**b**) the bar attachment should be placed vertically on the midline

The bar attachment could be made from a pre-milled castable plastic pattern (castable; the bar is cast with any alloy with coping; plastic wax burnout patterns are recommended when employing a rapid burnout technique) or prefabricated forms (it may be constructed by soldering prefabricated metal parts, usually from gold alloys). It can also be manufactured using CAD/CAM technology. The shape of prefabricated bars is either round, ovoid, or U-shaped. Frequently, soldering or laser welding is required to achieve the proper framework adaptation. In addition to compensating for the accuracy loss caused by clinical and laboratory errors, the prefabricated bars should reduce material distortion, fabrication time, and fabrication costs. The CAD/CAM bars are fabricated from a titanium or titanium alloy block. Typically, the denture is fabricated, and the stone cast and wax model are optically scanned to generate their exact 3D images. The data is transmitted to the milling machine, which then forms the bar. Because CAD/CAM technology reduces

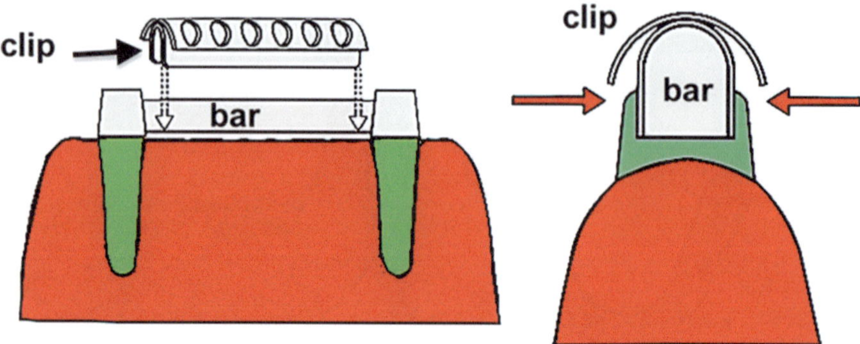

Fig. 4.4 The rigid Dolder bar form is U-shaped with parallel walls. Due to its U shape, this bar does not move

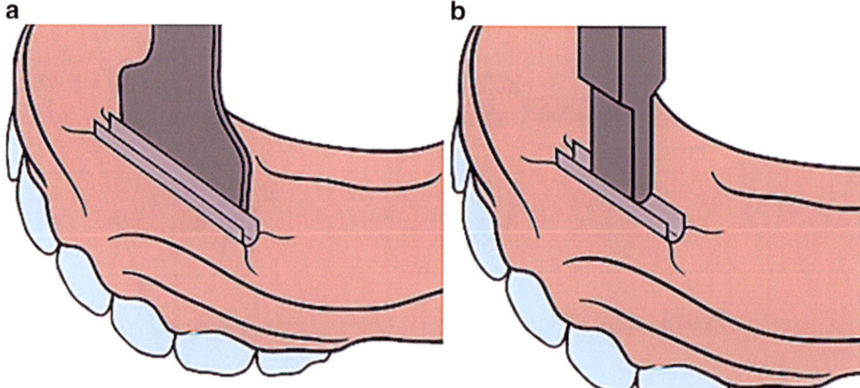

Fig. 4.5 (**a**) The activator tool is used to push the sleeve carefully inwards for activation, (**b**) the deactivator tool is pushed into the sleeve for deactivating

specific human errors, milled bars are typical of high quality and free of pores (Picture 4.1d). If the horizontal distance between the implants in implant-supported dentures is too short to permit the construction of a bar of adequate length, precision attachments may be incorporated into the bar to provide additional stability (Picture 4.1e). Short distal extensions may also be added to the bar attachment. The short distal extensions cause the flexible bar attachment to become rigid, contributing to the denture's stability and preventing rotation. Other in vitro and in vivo research has not confirmed these findings. In addition, neither the length of the cantilever nor the use of extensions (cantilevers) is possible without taking into account the restrictions they impose on rotational freedom.

Commonly used bar systems fall into three categories:

1. Hader or Dolder bar configurations with direct retainers.
2. Integrated into the bar, including Locator and Clix bar attachments.

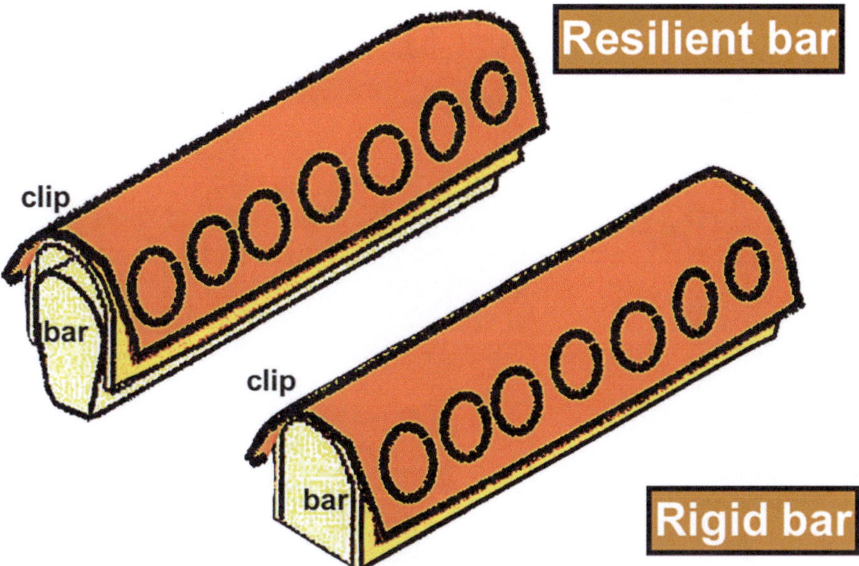

Fig. 4.6 Rigid and resilient Dolder bar

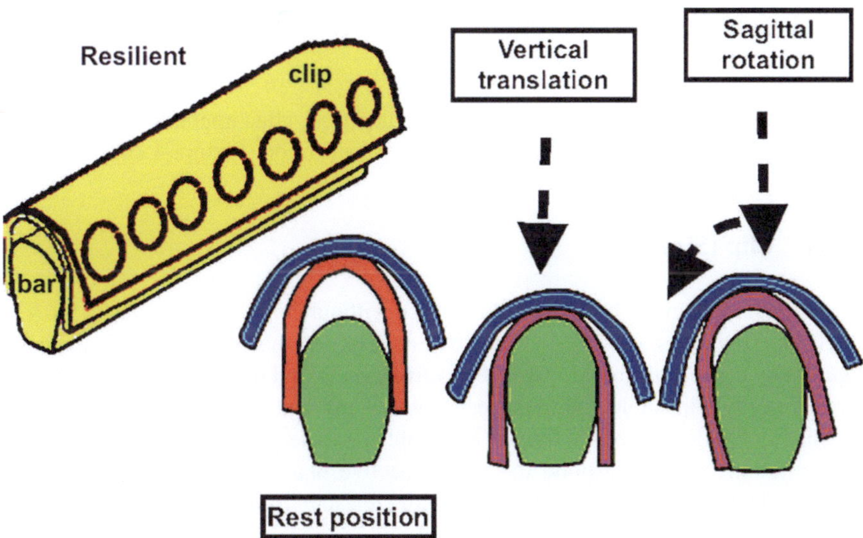

Fig. 4.7 Movement is seen in resilient Dolder bar

3. Offset attachments, such as the Plunger Loc, Sagix, and Vertix.

Typically, bar attachments, such as a Hader bar or Dolder bar attachment, are used as direct retainers. When vertical space is limited, Universal Plunger Loc,

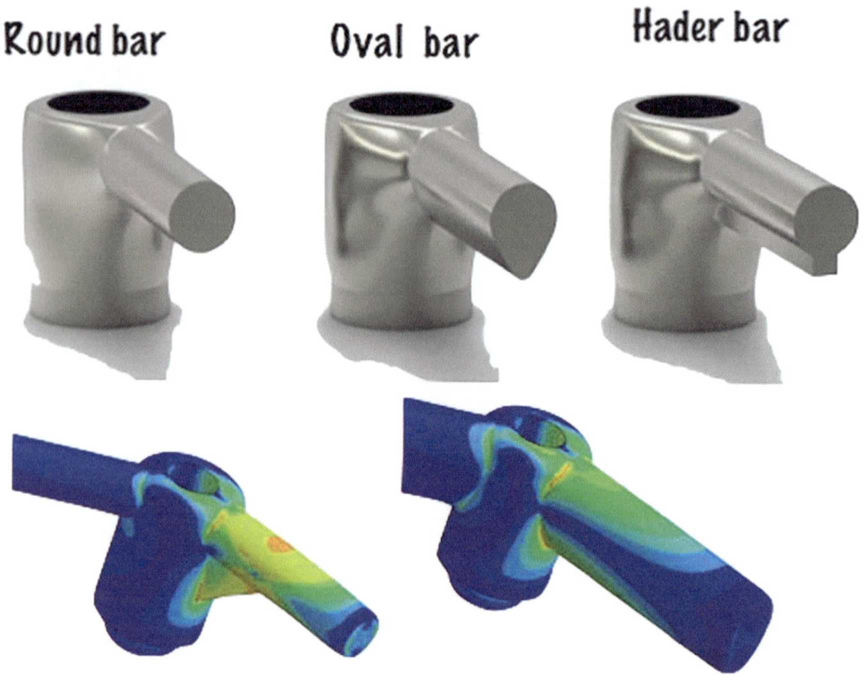

Fig. 4.8 The round, oval, and Hader bar cross-section

Sagix, or Vertix attachments are utilized. In addition, attachments such as a Clix, Locator, or Ceka are added to the bar to improve retention (Picture 4.1e).

4.1.1 Clip (Sleeve)

Clips are placed on the bar's superior surface without contacting the elastic flanges on its tapering sides. Clips are available in a variety of materials, lengths, and configurations that correspond to their respective plastic and metal bar systems. Metal clips are fully adjustable and more resistant to wear, and their elastic flanges allow for smaller bar dimensions. Clips are available in a variety of materials, lengths, and configurations that correspond to their respective plastic and metal bar systems. Clips made of metal are fully adjustable, more resistant to wear, and can be made in smaller sizes. However, removing a metal clip is more difficult than removing a plastic clip and requires more chairside time for prosthesis placement. The plastic clip is easily inserted into a metal housing with a light amount of pressure from a specific tool and is then integrated into the denture base. This makes their replacement simple and time-efficient. Plastic Hader/EDS clips cannot be adjusted, but they are easily replaceable at the chairside. For bar attachment overdentures, a metal housing with Hader or EDS plastic clips is typically recommended. They are

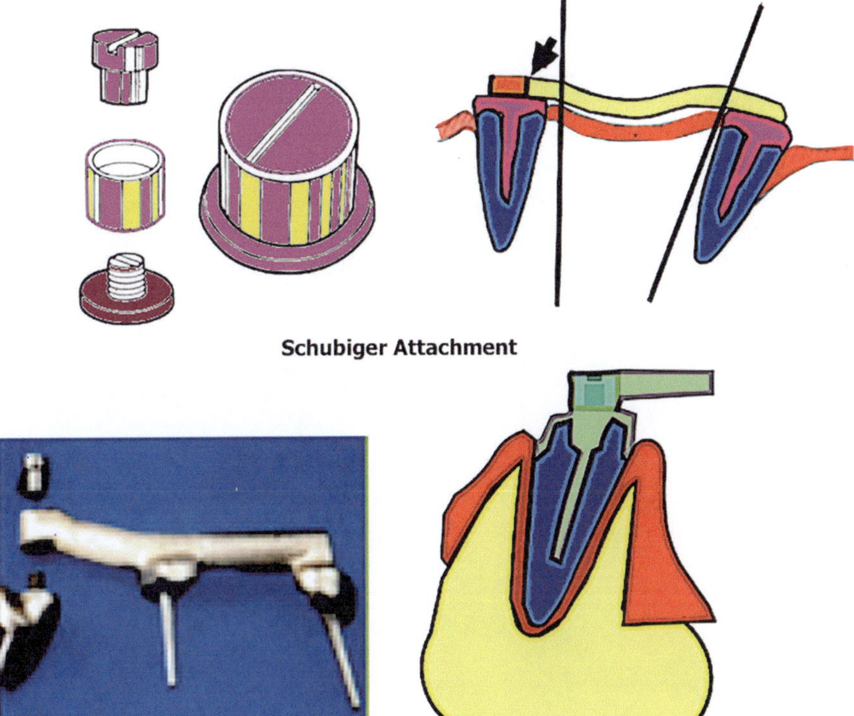

Fig. 4.9 The Schubiger attachment; if the post of the copings cannot be made parallel to seat the soldered bar, then a Schubiger unit is used

typically color-coded and come in a variety of hardnesses according to the desired retention force.

In general, resilient clips are easier and less expensive to replace than metal clips. As their retention decreases with clinical use, however, they should be replaced more frequently. The denture can be clinically placed using auto-polymerizing acrylic, while a metal clip can be easily replaced. However, the nylon clip cannot be adjusted or reactivated like the metal clip (Figs. 4.4, 4.6, and 4.7; Picture 4.2).

If the distance between the abutments is sufficient, a single clip is recommended. If the available length is limited, two shorter clips may be utilized. In contrast, a single long clip is typically preferred (Fig. 4.3).

4.1.2 The Processing Method of Clip to Denture

The clips are embedded in the denture base either directly or in a prefabricated "housing." The placement of the denture clip can occur either in the laboratory (indirectly) or chairside (direct). The direct technique necessitates extreme caution when positioning the clips, as no resin should flow beneath the bar; otherwise, it would be difficult to remove the denture after polymerization. During laboratory processing for the indirect technique, the clip is attached.

Presented is an alternative method for attaching the clip to a metallic superstructure. This method combines the benefits of direct and indirect techniques for attaching the nylon clip of the bar to the denture base. Some systems feature a spacer that can be connected during the processing phase. When the prosthesis is in place in the patient's mouth, the spacer creates a gap between the clip and the bar. During the function, the denture is capable of some vertical movement to provide occlusal load support in addition to abutment support (Picture 4.3).

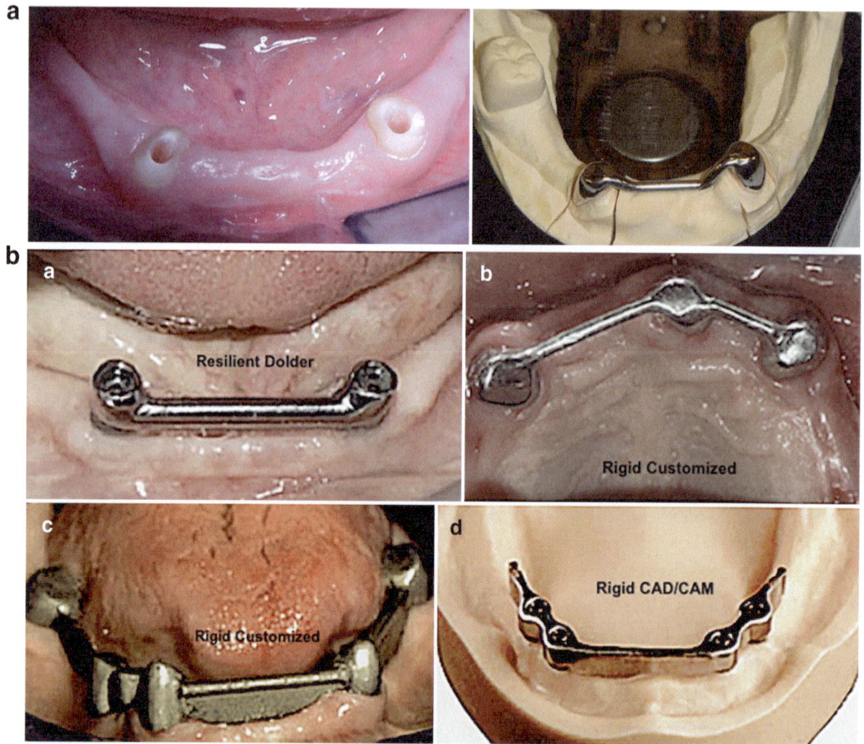

Picture 4.1 Different types of bar attachment using an implant and tooth-supported overdenture: (**a**) The customized round bar followed ridge contour; (**b**) *a* the Dolder bar using two implant-supported overdenture, *b* rigid custom bar cast CoCr alloys for maxillary TSO, *c* rigid custom bar cast CoCr alloys for mandibular TSO, and *d* rigid custom bar cast CoCr mandibular implant overdenture; (**c**) customized and prefabricated bar attachment; (**d**) CAD-CAM bar attachment for maxillary implant overdenture; (**e**) different types of attachment used with the bar attachment overdenture

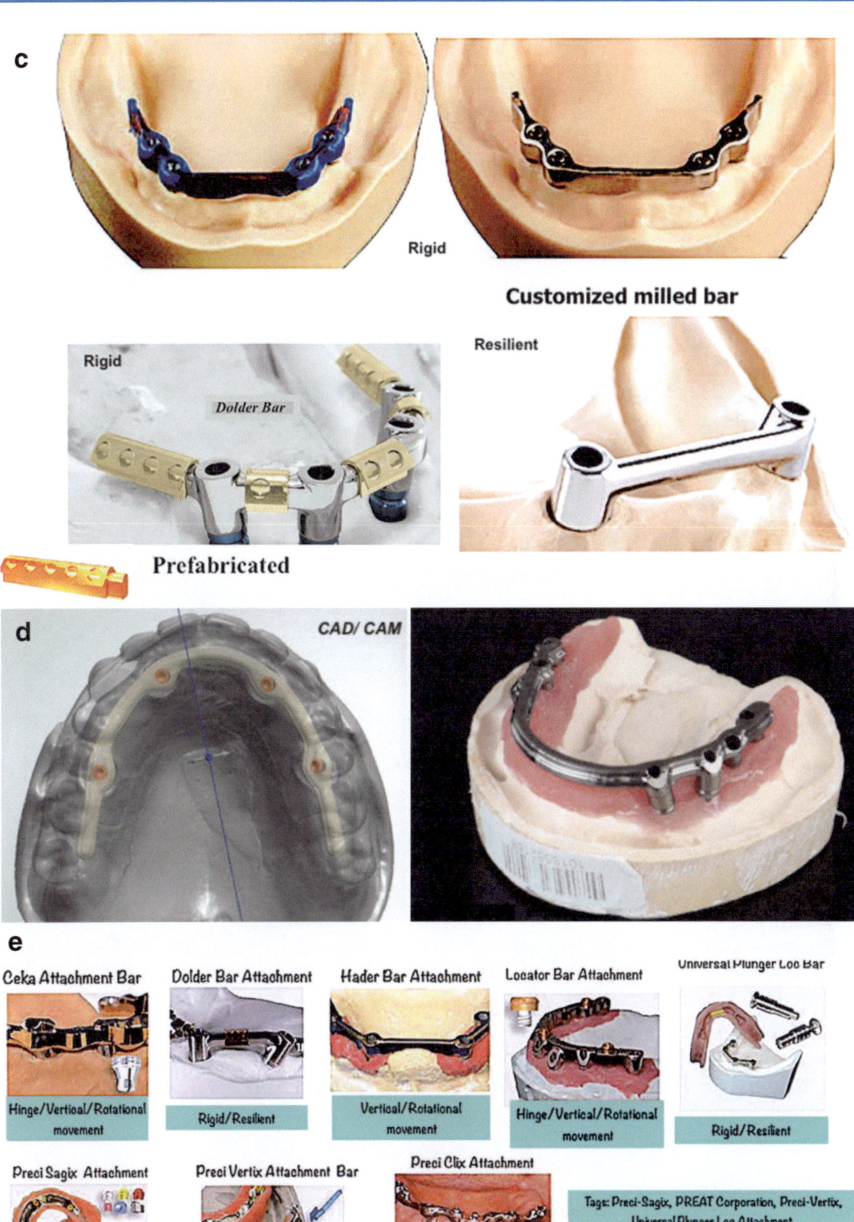

Picture 4.1 (continued)

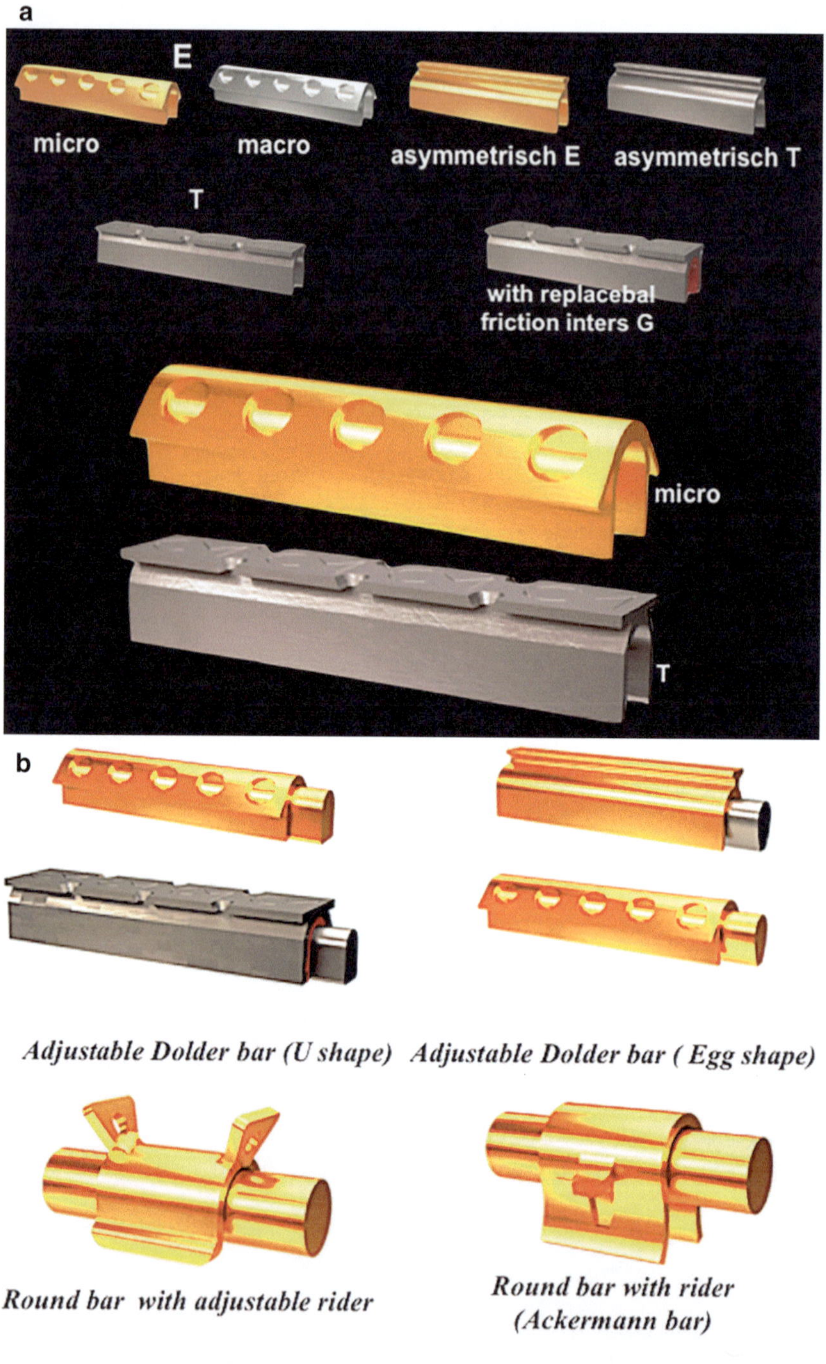

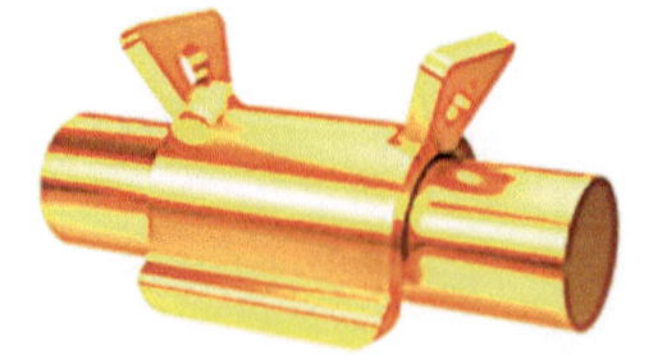

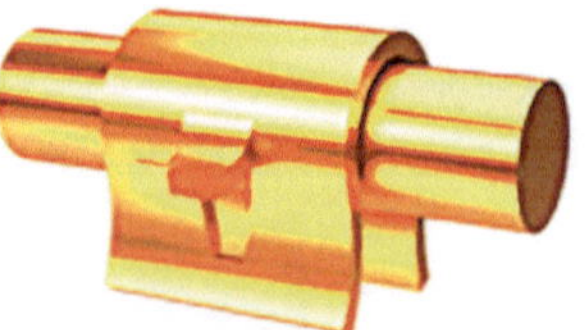

Picture 4.2 (**a**) Dolder gold/metal female part (rider), (**b**) adjustable rigid and resilient bars, (**c**) Hader bar plastic rider/metal house and CM gold rider, (**d**) Ackermann Gold clip (MD and BL version), (**e**) Hader plastic rider and metal house placed on the metal framework, (**f**) metal rider placed on zirconia partial denture framework and intaglio surface of the denture

c

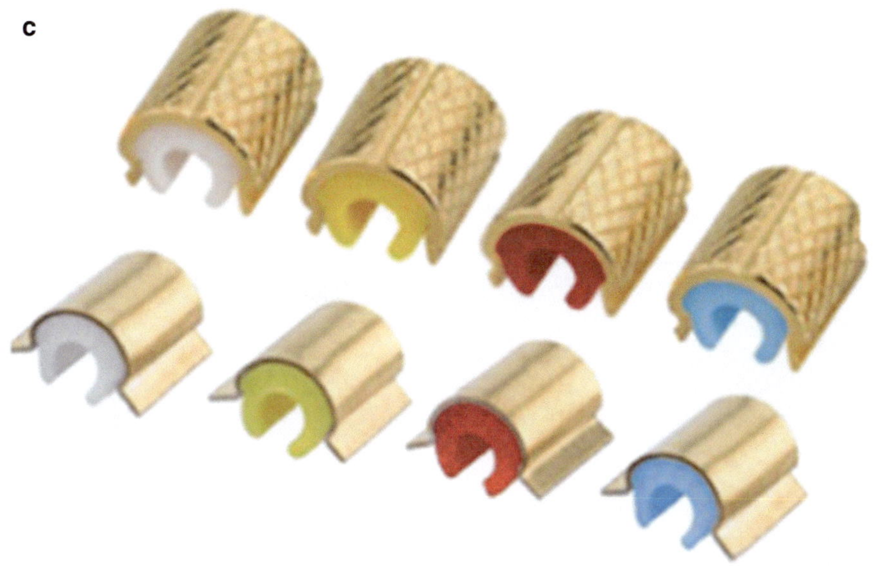

d

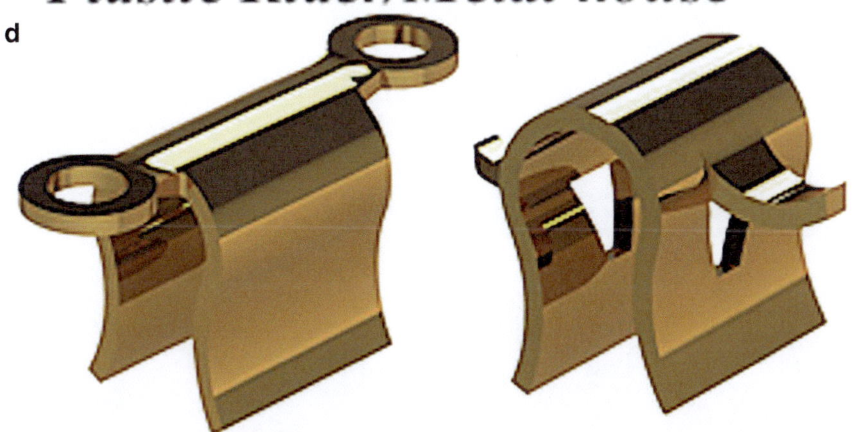

Picture 4.2 (continued)

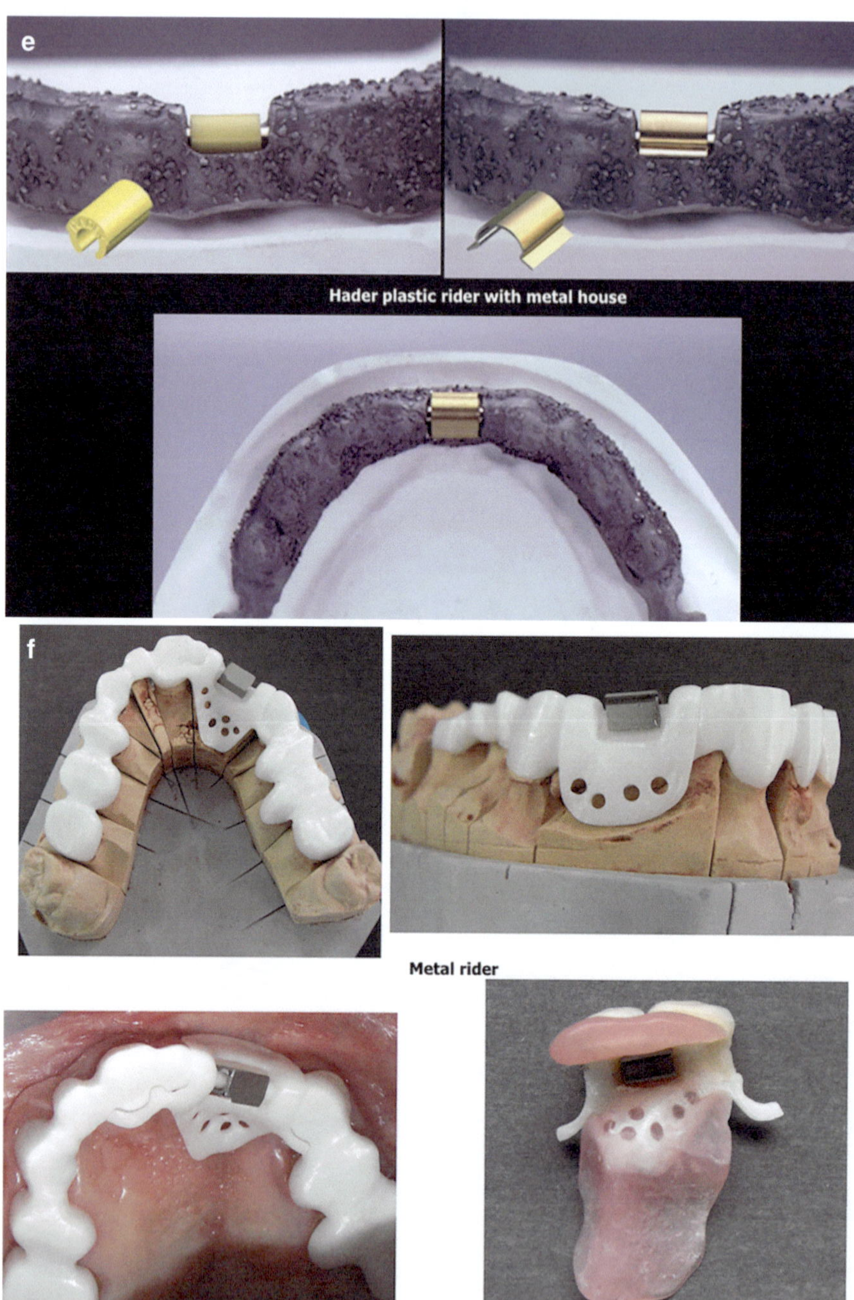

Picture 4.2 (continued)

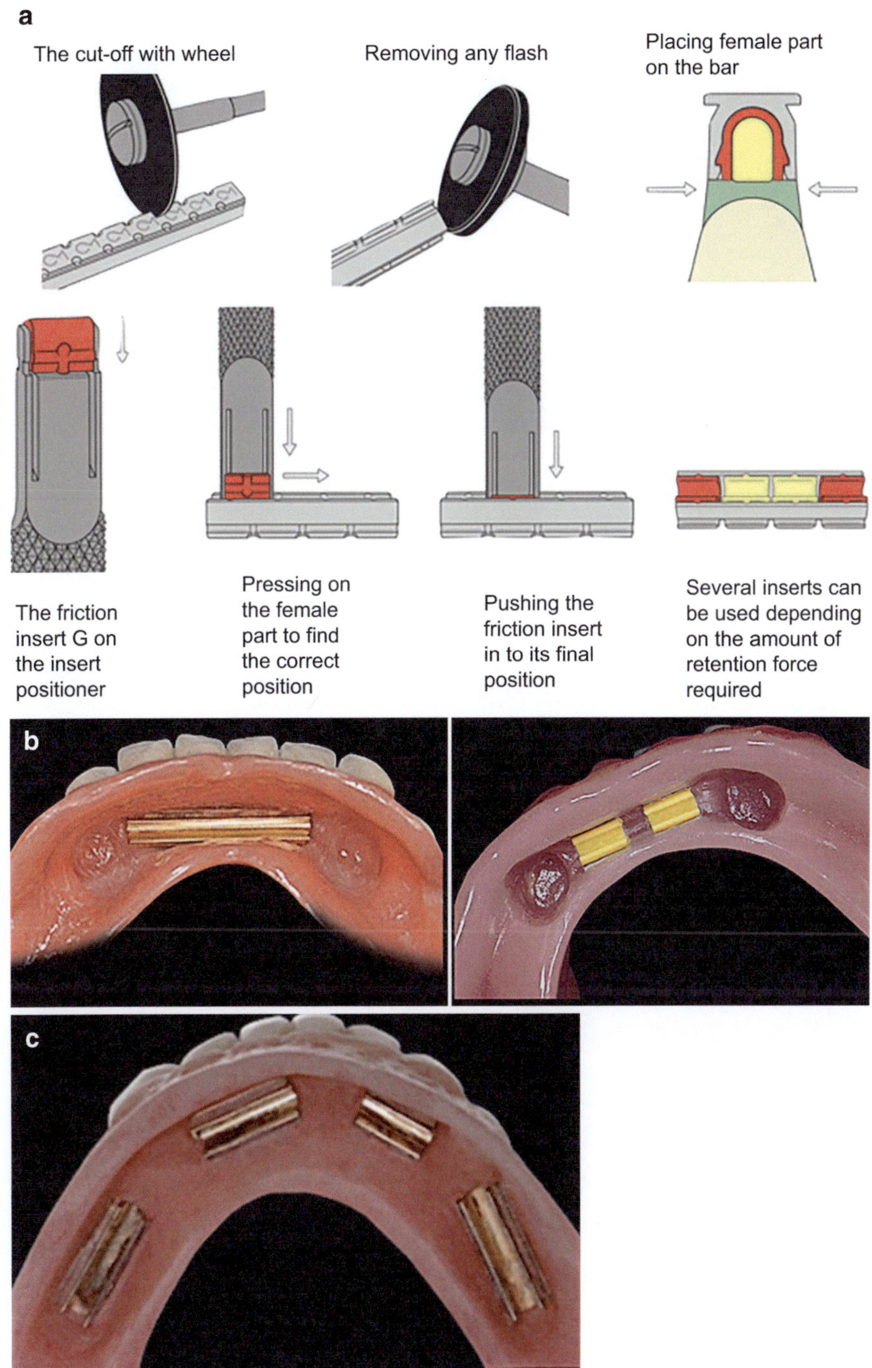

Picture 4.3 (**a**) The placing of the Dolder female part (the friction insert G) on the bar attachment, (**b**) the one and two clips placed in the intaglio of the denture, (**c**) the multiple clips placed in the intaglio of the denture

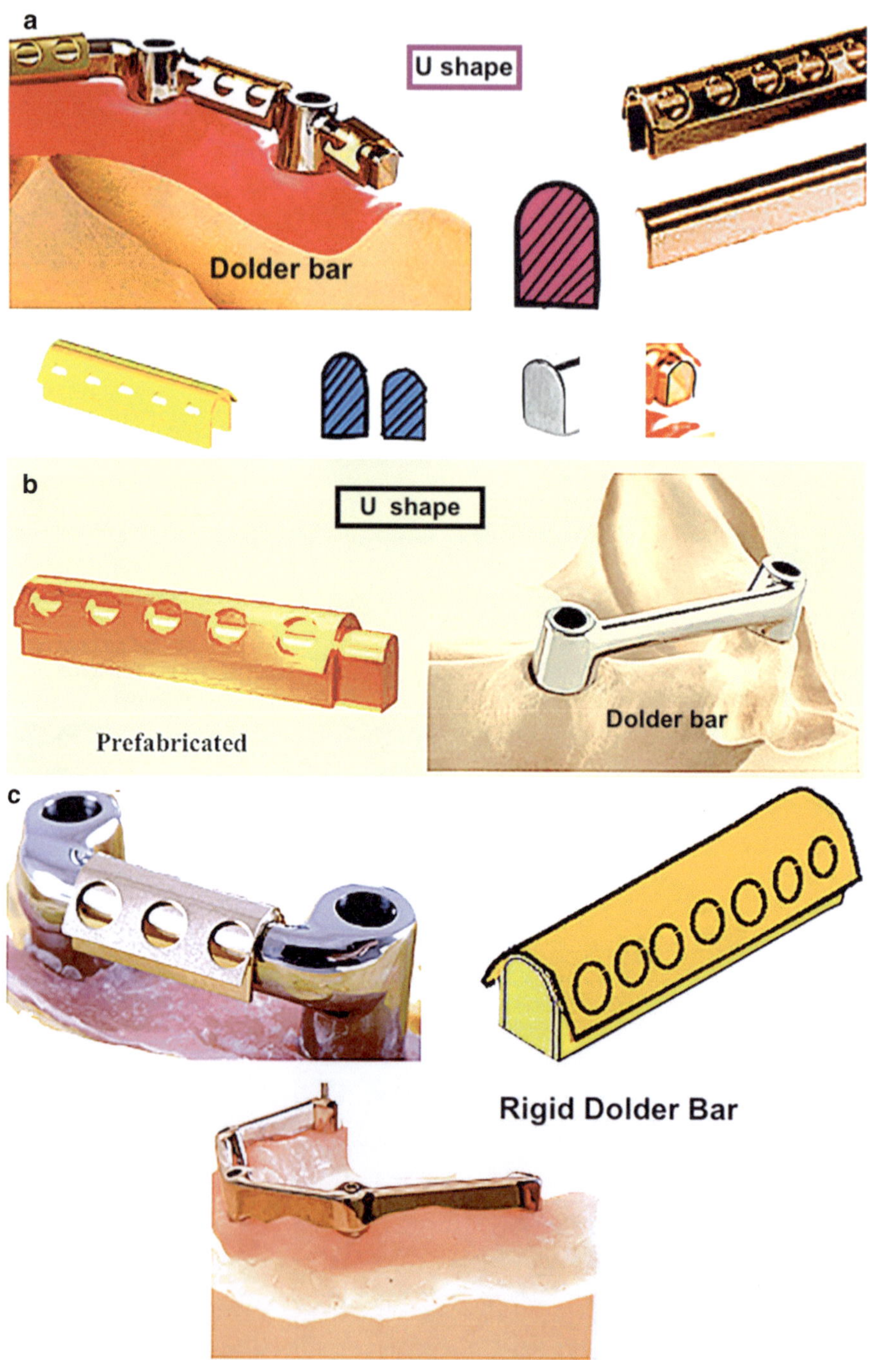

Picture 4.4 (**a–c**) Rigid Dolder bar (U-shaped bar)

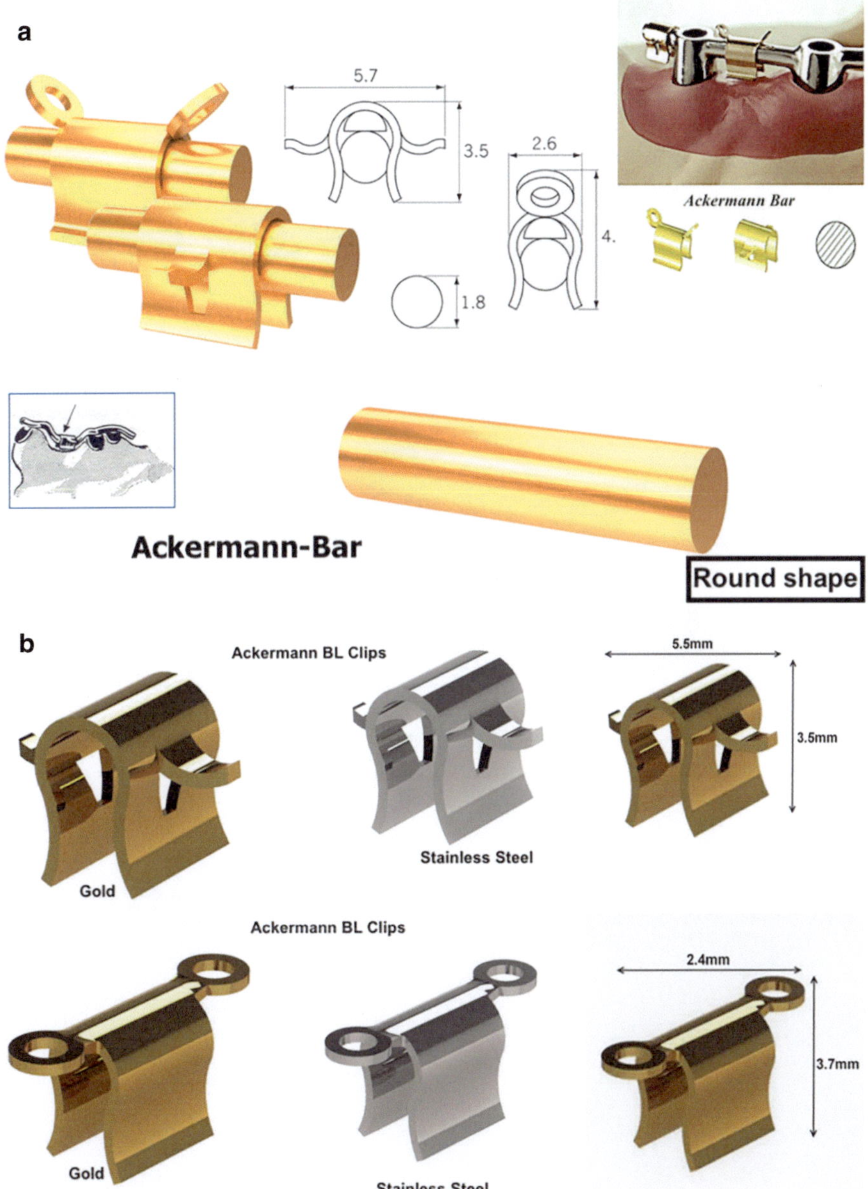

Picture 4.5 (**a**, **b**) Round-shaped bar (Ackermann bar/clips)

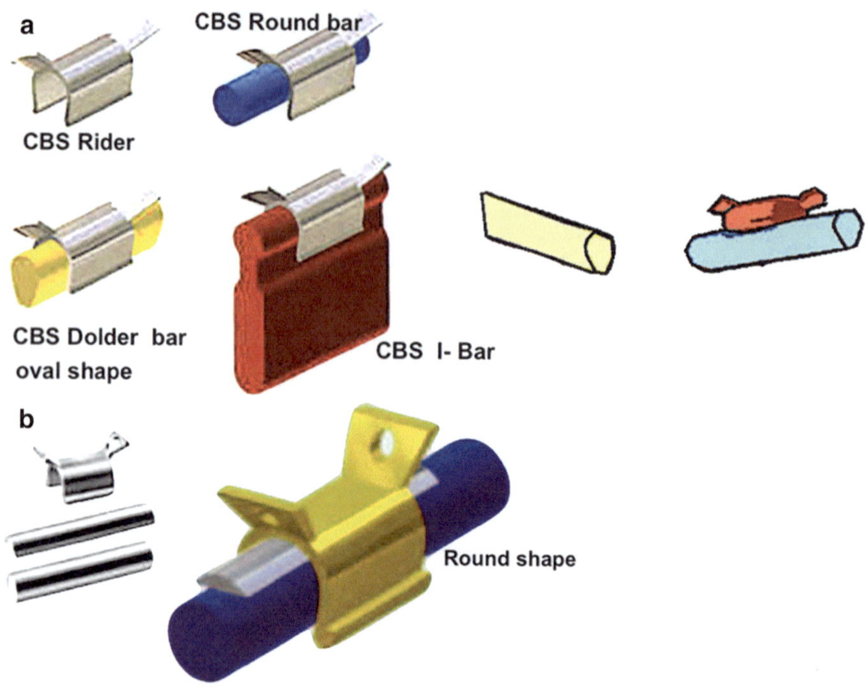

Picture 4.6 (**a**) The CBS bar system, (**b**) the CM Bar and Rider System (round-shaped bar), (**c**, **d**) MP clip/Ackermann Bar system (keyhole shaped)

c

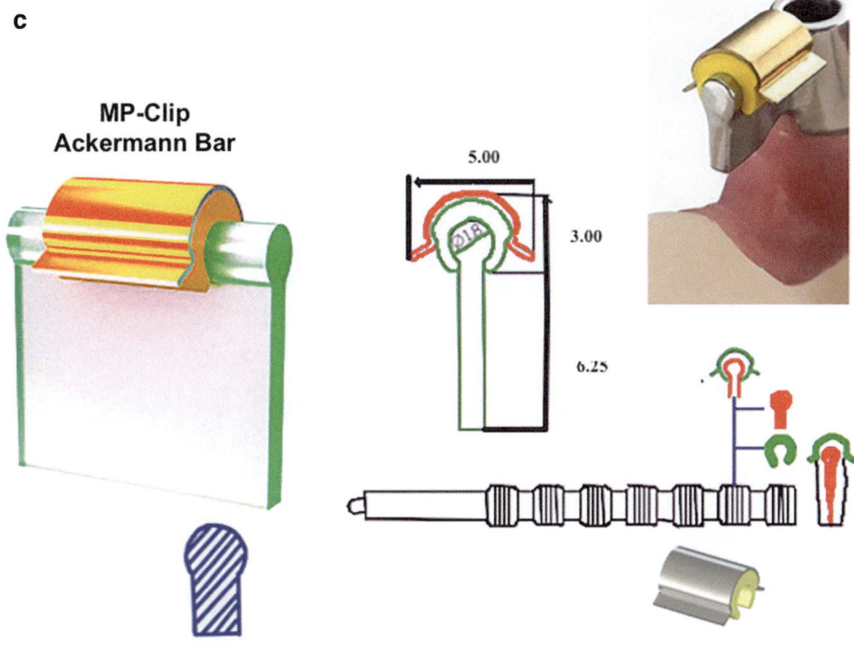

Picture 4.6 (continued)

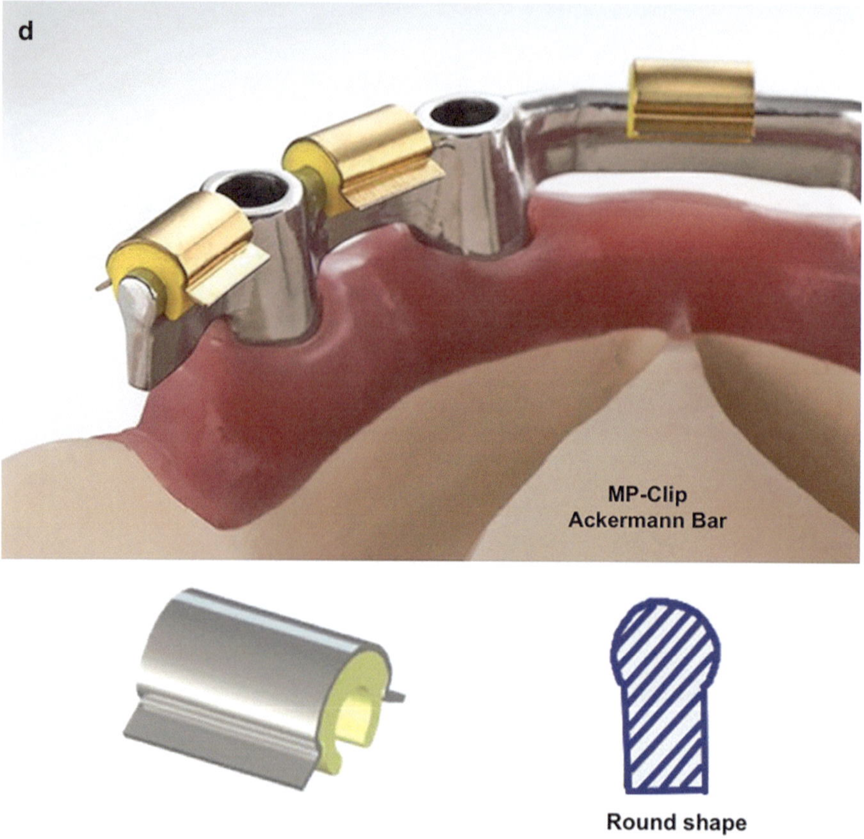

d

Picture 4.6 (continued)

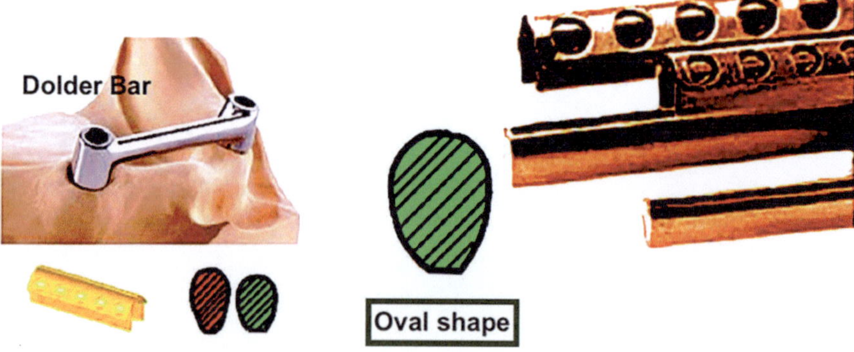

Picture 4.7 Resilient Dolder bar (oval-shaped bar attachment)

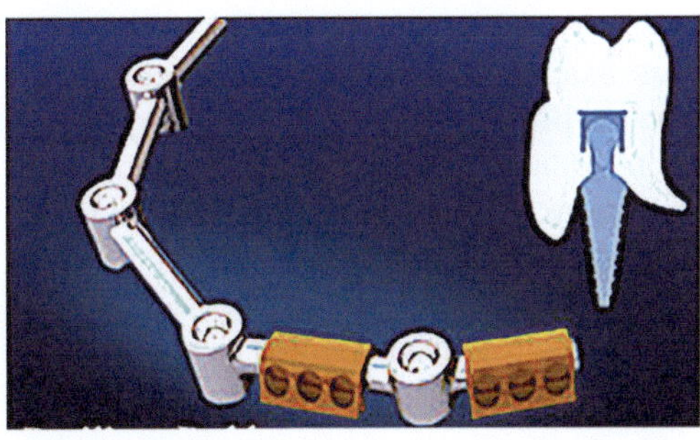 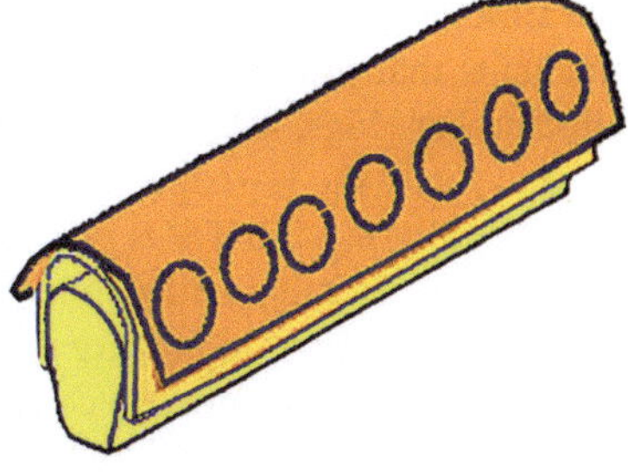

Picture 4.8 Resilient Dolder bar

4.1.3 Classification of Bar Attachments

4.1.3.1 Classification Based on Cross-Sectional Shape

U-Shaped Bar

The bar attachment is a rigid retentive unit with no rotational freedom, and its shape prevents movement. Overdentures that are rigidly supported (four or more teeth or implants in the arch) typically utilize rigid bar attachments (Picture 4.4).

Round-Shaped Section Bar

This bar allows for some limited movement and serves as a resilient attachment, depending on its configuration. Round bars provide greater denture rotation than rectangular bars, allowing for limited movement; they act as a stress-absorbing agent and prevent the transfer of excessive force to the supporting teeth or implants. A round bar is useful when the bar must be bent to accommodate the ridge anatomy or when there is a close bite. However, round bars require clip activation more frequently than U-shaped bars (Pictures 4.5 and 4.6).

Egg-Shaped Bar

This type of bar is resilient, which is advantageous for long-term retention. Its teardrop shape allows movement. It is primarily used between two roots, implants, or anterior posts and comes in standard and micro sizes (Figs. 4.7 and 4.8).

4.1.3.2 Classification According to Resiliency

1. Bar Units.
2. Bar Joints.
   (a) Single-part bar joints.
   (b) Multi-part bar joints.

Bar Units (Rigid)

Bar units that provide rigid overdenture fixation prohibit movement between the clip and bar (Figs. 4.1, 4.5, and 4.6; Picture 4.1b–g). With their parallel walls and friction force, the U-shaped (rigid or non-resilient) bars ensure rigid friction. They are generally used in TSOs with four or more teeth left in the arch. They provide outstanding retention and stability. In cases of TSOs with loss of posterior teeth, a bar unit can be used to prepare the parallel sides of a pear-shaped bar joint. Dolder bars and milled bars are also considered rigid attachments. Milled bars prevent the base of the denture from shifting and can provide relief to painful areas such as superficial mental nerves.

Pictures 4.9, 4.10, and 4.11 depict various bar attachments utilized in TSO cases.

In Picture 4.9, a rigid custom metal bar is fabricated for supporting the remaining weak mandibular teeth: seven teeth (11, 13; 17, 21; 22, 25) in the upper jaw and five teeth (33; 35; 38; 43; 48) in the lower jaw showed decreasing supporting ability. After a careful intraoral, extraoral, and radiographic examination, it was determined to splint teeth with a bar attachment for increased denture stability and retention.

The tooth was prepared by metal-ceramic restoration preparation guidelines: 1.2 mm of labial reduction, 1 mm of lingual reduction, and 2 mm of incisal/occlusal reduction with a 0.5-mm chamfer finish line. After impressions were made with polyvinylsiloxane (PVS), type IV dental stone was poured into the impressions to create the master casts. Horizontal and vertical maxilla-mandibular relation records were obtained with occlusal rims on acrylic base plates and transferred to a semi-adjustable articulator with the assistance of a facebow. Using auto-polymerized acrylic resin, provisional restorations were fabricated.

For economic reasons, custom rigid bar attachments were used in this case. On the model, the wax copings are prepared, and then the prefabricated plastic bar parts of 2 mm thickness and 3 mm height are adapted to the curvature of the ridge and connected to the wax copings. A space of two millimeters is left between the bar and the crest to promote oral hygiene. Using conventional casting techniques, metal crowns and bar attachments are cast together with base metal alloys. In the patient's mouth, the coping and bar assembly were tested after controlling the model for distortion and fit issues. After the try-on, the color of the ceramic layering of the metal copings was selected. After the application of ceramic, the entire assembly was completed and polished. Then, a second impression was taken of both jaws with a medium-body additional silicone impression material, utilizing individual acrylic resin trays on the bars and metal-ceramic restorations to obtain casts, on which a metal framework was fabricated (the authors preferred impressions with a bar and coping assembly instead of a cemented fixed bar assembly).

The final model, including the bar and coping assembly, was duplicated, the investment material was poured into the duplicate model, and the refractory cast was prepared. Just before duplicating, a thin layer of wax is placed on the saddle area (which will be replaced by acrylic resin), and in this way, a mechanical bond is enabled between the acrylic resin and metal construction. Using wax or self-adhesive plastic components, the metal framework components are fabricated. Co-Cr alloy was used to cast the framework wax pattern (Bellabond plus BeGo,

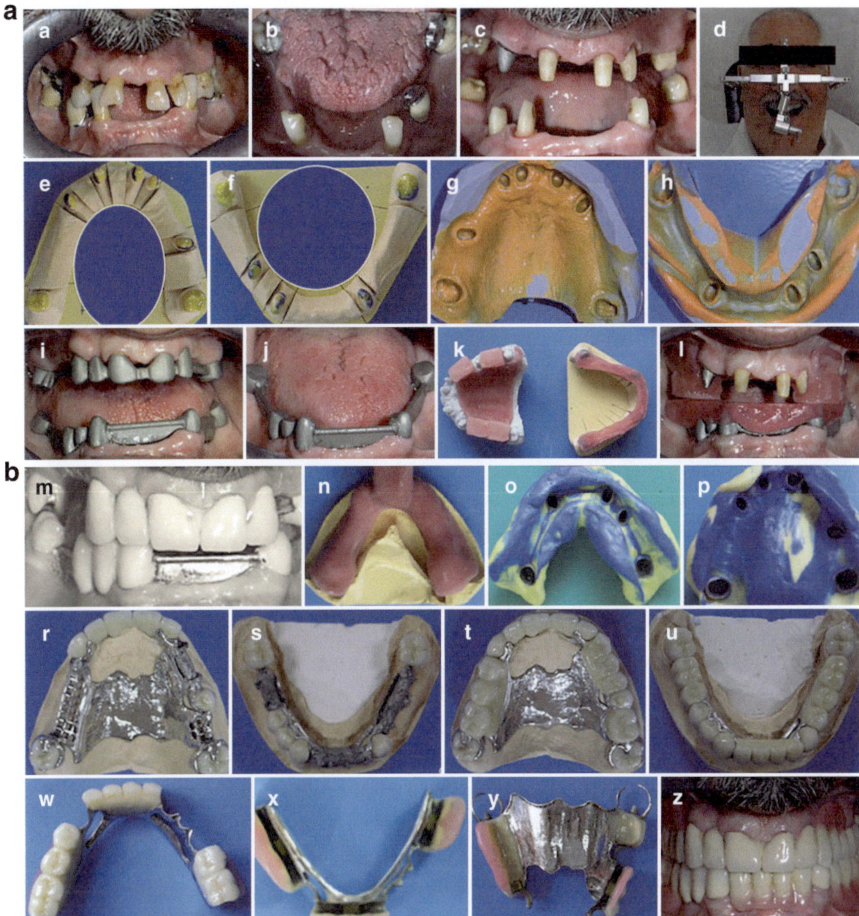

Picture 4.9 Rigid custom metal bar application for fixing the mandibular few and weak supporting teeth. (**a**) *a, b* Intraoral view of upper and lower jaw; *c* the preparation of upper and lower teeth; *d* face bow transfer; *e, f* primary model for controlling with surveyor the prepared teeth for paralleling and path of insertion; *g, h* impression is taken of prepared teeth with PVS impression material; *i, j* intraoral fitting of crown/bar assembly; *k, l* determination centric relation and vertical dimension of occlusion, (**b**) *m* metal ceramic try-in stage; *n, o, p* fabrication individual tray, and an impression is taken for metal framework fabrication; *q, r* fitting control of the metal framework on the cast; *s, t* resin teeth placed on the edentulous area on the model; *u, v, w* the extraoral appearance of prostheses; *x* bar-supported TSO in situ, (**c**) the intraoral appearance of patients before and after treatment, (**d**) panoramic radiographic image of bar-supported teeth

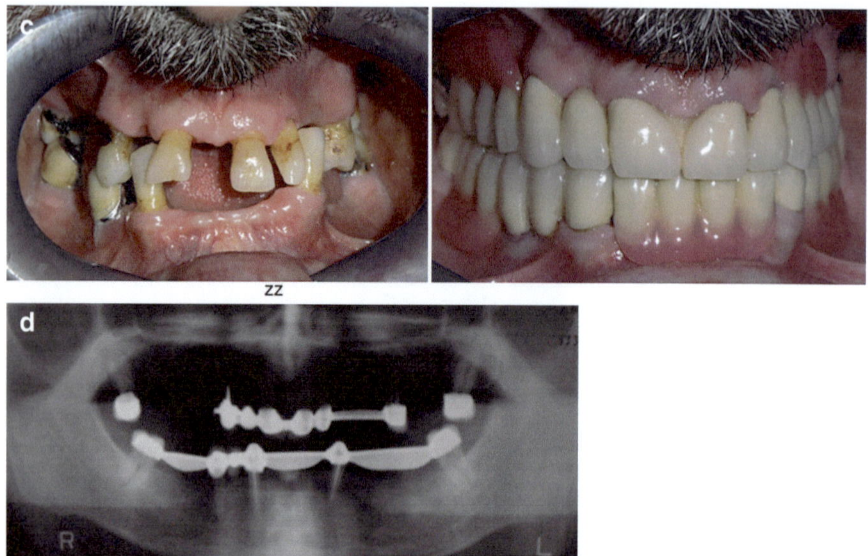

Picture 4.9 (continued)

Germany). After trimming and polishing, the framework was attached to the master mold. The framework is then tried for the final fit in the patient's mouth. For the prosthesis superstructure, special resin teeth are placed directly on the metal base of the edentulous area and tried in the mouth again. The gingival area is then coated with a pink, heat-activated acrylic resin and polymerized using a sectional mold and dental stone. The patient was instructed on how to insert and remove the TSO, as well as how to maintain proper oral hygiene. The primary benefit of this rigid bar attachment system is that it splints weak teeth to improve support and retention; aesthetics could also be enhanced.

Picture 4.10 shows the application of a rigid zirconium bar unit to a patient with a cleft palate. The author referred a 38-year-old woman with unilateral cleft lip and palate to replace the old restorations and achieve a more aesthetically pleasing facial appearance. After obtaining a medical and dental history, the patient was examined radiographically and intraorally. An intraoral examination revealed the loss of the maxillary left central and lateral incisors and the absence of the maxillary left anterior residual ridge (the patient has a central, canine, first and second premolar and first and second molar on the right side, and a canine, first and second premolar and first and second molar on the left side). The author chose to combine the existing teeth near the edentulous area with a sintered zirconia bar attachment system and a zirconia framework over the bar attachment system. Zirconia-based ceramic crowns were selected with a zirconia framework partial denture (ZPD) with precision attachments to create a natural gingival level for restorations, to compensate for tissue deficiencies, and to maintain oral hygiene.

The removal of old restorations caused gingival inflammation and an unattractive facial appearance. The initial periodontal treatment was then followed by the preparation of provisional restorations.

After completing tooth preparations with chamfer finish lines, PVS impression material was used to create an impression, and type IV die stones were used to obtain the master model. The milling program (Zeno Cam; Wieland Dental Technology, Germany) was utilized to create a plastic prototype for zirconia copings and bar attachments. The model was then used to evaluate the gingival margin and tooth contour, bar attachment height, and space for veneering restorations. After making the necessary adjustments, the zirconia framework was milled using the MAD/MAM (Manual Aided Design-Manual Aided Manufacturing) system and sintered furnace. The copings were veneered with lithium disilicate ceramic (IPS e-max Ceram, Ivoclar Vivadent). Then, the restorations were evaluated for their precision of fit on the teeth that had been prepared. Using PVS impression material, a new impression was taken for the zirconia framework following the temporary cementation of the crowns. Later, using the MAD/MAM system, the zirconia framework was milled from the wax pattern. After that, the prosthesis was completed with

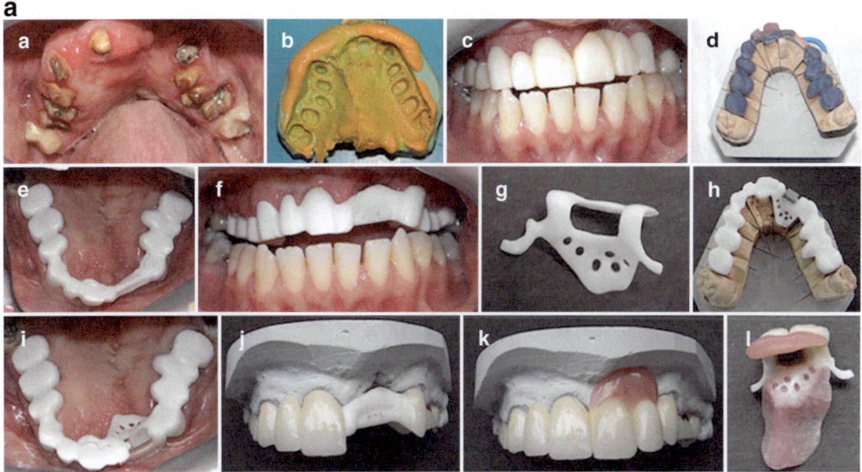

Picture 4.10 Rigid custom zirconia bar application for the patient has a cleft palate anterior region. It is essential in this case not to allow the movement of teeth after treatment because of cleft palate. (**a**) *a* clinical appearance of teeth; *b* PVS impression is taken after teeth preparation; *c* fixed provisional bridge temporarily cemented; *d* wax coping of zirconia (Amann Girrbach Ceramill MAD/MAM) structure; *e, f* zirconia bridge with zirconia bar assembly fit checked in the mouth; *g* zirconia framework of the removable part; *h* zirconia framework placed with metal rider on zirconia bridge with zirconia bar on the model; *i* zirconia framework and zirconia bridge with zirconia bar fit checked in the mouth; *j* porcelain-fused zirconia bridge; *k* finished denture on the model with fixed zirconia bridge; *l* intaglio surface of the denture, (**b**) *a* all assembly seen on the model (palatal view); *b* zirconia bridge with zirconia bar assembly cemented on the teeth; *c* zirconia framework placed on the bar; *d* all assembly seen on the model (facial iew); *e* intraoral view of denture

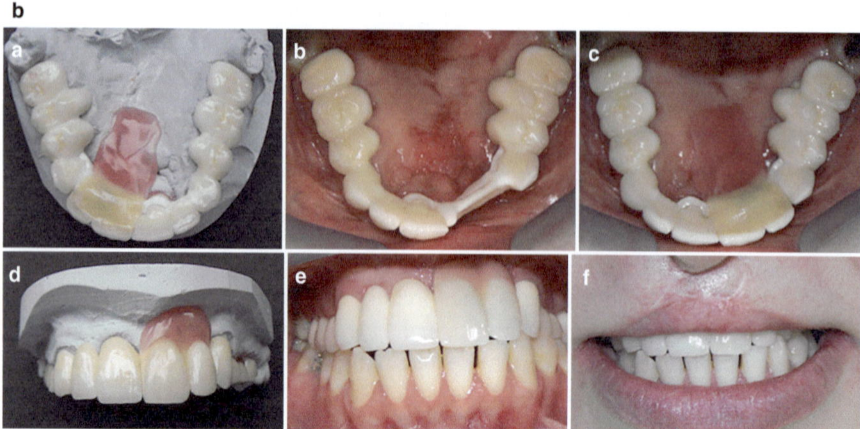

Picture 4.10 (continued)

acrylic resin teeth (Vitapan; VITA Zahnfabrik, Germany) and a heat-polymerized acrylic resin base material. The polished denture was inserted intraorally and evaluated for occlusion, retention, and stability.

Picture 4.11 shows an application of a rigid bar and post-coping to fix the mandibular and maxillary weak supporting teeth. The Schubiger attachment is typically screwed to the supporting tooth and provides denture retention and support with the bar attachment positioned between supporting teeth (Fig. 4.9). It is utilized when the supporting teeth are not parallel to one another.

This case describes the rehabilitation of a partially edentulous patient who was treated by TSO with a modified Schubiger attachment (Ozkan's design) for economic reasons.

A 31-year-old male patient in our department for esthetic rehabilitation is missing numerous teeth. The missing teeth were caused by periodontal disease. Intraoral examination revealed that the remaining teeth (teeth no. 13, 21, 23, 26, 27, 33, 37, 43, 45) were located in the cross arch as an advantage in stabilization, but the height of the clinical crowns was too high and bone support was insufficient to rehabilitate with a conventional removable partial denture. All situations were discussed with the patient, and a TSO treatment plan was chosen for both having the optimal esthetic and functional outcome and preventing the need for further extractions. As a result, both preventive treatments on existing bone and cost-effective treatment with prefabricated attachments were obtained. The applied treatment satisfied the patient's needs, including aesthetics and function. To achieve a low price, the Schubiger attachment design was modified and prepared from castings. The customized rigid bars connected the bonded metal post-coping to the teeth.

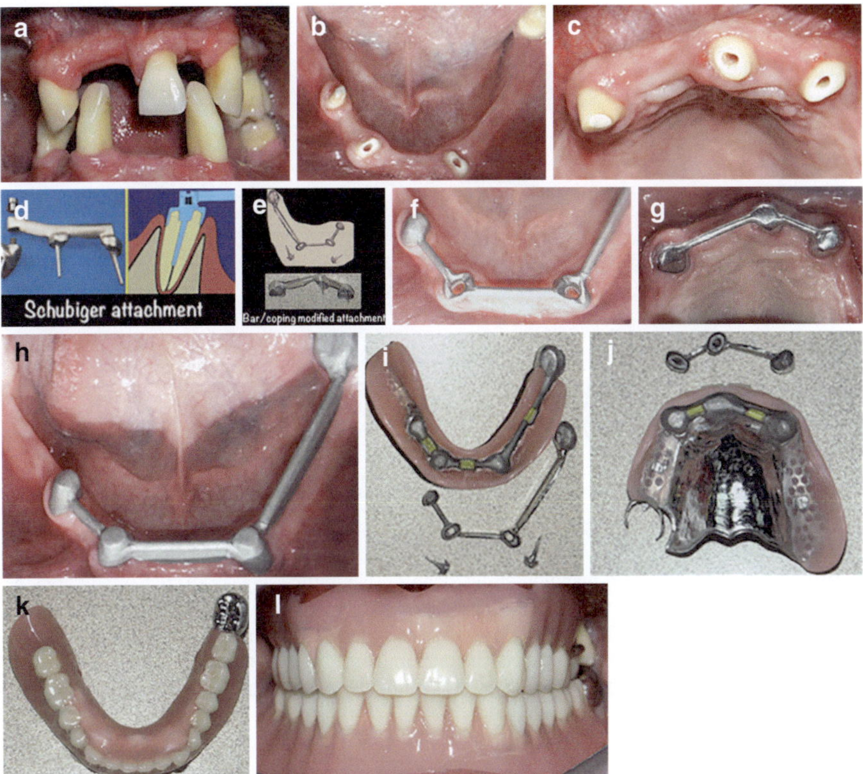

Picture 4.11 Rigid bar and post-coping application (Ozkan's design) for fixing the mandibular and maxillary few and weak supporting teeth. (**a**) Intraoral appearance of remaining teeth; (**b, c**) preparation of the upper and lower teeth; (**d**) original Schubiger attachment; (**e**) Ozkan design coping and bar assembly; (**f**) try-in bar and partial coping in the mandible; (**g**) conventional design of post/bar structure and adaptation (upper jaw); (**h, i**) intraoral and extraoral view of the bar units and modified copings (Ozkan's design); (**j**) conventional design of post/bar structure and upper denture intaglio surface; (**k**) mandibular TSO; (**l**) intraoral appearance of overdenture

4.1.3.3 Maintaining a Natural Tooth or Root in the Mouth That Is Healthy and Functional

To keep the natural tooth or root in the mouth as much as possible, it is essential to preserve the proprioceptive effect, prevent bone tissue loss around the supporting teeth, and provide psychological support to the patient by contributing to retention and stability.

Bar Joints (Resilient)

These bars have round, pear-shaped, and oval cross-sections. Bar joints are attachments that permit rotation or resilient movement between two components. Resilient bars reduce horizontal and transverse forces on supporting teeth, and their round or half-round section shape permits vertical and rotational motion. The oval shape

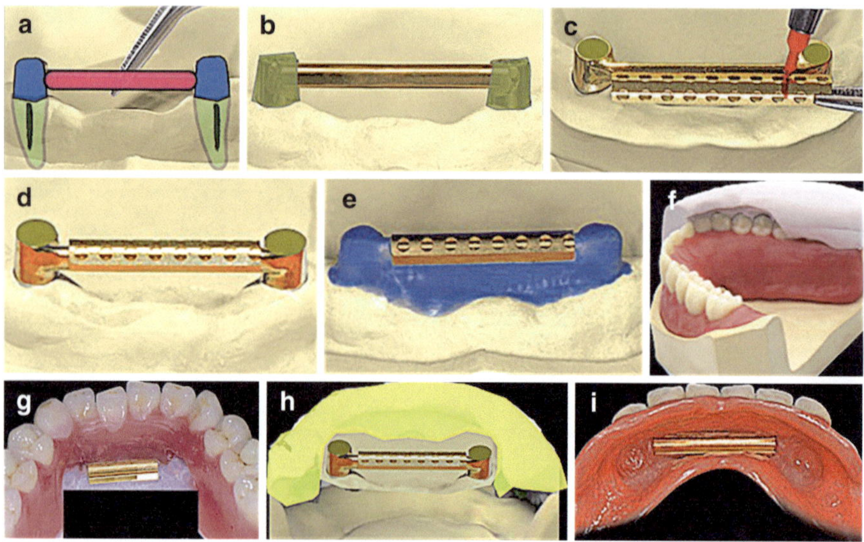

Picture 4.12 Bar-supported mandibular overdenture (laboratory stages): (**a**) Schematic drawing bar attachment assembly on the model, (**b**) prefabricated Dolder bar inserted between cast coping then soldered, (**c**, **d**) the Dolder metal clips and spacer measured and placed on the bar, (**e**) the block out wax material used to block out the undercuts of the bar, (**f–h**) controlling suitable bar space with try-in denture and silicone index, (**i**) mandibular overdenture with one metal clip (intaglio surface)

provides both vertical and rotational movement for resilient retention. When designed properly, resilient bars permit a single axis of rotation, provide greater mucosal support, and provide superior protection to the retentive attachments (Figs. 4.1a–c, 4.2, 4.3, 4.6, 4.7, and 4.8; Pictures 4.5, 4.6, 4.7, and 4.8).

Joints for bars can be utilized as single clips or multiple sleeves. In square arches, where the single clips must run straight without allowing the arch's anteroposterior curvature, they are utilized (Picture 4.12). Cross-sectionally, single-clip bar joints (Dolder bar joints) are pear-shaped. This type features an open-sided clip with a retention tag spacer to permit a small amount of movement in contact with the oral mucosa (Figs. 4.6 and 4.7; Picture 4.2a, b).

The multiple sleeves, on the other hand, can follow the curve of the arch and be utilized in more than one clip (Picture 4.5a, b). The system is referred to as a multiple-part joint if multiple short sleeves are used in place of a single long bar. If the distance between the abutments was too short, these types of bars would allow them to follow the arch's curve. The Gilmore, Ackermann, and derivative bars are examples of clip systems with multiple clips.

Regardless of the shape of the bars, the use of more than one clip could alter the rigidity of the prostheses. Regardless of the cross-section of the bar, the denture will be rigid (with no degree of space freedom) if multiple clips are placed in a single bar segment. If only one clip is placed on the anterior bar segment, a round bar creates one degree of space freedom, an egg-shaped cross-section creates three degrees of space freedom, and a bar attachment (or milled bar) creates none.

4.1.4   Selection Criteria for a Suitable Bar Joint Attachment

4.1.4.1 The Flexibility of Bar Attachment

The length of the bar between supporting teeth, the number of teeth supporting the bar, the height of the bar, the physical properties of the alloy, and the magnitude of the masticatory loads all influence the flexibility of the bar attachment. In the bar attachment system, the shape of the arch, the position of the supporting teeth, the shape of the supporting crests, and the vertical dimension for denture placement are also necessary. When selecting a bar attachment system, clinicians must consider all of the above factors.

4.1.4.2 Location of the Bar Attachment

- The bar should connect the roots with straight segments, without any curves. This bar type can therefore be utilized in square arch forms where the remaining roots or implants can be connected straight (Fig. 4.2). If the arch form is in the shape of a triangle or the supporting teeth are located on the lingual side of the crest, bar attachments would cause the denture to be excessively thick.
- In certain instances, the bar may conform to the anteroposterior crest's curvature. Nevertheless, the bar's anteroposterior inclination will prevent hinge movement and cause tilting movement.
- To ensure proper distribution of masticatory forces, the bar should be positioned horizontally concerning the ideal occlusal plane and the arbitrary hinge axis of the patient. They are positioning it at any other angle, resulting in improper implant loading and soft tissue compression (Figs. 4.2 and 4.3).
- The bar attachment should be vertically positioned along the midline (Fig. 4.3b). If the supporting tooth positions are located distally, a straight bar will obstruct the tongue space and create difficulties in denture fabrication. If the bar is positioned diagonally, it will prevent the anterior hinge from moving without friction. This condition causes excessive tilting stress on the supporting teeth.
- If a single bar is employed, 20–22 mm is the optimal bar length. If the abutments (supporting teeth and root) are too close together, the short bar cannot provide the overdenture with sufficient retention and stability.
- In certain instances, two short bar connectors will be used to attach the roots to this straight bar, but only the straight bar will be used for retention. In this instance, the force distribution on the roots will not be optimal (Picture 4.1a).
- Typically, a bar attachment system requires a minimum of 12 mm of vertical space for the restoration (Fig. 4.2b, c). The anteroposterior space bar attachment prevents accurate positioning of the anterior teeth when it is insufficient vertically.

- The space beneath the bar must permit efficient oral hygiene with interproximal brushes or special toothbrushes (Fig. 4.2b, c). When there is sufficient vertical space, leaving 2–4 mm of space between the bar and the mucosa facilitates cleaning and improves oral hygiene. Unfortunately, there is rarely sufficient vertical space, so the bar must be placed in even or passive contact with the mucosa in the majority of patients. Any compression of the mucosa by the bar will result in hyperplasia of the mucosa. It has been attributed to both inadequate oral hygiene and the negative pressure caused by the overdenture. For this reason, the bar should be placed at a distance from the gingival crest to permit the use of interdental brushes. Additionally, patients should be given specific instructions and a proper recall system should be implemented.
- If the anterior crest is straight, a Dolder bar joint (with three degrees of space freedom) should be used, as it places less force on the abutment regardless of the number of supporting teeth. When more than two supporting teeth are present in the anterior region, a bar attachment is used to connect all supporting teeth with several clips (the denture is called bar-retained); regardless of the cross-section of the bar, the prosthesis is a rigid type of retention.

Materials Used for Fabricating Bar Attachment

Attachments for bars can be prefabricated from type IV gold, such as the original 1.6 mm Dolder bar. Using a low-fusing solder, type IV gold bars should be soldered to the abutment (Pictures 4.4, 4.5, 4.7, and 4.8). Other types of bars are available as castable, pre-milled plastic patterns (Fig. 4.6). The bar castings must be made from hard alloy and must have a minimum Vickers hardness of 200 and a minimum ultimate tensile strength of at least 95,000 psi (Pictures 4.9, 4.10, and 4.11). Castable bars include round bars, plastic Dolder bars, I bar, EDS bars, and Hader bars. For telescopic milled restorations, these bars are available in 0, 2, and 4°.

4.1.5 Most Frequent Bar Attachments

4.1.5.1 Dolder Bar System

Dolder is one of the most widely utilized bar systems on the market (Figs. 4.2, 4.6, and 4.7; Pictures 4.4, 4.7, and 4.8). Dr. Eugen Dolder developed the Dolder bar, a prefabricated precision bar attachment, in Switzerland. This bar system is available in two distinct configurations: the U-shaped bar with parallel walls (for the rigid unit) and the egg-shaped form in cross-section (gingival taper for the resilient joint), which provides the previously described vertical and hinge resilience (Figs. 4.6 and 4.7). Due to the parallel walls and close adaptation, a U-shaped bar is not possible. It comes in standard and micro sizes (metal clips are only used on the regular version; titanium and plastic clips can be used on the micro version). The frictional retention of the denture is provided by the clips, which are embedded in the resin and rest over the bar. If the coping post cannot be made parallel to accommodate the soldered bar, a Schubiger unit is utilized (Fig. 4.8).

The Dolder bar joint reduces forces on the roots because it permits vertical and rotational movement (ovoid bar in cross-section). Although they have a small amount of lateral mobility, they are resistant to lateral forces. The height of the Dolder bar joint is manufactured in two sizes: 3.5 mm and 4.55 mm. The spacer permits vertical and rotational movement of the clips. During the clip attachment manufacturing process, a spacer may be added to the occlusal surface of the egg-shaped Dolder bar. When the spacer is removed, the retention clip no longer engages the top of the bar. As a result, the removable prosthesis may move down and then rotate around the bar. To allow PM-3 movements, the bar and clip must also be perpendicular to the direction of prosthesis rotation. In other words, a Dolder bar with a spacer and clip is constructed for movement in three planes. When there is no clip to facilitate prosthesis rotation, a more rigid system is produced (i.e., PM-2).

Typically, the Dolder bar is soldered to the abutments, and self-curing acrylic should be used to secure the clips to the denture base. Available sizes range in height from 2.3 to 3.0 mm and in width from 1.6 to 2.2 mm. The Dolder bar and its metal clips are made of gold alloy (Elitor) and are adjustable, allowing the clinician to control the amount of retention the bar provides. Dolder male components could be fabricated from Elitor (E), a warmly annealed, high-grade, yellow precious metal alloy with a robust structure. Casting materials include gold alloys, titanium alloys, and nonprecious metal alloys. To ensure that the cast male component has adequate strength, the casting alloy must have a minimum proof stress of 500 N/mm2 at 0.2%.

The female parts (sleeve) are compatible with gold, titanium, and cast bars that have been prefabricated. Female Dolder components could also be fabricated from Elitor, Doral (D, Au 15.00%, Pd 22.00%, Ag 49.30%, Cu 13.70%, TS-TL 930–1015 °C), Pure Titanium, and Galak (G, mouth-resistant plastic). The female component may be selected as type E (micro and macro) or type T (micro and macro). Female component T (with replaceable friction inserts G) is also supplied with six yellow (for light friction) and six red (for average friction) friction inserts (Picture 4.2e). The female component must not be less than 5 mm in length because it can be firmly anchored. Using the separating groove, the female portion of the bar can be shortened by 3.5 mm at regular intervals. When separating, the groove also serves as a guide for the cut-off wheel. After the friction inserts have been fitted, the female part is placed on the bar, and the space between the bar and the gingiva, as well as the root and implant caps, is blocked out. Resin is then bonded or polymerized into position.

On the insert positioner, the friction insert G is positioned. By pressing on the female component, the correct position of the friction insert can be determined. As soon as the friction insert engages in the groove (which is audible), it is pushed into its final position. For 2–4 weeks, only a few inserts, those with the least friction, should be used so that the patient can quickly adjust to the new restoration. The brass spacer is positioned between the pear-shaped or resilient bar and the female sleeve when employing the resilient bar. Place the clip in contact with the labial surface of the bar. The U-shaped, rigid bar does not utilize a spacer.

Picture 4.12 shows the use of a Dolder bar joint attachment with mandibular and canine abutments. When the bar attachment is used in TSO, the diagnostic setup should be useful for assessing aesthetics and overall dimensions. The diagnostic setup will aid the clinician and technician in evaluating the spaces with silicone masks and selecting the most suitable prosthetic solution. A TSO with stud attachment must be performed if the distance is short. Two canine teeth are used as supporting teeth in this case (abutments). After root canal therapy and post-space creation, teeth are prepared to create a common insertion path. Then, PVS impression materials were used to create an impression of the post space, teeth, and mandibular ridge, and a master cast was obtained. On the master cast, the post was made with plastic pattern resin, and the coping was made with wax resin. The entire assembly was invested, burned out, and cast in cobalt-chromium alloy before being finished and polished. Then, the prefabricated Dolder bar is inserted between the cast coping, cut at a suitable length on the model, and attached to the copings with sticky wax. Considering tooth placement and ridge contour, the bar is placed parallel to the occlusal plane and at a right angle to the midline to obtain hinge movement, and the bottom of the bar is relieved to follow the contour of the adjacent gingival papilla. Finally, the invested cast is assembled and the components are soldered. After soldering, the assembly was returned to the model and the passive fit was examined. The female component is adjusted along the length of the bar to achieve the greatest retention force possible (it must not be shorter than 5.5 mm). The bar and/or coping assembly is also examined for passive fit within the mouth of the patient. The bar clip is adjusted along the length of the model's bar to achieve the maximum retention force possible (it must not be shorter than 5 mm). Seat the clip on the spacer and rotate it into anterior contact with the bar. This position will provide a positive stop preventing undesirable posterior lift of the prosthesis. Then block out the space between the bar and gingiva, and over the copings with plaster. The block-out material should also cover both sides of the clip to approximately half its height and along its entire length.

After obtaining the patient's jaw relationship records, the cast was mounted on the articulator, the teeth were arranged, and the try-in was conducted. The wax setup was then applied to the master cast. By applying PVS material to the labial, buccal, and occlusal surfaces of wax, set-up indexes are obtained (the teeth should be adjusted with the clip in place to make enough space and proper contours). Reset the teeth using the silicon index and complete the final wax-up. Process the denture normally. Justify, complete, and polish the denture. Remove the obstructing material and spacer and adjust the clip retention as necessary (Picture 4.12).

4.1.5.2 The Activation and Deactivation of the Female Part

Using the Dolder activator or deactivator, the retention force can be precisely and individually adjusted. The lamella posterior, which is subject to greater loading, should be activated. The anterior lamella acts as a guide surface. The activator is used to push the clips inward to activate them. The deactivator tool is inserted into the clips to deactivate an overly tight bar clip until the required friction is reached (Fig. 4.5).

4.1.5.3 Hader-EDS Bar System/Hader Bar System/Preci-Horix Bar System

Helmut Hader developed the Hader bar system in the late 1960s, which is the most widely used bar system due to its affordability and simplicity. In 1992, English, Donnel, and Staubli altered the system to create the Hader EDS system. It resembles the Preci-Horix system (Figs. 4.13 to 15; Picture 4.13).

The height of the EDS bar is only 3 mm, whereas the original was 8.3 mm. The Hader bar and clip assembly has a total height of 4 mm, which may be less than the 5–7 mm required by the O-ring system. Consequently, a greater moment of force is applied to the bar during rotation, necessitating clearance beneath the denture base. However, for PM-2-type prostheses, the increased crown height above the attachment may decrease the denture's lateral stability. The bar can be cast in the alloy of your choice and is available in prefabricated plastic patterns. Depending on the available vertical space, the height of the plastic Hader bar can be easily adjusted on the master model before casting. In addition to plastic bars, this bar system offers titanium bars for laser welding and gold bars for soldering or laser welding. Also available are bars with round, ovoid, and keyhole-shaped cross-sections.

The standard EDS Hader bar has a round upper surface with a 13-gauge (1.8 mm) diameter and an apron toward the tissue below. With a total vertical bar height of 2.5 mm, a total vertical attachment height of 1.5 mm, and attachment widths of 4.2 mm, the patient may be provided with a stable and aesthetically pleasing restoration. The Hader bar is more flexible than other bar shapes because round bars flex to the fourth power of the distance, whereas other bar shapes flex to the third power. The apron serves as a stiffener to increase the bar's strength and limit its flexibility;

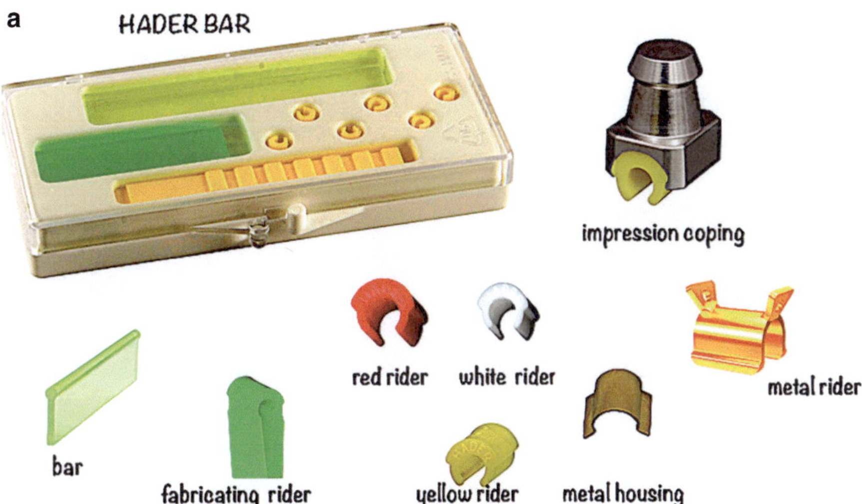

Picture 4.13 (**a**) Hader bar attachment assembly, (**b**) Hader/EDS bar attachment, (**c**) US Authentic Hader bar attachment

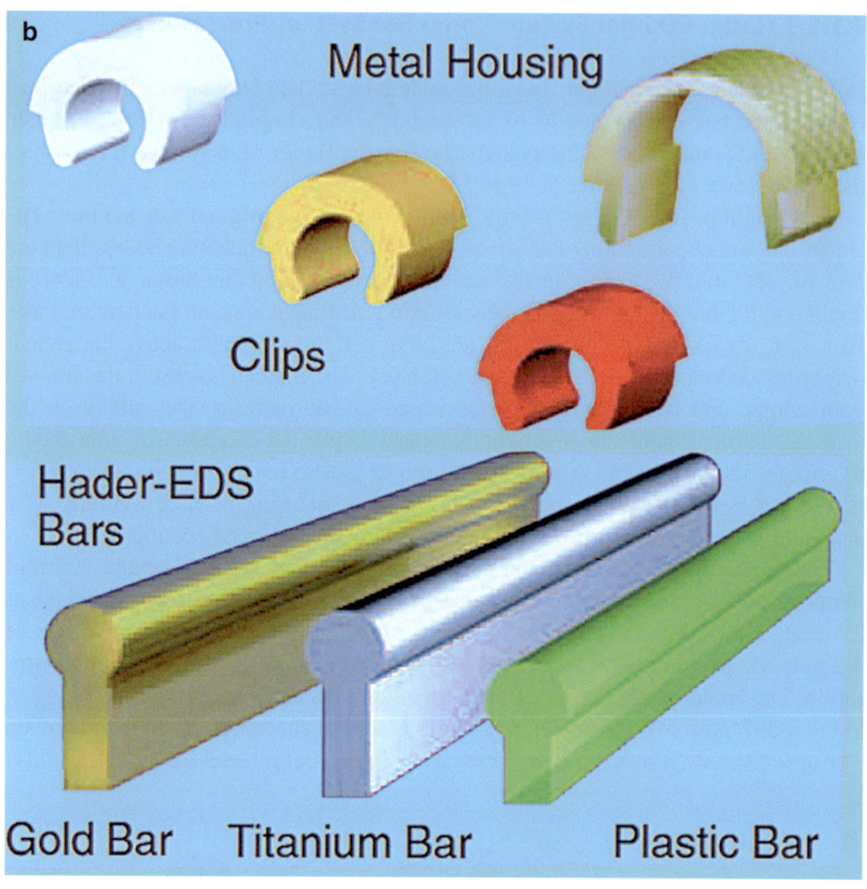

Picture 4.13 (continued)

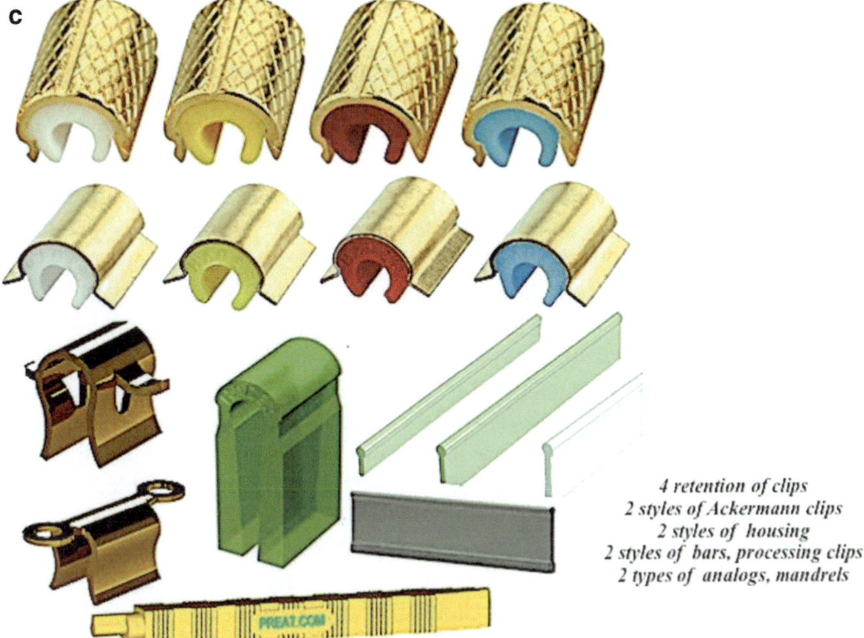

Picture 4.13 (continued)

it is added to the tissue side of the Hader bar to prevent metal flexure, which could lead to loose abutments or bar fractures. The clearance between the bar and the gingiva is proportional to the height of the apron.

From a biomechanical perspective, round bars permit more rotational movements with fewer fractures and complications; however, the round cross-sectional area permits greater bar deformation. Due to its inferior rectangular stiffener, the cross-section of a Hader bar with a keyhole shape is more rigid. This type of bar is known as a "resilient Dolder bar" when a particular rider engages a retention mesh attached to a bar with a pear- or oval-shaped cross-section.

Durable Hader-EDS clips are interchangeable with standard Hader clips and are available in three color-coded levels of retention strength and a 20° clip rotation, which significantly increases the system's adaptability to a variety of patient needs or preferences. In addition, a housing made of gold-plated stainless steel maintains the clip, reducing the need to cold-cure new attachments. This is a substantial advantage. In addition to fitting standard bar patterns such as the ABS, CBS (round, oval, and I-bar), and the original Hader bar, the clips were also compatible with standard ABS, CBS (round, oval, and I-bar), and Hader bars. Nylon clips for retention in processed denture acrylic sockets are also available; the optional metal housing is easily replaceable at the chairside if retention is lost. The gold-plated, machined metal Hader-EDS housing simplifies clip replacement and prevents acrylic degradation-induced looseness.

For the fabrication of processing models, plastic Hader-EDS impression clips and aluminum analogs of Hader-EDS bars are available. Each is 50 mm in length, is reusable, and can be shortened. Both are recommended for restorations and repairs.

Advantages of Hader Bar

- The Hader bar system is more affordable and widely accessible than other bar attachments. Depending on the available vertical space, the vertical height of the plastic Hader bar can be easily adjusted on the master cast before casting.
- The Hader clip and bar may have a lower profile for use in situations with limited crown height space (CHS). When a low-profile system is used in situations with a high CHS, the lateral stability of the prosthesis may be compromised.
- The system permits the rotation of the prosthesis around the bar. To accommodate anterior-to-posterior rotational movement, the clips protect the abutments by allowing the prosthesis to rotate around the bar. The rotation of the clip compensates for the resilience of the posterior soft tissue in the mandible, which is typically between 0.5 and 1 mm. Highly mobile tissue, which is typically found in the maxilla, necessitates an extensive range of clip movement.
- For a bar and clip to rotate, it is necessary to consider several design elements. For instance, the bar should be parallel to the occlusal plane and perpendicular to a line bisecting the angle between the posterior arches. It uniformly distributes force between the edentulous posterior crest and supporting teeth and reduces torque force on supporting teeth to the lowest possible level.
- Following the anteroposterior gingiva, the Hader bar can be positioned. The most important characteristic of this type of bar is its ability to minimize the distance between the bar and the gingiva.

Thayer and Caputo (1980) studied the various bar attachments and determined that the Hader bar produced less torque force and distributed forces more evenly between the posterior edentulous region and the abutments than the other bar designs.

Prosthesis Movement

Clinicians determine the amount of prosthesis movement (PM) a patient desires based on the condition of the supporting teeth and tissues. If the denture is rigid when in place, regardless of the attachments used, the PM is labeled PM-0. It is common knowledge that O-ring attachments facilitate movement in six different directions. If four O-ring attachments are placed on a full arch bar, however, a PM-0 restoration may result.

A hinge-like movement allows the denture to move in two planes (PM-2). Hinged attachments include the Dolder bar (egg-shaped) and clip without a spacer, as well as the Hader bar (round shape) and clip.

The Hader clip and metal encapsulator (three different retention clip strengths) are a class 2 attachment that is compatible with PM-0 to PM-2 systems. When the clips are placed parallel or at an angle to the desired PM, however, the prosthesis may become rigid.

A cross-section of the Hader bar with the apron is stronger than the round bar alone, and it also limits the amplitude of rotation of the clip (and prosthesis) around the fulcrum to 20°, resulting in a more rigid assembly of the prosthesis and bar. Therefore, the Hader bar and clip system may be utilized for a PM-2 when posterior ridge shapes are favorable and soft tissue is sufficiently firm to prevent prosthesis rotation.

Notably, to provide hinge movement, the hinge attachment must be placed perpendicular to the axis of prosthesis rotation, resulting in the PM existing in two planes (i.e., PM-2). If the Hader or Dolder bar is angled or parallel to the desired rotational direction, the denture is more rigid and may resemble a PM-0 system.

4.1.5.4 Preci-Horix Bar Attachment

Preci-Horix bar systems feature burn-out plastic bars with flexible plastic riders (clips). By compressing the plastic riders, the bar attachment enables rotational and minimal vertical motion. Riders are easily replaceable. The bars of plastic are cast from any hard alloy. The height, length, and diameter of the bar are, respectively, 4 mm, 50 mm, and 1.8 mm (Picture 4.14).

Picture 4.15 shows a mandibular TSO supported by two teeth using the Preci-Horix bar system. With a subgingival chamfer finish line, abutment teeth should be prepared to the desired height, which depends on the availability of the vertical space based on the clinical and radiographic evaluation. Using PVS elastomeric

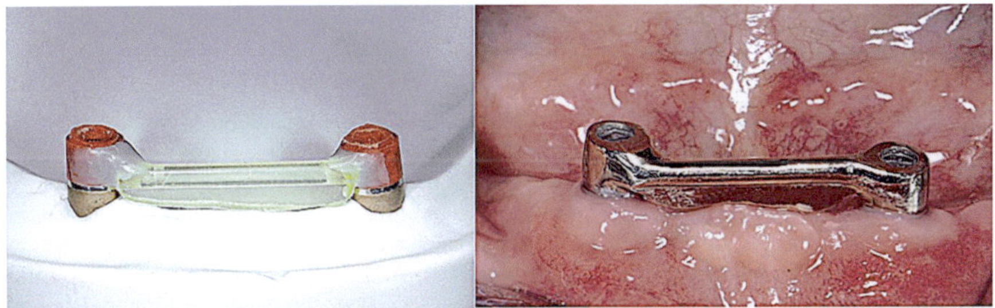

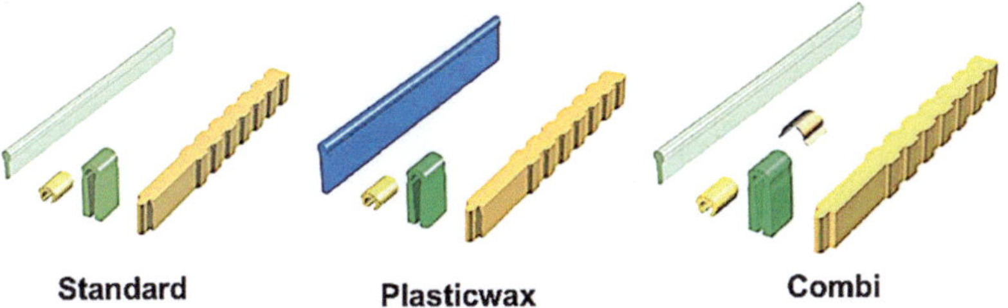

Picture 4.14 Preci-Horix bar system application on the mandibular TSO

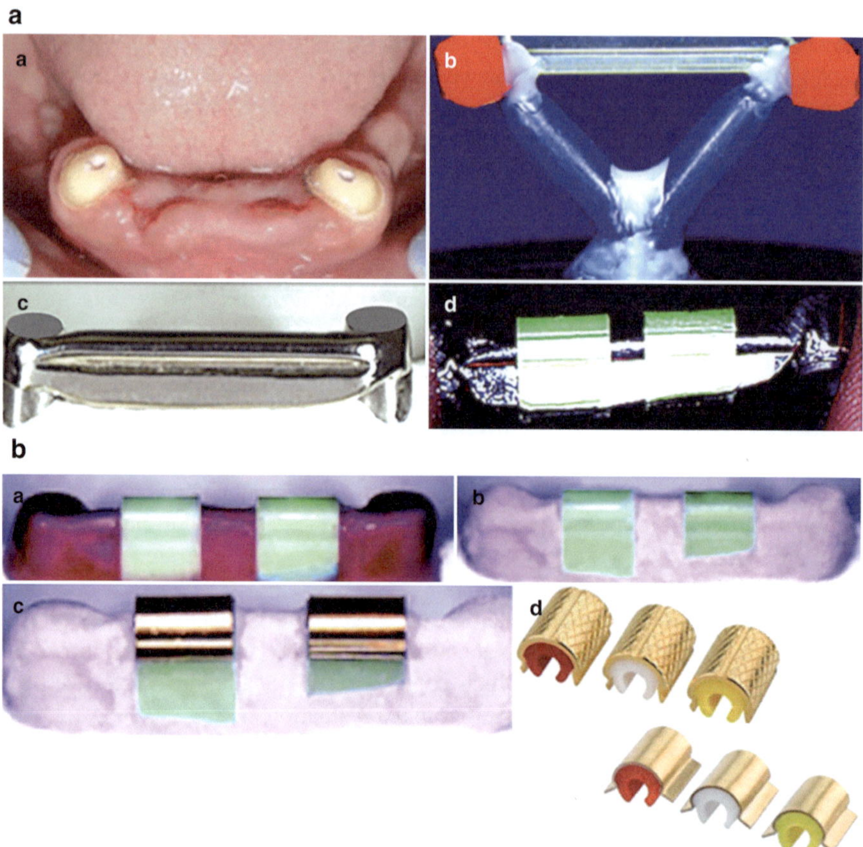

Picture 4.15 Mandibular TSO with Hader bar attachment. (**a**) *a* Preparation of two canine teeth, *b* spruing, *c* Hader bar and coping assembly controlling on the model, *d* the Hader processing spacers placed on the bar. (**b**) *a* Block out made on model the processing spacers placed, *b* refractory cast model obtained and the processing spacers placed on the model, *c* metal housing placed on green processing spacers, *d* two different styles of Hader metal housings. (**c**) *a* The cross-section of the metal housings with the plastic female rider; *b* the Hader clip, or female rider, is authentic Hader, as can be seen by the word "HADER" on end. The yellow clip is normal retention, orange is increased retention, and white is reduced retention; *c* the insertion of the white female rider. (**d**) Two metal housing seen in the prosthesis. (**e**, **f**) Insertion yellow clip in the metal house

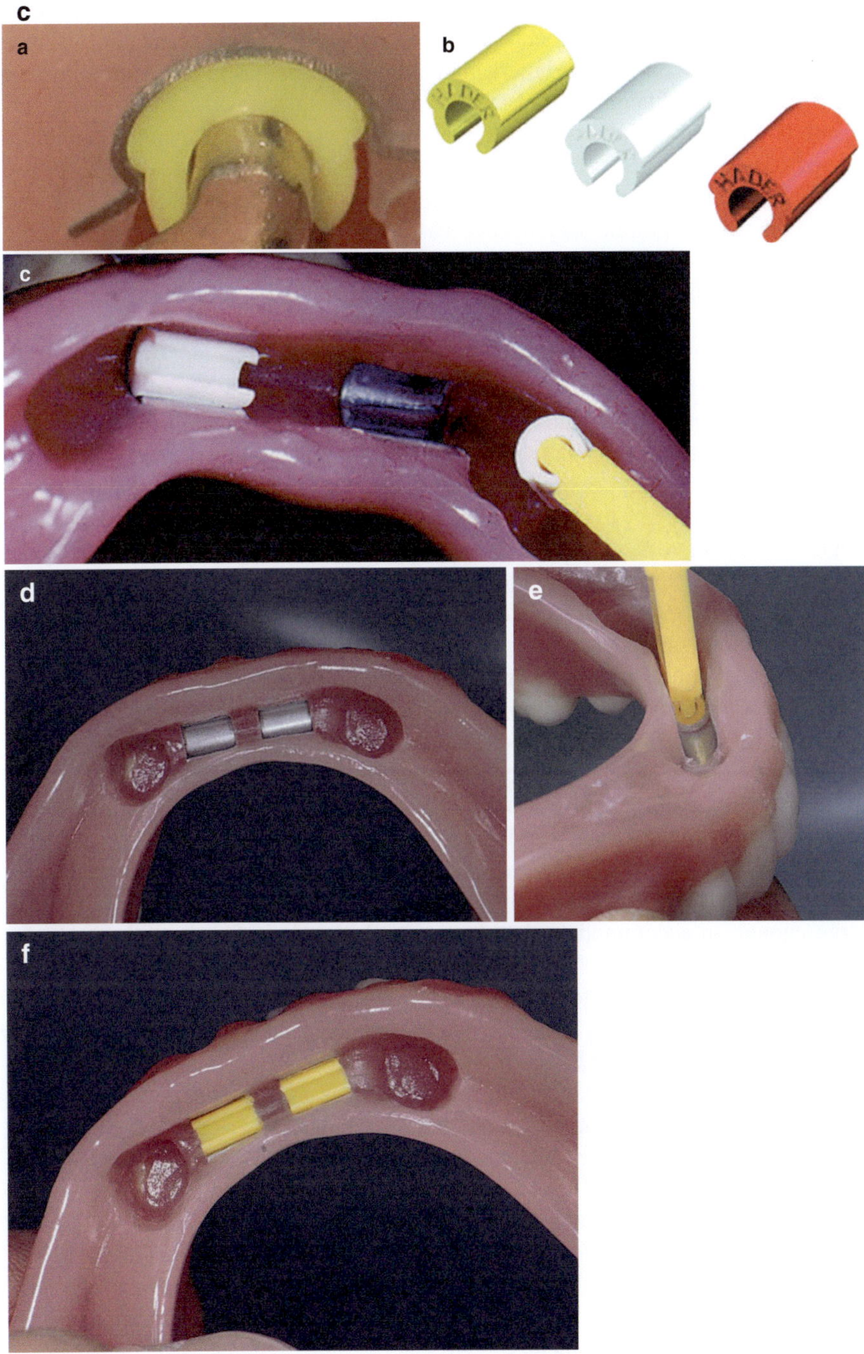

Picture 4.15 (continued)

impression material, a type IV dental stone is poured into the impression to create the master model. The abutments are fitted with wax copings, and the distance between them is measured and marked on a Preci-Horix plastic bar. After adjusting the bar's length and height, the plastic bar pattern adapted to anterior-posterior curvature is attached to the wax coping pattern with wax. The bar pattern is directly waxed onto the copings of the abutments and then cast with base metal alloys. Stones, burrs, or rubber wheels should not be utilized to grind the bar. This will reduce the diameter of the bar and alter the clip's fit and retention. The bar assembly is tried in the mouth, and the marginal fit of the copings and the relationship between the bar and the underlying ridge are evaluated and the passive fit is examined. The model was then placed in the place of the bar. The denture teeth must have adequate vertical space. If not, reduce the height of the bar further. The bar may be reduced to 2.5 mm, and the nylon rider extends occlusally to 0.9 mm. The nylon retention clips (fabrication clips) should be placed on the bar, positioned on the model, and tested on an articulator against the opposing model. Position nylon retention clips on the bar to the extent permitted by the spacer. This will allow additional clips to be inserted if necessary to increase retention. The undercuts of the bar are blocked-out and a new impression is created. In the duplicate model, the extensions of nylon clips embedded in the stone will hold the metal housing clips in the correct position. It should not shorten these extensions and mount the metal housing to the bar. The acrylic polymerization process is then concluded, and the fabricating clips are extracted using pliers or a hemostat. The retention sleeves/clips (the Hader nylon retainers) were then inserted into the metal housing using a seating instrument. When the clips are pushed into position, there should be an audible snap. The particular shape of the metal housing provides secure retention of the clips while allowing for some flex in the labiolingual direction during insertion and removal of the prosthesis (Pictures 4.14 and 4.15).

The spacer is crucial for the proper installation of bar retainers. This facilitates the insertion and removal of the actual clip and, more importantly, creates a "tunnel" large enough to accommodate the removal and insertion of the prosthesis. If the spacer is not placed on the bar, the clips will be fixed into the acrylic base and will only move within, leading to clip wear and fracture during denture insertion.

4.1.5.5 Ackermann Bar System

Similar to the Dolder bar system, the Ackermann bar system may be round or egg-shaped. It is possible to modify a round bar to fit the anatomy of the alveolar crest. It is an excellent option due to its small size and ease of installation (bar diameter, 1.8 mm). Similar to Hader-EDS and CM bars, it possesses resiliency classes 3–4. The CM gold rider is also commonly referred to as the "Gold Hader Clip." If the Hader clip does not fit the handlebar, the CM rider (Picture 4.5) must be used. The defining characteristic of this system is that the bar can be adjusted to follow both the vertical and anterior-posterior contours of the ridge. The spacer permitted both rotational and vertical movement.

The rider and clips of the Ackermann system are designed for vertical and rotational movement. The Ackermann clip (AC) is a clip or rider made of precious metal that fits Hader, Dolder, and Round bars (the AC fits standard 13-gauge, 1.8-mm bars). In addition, it has retention wings for securing the clip within the resin. Due to its horizontal or vertical retention tags, the AC requires less vertical space and offers adjustable retention and easy patient insertion and removal. The AC gold clips are available in BL and MD versions, with buccal-lingual and mesial-distal retention tags, respectively. BL types can be placed directly next to one another, whereas MD types require a certain distance between each rider. The BL rider is indicated for situations involving a deep bite. The BL retention tags provide a firm hold in acrylic while requiring no additional vertical space.

4.1.5.6 CBS Bar System

Since 1977, the CBS bar system has been successfully applied to non-precious bar restorations. This system is intended for bar restorations that require vertical and rotational motion. The CBS plastic bars are available in three different shapes: round, oval, and I-shaped. If the castable plastic bar restoration is cast in a precious alloy, the CM or Ackermann clips must be used. The Hader-EDS clips are compatible with CBS bars. Additionally, it has Class 3–4 durability and is adaptable (Picture 4.6a).

4.1.5.7 CM Bar and Rider System

This system is intended for bar restorations that necessitate vertical and rotational movement within a restricted vertical space. Similar to the Hader-EDS and Ackermann systems, it is adjustable and possesses Class 3–4 resilience. The CM gold clips are incorporated into the acrylic denture base. The CM gold round bar is a standard gold alloy of type 4, but plastic bars are preferable. The clips are adjustable in millimeters, and all bars are the standard 13 gauge, 1.8 mm diameter (Picture 4.6b).

4.1.5.8 MP-Clip

This system is more cost-effective than prefabricated metal bars. The diameter of the round bar is 1.8 millimeters. Adjusting the retention force is simple by exchanging the retention inserts (see Fig. 4.6c, d).

4.1.5.9 Schubiger Attachment

This attachment connects the supporting teeth to the bar joints via a screw system and used in when supporting teeth are not parallel (Fig. 4.9). The Schubiger screw (Cendres and Metaux SA, Bienne, Switzerland) system was described by Marquard.

The attachment complex is made up of a gold alloy screw base (OSV), Ceramicor clips, and a cap nut (OSV). The short Schubiger structure has a height between 2.80 and 3.05 mm and a circumference between 3.00 and 3.20 mm. The cylindrical metal sleeve is retained by a screw lock nut and slides over the threaded screw projection. The bar is then directly cast or soldered onto the metal sleeve.

If the bar attachment is not properly planned, it is known that the incidence of complications will be higher than with other systems. In bar attachments, clipping and matrix loosening are the most common complications. Table 4.1 lists the problems and solutions associated with bar attachment–supported overdenture.

Table 4.1 Problems and solutions: bar attachments

Problem	Possible Cause	Solution
Failure of abutments and bar to be a complete casting.	The plastic bar pattern did not adhere well to the abutment wax patterns or broke loose during investing.	Use adequate wax to adhere the plastic bar pattern to abutment wax patterns. Invest carefully without excessive vibration.
Failure of nylon clips to stay in a receptacle in the resin.	The fabricating clips were placed over the bar before taking the impression rather than the nylon retention clips. This causes the gingival extension of the fabricating clips to expand and causes an oversize receptacle to be processed in the resin.	Position the nylon retention clips, *not* the fabricating clips, on the cast bar before taking the impression for the processing model.
Insufficient retention of the nylon clips on the bar.	(a) The round bar was reduced in size due to over finishing. (b) The nylon clips are worn.	(a) Do not use stones or rubber wheels on the round bar when finishing. Polish only. (b) Replace plastic clips or use gold alloy clips that have retention adjustment capability.
The prosthesis is difficult to insert and remove.	(a) The nylon retention clips have been processed into the resin incorrectly. The denture acrylic is preventing the flanges of the clips from flexing. (b) The prosthesis was designed to engage a severe labial undercut. This causes the prosthesis to be positioned labially at the time of insertion; thus, the nylon clips are not correctly aligned to snap onto the bar.	(a) Use the rebasing procedure to replace clips. (b) Remove the labial flange area which engages the severe undercut from the prosthesis.

Further Reading

Abdel-Khalek EA, Ibrahim AM. Effect of bar cross-section and female housing material on retention of mandibular implant bar overdentures: a comparative in vitro study. J Indian Prosthodont Soc. 2017;17:340–7.

Bambara EG. The attachment retained overdenture. NYSDJ. 2004;70:30–3.

Bassi F. Comparing overdenture therapies with teeth and implant abutments. Int J Prosthodont. 2009;22:527–48.

Becerra G, MacEntee M. A classification of precision attachments. J Prosthet Dent. 1987;58:322–7.

Brewer AA, Morrow RM. Overdentures. 2nd ed. St. Louis, MO: CV Mosby Co; 1980.

Crum RJ, Rooney GEJR. Alveolar bone loss in overdentures; a 5-year study. J Prosthet Dent. 1978;40:610–3.

Dodge CA. Prevention of complete denture problems by use of "Overdenture". J Prosthet Dent. 1973;30:403–36.

Dolder EJ. The bar joint mandibular denture. J Prosthet Dent. 1961;11:689–707.

Dong J, İkebe K, Gonda T, Nokubi T. Influence of abutment height on the strain in a mandibular overdenture. J Oral Rehabil. 2006;33:594–9.

dos Santos MB, Caldas RA, Zen BM, Bacchi A, Correr-Sobrinho L. Adaptation of the overdenture-bars cast in different metals and their influence on the stress distribution: a laboratory and 3D FEA. J Biomech. 2015;48:8–13.

English CE. Bar patterns in implant prosthodontics. Implant Dent. 1994;3:217–29.

Evans DB, Koeppen RG. Bar attachments for overdentures with nonparallel abutments. J Prosthet Dent. 1992;68:6–11.

Alfred GH, Kundert M, Charles KC. Complete denture and overdenture prosthetics. New York: Thieme Medical Publishers Inc.; 1993.

Gotfredsen K, Holm B. Implant-supported mandibular overdentures retained with a ball or bar attachments: a randomized prospective 5-year. Int J Prosthodont. 2000;13:125–30.

Marquardt GL. Dolder bar joint mandibular overdenture: a technique for nonparallel abutment teeth. J Prosthet Dent. 1976;36:101–11.

Mensor MC. Removable partial overdentures with mechanical (precision) attachments. Dent Clin N Am. 1990;34:669–81.

Mericske-Stern R, Piotti M, Sirtes G. 3-D in vivo force measurements on mandibular implants supporting Overdentures. Clin Oral Implants Res. 1996;7:387–96.

Morrow RM, Feldmann EE, Rudd KD, Trovillion HM. Tooth-supported complete dentures. Approach to preventive prosthodontics. J Prosthet Dent. 1969;21:513–22.

Pacer FJ, Bowman C. Occlusal force discrimination by denture patients. J Prosthet Dent. 1975;33:602–9.

Pavlatos J. Root-supported overdentures. CDS Rev. 1998;91:20–5.

Preiskel HW. Overdentures made easy: a guide to implant and root supported prostheses. Chicago, IL: Quintessence; 1999. p. 189–232.

Reitz PV, Weiner MG, Levin B. An overdenture survey: preliminary report. J Prosthet Dent. 1977;37:246–58.

Rissin L, House JE, Manly RS, Kapur KK. Clinical comparison of the masticatory performance and electromyographic activity of patients with complete dentures, overdentures, and natural teeth. J Prosthet Dent. 1978;39:508–11.

Rudd K, Morrow R. Rhoads J Dental laboratory procedures Removable partial dentures, vol. 3. 2nd ed. St. Luis, MO: Mosby; 1985. p. 609–23.

Rutkunas V, Mizutani A, Takahashi H. Wear simulation effects on overdentures stud attachments. Dent Mater J. 2011;30:845–53.

Rutkunas V, Mizutani H, Takahashi H. Evaluation of stable retentive properties of overdentures attachments. Baltic Dent Maxillofac J. 2005;7:115–20.

Samra RK, Bhide SV, Goyal C, Kaur T. Tooth supported overdenture: a concept overshadowed but not yet forgotten! J Oral Res Rev. 2015;7:16–21.

Schuch C, Pinheiro de Moraes A, Onofre RS, Cenci TP, Boscato N. An alternative method for the fabrication of a root-supported overdenture: a clinical report. J Prosthet Dent. 2013;109:1–4.

Shah FK, Gebreel A, Elshokouki A, Habib AA, Porwal A. Comparison of the immediate complete denture, tooth and implant-supported overdenture on vertical dimension and muscle activity. J Adv Prosthodont. 2012;4:61–71.

Sposetti VJ, Gibbs CH, Alderson TH, Jaggers JH, Richmond A, Conlon M, Nickerson DM. Bite force and muscle activity in overdenture wearers before and after attachment placement. J Prosthet Dent. 1986;55:265–73.

Tanoue M, Kanazawa M, Takeshita S, Minakuchi S. Effects of clip materials on stress distribution to maxillary implant overdentures with bar attachments. J Prosthet Dent. 2016;115:283–9.

Thayer HH, Caputo AA. Photoelastic stress analysis of overdenture attachments. J Prosthet Dent. 1980;43:611–7.

Van Waas MA, Jonkman RE, Kalk W, Van't Hof MA, Plooij J, Van Os JH. Differences two years after tooth extraction in a mandibular bone reduction in patients treated with immediate overdentures or with immediate complete dentures. J Dent Res. 1993;72:1001–4.

Wang X, Ohkubo C, Hosoi T, Shimpo H, Kurihara D, Murata T. Retentive forces of 3 types of attachments for root-retained overdentures. Prosthodont Res Pract. 2007;6:104–8.

Williamson RT. Retentive bar overdenture fabrication with preformed castable components: a case report. Quintessence Int. 1994;25:389–94.

Telescopic Attachments Used in Tooth-Supported Overdentures

5

Yasemin Ozkan and Ulrich Heker

5.1   Introduction

Telescopic dental prosthesis (TDP) was launched in the United States at the close of the nineteenth century and refined in Europe during the twentieth century. The telescopic crowns, also known as the double crown, consist of an inner, primary telescoping coping and an outer, secondary telescopic crown. When telescoping crowns are used for tooth-supported overdentures (TSO), the denture is called a telescopic overdenture (TO). The TO enables the restoration of dentition utilizing a few residual teeth in undesirable situations for other prosthetic restorations (Fig. 5.1; Pictures 5.1, 5.2, 5.3, 5.4, 5.5, 5.6, 5.7, 5.8, 5.9, and 5.10).

The components of the TO are: *primary copings* composed of precious or non-precious dental metals that are cemented on the prepared abutment teeth. The primary copings provide retention and stability for the secondary crown as well as protection against dental cavities and thermal irritations for the tooth. *The secondary crown* that is slipping over the primary coping is designed to keep the prosthesis in place by exerting tight sliding friction on the teeth. The non-precious dental metal framework is embedded in plastic (acrylic resin) and supports the acrylic teeth that will replace the patient's missing natural teeth (Figs. 5.1, 5.2, and 5.3).

A force of 250–300 P (110–136 kg) is required to remove dentures. The maximum force necessary to remove a denture should not exceed 650 P (294.8 kg). The exact friction of the separate telescope components can only be achieved by the skills of the dentist, variations in milling speed, degree of cutter wear, polishing, casting procedure, and manner of setting retention forces resulting in a wide range

Y. Ozkan (✉)
Faculty of Dentistry, Department of Prosthodontics, Marmara University, Istanbul, Turkey
e-mail: ykozkan@marmara.edu.tr

U. Heker
Teeth ARE US, Essen, Germany

© The Author(s), under exclusive license to Springer Nature Switzerland AG 2023   279
Y. Özkan (ed.), *Treatment Options Before and After Edentulism*,
https://doi.org/10.1007/978-3-031-37582-8_5

of values. Additionally, the retention and stability of the TO are directly proportional to the number and distribution of abutments in the dental arch and the taper of the primary coping marginal walls. When at least two or three teeth are remaining in the jaw, TO should be fabricated; however, for optimal results, it should be placed on four to six teeth.

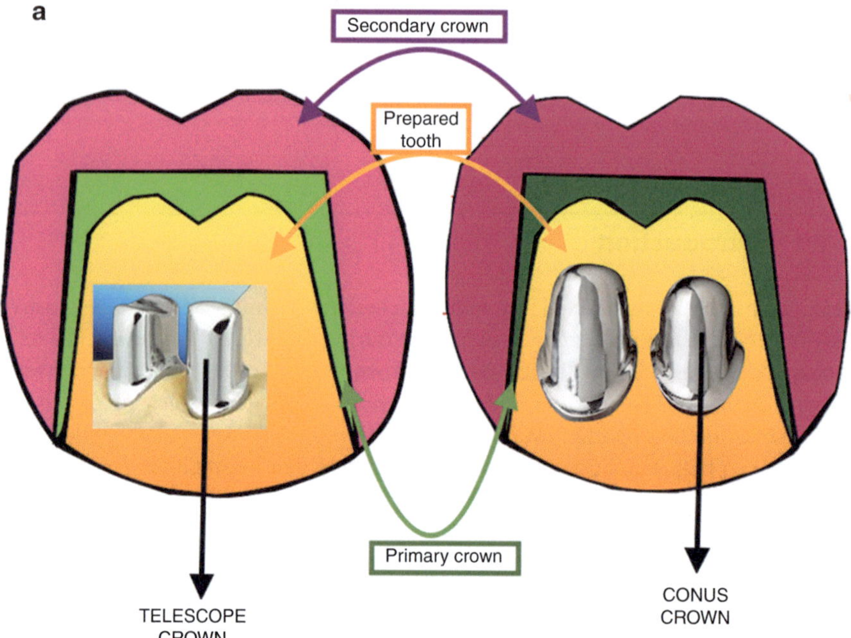

Fig. 5.1 (**a**) The telescope and conus crown assembly. (**b**) Classification of copings for TO. (**c**) The cylinder, conus, and resilient telescope crown (schematic view)

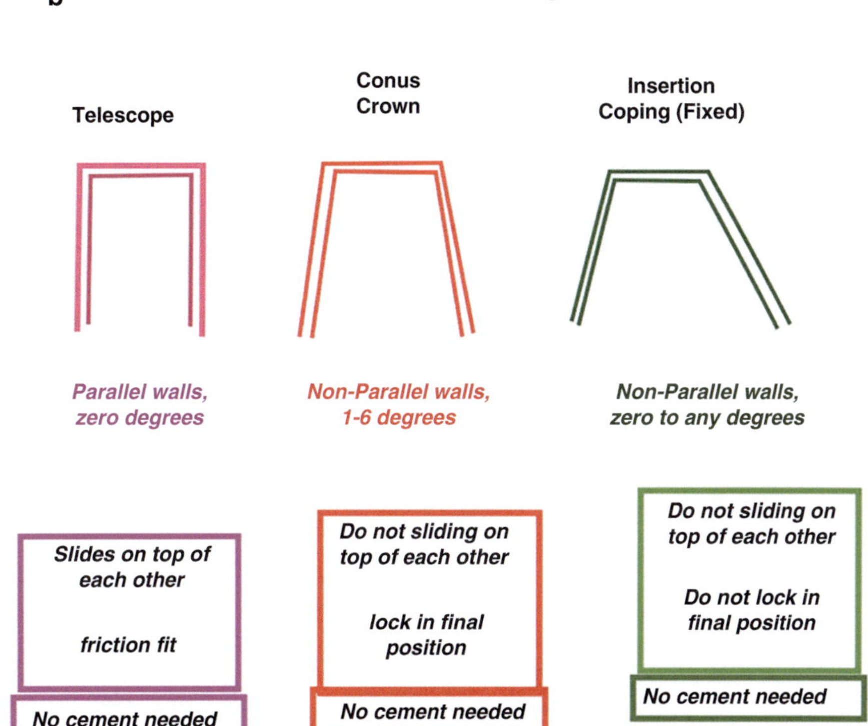

Fig. 5.1 (continued)

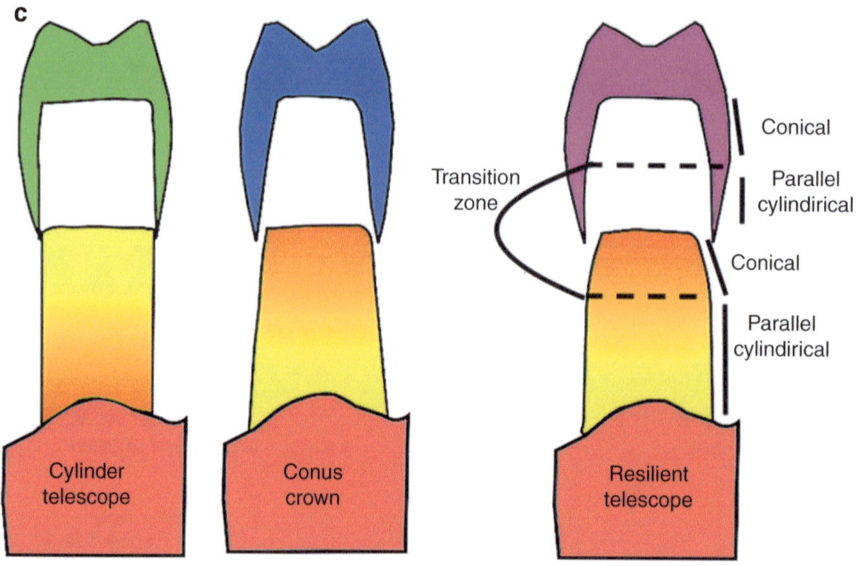

Fig. 5.1 (continued)

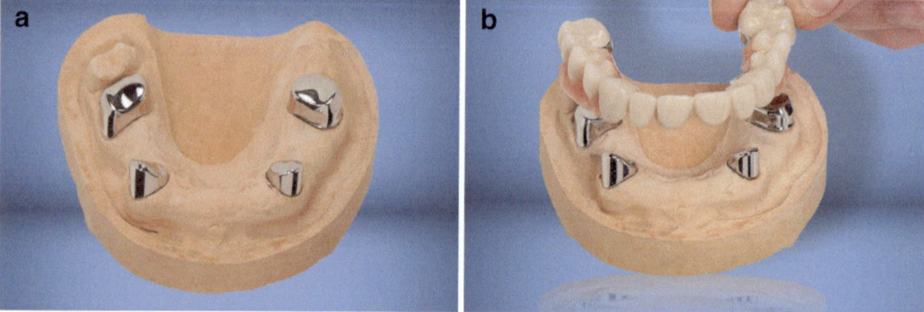

Picture 5.1 (**a**) The primary telescope crown placed on four abutments in the upper jaw. (**a, b**) The secondary crowns are cast with metal frame together as one piece (as the bridge in the anterior area) (Courtesy of Ulrich Heker)

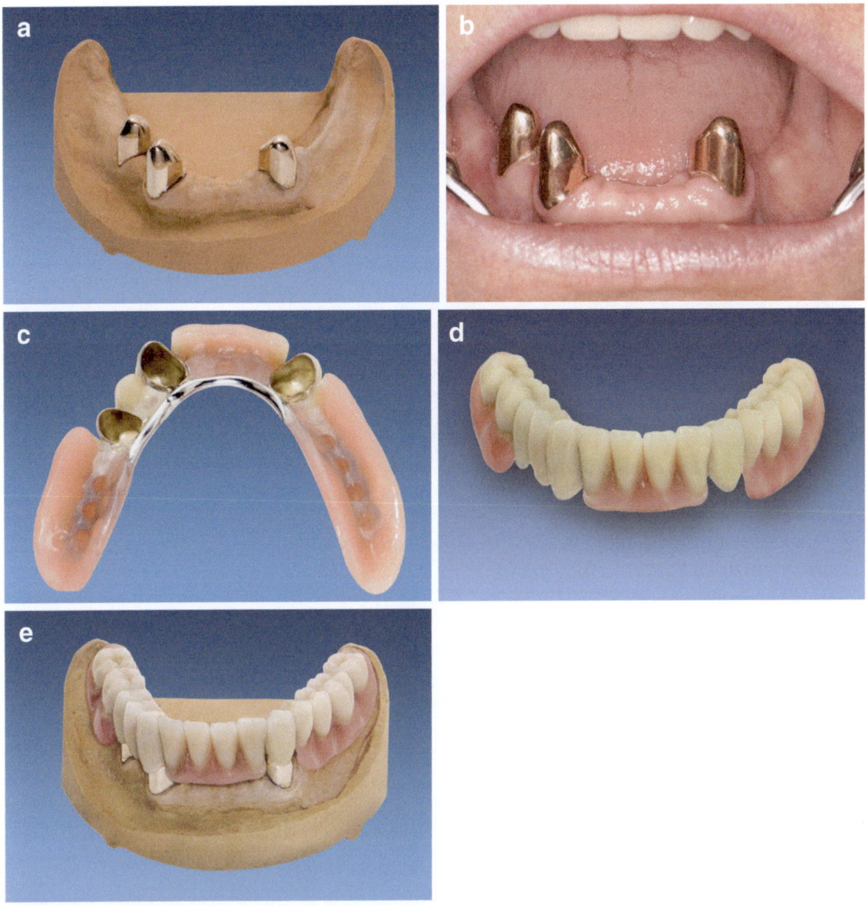

Picture 5.2 (**a**) The resilient telescope dentures are used on the mandibular jaw. The resilient primary coping cast with noble alloys on the lower canines and premolar tooth. (**b**) The primary coping cemented in the teeth. (**c, d**) The secondary crowns are cast as one unit with a metal framework and secondary coping veneered with porcelain materials; the rest is produced as dentures with acrylic teeth. (**e**) The prosthesis is seated on the primary coping (Courtesy of Ulrich Heker)

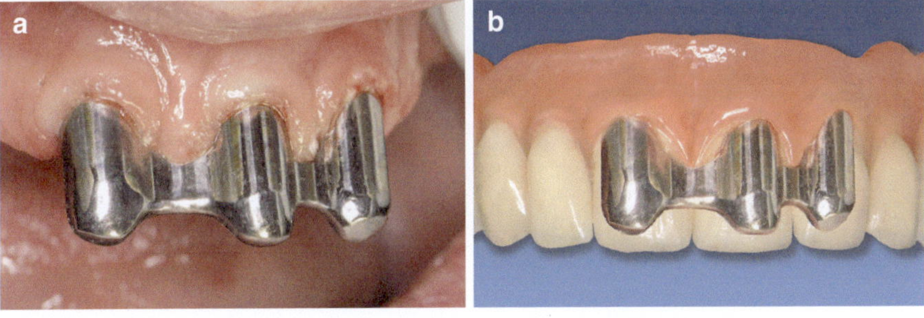

Picture 5.3 (**a**) In the upper anterior teeth, telescopic abutments and primary coping cast with Co-Cr alloy as adjacent copings are used. (**b**) The primary coping is directly placed in an acrylic denture (Courtesy of Ulrich Heker)

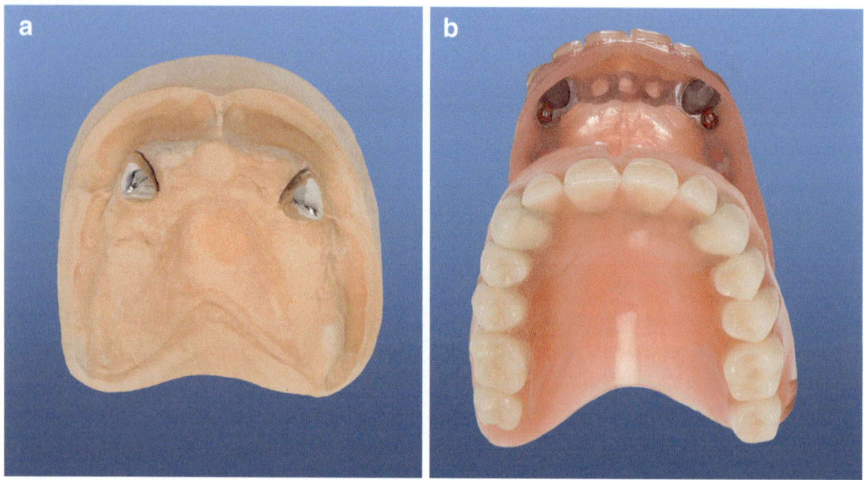

Picture 5.4 (**a**) Two upper canines were used as an abutment for upper TO and the primary coping was cast with Co-Cr alloy. (**b**) Two secondary crowns are attached to the metal framework (Courtesy of Ulrich Heker)

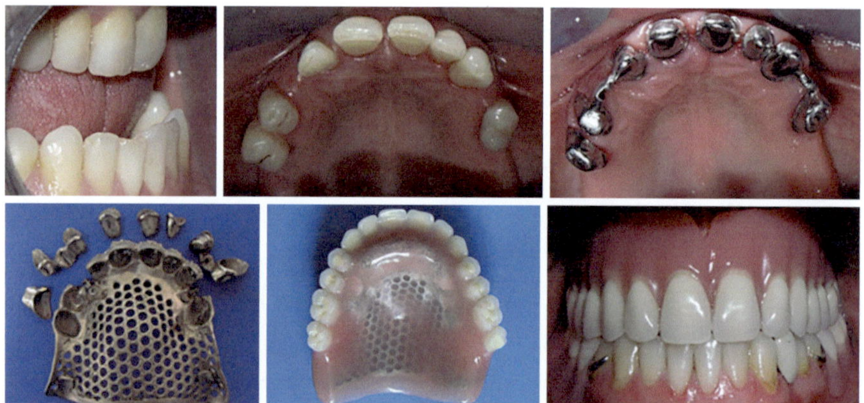

Picture 5.5 Intracoronary attachment is used as a modification of the telescopic crown-and-sleeve coping retainers for a Class III patient treatment

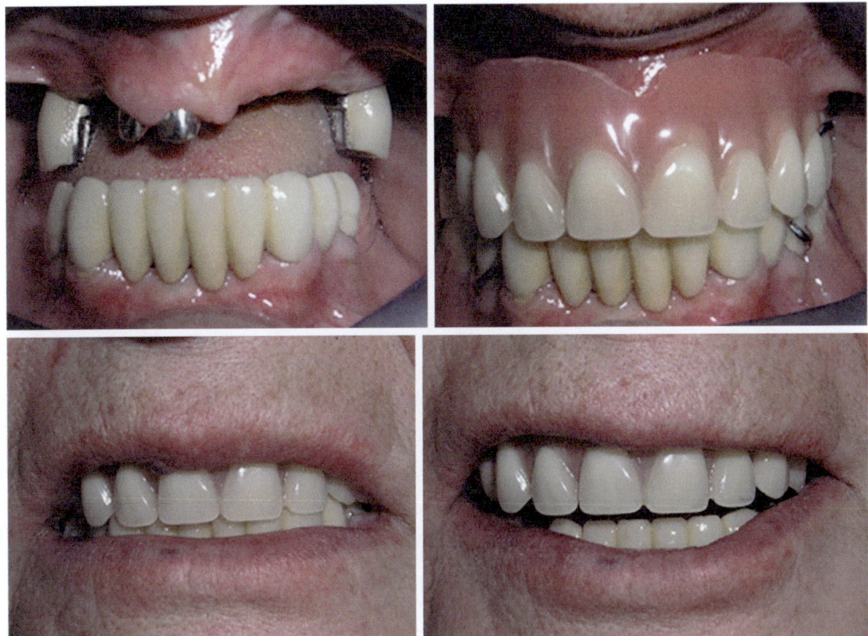

Picture 5.6   Poor design of the TO results in an unfavorable aesthetic appearance. When the abutment teeth have an undercut and teeth preparation is made not taking into consideration this undercut, the bulk of the double crowns could create an esthetic problem

Picture 5.7   The support provided by the abutment teeth is in addition to that supplied by the residual ridges; and after teeth extractions, residual ridges should be used easily for implant placement

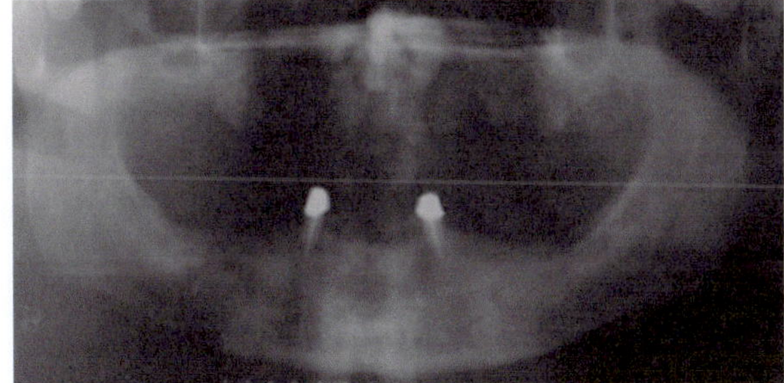

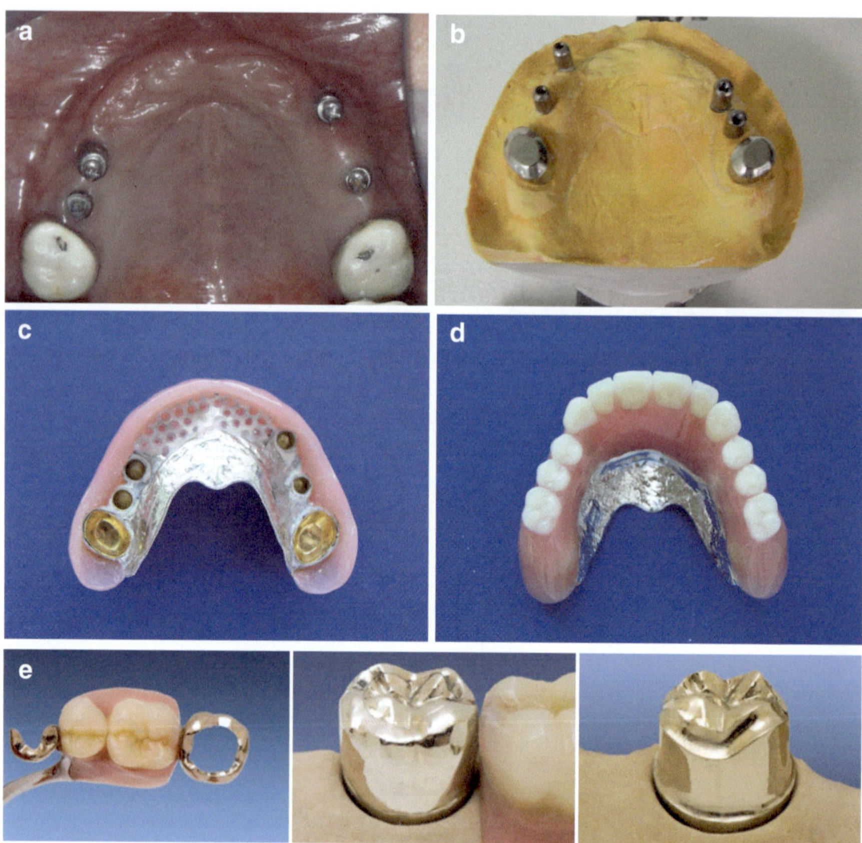

Picture 5.8 (**a**) Telescope crown on natural teeth and implant-retained overdenture. The molar teeth served as supporting elements along with four implants placed in the upper jaw. (**b**) The primary metal crown cast with non-precious alloys on the molar abutment teeth and telescope abutments placed on the implant seen in the model. (**c**) The TO denture intaglio surface. The metal framework is cast together with secondary crowns. Galvano coping produced on primary coping luted with metal framework. (**d**) The external view of TO. (**e**) The ring telescope crown (Courtesy of Ulrich Heker)

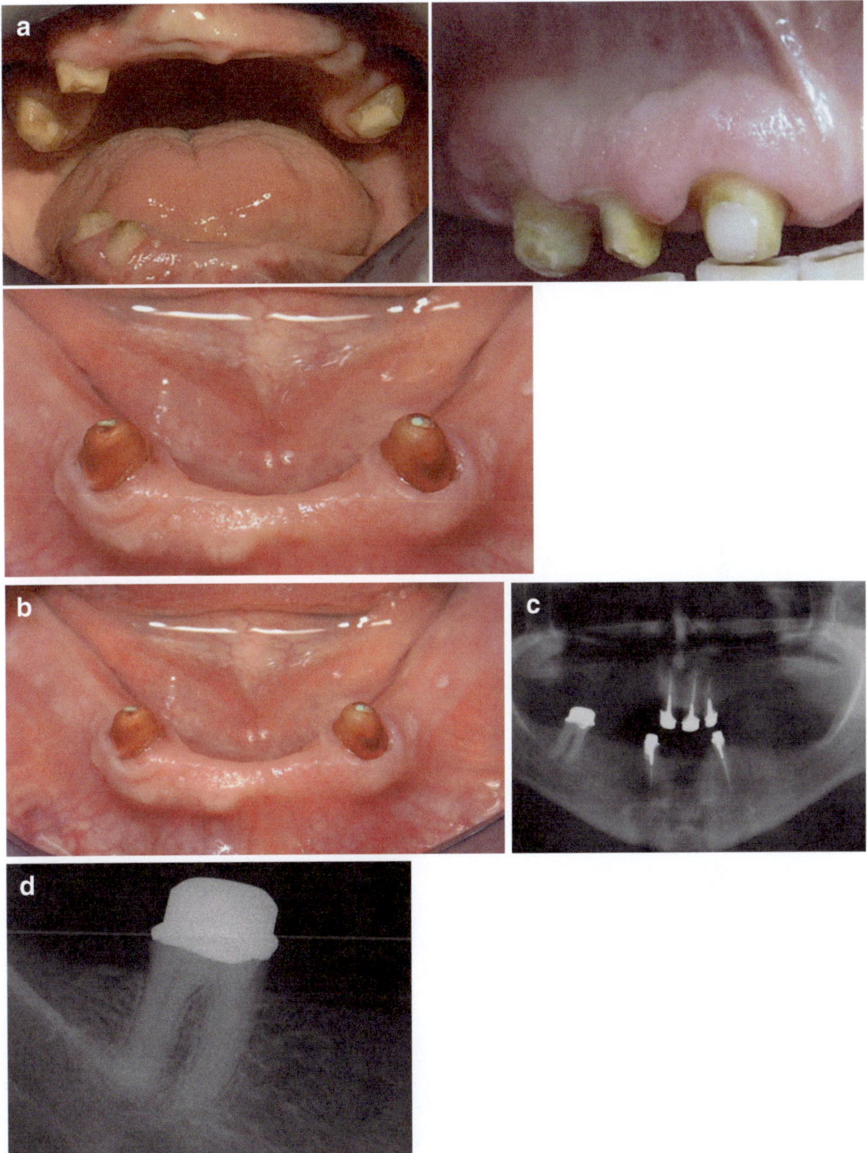

Picture 5.9 (**a**) The selected abutments should be periodontally sound (clinically assessment). (**b**) The preparations should be done with a circumferential shoulder margin. (**c**, **d**) The abutments should have adequate bone support and no/minimal mobility (radiological assessment)

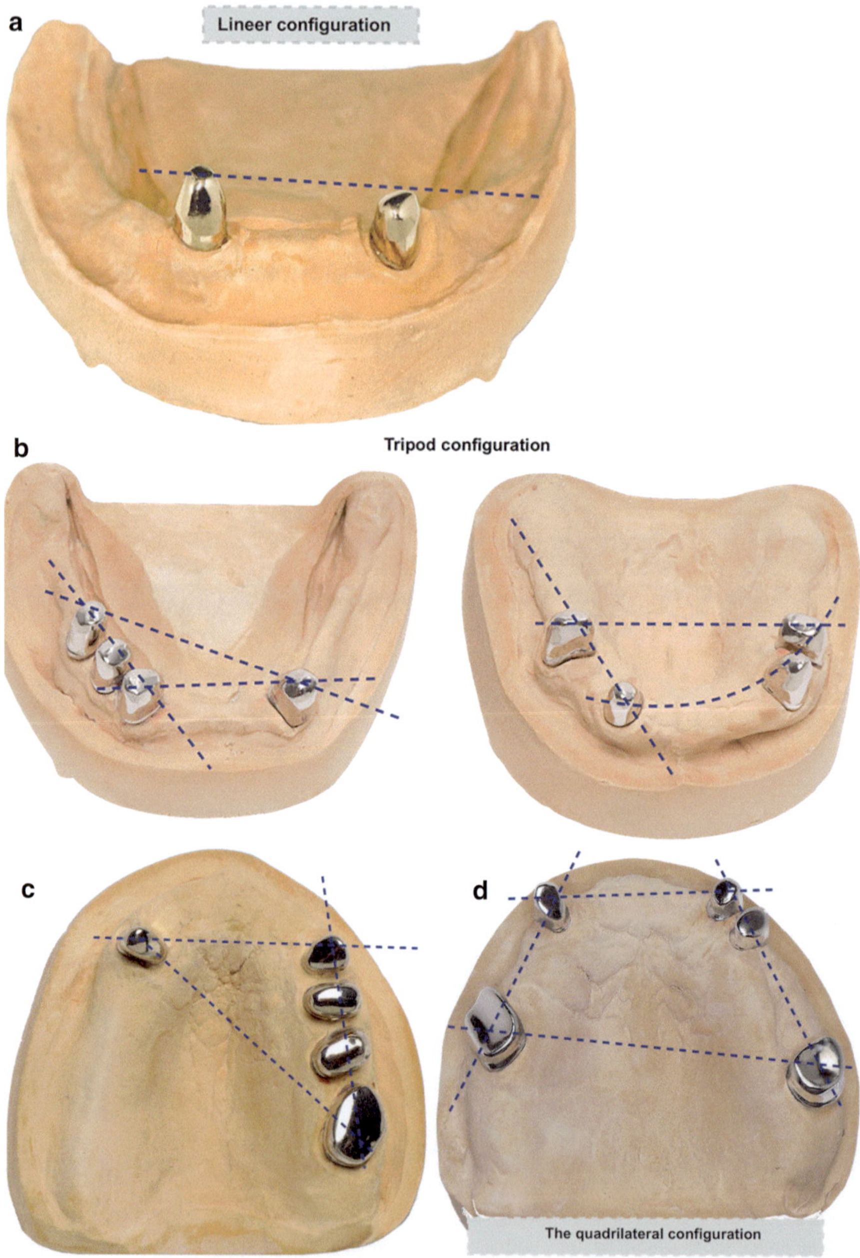

Picture 5.10 (**a–e**) Different configurations (linear, tripod, quadrilateral) abutment for TO: (**a**) linear configuration. There should be at least one healthy abutment in each quadrant; (**b**, **c**) tripod configuration: leverage controlled to some extent by creating tripod configuration; (**d**) the quadrilateral configuration; (**e**) different configurations (Courtesy of Ulrich Heker)

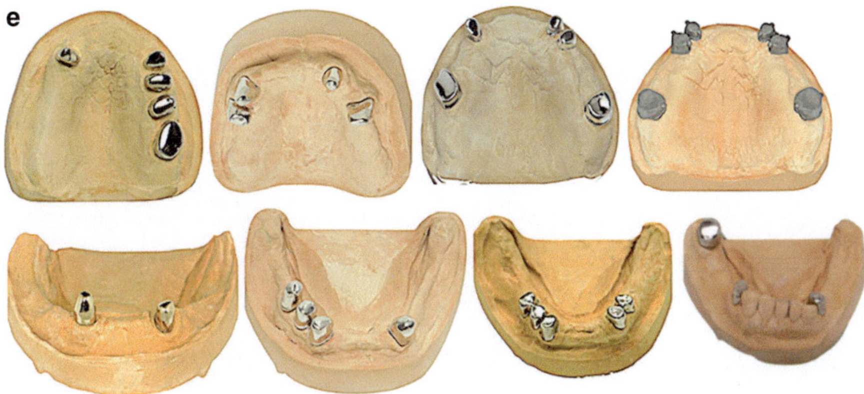

Picture 5.10 (continued)

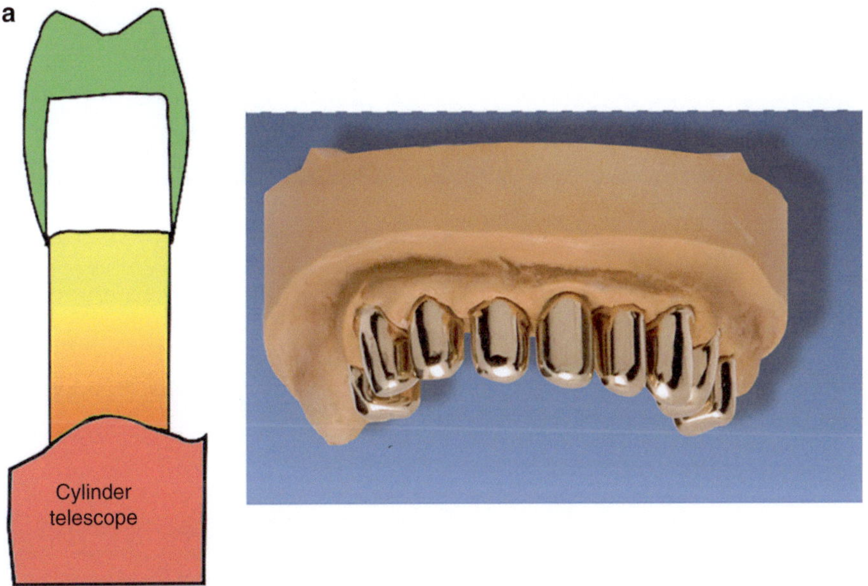

Fig. 5.2 (**a**) The cylinder telescope (schematic view) and the casted model. (**b**) The cylinder telescope crown assembly (schematic view). (**c**) *a* The prepared tooth, *b* primary cylinder telescope, and *c* cast with noble metal alloys (schematic view)

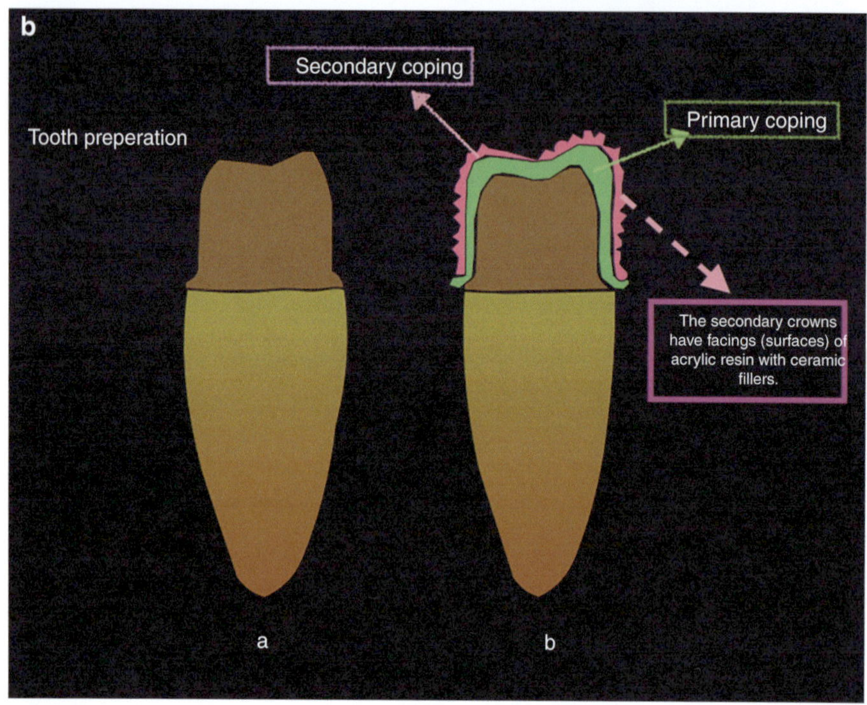

Fig. 5.2 (continued)

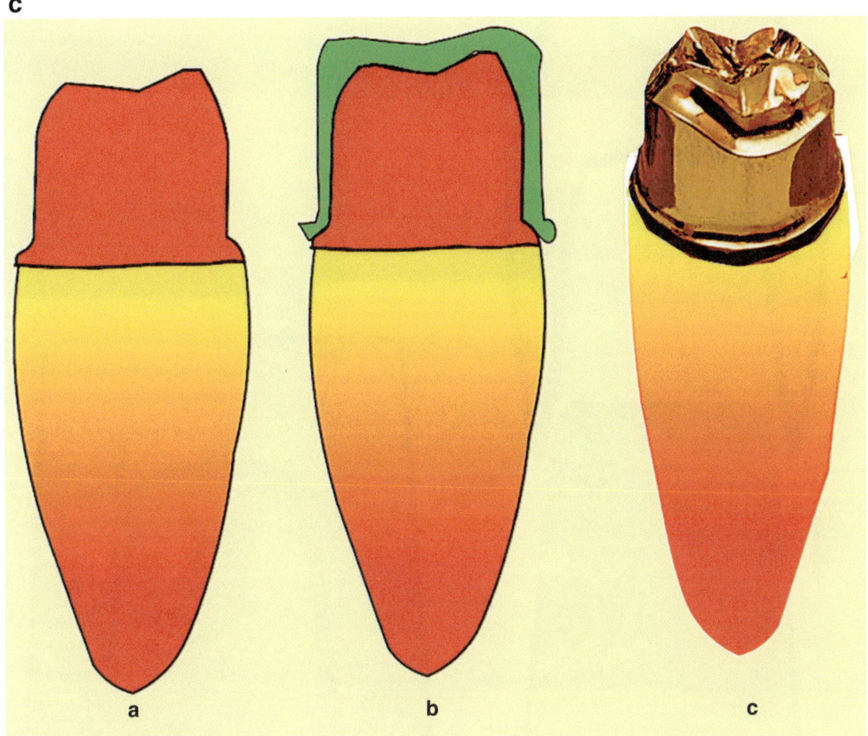

Fig. 5.2 (continued)

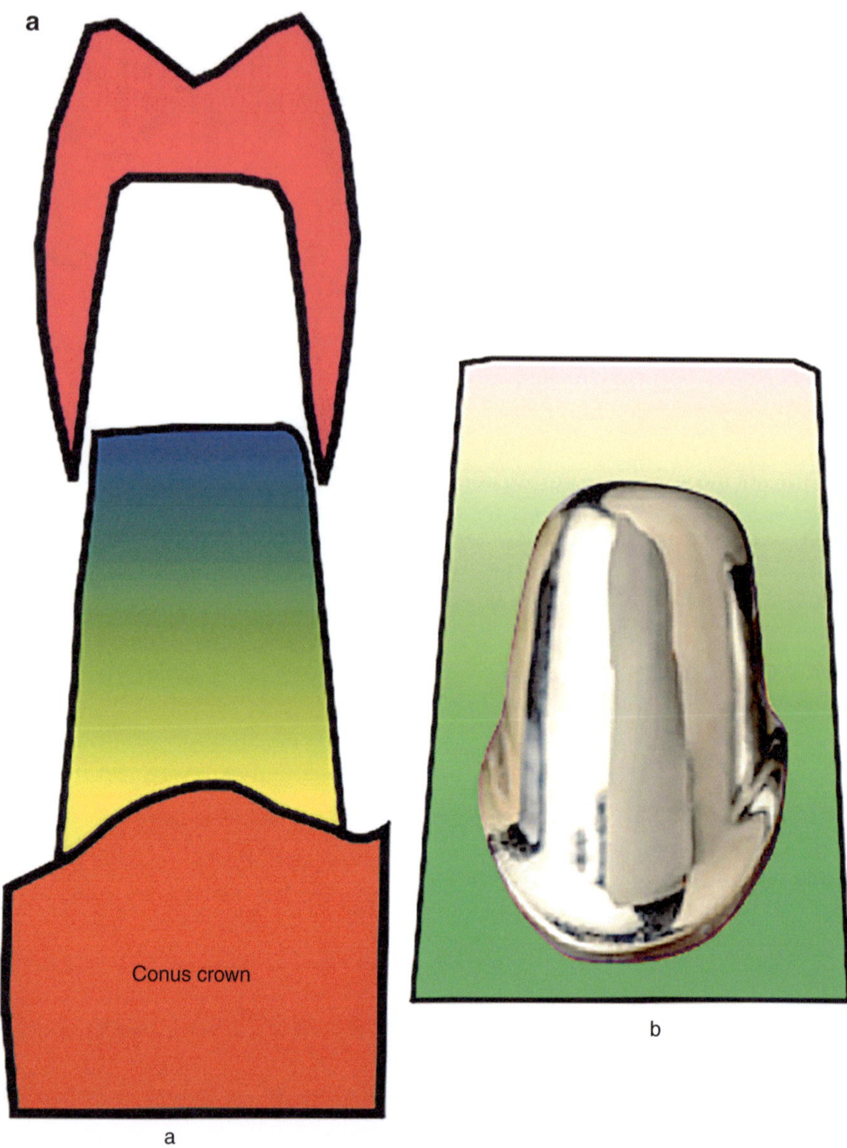

Fig. 5.3 (**a**) *a*: The conus crown in schematic view and *b*: cast with noble metal alloys. (**b**) The conus crown in schematic view. (**c**) The primary coping with 6° taper angles. (**d**) The primary copings with three different taper angles. (**e**) The milling waxes primary coping with 60 taper angle and conus crown

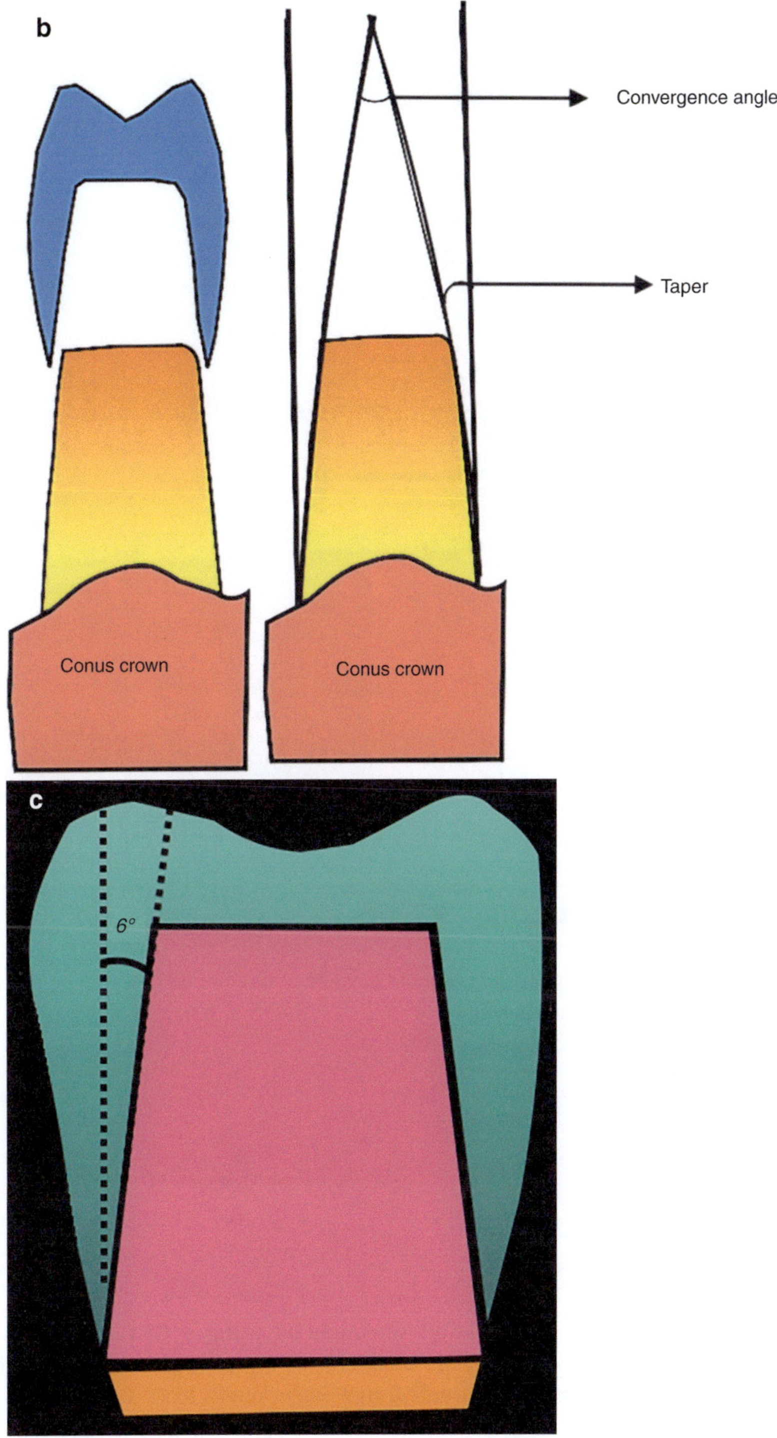

Fig. 5.3 (continued)

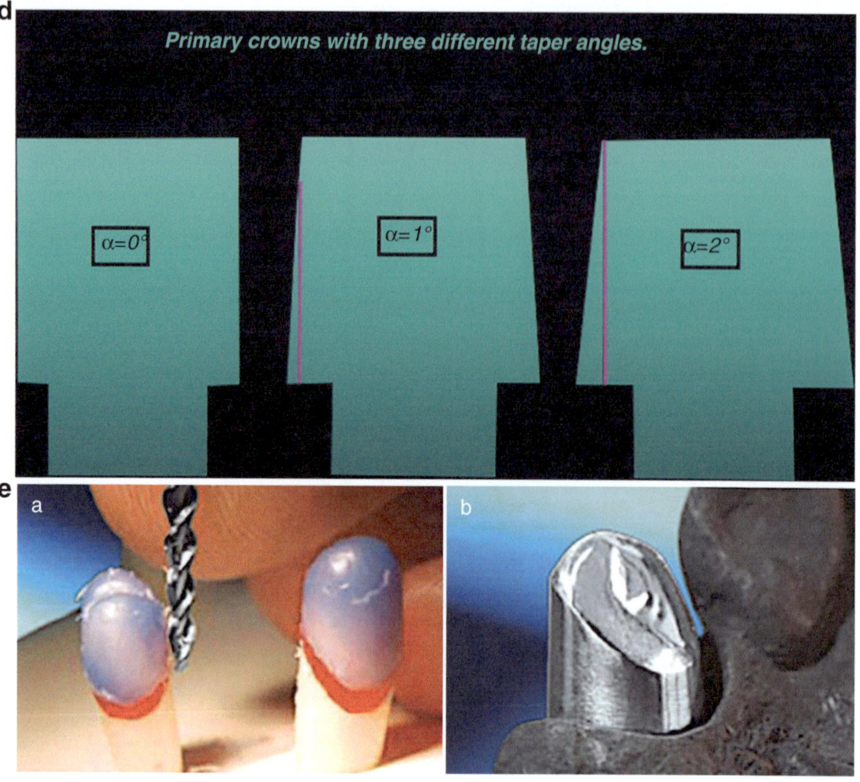

Fig. 5.3 (continued)

5.2 Telescopic Attachment Types

Numerous types of telescopic attachments have been developed to meet the particular needs of clinical scenarios (Figs. 5.1, 5.2, 5.3, 5.4, 5.5, 5.6, and 5.7):

1. Cylindrical crowns.
2. Conus crowns.
3. Robust designs.
4. Modified designs.

5.2.1 Cylindrical Crowns

The telescopic crowns (TC) achieves retention by using a friction mechanism (Figs. 5.1 and 5.2; Picture 5.1). These crowns have a predetermined end position, meaning they do not permit more vertical movement under load. The primary and

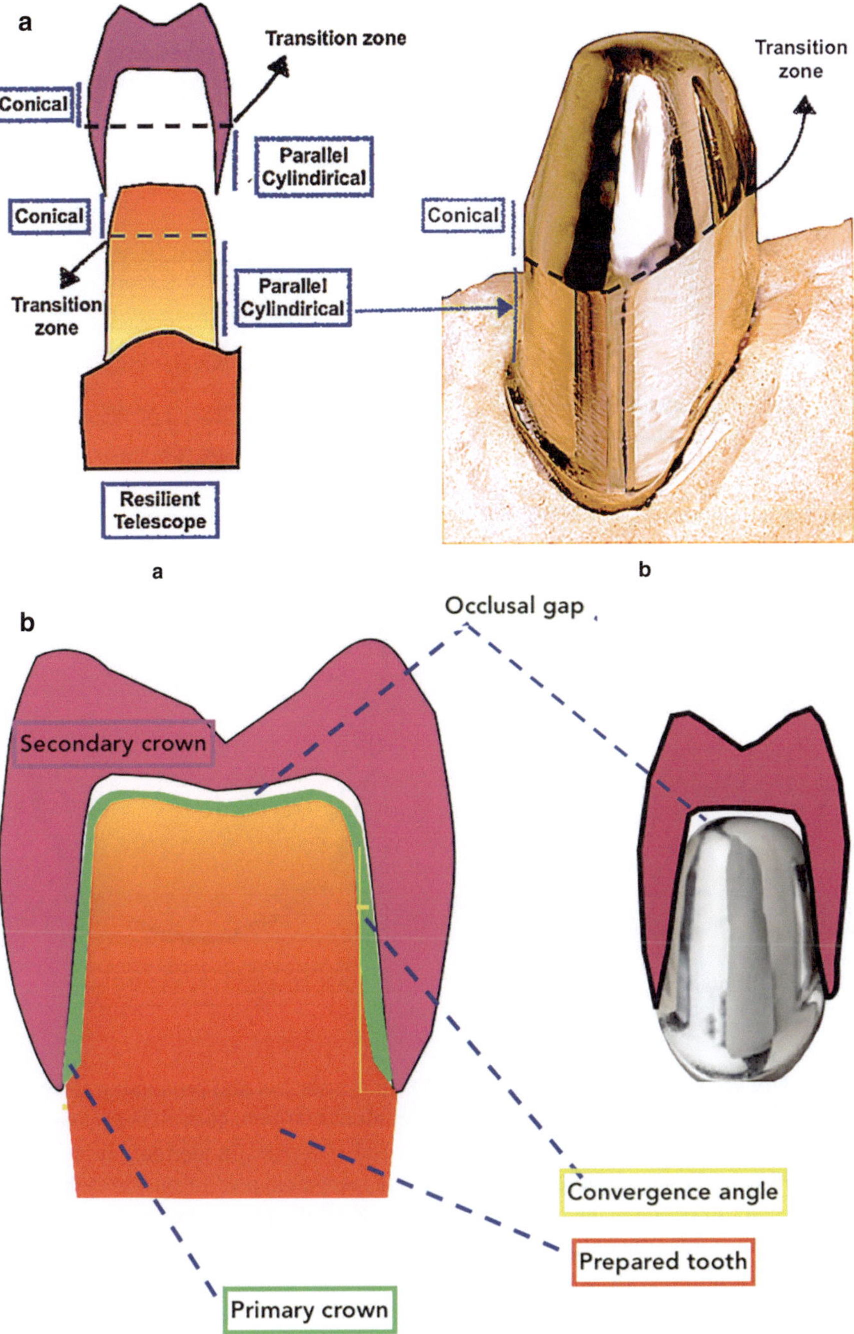

Fig. 5.4 (**a**) The resilient telescope designs. (**b**) The resilient telescope design is characterized by built-in occlusal space (0.3 mm) between the primary coping and secondary crown for compensation of soft tissue resiliency. (**c**) The primary coping with 6° taper angle and 0.3 mm occlusal space

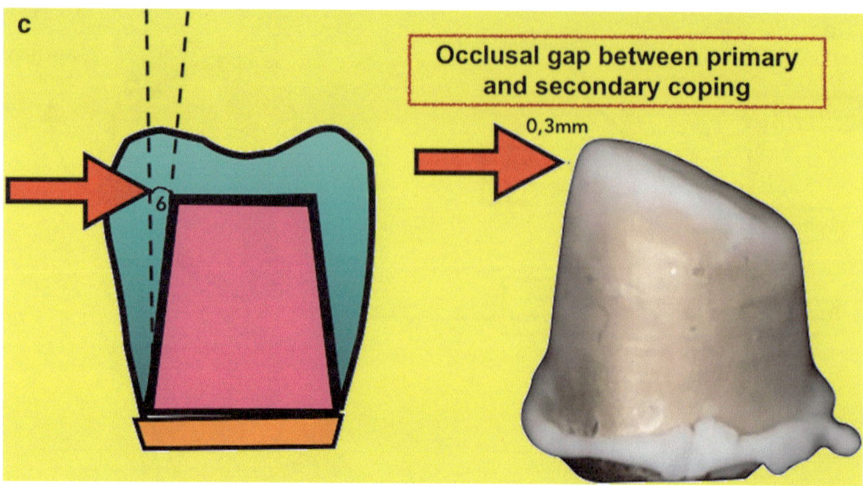

Fig. 5.4 (continued)

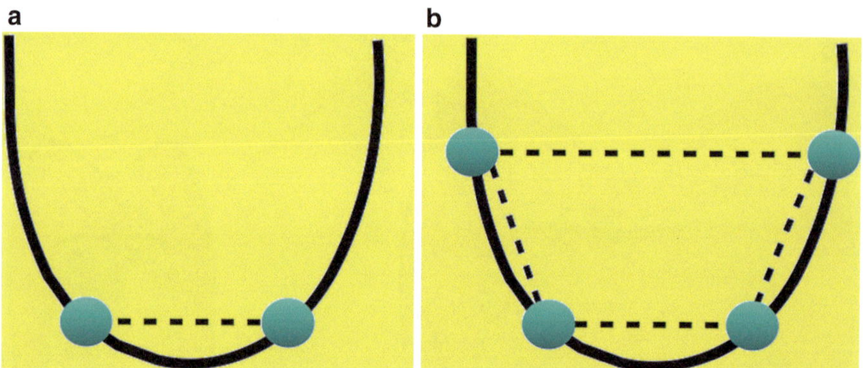

Fig. 5.5 Distribution of abutment teeth for TO: (**a**) linear configuration and (**b**) quadrilateral configuration

secondary crowns are linked by friction. During insertion and removal of the prosthesis, interfacial friction occurs as the two components engage and disengage. This design has the benefits of superior retention and aesthetics in the margin area. The fabrication of these types of crowns necessitates technical perfection due to the need for a perfect fit between the crowns, as they have a definite end position and friction levels that are low enough to facilitate easy removal of the overdenture, but high enough to minimize movement during function. In TC, friction is a difficult-to-measure parameter. It is principally dependent on the technical construction of the crown, which is influenced by the following factors: the number of telescopic crowns, the length of the friction surfaces, and the placement of the friction surface relative to one another. Only opposing-facing parallel surfaces can provide the

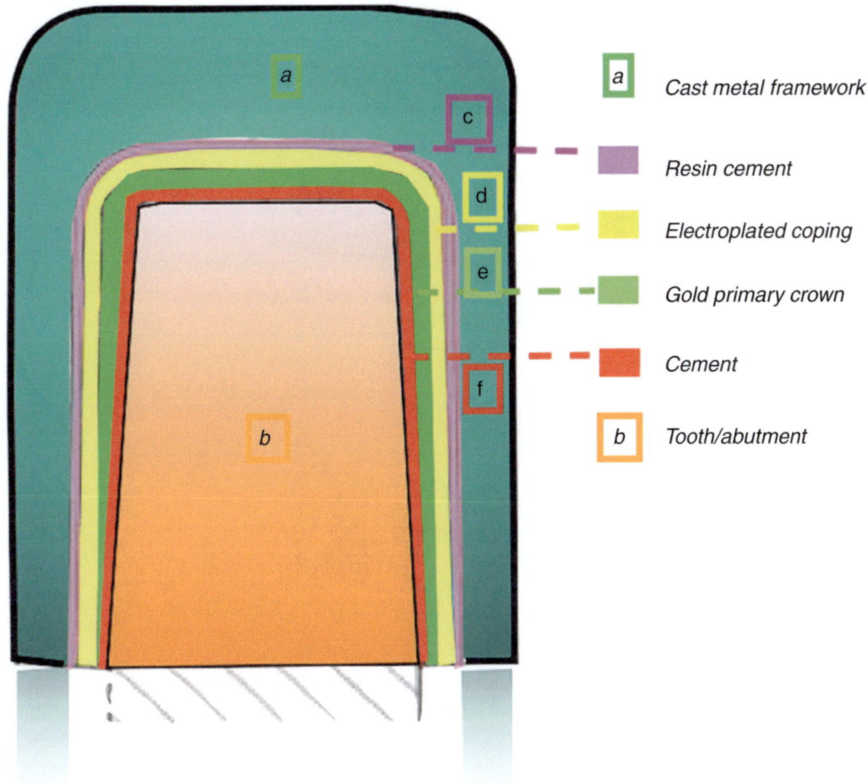

Fig. 5.6 The layer of telescope crown using the Galvano technique: (**a**) The cast metal framework (secondary coping), (**b**) the prepared tooth, (**c**) resin cement, (**d**) electroplated coping, (**e**) gold primary coping, (**f**) cement

required friction of telescopes, which is related to the elasticity of the materials used, so gold alloys are often used. Also, parallel surfaces can generate the necessary friction for telescopes, that is proportional to the elasticity of the materials in which gold alloys are frequently employed (Figs. 5.1 and 5.2; and Pictures 5.1, 5.2, 5.3, and 5.4).

5.2.1.1 Characteristics of Telescoping Crowns

-As with a shock absorber, the primary and secondary crowns slide over each other without a final locking position.

- The milling telescope is a wall coping with a 0° angle, and the second crowns (superstructure) are not cemented, with retention improved by a friction fit.
- The denture can be readily removed and cleaned by the patient.
- If the crowns are too bulky, esthetic problems occur.
- When three to four abutment is used palatal coverage can be minimized.
- A 1 mm chamfer preparation is required for primary coping.

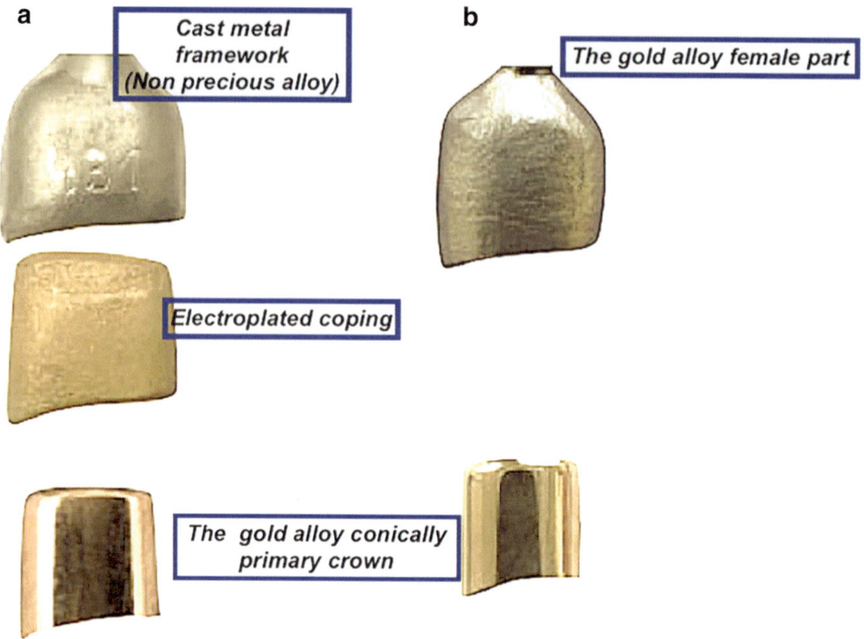

Fig. 5.7 The primary coping and secondary crown fabrication types: (**a**) The electroplated method; primary coping produced with gold alloy, secondary crowns cast with non-precious alloy and electroplated cooping and (**b**) primary coping and secondary crown produced with gold alloy

5.2.2 Conical Crowns

Professor Karl Heinz Korber described the conical shape design. Due to expansion issues with investments and casts, the fit of telescopic crowns was frequently too tight which resulted in retention problems for patients wearing TO. The conical approach is based on the straightforward concept of a pressed fit. Conical crowns or tapered telescope crowns only exhibit friction when fully seated through a "wedge" effect (Figs. 5.1 and 5.3). The operation of this system is illustrated by utilizing plastic cups. The working principle of this system is explained with plastic cups. Plastic cups are put half-together. If one cup is wholly put into another, there is a close fit, and they become wedged together. The inner crown has a cone-like shape. So, the axial surfaces of it are tapered occlusally at a specific angle called the convergence angle (or taper). Retention is obtained by the wedging action. The smaller the convergence angle the greater the retention force will be.

In combination with a removable denture, the conical crown has become widely used in Germany and Sweden, since the system enables modifications with maintained function if abutments are lost. So, the axial surfaces of it are tapered occlusally in a specific angle called the convergence angle (or taper), and retention is obtained by the wedging action (Fig. 5.3c). The tapered configuration of the contacting walls generates compressive, tensile stress. The tension should be sufficiently strong enough to sustain the denture in its place. The smaller degree of the taper provides a higher frictional rate (Fig. 5.3d). An increase in the tapering of the coping walls reduces the retention between the copings. A taper of 6 degrees is recommended to achieve a retention force between 5 and 10 N when using high precious alloys (Fig. 5.3e). It is mentioned that a 40–80° angle may be used according to crown length and the physiologic movement of the abutment. It is generally stated that the walls of the abutments with short clinical height should be kept parallel to each other, or the taper of the wall should be reduced (2–5°) to improve retention. Many laboratories tend to produce crowns with a slightly conical angle of 1–2° to facilitate preparation during the milling process. It also has to be recommended that minimal conicity of the primary crowns can occur very quickly, as milling parallel surfaces are challenging.

Ohkawa et al. [1] mentioned a 2° taper angle to be used as a maximum angle for double crown systems in long-term clinical use. Kiyama et al. [2] reported that as the axial angle decreased and the height of the inner crown increased, the retentive force increased.

When placing a conus telescope partial denture in the mouth, retentive force is achieved by applying a load. The retentive force of the conus crown was performed by a slight deformation of the outer crown based on the wedge effect. If the applied load increases, expanding deformation of the outer crown will also occur, thereby leading to an increase in the retentive force of the conus telescope crown. For the deformity of the outer crown, a gap needed to exist between the inner crown and the outer crown. If the reverse side in the occlusal area of the outer crown were in contact with the occlusal surface of the inner crown, then no retentive force would be exhibited. In other words, it was suggested that if the gap were 0 μm, the reverse side of the outer crown would already be in contact with the occlusal surface of the inner crown, which meant that retentive force would not increase even if more load were applied. In sharp contrast, when the gap was more than 50 μm, the deformation amount of the outer crown would remain the same when the same load was applied.

The conical type is used more widely than the cylindrical design because it is less complicated in fabrication and less harmful to abutments and their supporting tissues. This design also has the advantage of determining the forces that would be applied to each abutment by selecting the convergence angle according to the clinical situation. However, the conical design has the disadvantage of retention decreasing after a period of use. Hulten al. [3] treated 78 patients with conical crown-retained dentures and followed up for 4 months (1983–1988) using the CDA quality evaluation system. They reported that more than 80% of the removable dentures and abutments were in function at the time of examination. Forty-four percent of the conical crown-retained dentures were considered to have acceptable quality while 56% were not adequate, mainly due to caries at the margins of the abutments.

5.2.2.1 Characteristics of the Conus Crown

- When the primary coping is tall and the applied load increases, the retentive force also increases.

- As the space between the inner crown and outer crown increased at the occlusal region, the retentive force of the conus telescope crown also increased.
- The walls of the conus should be conical, with an angle between 1 and 6°.
- When the conical surfaces reach their final position, the terminal lock occurs. There is no contact between the two components until they have been completely seated.
- If the abutment teeth number increases, the patient will have difficulty removing dentures.
- There is no need for cement between copings.

5.2.3   Resilient (Non-rigid) Designs

Resilient TC does not have a definite apical endpoint; hence they permit some vertical movement under load (Fig. 5.1). Since 1989, resilient TC has been used to support mandibular overdentures. That may be achieved by some modifications in the inner crown, the outer crown, or both. These modifications result in a reduction of intimate contact and the creation of a space between the inner and the outer crowns. The Marburg double crown is a well-known resilient design. It is based on the clearance fit system where only the cervical third of the inner crown is parallel to the outer crown providing a space between the crowns. This space allows a minor lateral movement between the crowns and prevents stress occurrence. This design as incorporating occlusal space (0.3 mm) between the primary coping and secondary crowns is to compensate for soft tissue resiliency (Fig. 5.4). Additionally, a little space (0.3 mm) could be provided between the primary and secondary crowns to reduce the moment loading of the abutments during chewing. This perfect clearance between the primary and secondary crowns permits minimal, undetectable lateral movement and smooth, frictionless sliding throughout the insertion path. In addition, an occlusal space between the primary coping and secondary crown allows for resilient support. Once the occlusal load is eliminated, the denture returns to its previous place. Therefore, the secondary crown was functionally coupled to the primary coping to compensate for the mucosal resilience potential during functional loading, and the occlusal-apical movements of the denture will not increase the load to the attachment.

Four to six degrees convergence angles to retain implant-supported overdentures were suggested as an alternative method. The use of a 6° occlusal convergence taper for robust telescopic attachment to hold two implants and a mandibular overdenture is a potential prosthodontic modality if rigorous prosthodontic procedures are taken to reduce the lingual component of force.

It was reported that the non-rigid telescopic attachment provides excellent horizontal stability, increased implant stability over time, ease of use, and hygiene, which makes it ideal for those with handicapped patients.

On the other side, it was stated that rigid TO generates a stable occlusal plane and denture position, hence decreasing the possibility of posterior mandibular and anterior maxillary jaw resorption. In comparison to resilient stabilization, rigid prosthesis minimizes the frequency of implant denture prosthodontic maintenance for removable dentures. The non-rigid telescope attachment is still mostly unknown, and studies comparing it to other connectors are scarce.

The Marburg double crown is a well-known resistant structure. It was first reported in 1988 by Lehmann and Gente and employs extra prefabricated pieces (TC-Snap System, Si-Tec) to enhance the retention of telescopic crowns. It is a versatile approach for reconstructing partially edentulous arches in which either natural teeth or dental implants can be utilized as abutments. Its application is independent of the quantity and positioning of abutments. The denture base does not cover the abutment teeth's marginal periodontium. The denture adjacent to the abutment teeth is perioprotective. The distal extension base is functionally extended to give optimal support. Through extra attachment or a functional border seal, retention is achieved. The denture base is in touch with the denture-bearing mucosa following the cementation of the primary copings and placement of the removable partial denture (RPDs), while there is a gap between the primary and secondary crowns due to the clearance fit system. When an occlusal load is applied, the denture moves downward; the degree of movement relies on the elasticity of the mucosa supporting the denture.

In addition, the perioprotective characteristic is essential for maintaining periodontally healthy abutment teeth. These designs provide a durable connection between the abutment and the denture and, according to their proponents, prevent negative effects, and harmonize with tissue elasticity, resulting in a better distribution of forces and increase abutment survival rates. In cases of a few remaining or weak abutments and distal extensions, resilient designs may be useful.

In Hofmann and Ludwig's design, the cervical half of the inner crown is parallel-sided while the occlusal half is conical with a space of 0.2–0.5 mm between the crowns in the occlusal region. Yalisove produced a conical design in which the contact between crowns was restricted to the two occlusal thirds, while there was a space of 0.003–0.010 in. between the crowns in the cervical third, allowing rotation of the outer crown and preventing friction. Heckmann et al. (2001) [4] discovered that robust telescopic attachments hold the denture in place and act as a stiff lever, exerting significant moment forces on the implant, which induces a triaxial stress state in the surrounding bone. This stress state maybe five times the value of a non-rigid telescope. Hofmann et al. (2006) [5] also reported that the resilient telescopic attachments compensate for soft-tissue elasticity, resulting in reduced stress transmission to the implant surface.

5.2.4 Modified Designs

Some systems were developed with significant modifications in the TC concept. They mostly depend on merging the telescopic system with another type of attachment.

Magnotelescoping spires.

O-ring attachment for coping.

Telescopic attachments that are prefabricated.

Clinical experiences for the past 9 years have demonstrated the practicability of the O-ring coping attachment, a modification of the telescopic crown-and-sleeve coping retainers, for removable partial dentures. A circumferential groove placed in the primary coping receives an elastomeric O-ring that fits into a corresponding groove made on the internal surface of the telescopic crown. The O-ring not only provides controllable retention but also acts as a shock absorber. Long-term retention of the prostheses can be easily maintained by periodic replacements of the O-rings; sophisticated procedures and expensive machines are not required to make the prostheses. Excellent patient acceptance and versatility in clinical applications make this system one of the winning designs for removable partial prosthodontics. The author used the intracoronal attachment, a modification of the telescopic crown-and-sleeve coping retainers for a Class III patient treatment (Picture 5.5).

5.3   The Advantages of TC

- Better force distribution. Telescopic crowns also provide better force distribution due to the circumferential relation of the secondary crown to the abutment which makes the axial transfer of occlusal load that produces less rotational torque on the abutment by improving the crown-root ratio so preserving the tooth and alveolar bone.
- Good retention and stabilization. The great retentive force results from the fitting and extensive contact between the surfaces of the inner and the outer crowns.
- Secondary splinting action. They also provide an indirect splinting effect, easy oral hygiene maintenance, and easy ways of repair. This is due to the accurate relation between the primary and the secondary crowns, as they are rigidly connected to the denture base.
- Transferring occlusal forces through the long axes of abutments.
- One of the main advantages of the TC is that being pericoronal retainers, they transmit the occlusal forces in the direction of the long axes of the abutment teeth. The axial forces stimulate periodontal tissues and alveolar bone.
- Creation of a common path of insertion. That can be easily provided by the parallelism of inner crowns even if the abutments are tilted.
- Hygienic advantages. The TC also has the advantage of ease of removability. This encourages the patient for cleaning and maintaining the hygiene of TSO. Moreover, the excellent fitting of the inner crown on the abutment protects it from caries and thermal irritation. The TC also has a significant advantage for the peri-implant soft tissues, since they allow more comfortable and more effective oral hygiene compared to the bar attachment. There will be inflammation on the peri-implant tissue surrounding the bar anchors and light hyperplasia under the bar timely. In contrast, the condition of the soft tissues around the telescopic copings will be significantly healthier.
- Esthetic advantages. Using double crowns as the retentive element allows better esthetics than clasps for removable partial dentures. Excellent esthetics can be provided by using ceramic faces and a suitable color selection.

- Patient satisfaction. TSO with TC retainers has also a self-fit mechanism due to telescopic constructions facilitating denture insertion considerably. This type of TSO seems to be an effective treatment modality for geriatric patients with severe systemic diseases as in Parkinson's disease. Many authors reported reasonable patient satisfaction rates with telescopic dentures.
- Repair and adjustment ability. Telescopic TSO can be easily repaired even when an abutment is lost.

5.4   Disadvantages of TC

- Technical complications. Telescopic TSO fabrication requires very complicated clinical and laboratory procedures. The technique-sensitive procedure must be followed, which requires a skilled and experienced dental laboratory.
- Cost problems. The cost is also increased, due to technical complexity, the need for prefabricated abutments (requiring precision milling), and the casting of the secondary crown. Telescopic copings are the most expensive retention system, followed by cast bars. The magnets, balls, and locators need minimum additional laboratory stages. Furthermore their maintenance is easier and more comfortable to accomplish at the chairside.
- Retention-related problems. It may be challenging to achieve the exact retention required between the primary coping and the secondary crown. Also, the retentive force between the crowns decreases after a period of use. That results from the repeated insertion and removal of the denture, and the wears of metals occur. Various tribological processes are a result of the effects of crown parts on surface changes. The most common four tribological factors are tribochemical reaction, abrasion, adhesion, and surface deformation. They can occur separately or in combination. Interaction, appearance, and combination of these factors are affected by the structure of the retentive components as well as the material. In vitro studies for wear tests set up a saliva substitute as a necessary component. It is needed as part of the tribologic system comprising the primary coping, intermediary (saliva), and secondary crown. The absence of such an intermediary leads to significant changes in frictional wear. The effects can be determined by analyzing the surface structures and by the changes in the retention force.
- Cervical caries. Failure in providing the accurate fit of the crowns or poor oral hygiene may lead to the occurrence of cervical caries.

Esthetic problems. The over-contouring of the crowns is the most common esthetic problem (Picture 5.6).

For ensuring the esthetic outcome of the denture, a temporary denture setup must be made and the space must be determined for the primary coping and the secondary crowns. The preparation of the teeth should be more aggressive which may need endodontic treatment (higher loss of dentin material in the supporting teeth due to preparation (approximately 1.8 mm)) to obtain a better result from an aesthetic point of view. In any case, shoulder preparation is the best precondition.

- Technical failures. Technical failure is one of the primary problems associated with the TO. Many studies reported high rates of technical shortcomings in this type of prosthesis. Technical failures may be loss of cementation; loss of veneering material; or fracture of artificial teeth, the metal framework, or the denture base.
- Critical need for follow-up. Follow-up, periodic evaluation, and maintenance are necessary to overcome the problems related to technical failures, cervical caries, and retention.

5.5   Indicators of TC

TC-retained TSO or telescopic overdenture may be preferred in the rehabilitation of partially edentulous patients to the conventional removable dentures, because of their advantages such as better retention, stability, stable occlusion, and good chewing ability due to the conservation of proprioception feedback, especially when patients have a few remaining or unfavorably distributed abutment teeth (Pictures 5.1, 5.2, 5.3, and 5.4).

Other treatment options include extraction of the remaining teeth, followed by a conventional complete denture. This option should not be selected because extraction would have decreased the available support and proprioception provided by the teeth and their periodontal ligaments.

Also, implant-supported dentures should be another option for this type of patient; however, this treatment could not be suitable for medically compromised patients and also because of the cost involved in the procedure.

The clinical longevity of a TO is primarily influenced by the applied restorative concept of connecting the removable denture with the remaining teeth. Concerning the number, alignment, and periodontal status of the remaining teeth, the clinician needs to select the appropriate retainer for a successful long-term restoration.

- Patients with advanced resorption of the ridge are suitable for a bar or telescopic attachment assemblies that offer horizontal stability. The support provided by the abutment teeth is in addition to that supplied by the residual ridges. The retained tooth or root's vertical component in the alveolar bone increases stability (Picture 5.7). The factors of border seal and tissue adaptation are more constant during the function in overdentures than in conventional dentures, and the increased support and stability enhance retention.

Telescopic overdenture offers a solution in cases of limited vertical space where a bar cannot be properly formed. In these cases, remaining teeth with a good or doubtful prognosis can serve as supporting elements along with implants placed in strategic positions. If a tooth fails and has to be extracted, the overdenture can remain in function with minimum repair by the rest of the teeth or implant (Picture 5.8a–d).

- Telescopic overdenture is often used when it is difficult to arrange a suitable path of insertion as in the case of unparallel abutment teeth.

5.6 Clinical Considerations

The TO should be kept in mind during treatment planning of cases requiring prosthodontic rehabilitation. It has many advantages and some disadvantages which must be evaluated carefully according to the clinical situation.

5.6.1 Careful Assessment of the Interarch Space

Careful evaluation of the interarch space is very important for the successful fabrication of TO. Sufficient space must be present to accommodate the primary coping and secondary crowns, to have an adequate denture base thickness to avoid fracture, for the arrangement of the teeth to fulfill the aesthetic requirements, and to have an interocclusal gap. The interocclusal gap/interarch distance should be ≥ 10 mm, to have sufficient space for the double crowns, denture base, teeth placement, and adequate freeway space. Space consideration usually requires devitalization of the abutments. A solution to solve problems caused by missing occlusal space in the premolar and molar area is the use of the so-called ring telescope, where the primary copings occlusal surface and the secondary crown part is constructed as a ring completing the form of a full metal crown (Picture 5.8e).

5.6.2 Intraoral and Radiologic Examination

During the intraoral examination, the potential abutments should be evaluated clinically to determine periodontal condition, pocket depth, mobility, caries, vitality, abrasions, and supraeruption. The radiographs should be evaluated for the supporting situations of the teeth in the bone. The periodontal tissues' health, bone support, and patient expectations/benefits should be considered. The selected abutments for TO should be periodontally sound with adequate bone support and no/minimal mobility (Picture 5.9).

5.6.3 Tooth Preparation

On the remaining teeth, the necessary endodontic and periodontal treatment should be done. Tooth preparations should be done with a circumferential shoulder margin configuration shown with tapered walls (2–5°) (Picture 5.9a, b).

5.6.4 Distribution of Abutments

There should be at least one healthy abutment in each quadrant. An even distribution of the abutment in each quadrant of the arch is preferable for better stress distribution and increased retention and stability of the denture (Fig. 5.5; Pictures 5.8, 5.9, and 5.10). If a total of four abutments for telescopic copings were utilized to support the overdenture, generating a quadrilateral configuration, at least two abutment teeth should be splinted for optimal stress distribution in TO, according to reports. The benefit of this treatment strategy was that it acted as a hard splint by distributing the load over the remaining periodontally compromised teeth. This approach was believed to have a more favorable prognosis for the remaining teeth and a more secure denture.

- *The Determination of the Direction for the Path of Insertion*
      If more than three abutments are utilized for TO, the surveying process becomes significant. During the surveying of the model, the objective is to locate an insertion direction that satisfies the following conditions:
- There must be at least two opposing parallel surfaces on all principal copings.
- The spacing between individual die stumps or surviving teeth should be sufficient for secondary components.
- The predicted friction surfaces should not be shorter than 3.5 mm in length.
- The material thickness of the pre-milled wax copings must be chosen so that minor adjustments can be made without perforating the primary coping after the impression is taken (Picture 5.11).

5.6.5   Retention Effect of Telescopic Overdentures

Clinically, the secondary crown seats the primary coping with a chewing force. This chewing force value can vary based on the opposite arch situation, the location of the abutment, the occlusion relationship, and personal factors.

The retention force of a TC is also influenced by the abutment preparation, such as taper angle, the height and size of the inner coping, marginal design, and even by factors associated with the fabrication process (milling speed, degree of cutter wear, polishing, casting technique). The contact surface pressure, surface roughness, and the static frictional coefficient also have a significant influence on the retention thus it could be controlled by changing the taper angle of the double crown and the thickness of the secondary crown.

For the TO to have a long service life, it must have a suitable vertical wall height (at least 4 mm), sufficient coping thickness (never less than 0.7 mm for each casting), and a taper of around 6 degrees (Picture 5.11).

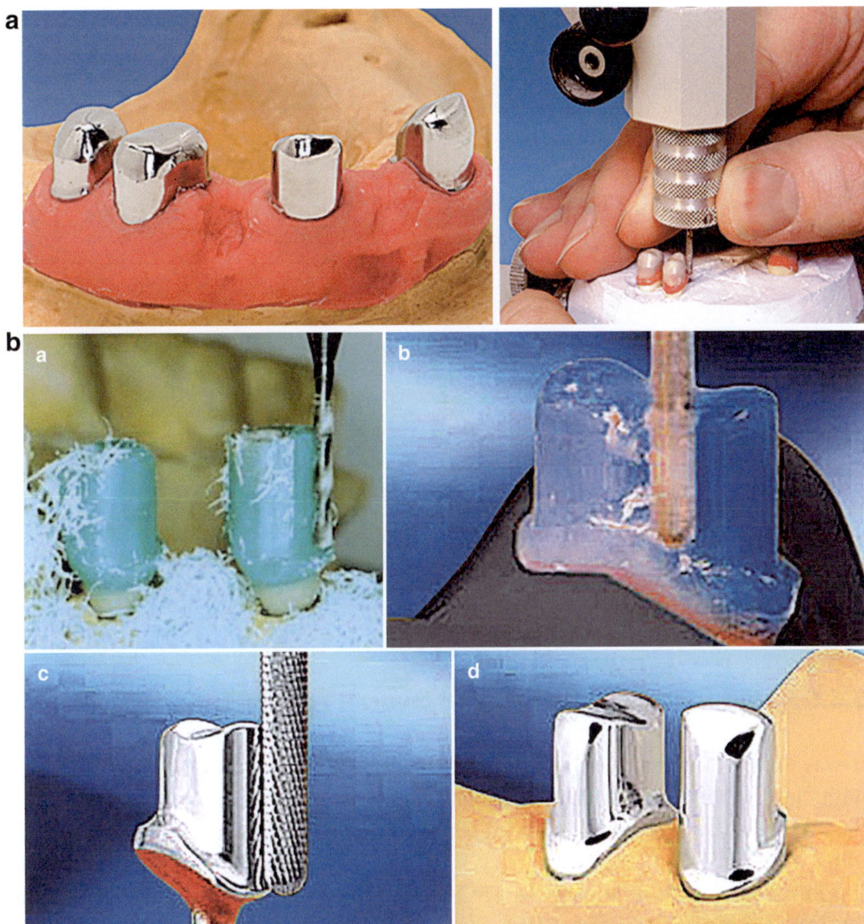

Picture 5.11 (**a**) The essential requirements for the long service of the telescopic prosthesis are to provide an adequate height of the vertical walls (at least 4 mm) (Courtesy of Ulrich Heker). (**b**) The height of the vertical walls prepared on the wax copings. The primary coping should be at least 4 mm and parallel each other, and the gingival chamfer prepared for cylinder design (casting appearance). (**c**) The sufficient thickness of the copings should be at least 0.7 mm and the conus crown should be with the 6° taper

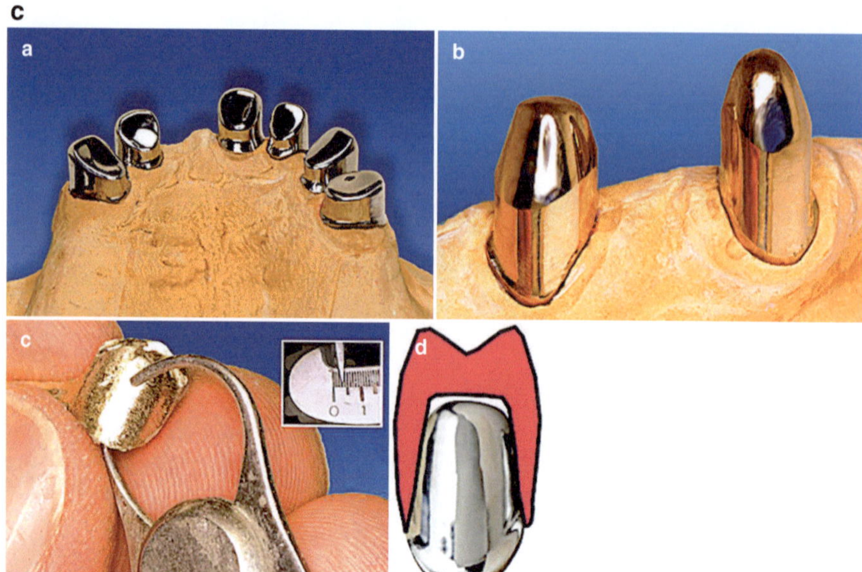

Picture 5.11 (continued)

5.6.6 Number of Abutments and Overall Withdrawal Force

It was established that the overall withdrawal force of dentures does not correlate with the number of telescope abutments. Sometimes the overall withdrawal force of dentures with two TC was much higher than that of dentures with twice or three times as many TC.

On the one hand, removing the TSO with many abutments will be a problem in the initial period after fitting. This considerable increase in the withdrawal force could be caused by the tipping of the telescopic crowns. Frequently relieving the telescopic crowns by polishing the frictional surfaces can subsequently lead to a considerable reduction in the overall withdrawal.

It is also questionable whether any frictional wear is more likely to be caused by the fact that the telescopic crowns were not parallel initially. This would mean that the secondary crown was only able to slide smoothly over the primary coping after the abutment teeth became aligned due to minimal tooth migration. If this happens, the overall retentive force of the telescopic crowns is reduced, though sometimes only very slightly, as demonstrated in studies.

5.6.7 The Number and Distribution of Abutment Teeth

It can be anticipated that the long-term success of TO is highly dependent upon the number and topographic distribution of the remaining abutment teeth. Moreover, the integration of one to three telescopic abutment teeth was less favorable concerning the prosthetic loading forces, especially if the distribution of these abutments was arranged in a tangential or cross-linear arch relation to the arch. Four or more telescopic abutments can have a positive impact on the survival of the complete restoration (Picture 5.10). In a retrospective longitudinal study, it was shown that the 5-year survival rate of the double crown–retained RDPs was dependent on the number of abutment teeth. It is indicated that only a few abutment teeth (one to three abutments) and large extensions are less favorable for the distribution of loading forces and are a predictor of early failure. It seems that three or more teeth supporting double crown–retained dentures can have a positive impact on the survival rate of teeth.

5.6.8 Abutment Number Effects on Survival Rate

It was shown that the survival rates of the tooth-supported double crown–retained prostheses were 90.0% and 95.1% after 4 and 5.3 years, respectively. Despite these high survival rates, the long-term prognosis TO depends on the number of the abutment. Several clinical investigations reported that the failure rates of abutment teeth and telescopic prostheses in severely reduced dentitions differed significantly from those in patients with more than three remaining natural abutments. Four or more telescopic abutments can have a positive impact on the survival of the complete restoration.

Wo ̈stmann et al. evaluated 554 TO on 1758 primary coping in 463 patients. After 5 years of recall 66 (3.8%) abutment teeth were extracted, and 26 (4.7%) TO were reported as failures. The survival rate after 5 years was 95.3% for the abutment teeth and 95.1% for the TO. The estimated 5-year survival probability for dentures with only one abutment was 70.9% compared to 90.4% with two, 95.0% with three, and 97.9% with four abutments. It was summarized that the number of abutments supporting the prosthesis had a considerable impact on the survival of the denture.

5.6.9 The Effect of Root Canal Therapy on the Telescopic Overdenture Survival Rate

The influence of root canal treatment on the survival rate of TO is also controversial. After an observation period of 6.3 years, significantly higher failure rates were reported for teeth with root canal treatment (20%) compared to vital teeth (5.7%). The fracture and extraction rates for non-vital teeth were shown to be twice as high as those of important ones supporting TO after an observation period of 3 years. Although the survival rates of endodontically treated teeth are reported to be less than those for vital teeth in most studies, the current evidence is weak.

5.6.10 Fabrication Methods and Materials Use of Telescopic Overdenture

There are many laboratory methods used to fabricate these TOs (Figs. 5.5 and 5.6). In conventional technology, the primary and secondary crowns are manufactured using a casting technique. Secondary crowns can also be made from pure electroplated gold, and this technique can be used in a variety of ways. The secondary crowns are luted or soldered to the denture framework or may be cast as a homogenous unit together with the framework.

5.7   Components of TC

The use of a harder and more wear-resistant main coping material against a softer secondary crown material is favorable because the changes in the fitting surface of the secondary crown enhance the adaptation between the primary coping and secondary crowns. Material options for telescopic crowns include precious and non-precious metal alloys, zirconia, and polyetheretherketone (PEEK) (Pictures 5.12, 5.13, 5.14, 5.15, 5.16, 5.17, 5.18, and 5.19).

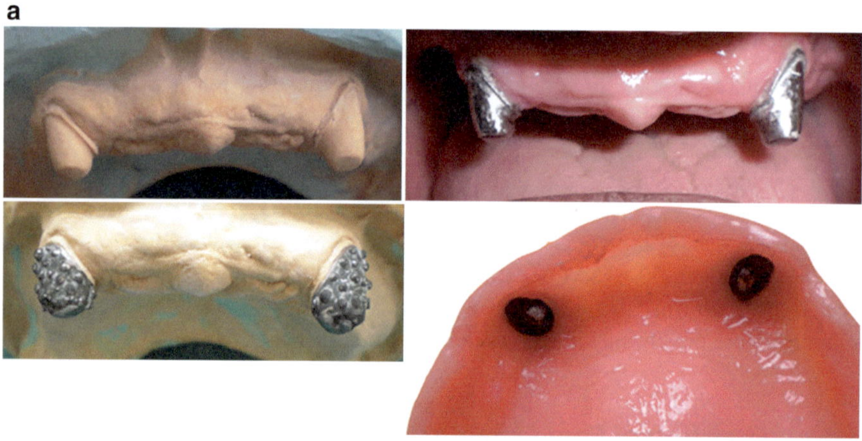

Picture 5.12 (**a**) The simple solutions of TO; primary coping produced with Co-Cr alloys and secondary crown produced with Co-Cr alloys with retention beads and which are directly embedded in acrylic dentures. (**b, c**) One-piece casting for TO: (**b**) The primary copings; (**c**) secondary crowns are fabricated using a casting technique (Co-Cr alloys). Secondary crown casting with the framework as a homogenous unit together with the metal framework. (**d**) One-piece casting for TO: *a* The primary coping; *b* secondary crowns are using a casting technique (Co-Cr alloys). Secondary crowns cast with the metal framework as three units crowns and porcelain veneering on crowns; *c* the intaglio surface of TO consists of three metal-ceramic porcelain crowns together with a metal framework in acrylic denture. (**e**) One-piece casting for T. *a, b* The primary wax coping prepared and cast with Co-Cr alloy; *c–e* the duplicated model for preparing the metal framework and wax prepared and cast as one unit with secondary crowns; *f* the secondary crown and metal framework cast together as one piece. (**f**) The primary coping cast with Co-Cr alloy in the right canine and left canine, premolars, and first molar teeth. (**g**) The secondary crowns and frameworks were fabricated as a homogenous unit consisting of eight units of the metal-ceramic bridge (*left* side) and free and saddle acrylic resin teeth and denture flange on the metal mesh (Courtesy of Ulrich Heker)

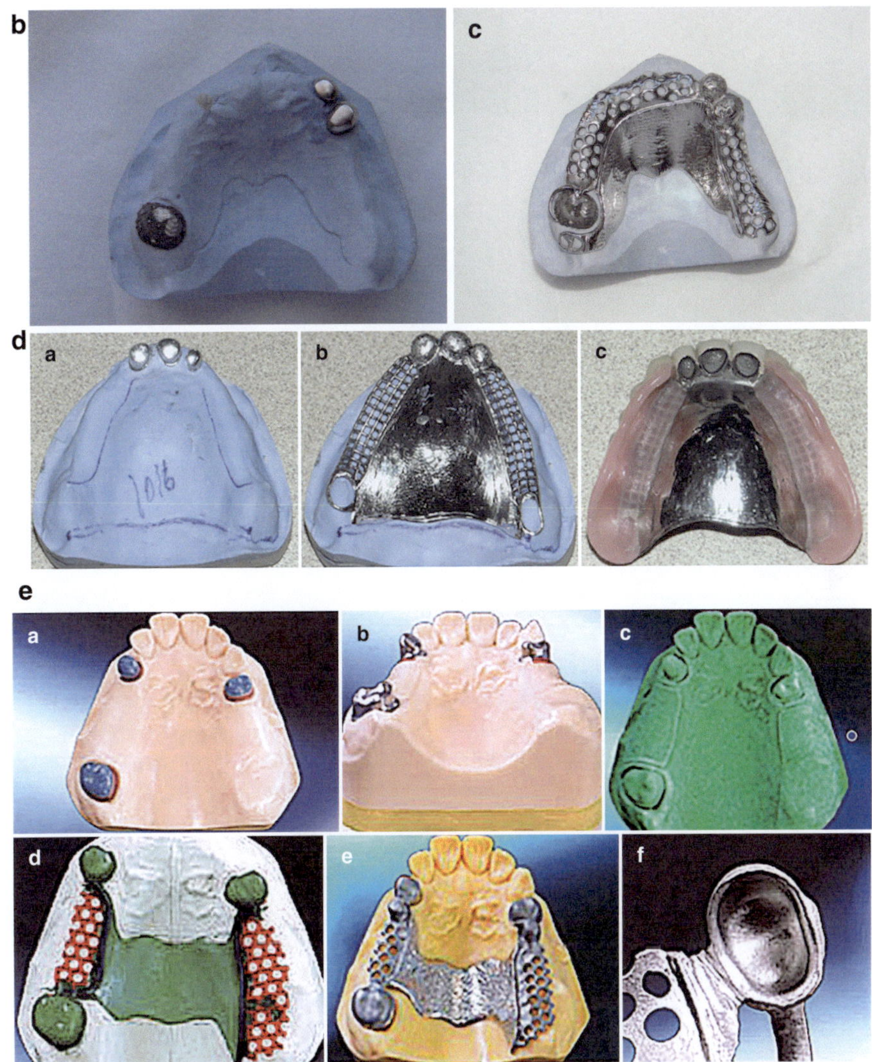

Picture 5.12 (continued)

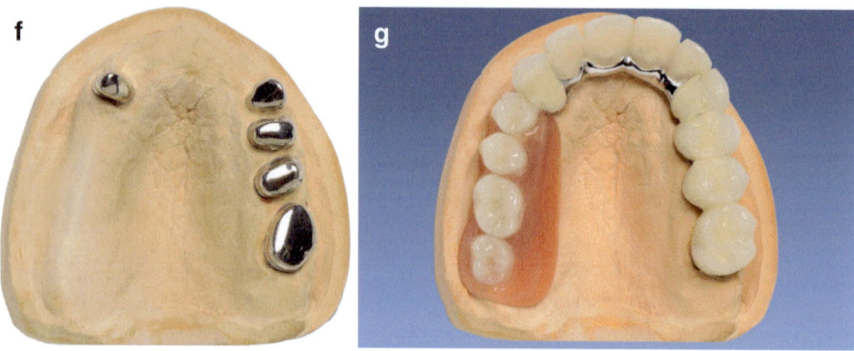

Picture 5.12 (continued)

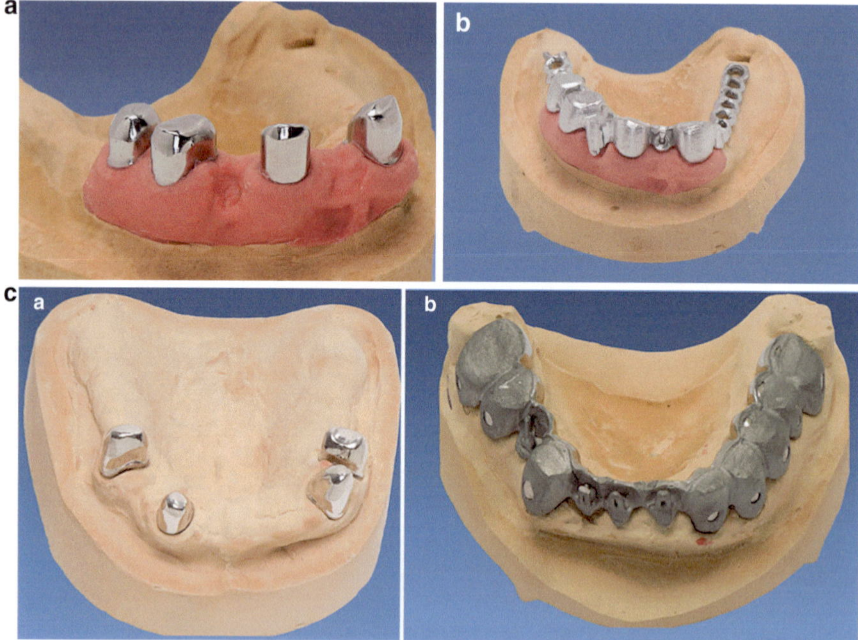

Picture 5.13 (**a**) The four primary copings are cast with Co-Cr alloys. (**b**) The secondary crowns cast a homogenous unit as a metal framework and fixed bridge restorations (Courtesy of Ulrich Heker). (**c**) *a* The four primary copings are cast with Co-Cr alloys and *b* the secondary crowns are cast with Co-Cr alloys as a fixed bridge. (**d**) One-piece casting for TO: *a* The primary copings cast Co-Cr alloys cemented on the teeth; *b* the secondary crowns and metal framework (secondary crowns cast as veneer crown) and the rest finished as acrylic resin teeth and acrylic flange as conventional denture; *c, d* the intaglio and external surface of the denture

d

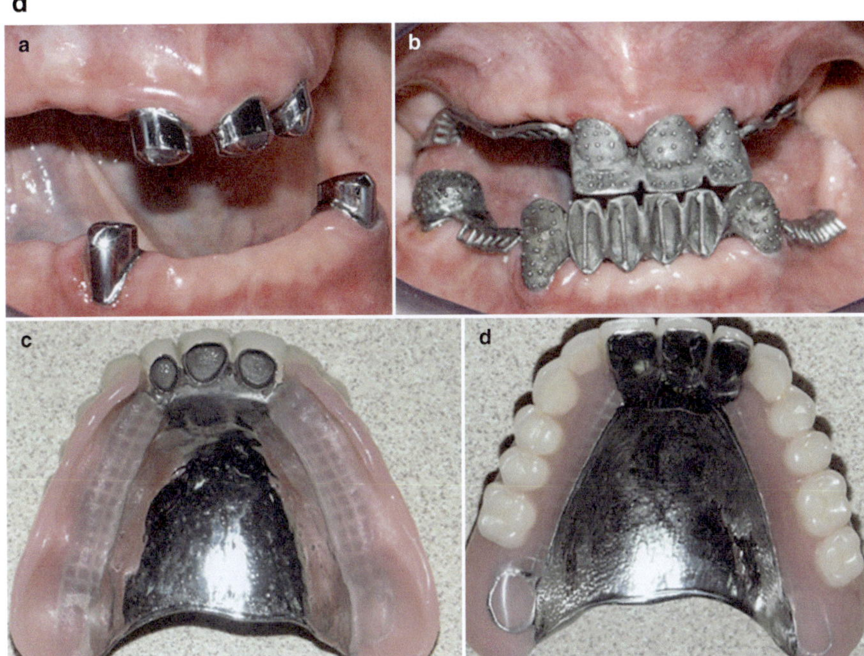

Picture 5.13 (continued)

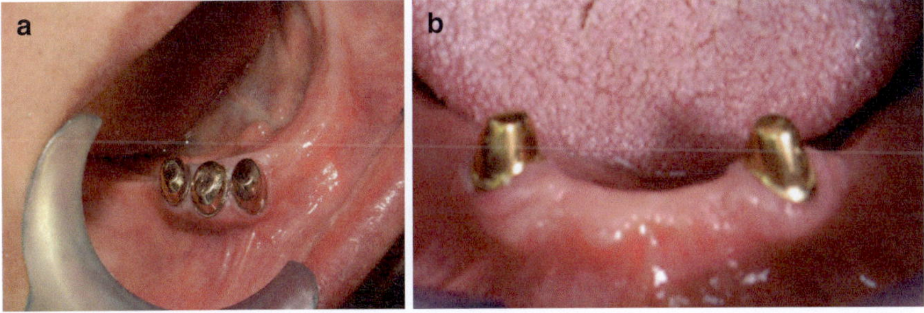

Picture 5.14 (**a**) The primary coping is cast with gold alloys and (**b**) the secondary crowns are cast with gold alloys as a fixed bridge

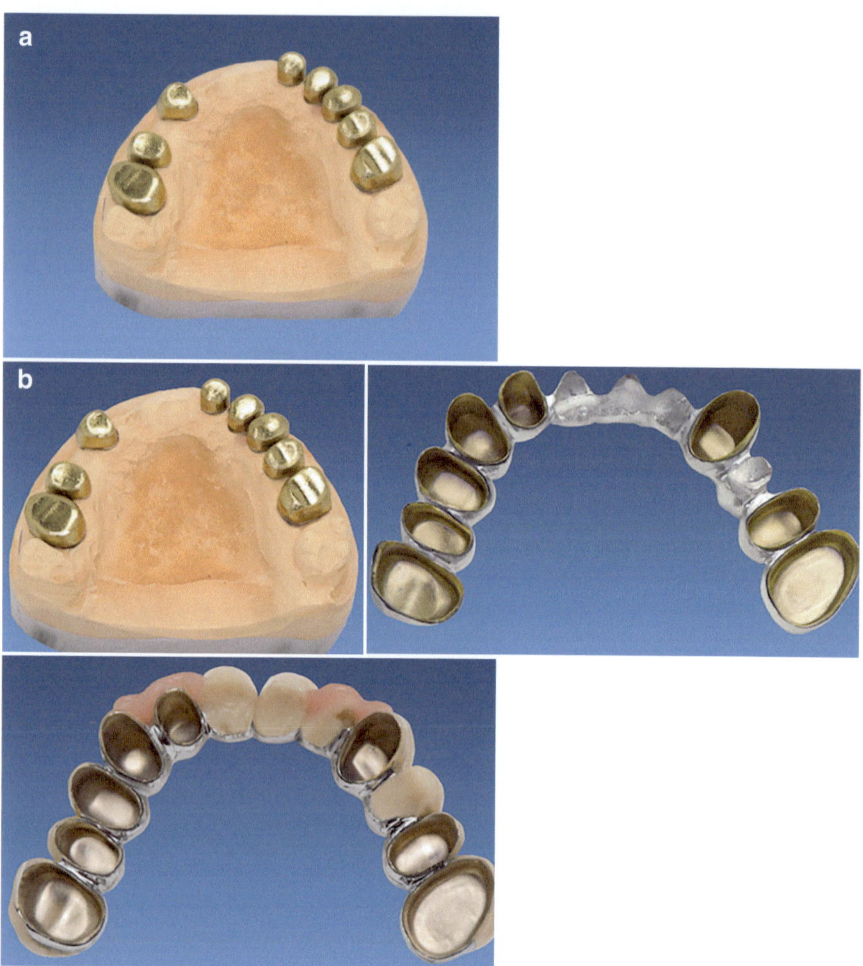

Picture 5.15 (**a**) The primary copings were cast with gold alloys; (**b**) the secondary crowns and framework were also cast with gold alloys as a metal-ceramic fixed bridge and only the anterior area added pink porcelain as gingiva (Courtesy of Ulrich Heker)

5.7.1 Metal Alloys

The recommended alloys for the fabrication of copings are highly noble (ADA type IV). Ag-Au-Pd alloys have better precision and better retention but are technique-sensitive and costly (Picture 5.14). Gold alloys are ideal for the casting of secondary crowns due to their biocompatibility, precision casting, and sufficient friction, but they are costly. Base metal alloys may also be utilized, but they must be cast with extraordinary care to produce the required friction coefficient (Picture 5.15).

Primary copings of telescopic systems are produced with precious or non-precious alloys via the lost-wax technique by conventional methods. Base metal

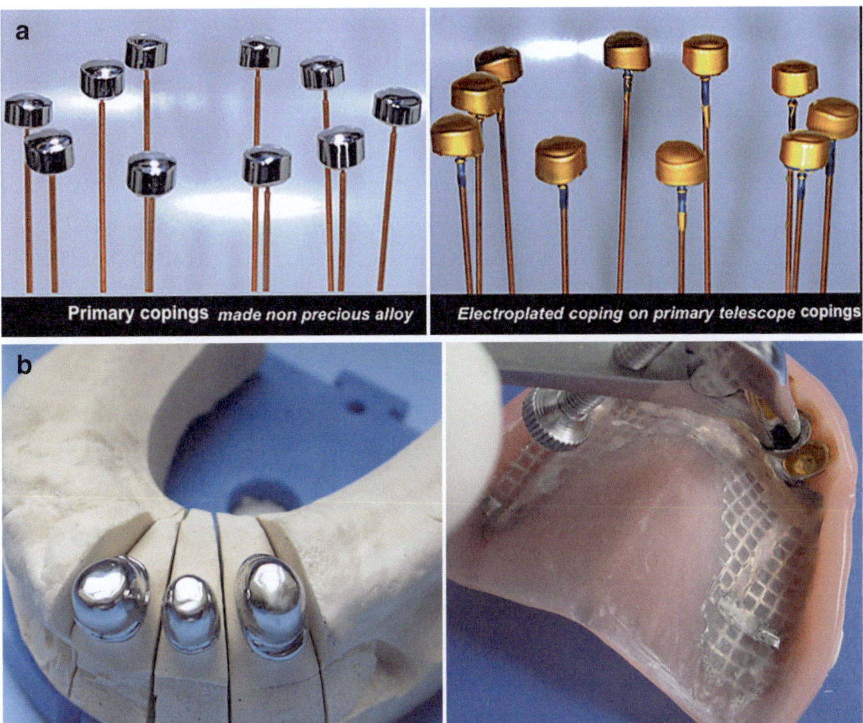

Picture 5.16 (**a**) The primary telescope copings and electroplated coping on the primary coping (experimental design). (**b**) The primary copings are cast with Co-Cr alloys. Secondary crowns also cast the same metal alloys. The electroplated gold coping fabricated and luted the secondary crowns in the denture framework

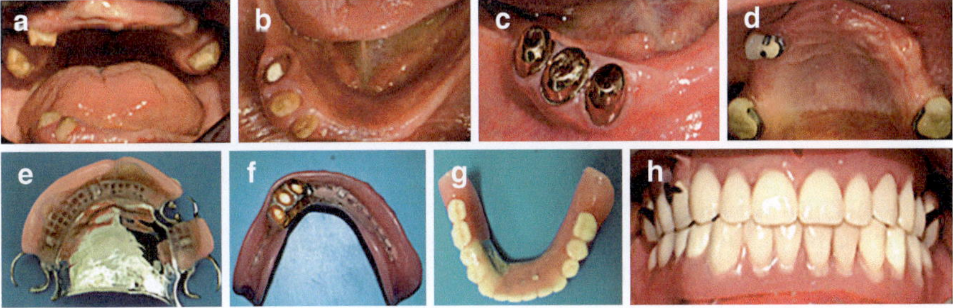

Picture 5.17 The TO produced by electroplating methods: (**a**) In the upper jaw three abutment teeth prepared as metal-ceramic crown preparation rules; (**b**) in the lower jaw three teeth (canine and premolars) in the right side prepared as TC abutment; (**c**) the primary telescope coping cast gold alloys and cemented on abutment teeth; (**d, e**) metal-ceramic crowns cemented on the abutment tooth in the upper jaw and removable partial denture prepared; (**f, g**) in the lower jaw the secondary coping cast with the metal framework as one unit and electroplated gold alloys coping luted the secondary coping; (**h**) maxillary removable denture and mandibular TO in situ

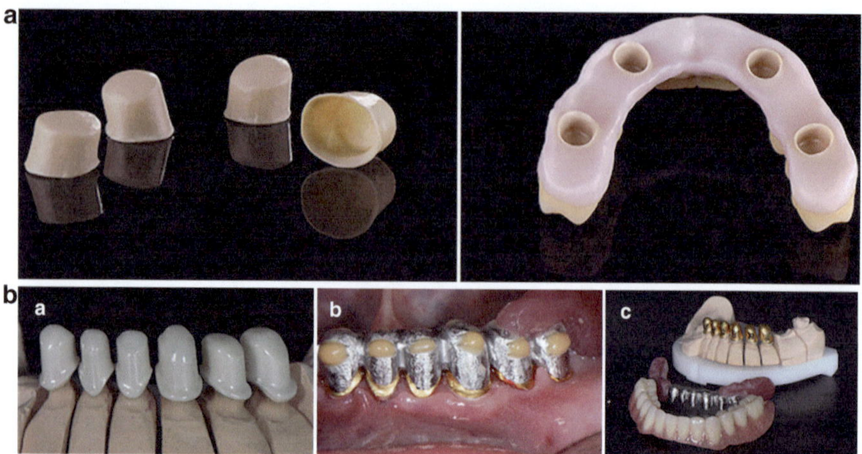

Picture 5.18 (**a**) Primary copings and secondary crowns produced zirconium material. (**b**) *a*: Primary copings produced zirconium material; *b*: secondary crows cast with Co-Cr alloys and electroplated gold coping produced on primary copings (acrylic denture, secondary crown cast Co-Cr alloy, and electroplated gold coping assembly)

alloys (Co-Cr) are used because they have low thermal conductivity. Thus the patient does not experience unpleasant thermal sensations caused by excessive tooth preparation. Moreover, they are easy to fabricate and more economical (Pictures 5.12 and 5.13).

The Computer-Aided-Design and Computer-Aided-Manufacturing (CAD/CAM) systems also used for the fabrication of telescopic crowns have recently been introduced, but there is not yet sufficient clinical data to compare the conventional casting procedure with the newly introduced technology. Recently, direct metal laser sintering (DMLS), a fast method of prototype production, can be defined as an additive fabrication technique that involves binding powdered metal together to form a solid structure using a laser as a power source.

Due to their lower density, Co-Cr alloys have a lower weight compared to gold alloys. This material presents high biocompatibility and corrosion resistance. A few different fabrication methods, based on laser sintering, casting, or milling, are known to produce Co-Cr alloys. The laser sintering process, a relatively new way of bringing Co-Cr alloy into its final form, fuses Co-Cr granules in layers by using a carbon dioxide laser beam. This procedure impresses with its little material wear, but the costs and technical effort seem to be difficult for routine use. Co-Cr alloy is cast with the lost-wax technique depending on technical skills and hand-made fitting, whereas the milling process allows using industrial prefabricated homogenous blanks.

As a result of their reduced density, Co-Cr alloys are lighter than gold alloys. This substance is very biocompatible and resistant to corrosion. Co-Cr alloys can be manufactured using a variety of processes, including laser sintering, casting, and milling. Using a carbon dioxide laser beam, the relatively new laser sintering

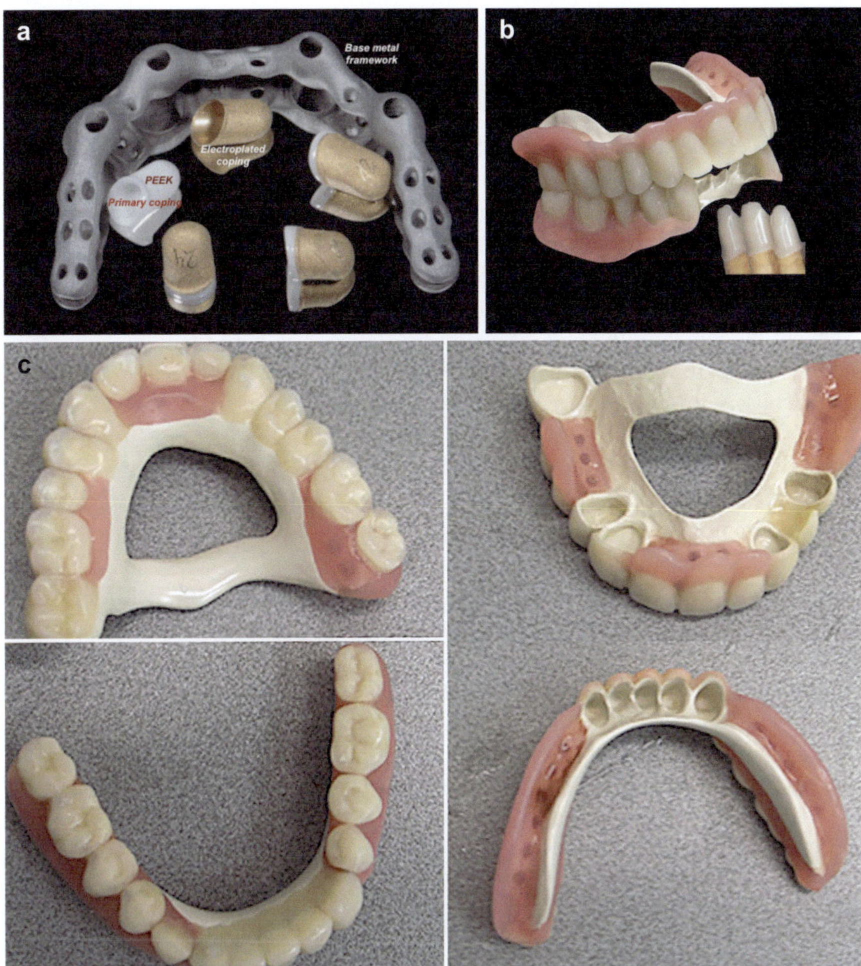

Picture 5.19 (**a**) The PEEK primary coping, electroplated coping, and base metal framework. (**b**) The PEEK primary coping and the PEEK base framework and superstructure. (**c**) The TO consists of the PEEK base framework and superstructure

technique fuses Co-Cr grains in layers to create the final form of Co-Cr alloy. This process is remarkable for its low material wear, but its expenses and technical effort make it difficult to use it consistently. Co-Cr alloy is cast using the lost-wax method, which requires technical expertise and hand-made fitting, whereas the milling process permits the use of industrially produced homogeneous blanks.

In contrast to casting, the milling process is affected by the design program and milling settings of the CAD/CAM procedure. It can be machined from a prefabricated homogeneous block using CAD/CAM technology. After milling, the framework is sintered to impart the final density, dimension, and mechanical qualities to the material. To simplify the milling process for Co-Cr alloy, the blocks are milled in dry conditions with smaller CAM machines before being sintered.

5.7.1.1 Titanium

It has even emerged as the new metal processing method substitute for the conventional lost-wax method. However, when manufacturing crowns using a CAD/CAM system, an expensive precious metal alloy is unsuitable because the quantity of ingot required for cutting far exceeds that needed for the completed crown. Titanium, on the other hand, is considered to be a suitable material for the CAD/CAM system because of its many significant advantages such as being inexpensive and having excellent biocompatibility and corrosion resistance. The pure titanium conus telescope crowns are fabricated with CAD/CAM technology. The density of titanium (4.2 g/cm^3) is lower compared to conventional alloys, such as cobalt-chromium (8.9 g/cm^3) and gold (19.3 g/cm^3), allowing the fabrication of prostheses with a lightweight without compromising critical mechanical properties [tensile strength and hardness and high melting point (1720 °C)]. Moreover, the high chemical reactivity of titanium with elements in the investment has produced many defects, including porosity and castability.

Al Wazzan and Al-Nazzawi [6] evaluated the marginal and internal fit of CP Ti and Ti-6Al-4V crowns and showed that Ti-6Al-4V had less fit discrepancy than CPTi. However, both castings were considered clinically acceptable. On the processing accuracy of the CAD/CAM system, the new technique produced titanium crowns with delicate marginal fit form and high working accuracy, where accuracy was in the order of tens of micrometers. Therefore, even if the gap in the occlusal area between the inner crown and an outer crown was set to 0 μm on the computer, a gap was produced in this area.

5.7.2 Electroforming

The electroforming process with pure gold was first used in conservative dentistry for inlays in 1961. The process itself has been known for more than 150 years within the electroplating industry, particularly in the production of jewelry, decorative items, and watch fabrication. Electroformed copings used in modern telescopic removable prostheses and fixed dentures play an essential role as a secondary structure. Galvano system aims to obtain a thin gold substructure with electrolysis (the galvanic copings thickness of approximately 0.25 mm is made of 99.9% pure gold with an elastic modulus of 78.5 GPa). Electroforming baths suitable for dental restorations are non-cyanide and contain a gold sulfite electrolyte corresponding to the chemical formula. A thin layer of silver conductive lacquer applies on the outer surface of the primary crown, and the automatically running electroplating process creates precise secondary coping. The electroplated gold was assumed to improve wear resistance compared to the conventional cast metal double crowns, and so leading to more predictable and constant retentive forces of the overdenture.

Producing secondary crowns using electroforming also eliminates the hand-modeling phase and fitting and even demands no adjustment like conventionally cast ones do. These galvanic crowns are captivating due to their highly precise fitting. This fitting is essential for proper retentive force and indispensable for the normal function of double crown dentures (Pictures 5.8, 5.16, and 5.17).

Between the primary coping and secondary crown, there is always a space of 8–12 μm. This space is always filled with saliva, there is an adhesive power inside, and friction does real work. Galvanized telescopic crowns also have a homogenous structure made of gold cations that are tightly packed. Since Galvano uses 24-carat gold, it is a tissue-friendly technique, and it is much more esthetic than conventional metal alloys when used as a core material in ceramic treatments.

The data concerning the wear behavior of electroplated copings on conical crowns are sparse.

It is stated that the electroformed double crown systems showed different values of retention forces both higher and lower compared to non-electroplated crowns. Therein, the electroplated secondary crowns on their cast primary copings with a taper angle of 2° showed lower retention force values than the cast secondary gold crowns on their cast primary copings.

Weigl et al. [7] showed the advantages of electroplated copings on empress ceramic crowns in denture retention and wore development compared with the combination of gold/gold and titanium/titanium. All three combinations showed clinically acceptable results, but the gold copings on ceramic conical crowns showed less tribological effects and constant retentive forces. They reported that double-crown assemblies with electro-formed secondary crowns have more stable retention forces than double-crown assemblies with cast secondary crowns.

Beuer et al. [8] found that electroformed galvanic crowns showed a higher retention force, whereas Engels et al. [9] also found that electroformed crowns showed a lower retention force compared to cast ones. Wagner et al. [10] compared the initial retention values of the double-crown systems produced by the Co-Cr milling and Co-Cr casting methods and found the retention force values to be similar. They showed that double crowns produced with new fabrication methods for Co-Cr materials, for example, milling under dry conditions and later sintering, showed positive values considering retention forces in comparison to conventional cast secondary crowns and electroforming secondary crowns. The retention force values of the electroformed secondary crowns confirmed their clinical use for conical crowns as well as telescoping crowns. However, further investigations regarding fatigue testing and thermo-mechanical loading will be beneficial to improve this.

Conical crown-retained TO made by use of the electroforming technique should be devoid of the problems mentioned previously since the outer crown has an ideal fit for its inner component. However, the construction becomes more complicated since the electroplated copings have to be luted to the separately fabricated framework.

It is stated that mechanical defects have been shown in dentures with secondary crowns fabricated by electroforming. Depending on the material used for fabrication of the primary copings (gold alloy or chromium-cobalt alloy), veneer chipping was in 42.86% and 71.43%, whereas loss of retention was noted in 30.95% and 57.14% of dentures, respectively. Also, the non-precious primary coping has shown documentation (57.14%) as compared to a precious one (4.76%).

5.7.3 Ceramic

The recent improvement of the CAD/CAM technology offered easier manipulation of different materials of high quality, especially ceramics. Weigl et al. [7] first described the use of all-ceramics for the construction of double-crown attachment systems. This so-called ceramic-galvanic double-crowns (CGDC) consists of tapered all-ceramic primary coping and secondary crowns made of Galvano-formed gold which is cemented to a reinforcing cast metal denture framework. When the primary copings were fabricated from reinforced glass ceramics, this material exhibited increased rates of fracture, and therefore it was later replaced with zirconia.

Groesser et al. (2014) [11] suggested that although the system of ceramo-galvanic double-crown offered favorable tribological characteristics and was widely reproducible because of its automated electroforming process of manufacturing, it must be considered that many different materials in the form of ceramics, electroplated-gold, bonding material, and Cr Co Mb alloy of the denture framework are included in this system. Consequently, they introduced the design of all-zirconia double-crowns without the presence of any galvanic elements. They reported that retention forces of all-zirconia double-crowns are reproducible. Rinke et al. [12] published the successful function, high survival rates, and rare biological complications of CGDC-retained implant overdentures over a prolonged period. The zero degrees taper of the primary coping is of great importance for ceramic because a tapered angle of the primary coping leads to tension within the walls of the secondary coping. In contrast to gold alloys, ceramics are susceptible to tensile stress that may induce the formation of cracks within the secondary crown.

5.7.4 Zirconia

To date, zirconia has been evaluated exclusively as a framework material for crowns and fixed partial dentures. It has demonstrated high reliability and low fracture rate for functional periods of up to 10 years for these indications. CAD/CAM technology offers the fabrication of primary and secondary zirconia crowns. ZrO_2 has also been demonstrated as a material for primary copings in the double crown technique and has featured itself as an alternative to a gold alloy (Picture 5.18).

It was shown that double crowns with different conus angles of 0°–6° concluded that ZrO_2 primary copings result in more predictable and less excursive retention loads and that the retention load increased as the conus angle decreased. In addition to the taper, the surface roughness also has an impact on retention load, and ZrO_2 with its low surface roughness is therefore well suitable.

Moreover, the low surface roughness and low surface energy result in low biofilm accumulation, which not only applies to ZrO_2. The physical properties of the ZrO_2 material can be improved by stabilization with the metallic oxide yttrium (Y_2O_3). The resulting yttrium-stabilized tetragonal zirconium oxide (Y-TZP) shows even better mechanical properties than other zirconia oxides, which is a result of the crystalline modification from a tetragonal (T) to monoclinic (M) arrangement. Most of the studies assessed assemblies with Y-TZP primary copings and secondary crowns of a different material, especially gold alloy. It was stated that the combination of a ZrO_2 primary coping with a galvanic-formed gold coping showed more a predictable and less excursive retention load than conventionally cast telescopic crowns.

A more predictable and less excursive retention force can be obtained using a hard and rigid primary coping material like zirconia. Zirconia (1250 HV) is a harder material than a gold alloy (295 HV), the adaptation of the double crown takes place with the deformation of the secondary crown to fit the primary copings, without any wear on the primary copings. Therefore, the use of a hard and wear-resistant primary coping material against less hard secondary crown materials seems to be advantageous.

The Co-Cr alloy is also a much stiffer metal with an elastic modulus similar to that of Y-TZP and can be used for primary copings. According to the manufacturer's specifications, the value is 204 GPa for Y-TZP, and 200 GPa for Co-Cr alloys. The latter one, assembled with the electroformed secondary crown, was investigated and it was shown that Co-Cr alloys have higher retention load values as compared to gold or ZrO_2 crowns.

Besimo et al. [13] observed no significant influence of the primary coping materials; a contrary outcome has been documented. In recent studies, it was assumed that different hardness levels and surface treatments such as polishing might have an impact on the retention load values. The retention forces of all-zirconia double-crown systems are reproducible as demonstrated by Groesser et al. (2014), and Rinke et al. [12] reported that no fractures of the zirconia copings were observed during the entire observational period of their study.

Turp et al. [14] investigated double-crown systems consisting of gold alloy primary copings with electroformed gold secondary crowns, zirconia primary crowns with electroformed gold secondary crowns, and zirconia primary copings with cast secondary crowns of non-precious alloy. They showed decreasing retention force values with an increased taper angle from 2° to 4° up to 6°. They stated that a more predictable and less excursive retention force could be obtained using a hard and rigid primary coping material like zirconia. Moreover, they also reported that despite a lack of knowledge about the aging of zirconia without a veneer layer in the oral environment, zirconia primary copings are more advantageous in terms of retention force development and wear.

Guven et al. [15] investigated many types of double crowns, such as casting gold alloy primary coping/casting gold alloy secondary crown (AA), laser sintering primary coping/laser sintering secondary crown (LL), casting Cr alloy primary coping/casting Cr alloy secondary crown (CC), primary zirconia coping/electroformed secondary crown (ZA), and CAD/CAM titanium alloy primary coping/CAD/CAM titanium alloy secondary crown (TT) groups at conus angles of 4° and 6° for retention force values. They showed that the retention forces increased when the conus angle decreased. They found the highest initial and final retention force values in the LL-4° group and the lowest retention force values in the ZA-6° group. They showed that the ZA group samples showed the least change in the retention force, and no wear was observed. In the other groups, wear was seen mostly in the primary coping. They showed that a more predictable, clinically relevant, and less excursive retention force was found in the ZA groups. The retention force values of the LL groups were statically similar to those of the other groups, except for the ZA groups. Also, they stated that the LL group's retentive forces were higher than the clinically suggested values. However, the retentive force values are similar among all groups except for the ZA groups.

These copings proved to be a successful alternative to classic gold copings, especially when the patient's esthetic demands are high. However, the preparation angle of the natural abutments, the thickness of the zirconia, and the occlusal load must be considered.

5.7.5 Polyetheretherketone

Recent articles have reported that PEEK is a good material for twin crown systems (Picture 5.19). PEEK, a modified polyaryletherketone (PAEK), is a thermoplastic high-performance polymer with a melting temperature of roughly 343 °C. PEEK material is soft and ductile (110 HV 5/20) and has a low elastic modulus (4 GPa); nevertheless, Co-Cr and ZrO_2 both present a high elastic modulus (200 GPa) and are robust and stable (280 HV 10; 1200 HV 10). Both PEEK as well as ZrO_2 represent very biocompatible materials and are used for several applications, for example, for dental implants, temporary abutments, fixed dental prostheses, and removable dental prostheses. However, it is necessary to connect PEEK with other resin composite materials. Despite the resistance to surface modification, a suitable bond can be reached via etching and the use of Methyl Methacrylate (MMA)-containing coupling agents. The examined physical properties, abrasion resistance, high hardness, and low water absorption and solubility render this material new material for dentistry. In dentistry, there are three ways of converting the PEEK material: milling from blocks with CAD/CAM software, pressing from granules, or pressing from pellets with the unique vacuum-pressing device. Blanks and pellets are pressed forms from the raw material PEEK granules. Primary copings are made of zirconia, and secondary crowns as well as framework and clasps are created of one piece of high-performance plastic PEEK. There are no variety of materials in the mouth since secondary crowns and frameworks are manufactured from one piece. Thus, the highest break resistance is achieved.

It is stated that a gold alloy with its ductility already affects good results in combination with ZrO_2. Therefore, a new concept could be the combination of these two biocompatible materials, that is, ZrO_2 and PEEK, to produce metal-free fixed dental prosthesis (FDPs) such as telescopic crowns.

In cases where the primary coping is made of metal and the secondary crown is made of PEEK, it was proven that the secondary crown is the determinant of the retentive forces. Whereas the hardness of the primary coping (metal; 455.88 HV) is more than that of the secondary crown (PEEK;110 HV), therefore, the use of a hard and wear-resistant primary coping material against a less hard secondary crown material is advantageous. Thus, the adaptation between primary coping and secondary crowns will be achieved by the changes in the fitting surface of the secondary crown. Another potential explanation is that PEEK is a soft and ductile material that yields and adapts well. The adaptation process resulted in an excellent marginal fit.

Merk et al. [16, 17] investigated the retention load (RL) between ZrO_2 primary copings (with three different tapers as 0°, 1°, and 2°) and polyetheretherketone (PEEK) secondary crowns made by different fabrication methods [milled from breCam BioHPP blanks (PM), pressed from industrially fabricated PEEK pellets (PP) (BioHPP Pelle), and pressed from granular PEEK (PG) (BioHPP Granulat)]. They reported that the fabrication method of the secondary PEEK crowns showed no consistent effect within all tested groups.

Putting a Co-Cr or ZrO_2 secondary crown on a PEEK primary coping could lead to strong wedging due to the flexibility of PEEK and the differences in elastic modulus.

Uniting the advantages of PEEK with these materials, Co-Cr and ZrO_2 materials, seems feasible in telescope-retained overdenture as CAD/CAM produce PEEK materials suitable for the primary coping in combination with CAD/CAM-produced Co-Cr and ZrO_2 materials as secondary crowns. So, the primary coping can be cast using a traditional lost-wax technique or fabricated from zirconia using CAD/CAM. The precision of conical crowns made with the lost-wax technique affects the retentive value of the denture. Both low and too-high retentive forces are not desirable. The former hinders normal function, whereas, with the latter, complications may occur, including periodontal injury, primary coping decementation, and abutment fracture.

5.8 Joining the Secondary Crown with the Denture

5.8.1 Laser Welding, Soldering/Adhesive Bonding

For joining the secondary crowns with the partial cast denture, laser welding is "state of the art." Alternatively, the parts can be joined by soldering or adhesive bonding. With soldering, one should strive for uniform heating of the soldering block. If the accuracy of the tooth placement has already been checked in the patient with a wax-up, this is transferred to the metal framework, and the denture is assembled for a full test fitting.

5.8.2 One-Piece Method

Another cheaper way is to produce both the secondary crown and metal frame/denture base plates as one piece. This technique is mostly used in daily practice. If TO is made of non-precious alloys, it is obvious to cast the secondary parts and the partial cast denture together in one piece, therefore called one-piece cast. There is no need to cast the secondary crowns separately and to join the double crowns along with the cast partially by soldering, laser welding, or adhesive bonding. This process saves a lot of time and material. A further advantage is biological compatibility due to the usage of only one alloy for all metal parts of the denture. However, clinicians have to get the discrepancy between the single fit of the telescopic crown and the fit in the span of the complete prosthetic work under control. That is a matter of casting expansion and can be regulated by the well-aimed use of different investment concentrations (Pictures 5.12 and 5.13).

As a result, in TO, where primary coping and secondary crowns were fabricated by casting using a precious alloy, the ratio of the mechanical defect was highly low.

- If the secondary crowns and frameworks were assembled as a homogenous cast since such a construction consists only of the structure and veneer material, there is only one junction.
- Analysis of the clinical material showed the lowest percentage of faulty dentures when both the primary copings and secondary crowns were fabricated by casting using a precious alloy, and the secondary crown constituted a homogenous cast with the denture framework. Dentures of this type exhibit the best and most stable retention over time.
- The rigidity of the framework and secondary crowns have an indirect effect on the stability of retentive force. The greater rigidity of the secondary crown and the lower vulnerability to lateral load and the action of the forces operating during non-symmetric load distribution occurs in the denture on mastication. The

secondary crowns were fabricated by electroforming and show lower resistance to lateral forces (balancing forces) can result in permanent deformations, thus leading to a reduction in the contact area between the crowns and a decrease in retention.

- A more complicated denture construction is seen when secondary crowns are fabricated by electroforming. In these types of constructions, there may be as many as six layers in the vicinity of the abutment tooth (i.e., the primary crown, the secondary crown, glue, denture framework, bonding material, and veneer). With that many layers and junctions, there is a higher risk of errors. The retention force values achieved with electroplated secondary crowns were still sufficient and reproducible. It should be considered that additional parameters such as the viscosity of the used saliva, the chamfer design, and details during the manufacturing process of electroplating could influence the retention force.

- However, the high rigidity of the cast crowns may also have negative consequences. In the process of wearing the denture and resulting from multiple insertions and removals, dentures gradually adjust, and the contact surface increases, thus increasing the adhesion interactions that in extreme cases may cause denture impaction. It can be assumed that with a more extended period of functioning of cast crowns, such situations are likely to be more frequent.

5.9   Steps for Telescopic Overdenture Fabrication

5.9.1   Planning the Case

Every TO must be preceded by careful planning with clinical and laboratory procedures. In most cases, the patient and the clinician will consider several restorative options based on the clinical status, photos, and primary models. After intraoral examination, the bone support of the tooth to be selected as abutments is assessed using an intraoral periapical radiograph. The teeth should be periodontally sound with no mobility. If required, root canal treatment of the abutment tooth should be performed. Careful assessment of the interarch space is very important for the successful fabrication of telescopic dentures. Maxillary and mandibular impressions are made with irreversible hydrocolloid impression material followed by fabricated record base and wax rims. Tentative jaw relation is recorded to view if there is sufficient interarch space for the copings, the denture base, and the teeth. Adequate space must be present to accommodate the primary copings and secondary crowns, to have an adequate denture base thickness to avoid fracture, for the teeth arrangement to fulfill the aesthetic requirements, and to have an interocclusal gap. Pictures 5.20, 5.21, 5.22, 5.23, 5.24, 5.25, 5.26, 5.27, 5.28, 5.29, 5.30, 5.31, 5.32, 5.33, 5.34, 5.35, 5.36, and 5.37 depict the treatment steps of a case treated with TO.

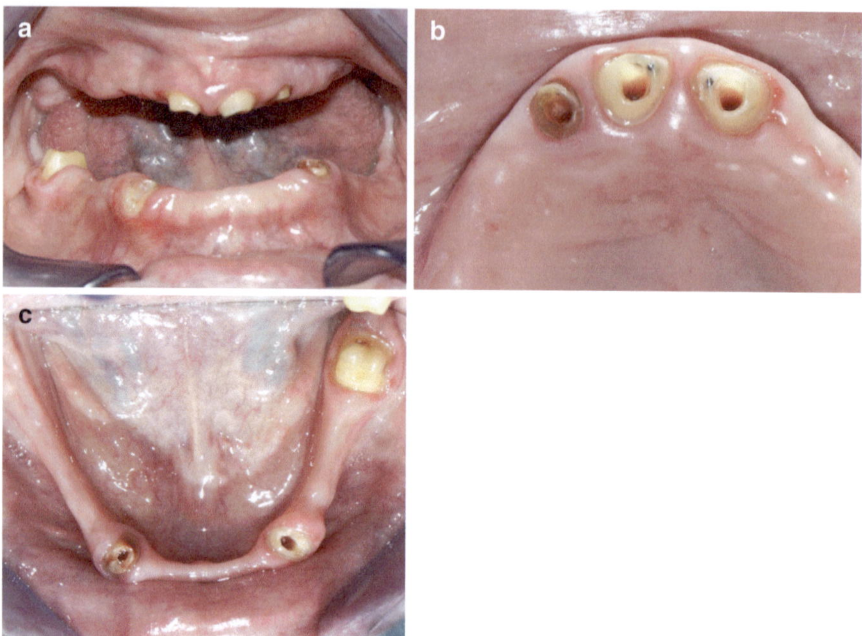

Picture 5.20 Maxillary and mandibular TO: (**a–c**) Prepared teeth for the upper and lower jaw. Three teeth (right central and left central and lateral teeth) in the maxilla and two teeth in the mandible (canines) are treated with root canal treatment, and primary coping is planned with a post and right first molar in the mandible tooth is sound and only primary coping is planned

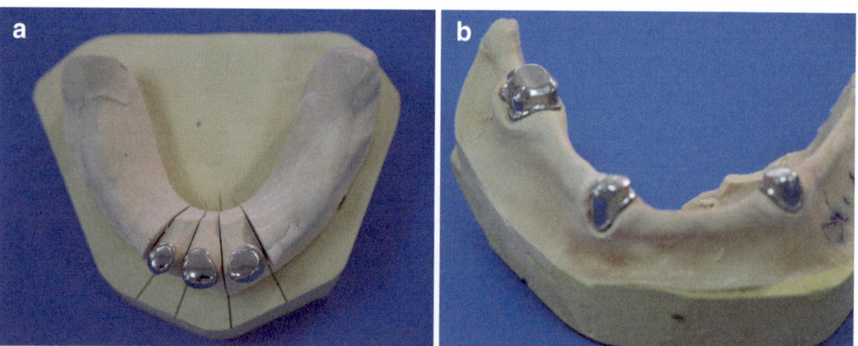

Picture 5.21 (**a, b**) The upper and lower primary copings cast with Co-Cr alloys on the model

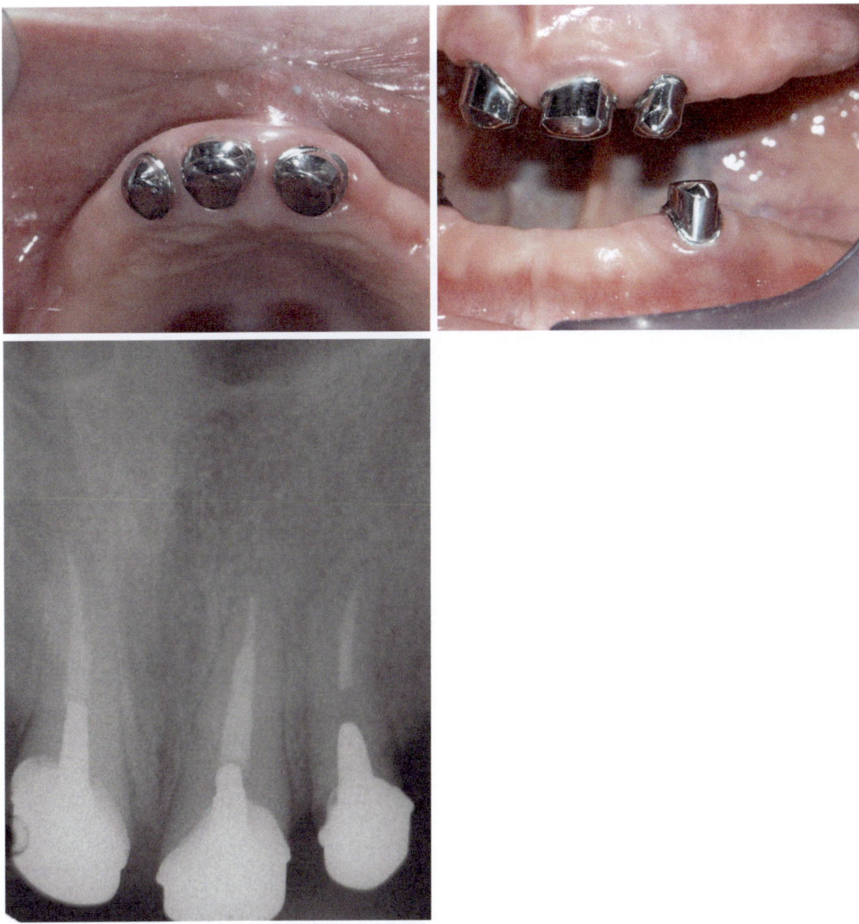

Picture 5.22 The upper primary coping was checked intraorally and radiologically

5.9.2 The Preparation of the Abutment

Following endodontic treatment, the teeth are prepared for primary coping with a tapered round-end diamond rotary bur with a chamfer finish line (Picture 5.20). Then impressions are made with a polyvinyl siloxane elastomeric impression material (Elite HD, Zhermack, Italy) in a two-stage putty wash technique by using metal trays. The silicone impression was poured into a die material to obtain the model. Interocclusal record is made by using the face bow transfer. The vertical dimension of occlusion determines the size of the copings.

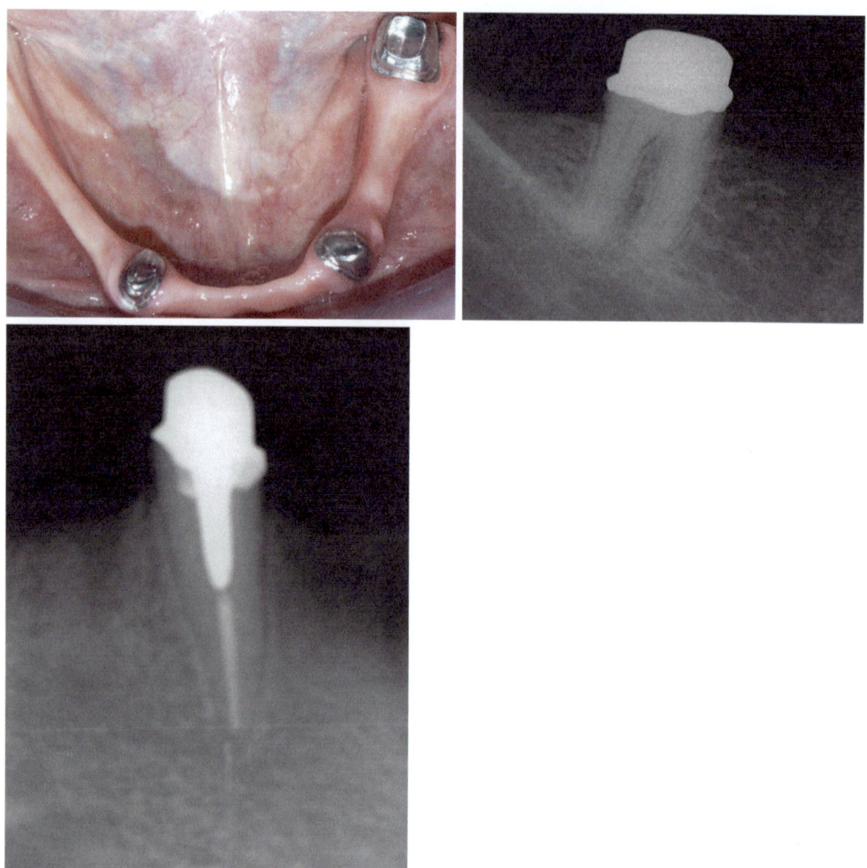

Picture 5.23 The upper primary coping was checked intraorally and radiologically

5.9.3 Casting Main Crowns

On the model, the milling wax that can be milled by a power system should be used for the primary copings. The wax copings are milled at the determined angle as already set on the surveyor model table, using the milling cutters and wax patterns of primary copings were milled following an appropriate path of insertion. The wax coping must not mill too thinly, that is, >0.6 mm. Then, primary copings are cast using a non-precious cobalt-chromium alloy. The cobalt-chromium alloy is generally preferred for easy processes due to its low hardness (HV 280), which also

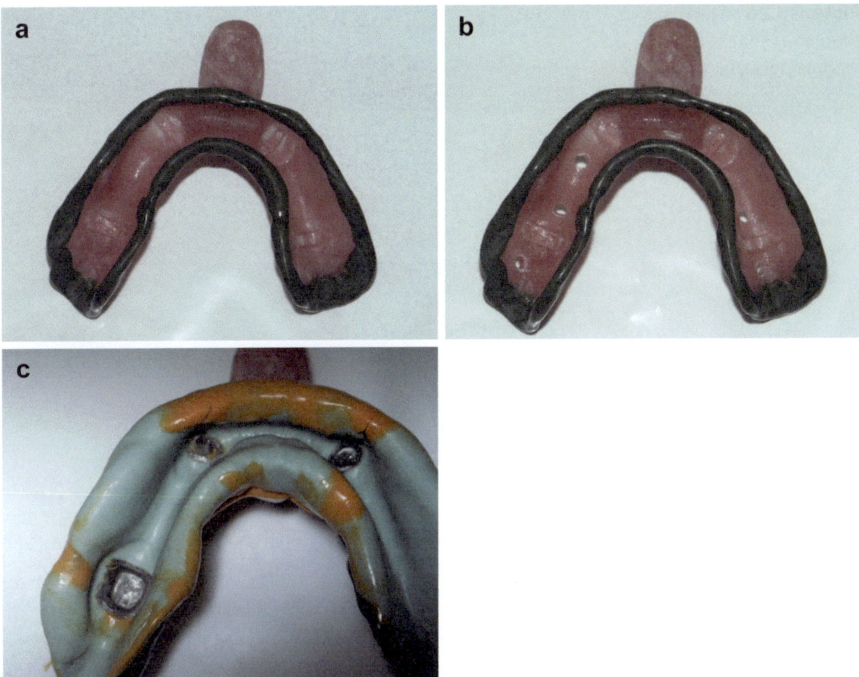

Picture 5.24 (**a**, **b**) The lower acrylic individual tray border was molded, completed, and drilled for ready impression; (**c**) the impression was taken with PVS impression materials (primary copings seen in the impression)

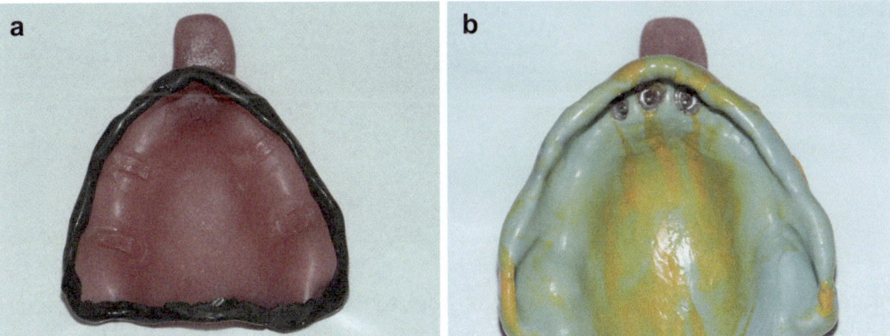

Picture 5.25 (**a**) The upper acrylic individual tray border was molded and completed for ready-to-impression; (**b**) the impression was taken with PVS impression materials (primary copings seen in the impression)

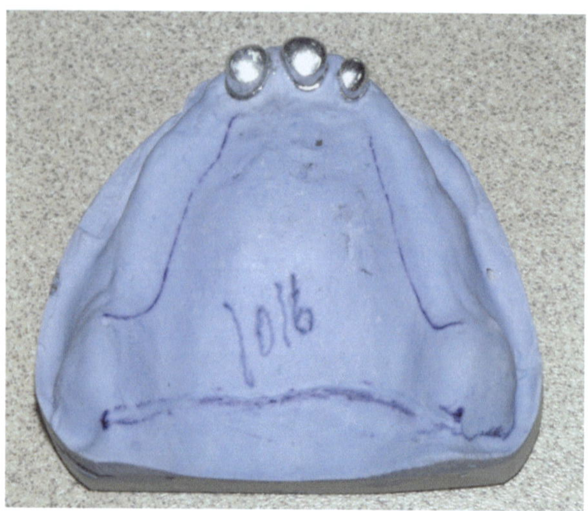

Picture 5.26 The upper primary copings seen on the final model

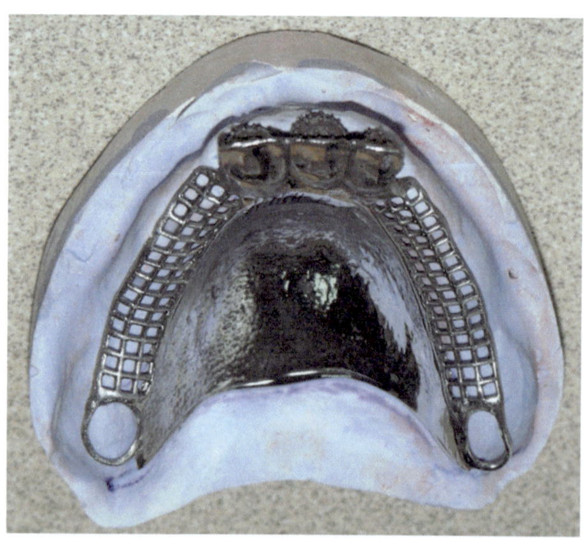

Picture 5.27 The maxillary framework cast in Co-Cr alloy combined with secondary crowns placed on the primary copings on the model

prolongs the lifespan of high-priced milling tools. The primary copings are controlled on the model and in the mouth, respectively, controlling fitting and accuracy and controlled periapical radiography. The perfect fit of every coping is required at this stage. One of the advantages of TO as the axial inclination of the individual teeth that create divergences and undercuts can be compensated by the primary copings. The clinician also needs to ensure that the primary part of the coping has sufficient space buccally to allow room for the manufacture of secondary crowns over it. It is also necessary to ensure that the preparation is designed in such a way that a unique fit is created for each primary coping to prevent twisting of the crowns during the try-in and when taking off the over impression (Pictures 5.21, 5.22, and 5.23).

Picture 5.28 The lower primary copings are seen on the final model

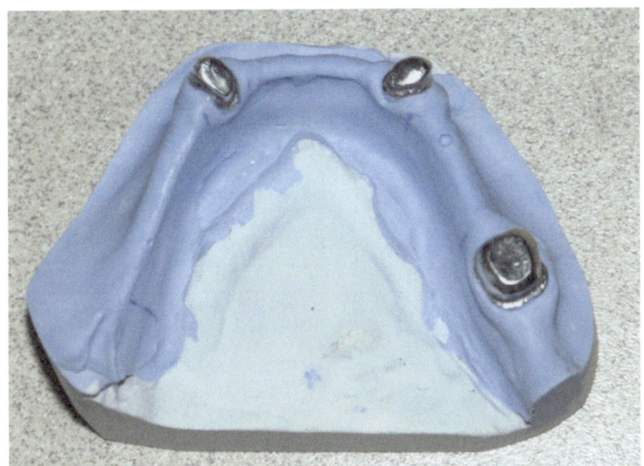

Picture 5.29 The mandibular framework cast in Co-Cr alloy combined with secondary crowns placed on the primary copings on the model

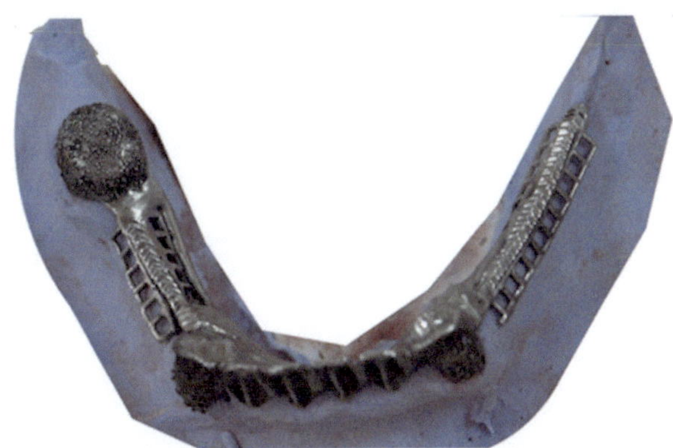

Picture 5.30 The maxillary framework on primary coping evaluated intraorally

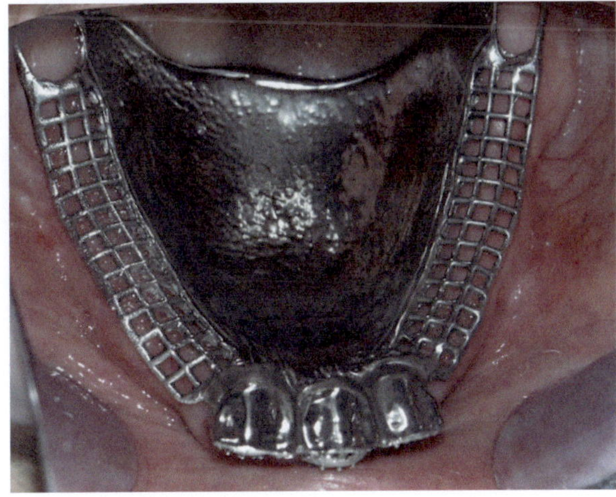

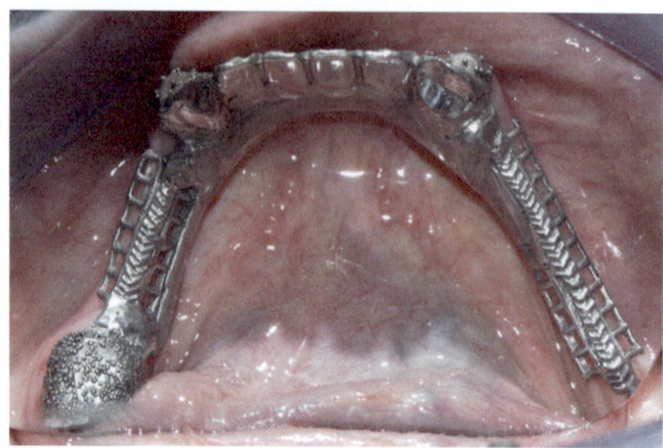

Picture 5.31 The mandibular framework on primary coping evaluated intraorally

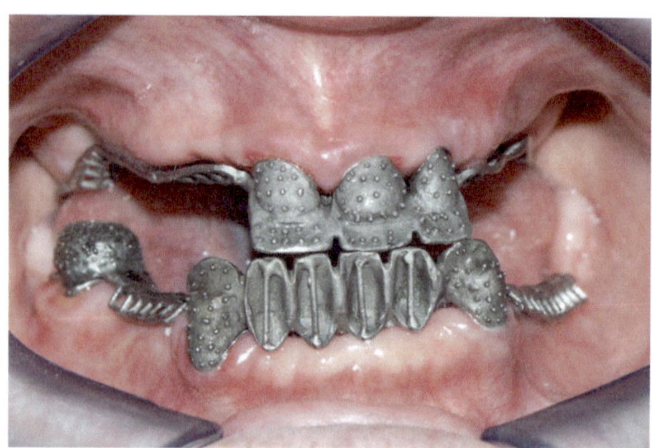

Picture 5.32 The maxillary and mandibular framework in situ

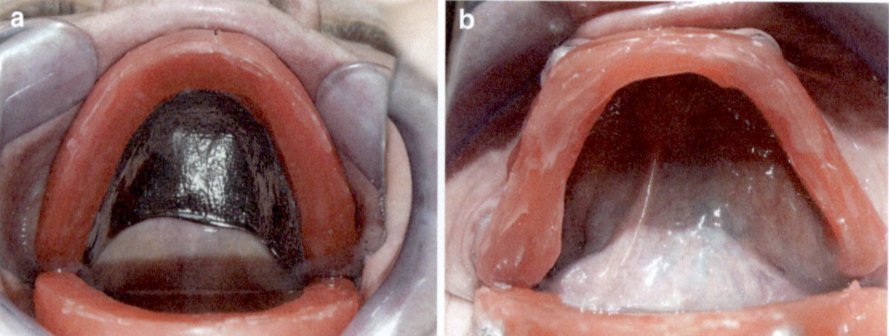

Picture 5.33 (**a, b**) The jaw relation record is made with occlusal rims on the framework

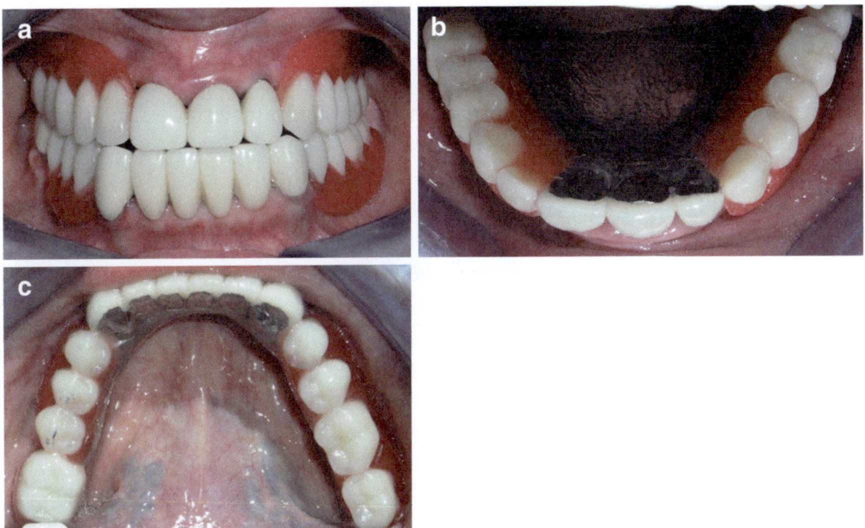

Picture 5.34 (**a–c**) The upper and lower teeth arrangement try in the mouth (secondary crowns veneered with porcelain veneers)

5.9.4 Fabrications of the Special Tray for Pick-Up Impression

After all the crowns are carefully adjusted on the model, the primary coping is blocked out to guarantee an equal spacing of the impression material for the pick-up (second) impression. The individual acrylic tray should extend over the potential denture-bearing areas. When all primary copings are fitting well on the prepared teeth, an over-impression or pick-up impression is taken by the dentist. The custom tray is tried in the mouth and checked for fitting, border molding is performed, and final impressions are made by medium body impression material, and the master model is poured (*The authors preferred impression with primary coping instead of cemented primary coping*) (Pictures 5.24, 5.25, and 5.26).

The accuracy of the master model is crucial because it is responsible for the fit of the whole assembly (chrome and acrylic design). This model would be used for the fabrication of the partial cast superstructure. The final model together with the primary copings was duplicated, and the refractory model was prepared. Smooth surface preparation is made on copings by using a surveyor (created a minimum 4 mm smooth surface for friction for the primary telescope crown). Then a small amount of baseplate wax is placed in the undesirable undercuts on the model and duplicated for refractory cast by using an agar impression material. The investment material (the type of investment depends on the type of alloy used) is poured into the duplication model. On the refractory cast, metal framework waxed up with secondary crowns and framework. The design of the framework included secondary copings on primary crowns and meshed for the acrylic spanning anterior edentulous segment. The prepared wax pattern was cast using Co-Cr alloy (Bellabond plus BeGo, Germany). After trimming and polishing, it is fitted onto the master cast (Pictures 5.26, 5.27, 5.28, and 5.29). The framework is tried in the patient's mouth for the final fit (Pictures 5.30, 5.31, and 5.32). The friction between the parallel surfaces of primary and secondary copings obtains retention in telescopic attachment retained overdenture. Horizontal and vertical maxilla-mandibular records were obtained again with the wax rim on the framework for controlling the vertical dimension of occlusion and centric relation. Then, it is transferred to a semi-adjustable articulator help of a facebow (Picture 5.33). Traditional porcelain veneering was made on the secondary crowns, and acrylic teeth were set with the same shade as were veneered on the edentulous areas. The teeth arrangements were evaluated intraorally according to phonetics, aesthetics, vertical dimension, and centric relations, and patients' approval is taken (Picture 5.34). Then a conventional method was applied for polymerization of the dentures using heat-activated acrylic resin. After evaluating the fit of the dentures on the primary copings in the mouth, the primary copings were cemented with glass ionomer luting cement or resin cement, and TO was delivered to the patient after occlusal adjustments (Pictures 5.35, 5.36, and 5.37).

5.9.4.1 Counsel for the Patients

Postinsertion instructions were given to the patient that included maintenance of meticulous oral hygiene, and the patient's recall on a 6-month follow-up recall. At each follow-up visit, the patient was evaluated for the effectiveness of oral health, retention, and stability of the denture and radiographic control of teeth (Picture 5.38). For TO, insertion and removal of the denture and routine oral hygiene are easy to perform, even for patients with limited manual dexterity. As a full-arch reconstruction, the double crown denture system enables easy adjustment, modification, and relining with low follow-up costs. The patient also plays a vital role in

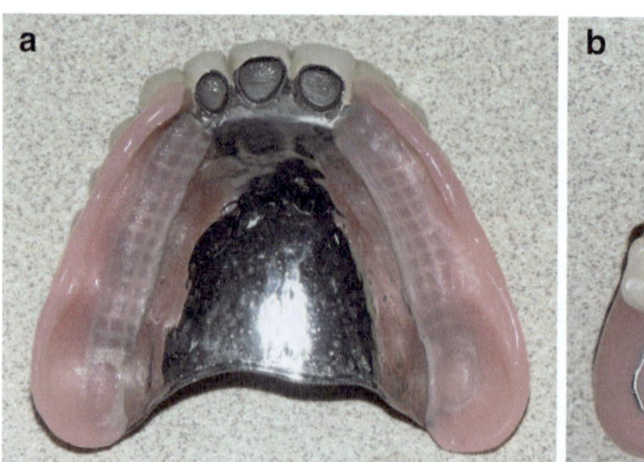
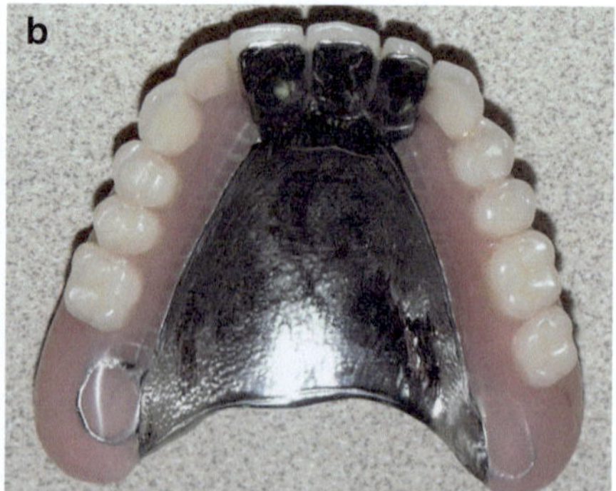

Picture 5.35 (**a, b**) The intaglio and external view of the upper TO

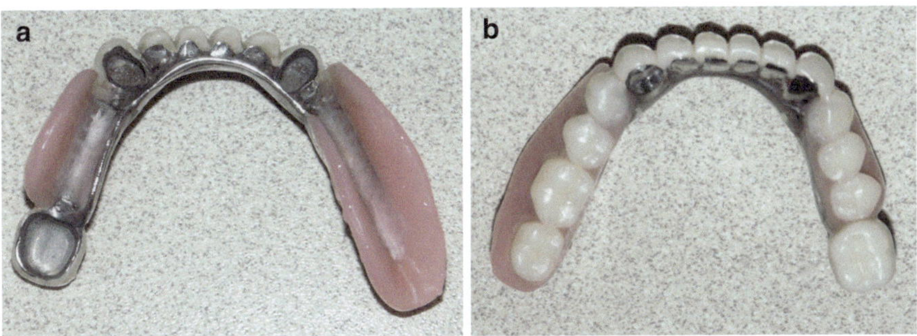

Picture 5.36 (**a**, **b**) The intaglio and external view of lower TO

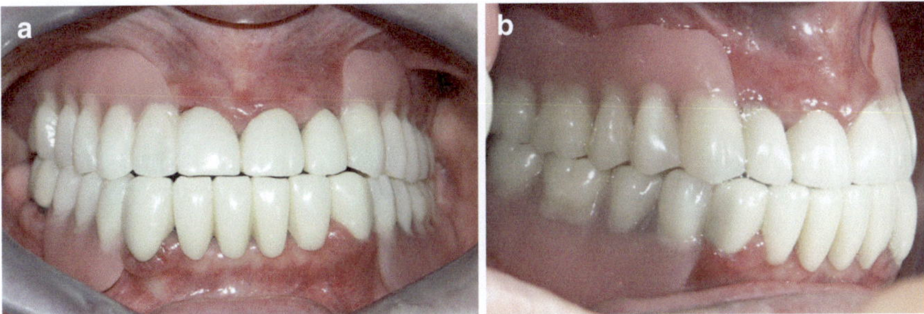

Picture 5.37 (**a**, **b**) The TO in situ

Picture 5.38 Panoramic radiograph taken after 3 years

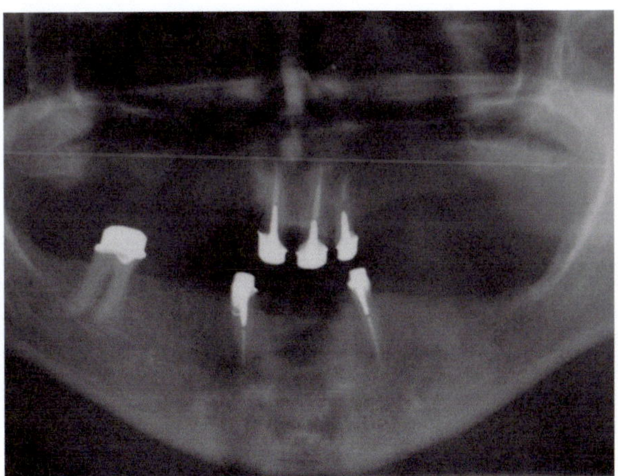

the longevity of the denture. The patient, therefore, can also contribute to ensuring the success of such quality work by providing a commitment toward oral and dental hygiene, regular checking of the denture for intactness, freedom from stresses, adaptation of the gingival surfaces, and ease of the removing and inserting the denture. For ensuring proper care and appropriate handling of the denture after instruction by the practitioner, follow a short "instruction manual."

Pictures 5.39, 5.40, 5.41, and 5.42 depict the steps of two distinct cases addressed using distinct TO techniques.

Picture 5.39 A few teeth remained in a patient treated by TSO instead of implants-retained over-denture because of his systemic complications. (**a**) Frontal view of a patient with denture; (**b**) panoramic X-ray and view of dentures in situ (the patient had upper clasp retained removable denture and lower attachment retained removable denture); (**c**) in the upper jaw lateral and canine teeth and in the lower jaw right premolar, left central, lateral, canine, first and the second premolar remained; (**d**) all crowns removed and teeth evaluated clinically; (**e**) in the lower jaw, second pre-molar teeth saw root fracture under the gingival level and the central and lateral teeth showed mobility and decided to extraction; (**f**) in the upper jaw, lateral tooth showed mobility and decided to extraction; (**g**) after extraction of teeth; (**h–j**) after a healing period, teeth preparation was made; (**k, l**) pouring cast model for preparing primary coping; (**m, n**) primary copings; (**o**) intraoral check of primary copings (impression taken with copings for metal framework); (**p, q**) metal framework cast with secondary coping as one unit for mandible; (**r**) internal view of the metal framework and primary copings; (**s, t**) metal framework cast with secondary coping as one unit for maxilla; (**u**) internal view of the metal framework and primary copings; (**v**) adjustment of the metal framework onto the copings and checked intraorally

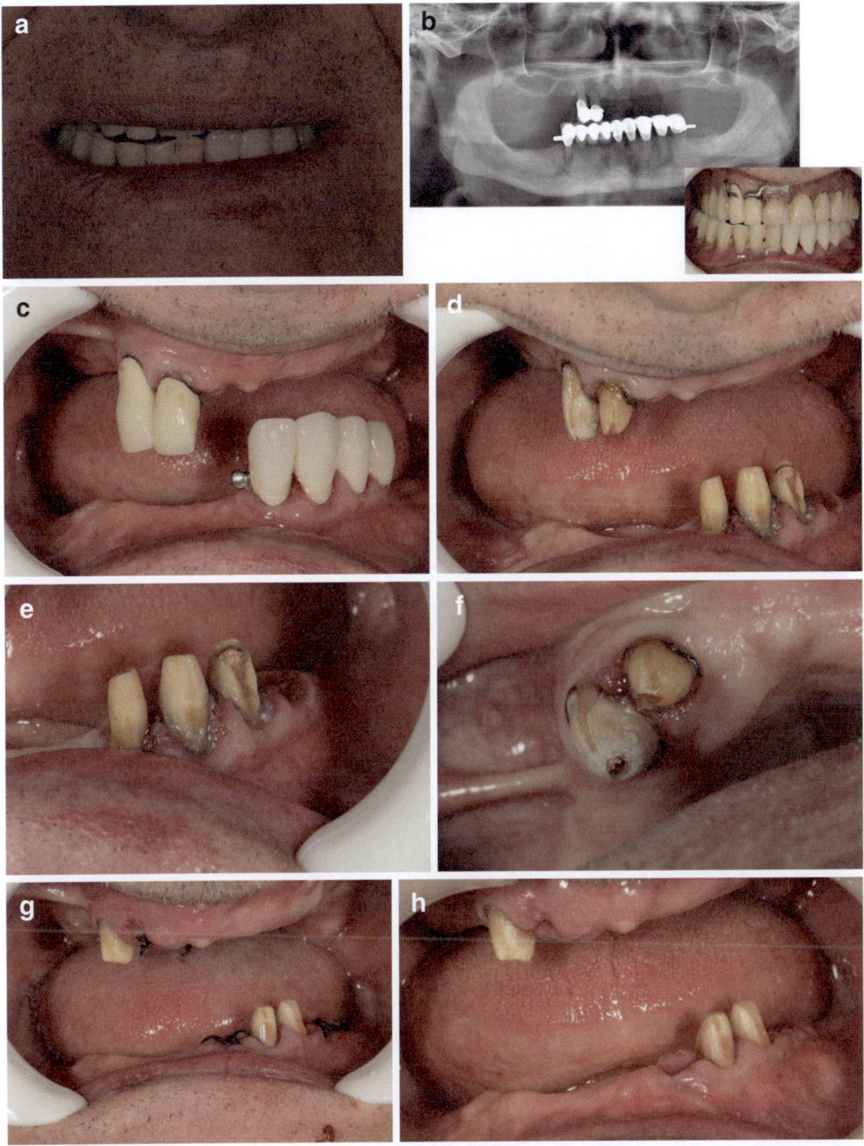

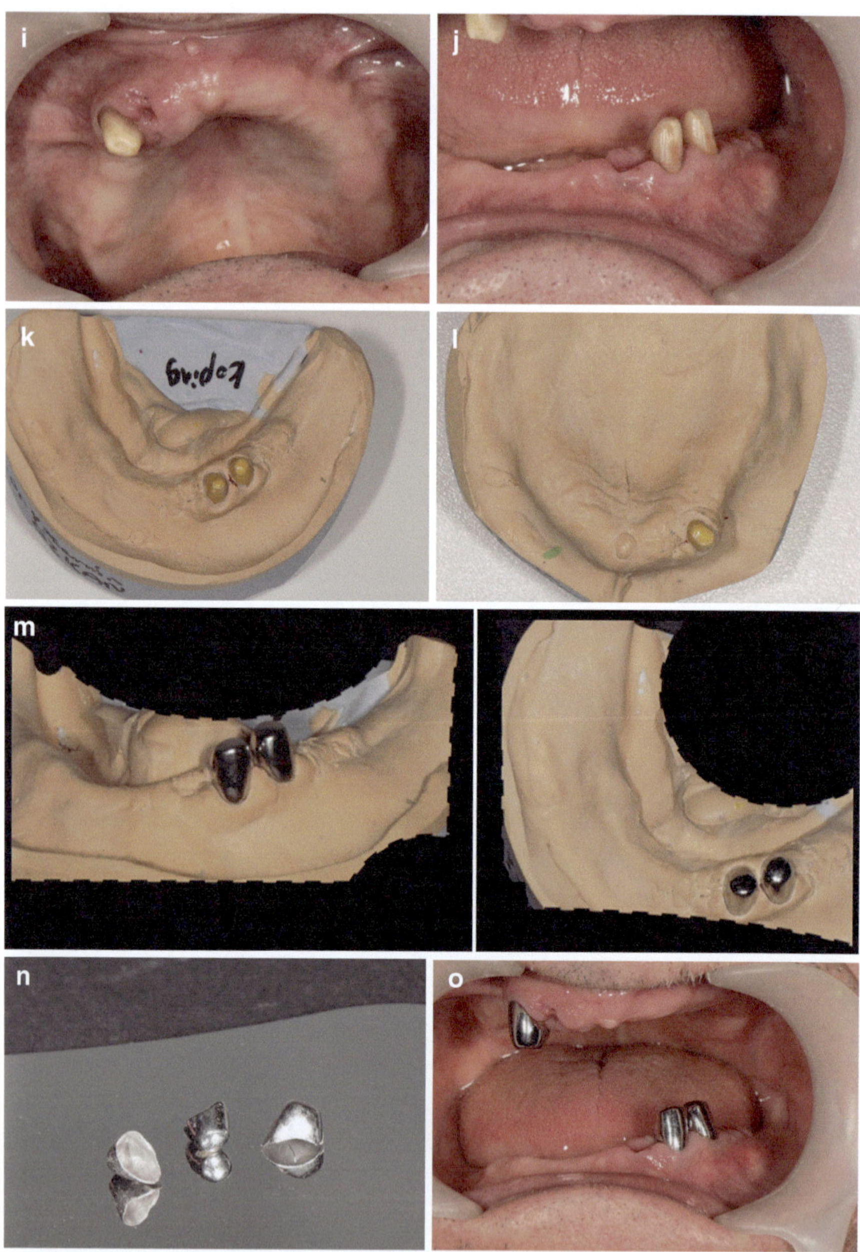

Picture 5.39 (continued)

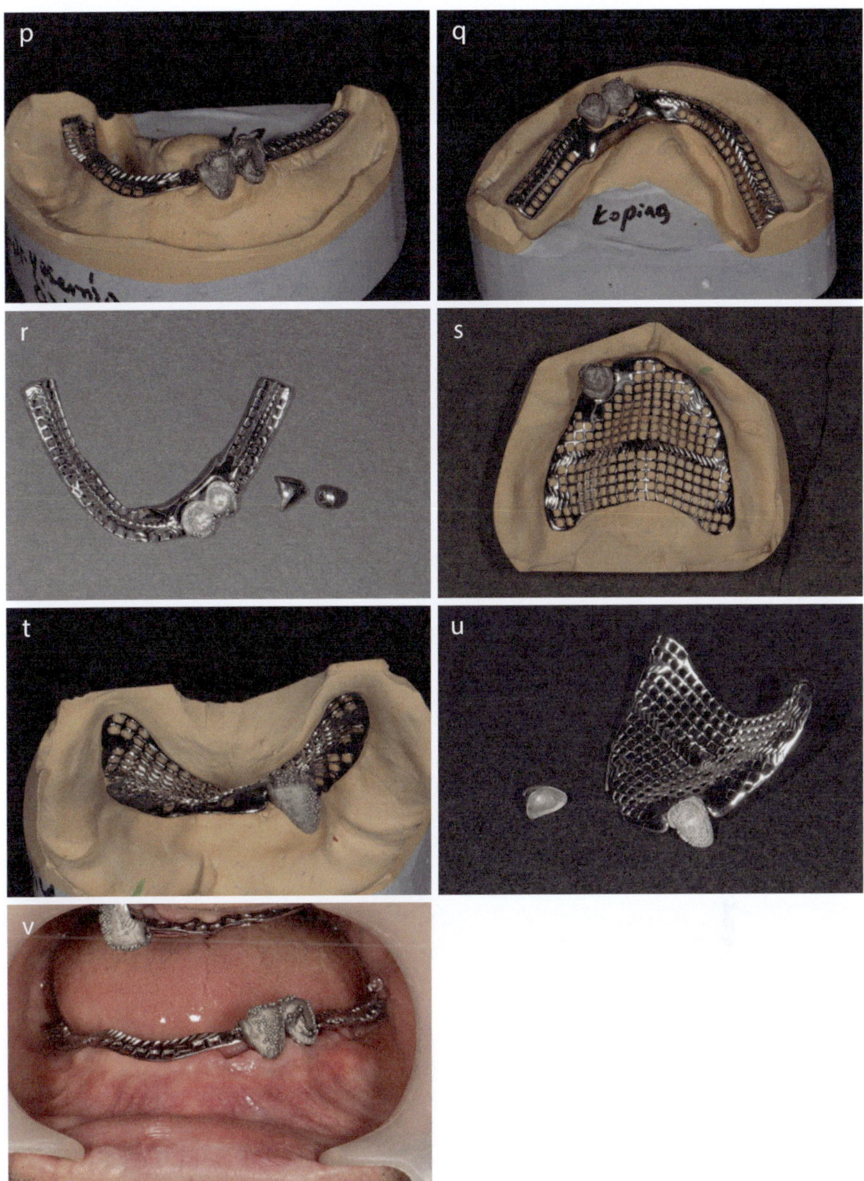

Picture 5.39 (continued)

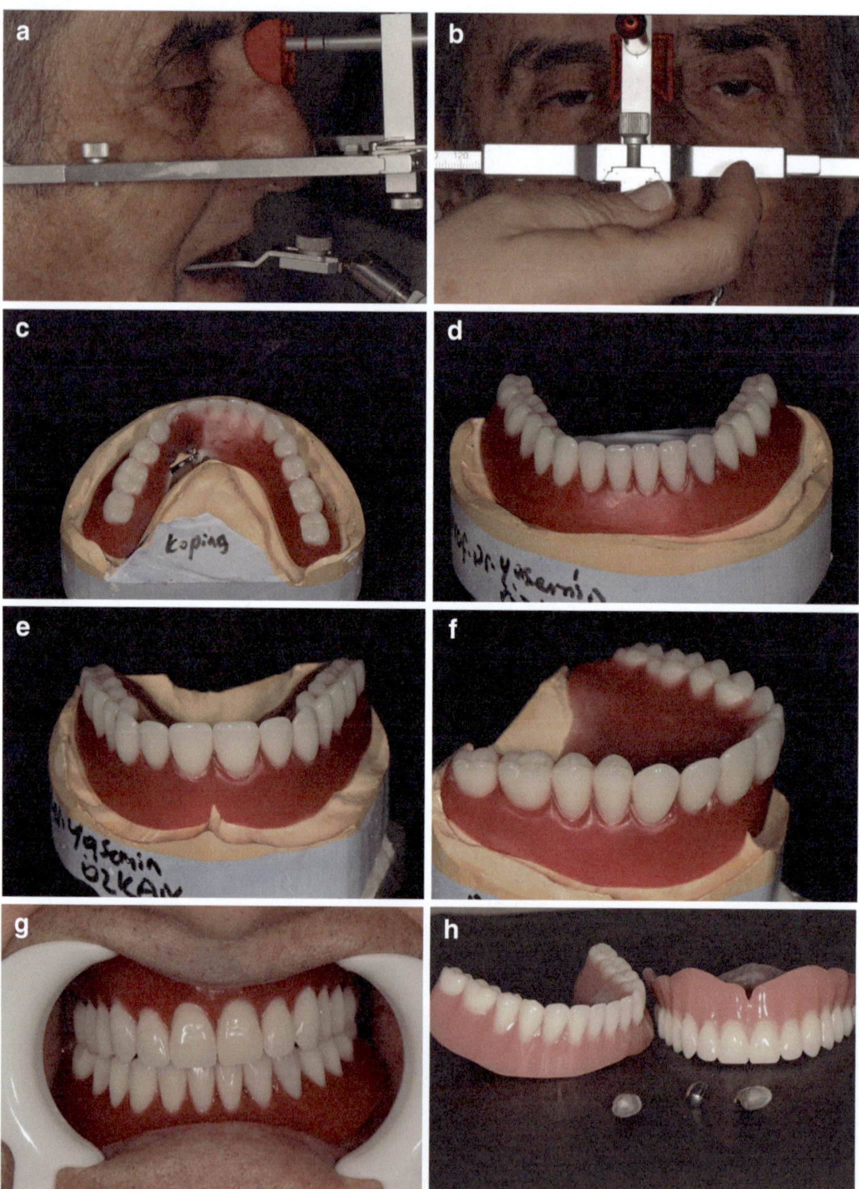

Picture 5.40 A few teeth remained in a patient treated by TSO instead of implants-retained over-denture because of his systemic complications. (**a**, **b**) Determined centric relation and face bow record; (**c–g**) mandibular and maxillary teeth arrangement; (**h**) try-in stage; (**i–k**) extraoral view of dentures and copings; (**l**, **m**) teeth-supported overdenture in situ

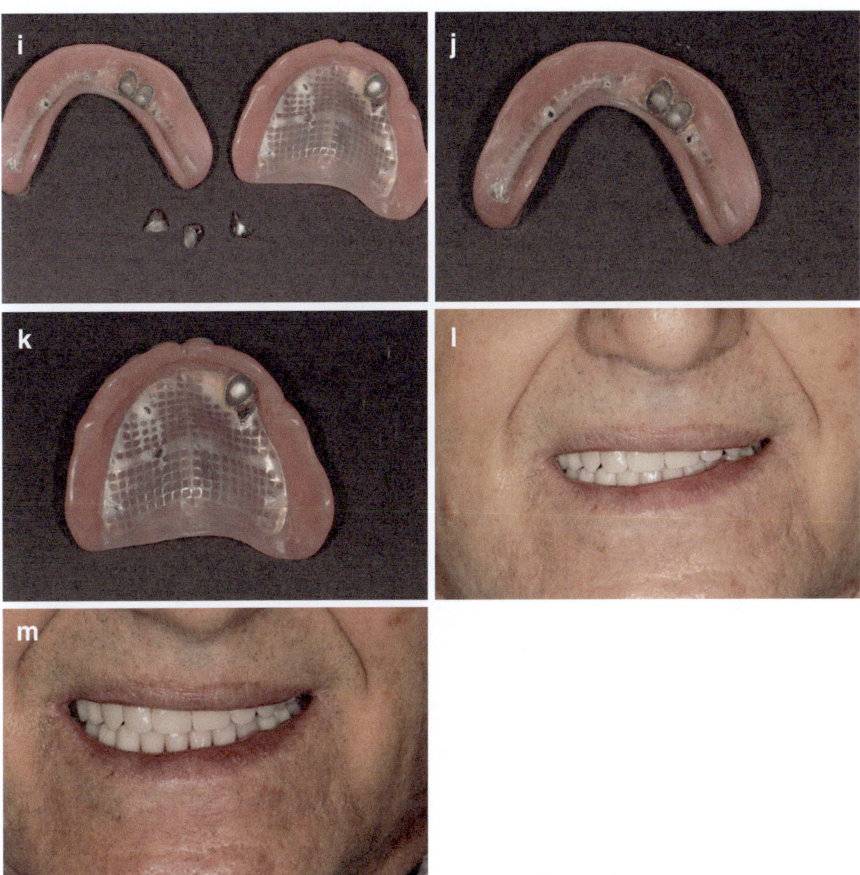

Picture 5.40 (continued)

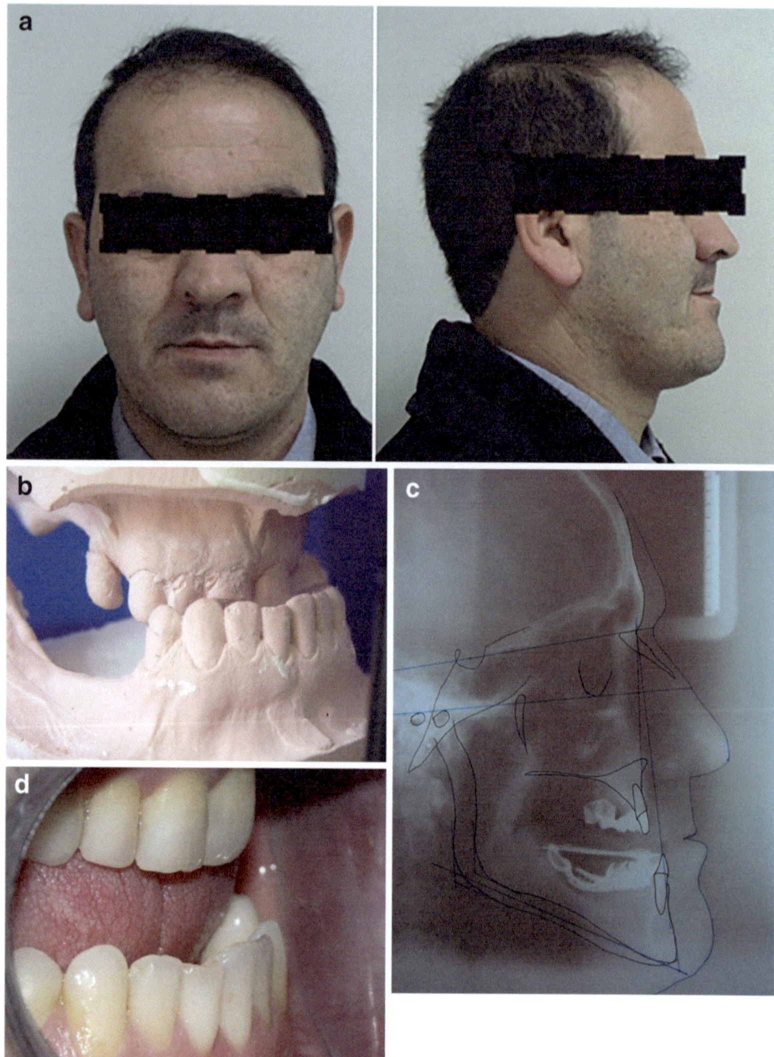

Picture 5.41 Severe Class III patients treated by overdentures instead of surgical interventions: (**a**) Front and profile view of Class III patient; (**b**) diagnostic cast evaluation; (**c**) cephalometric examination of the maxillomandibular relation; (**d**) anterior teeth relation; (**e**) intraoral view of maxillary dentition; (**f, g**) temporary prosthesis on the cast and mouth; (**h**) maxillary teeth preparation for telescopic crowns according to the temporary prosthesis; (**i**) intraoral check of the primary crowns (attachments were used between copings at the right and left sides); (**j**) impression including copings made for the metal framework; (**k**) a metal framework for the lower jaw; (**l**) metal framework and secondary coping cast as one unit on the copings for the upper jaw; (**m**) a metal framework with secondary crowns and primary copings; (**n**) adjustment of the metal framework onto the copings; (**o, p**) aluminum sheet placed on the wax rim for the record of accurate vertical and centric relationship with cephalometric X-ray; (**q**) try-in stage of teeth arrangement; (**r, s**) extraoral view of upper TO and lower clasp-retained RPD; (**t**) intraoral appearance of the prosthesis; (**u, v**) extraoral and facial appearance of patients with dentures

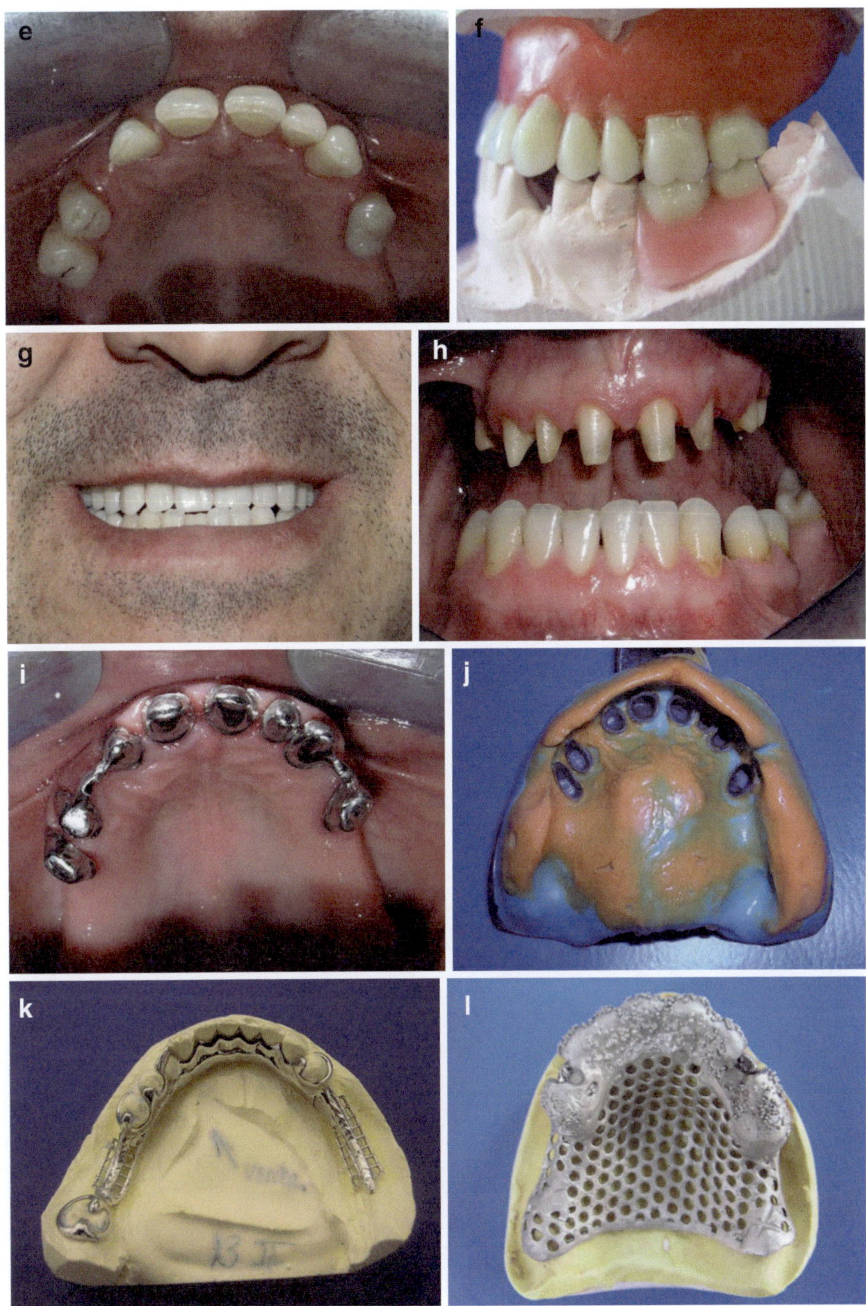

Picture 5.41 (continued)

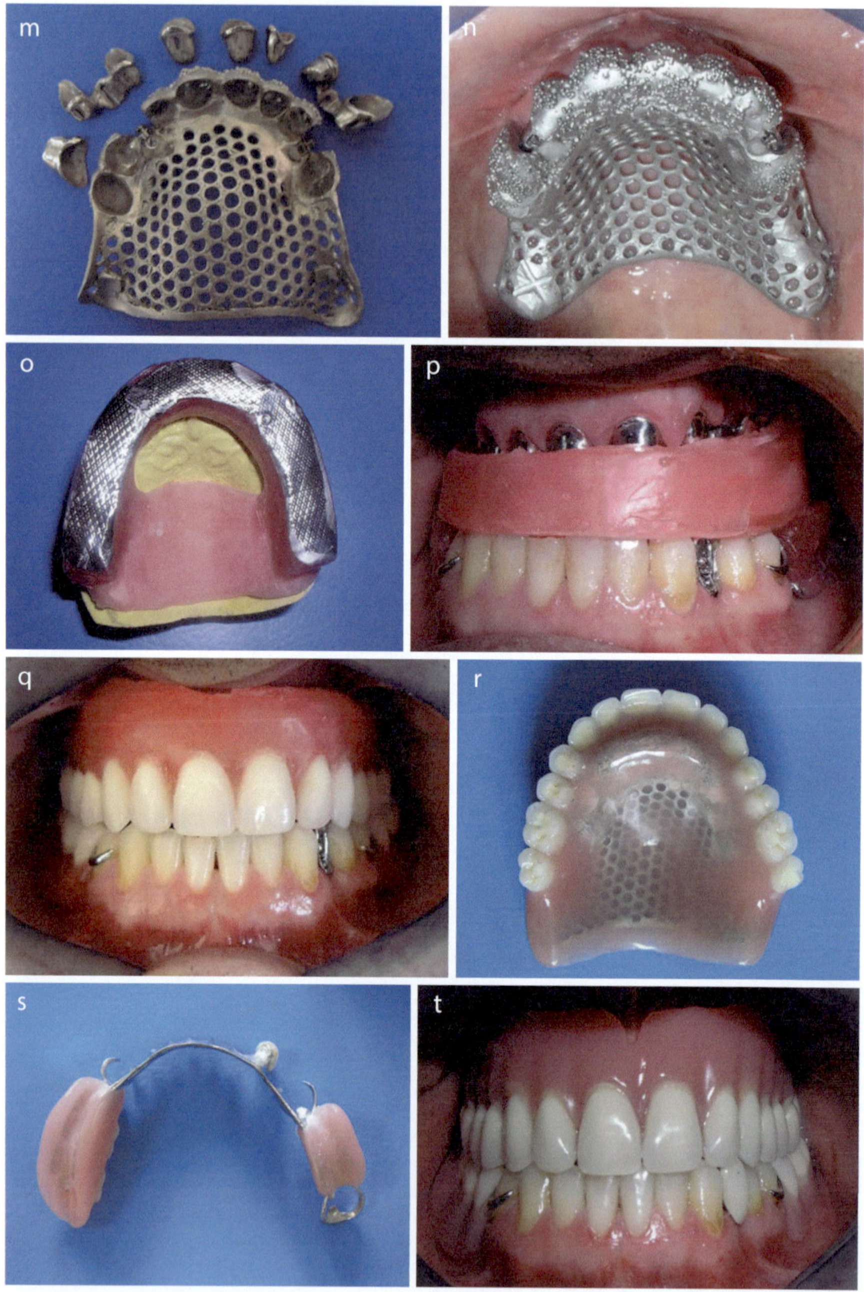

Picture 5.41 (continued)

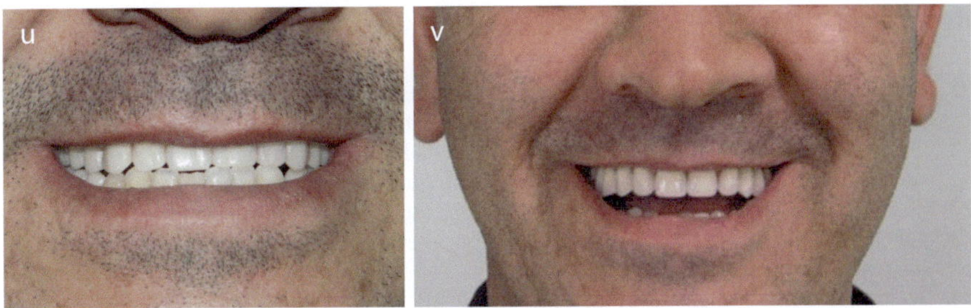

Picture 5.41 (continued)

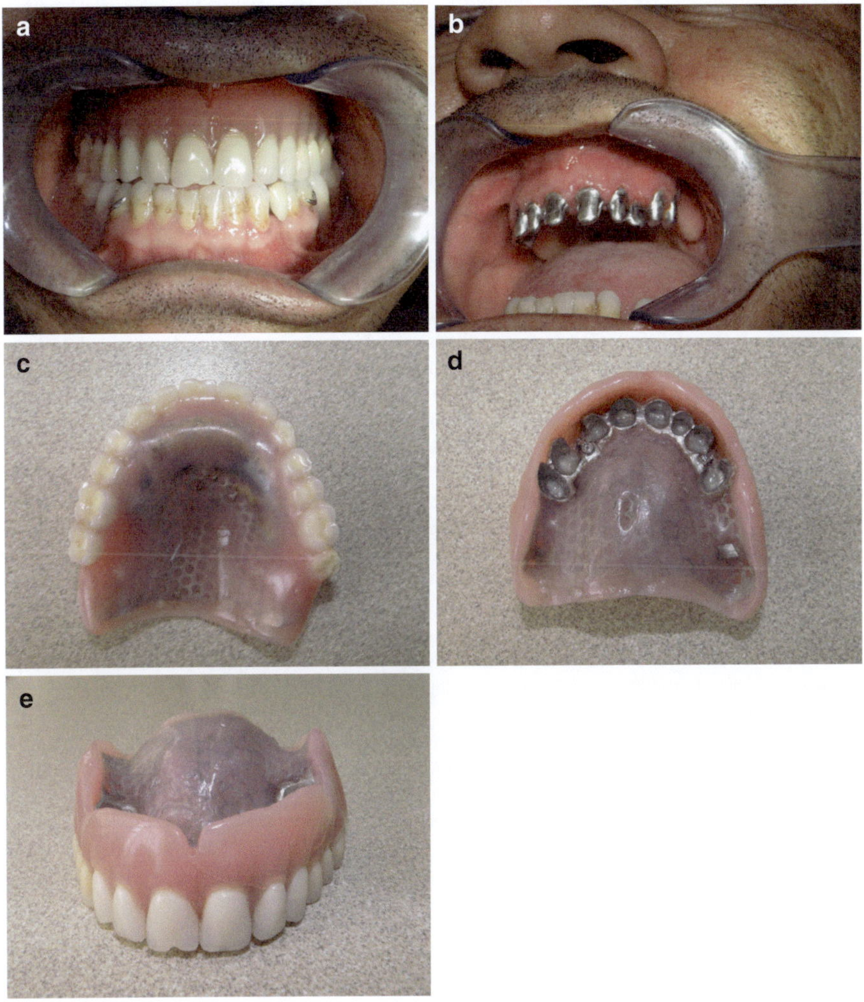

Picture 5.42 (**a–e**) Seven years later. The patient was very happy with his overdenture. There were only minor changes in both soft tissue and dentures

References

1. Ohkawa S, Okane H, Nagasawa T, Tsuru H. Changes in retention of various telescope crown assemblies over long-term use. J Prosthet Dent. 1990;64:153–8.
2. Kiyama M, Shiba A, Takayanagi Y, Suzuki M, Ikeda M. Studies on the retentive force of conical telescopic double-crown. Part 2. The retentive force of conical telescopic double-crown is related to the diameter of the cone. J Jpn Prosthodont Soc. 1997;41:71–9.
3. Hultén J, Tillström B, Nilner K. Long term clinical evaluation of conical crown-retained dentures. Swed Dent J. 1993;17:225–34.
4. Heckmann SM, Winter W, Meyer M, Weber HP, Wichmann MG. Overdenture attachment selection and the loading of implant and denture-bearing area. Part 2: A methodical study using five types of attachment. Clin Oral Implants Res. 2001;12:640–7. https://doi.org/10.1034/j.1600-0501.2001.120613.x.
5. Hoffmann O, Beaumont C, Tatakis DN, Zafiropoulos GG. Telescopic crowns as attachments for implant supported restorations: a case series. J Oral Implantol. 2006;32:291–9. https://doi.org/10.1563/0-815.1.
6. Al Wazzan KA, Al-Nazzawi AA. Marginal and internal adaptation of commercially pure titanium and titanium-aluminum-vanadium alloy cast restorations. J Contemp Dent Pract. 2007;8:19–26.
7. Weigl P, Hahn L, Lauer HC. Advanced biomaterials used for a new telescopic retainer for removable dentures. J Biomed Mater Res. 2000;53:320–36.
8. Beuer F, Edelhoff D, Gernet W, Naumann M. Parameters affecting the retentive force of electroformed double-crown systems. Clin Oral Investig. 2010;14:129–35.
9. Engels J, Schubert O, Güth JF, Hoffmann M, Jauernig C, Erdelt K, Stimmelmayr M, Beuer F. Wear behavior of different double-crown systems. Clin Oral Investig. 2013;17:503–11.
10. Wagner C, Stock V, Merk S, Schmidlin PR, Roos M, Eichberger M, Stawarczyk B. Comparison of retention forces of different fabrication methods of Co-Cr crowns: pre-sintered and milled, cast and electroforming secondary crowns with different taper angles. Int J Dent Oral Sci. 2015;3:15–20.
11. Groesser J, Sachs C, Heiß P, Stadelmann M, Erdelt K, Beuer F. Retention forces of 14-unit zirconia telescopic prostheses with six double crowns made from zirconia--an in vitro study. Clin Oral Investig. 2014;18:1173–9. https://doi.org/10.1007/s00784-013-1093-1.
12. Rinke S, Buergers R, Ziebolz D, Roediger M. Clinical outcome of double crown-retained implant overdentures with zirconia primary crowns. J Adv Prosthodont. 2015;7:329–37.
13. Besimo CH, Graber G, Flühler M. Retention force changes in implant-supported titanium telescope crowns over long-term use in vitro. J Oral Rehabil. 1996;23:372–8.
14. Turp I, Bozdağ E, Sünbüloğlu E, Kahraman C, Yusufoğlu I, Bayraktar G. Retention and surface changes of zirconia primary crowns with secondary crowns of different materials. Clin Oral Investig. 2014;18:2023–35.
15. Guven MC, Tuna M, Bozdağ E, Ozturk GN, Bayraktar G. Comparison of retention forces with various fabrication methods and materials in double crowns. J Adv Prosthodont. 2017;9:308–14.
16. Merk S, Wagner C, Stock V, Eichberger M, Schmidlin PR, Roos M, Stawarczyk B. Suitability of secondary PEEK telescopic crowns on zirconia primary crowns. Materials (Basel). 2016;11:908.
17. Merk S, Wagner C, Stock V, Schmidlin PR, Roos M, Eichberger M, Stawarczyk B. Retention load values of telescopic crowns made of Y-TZP and COCR with Y-TZP secondary crowns: impact of different taper angles. Materials. 2016;9:354.

Further Reading

Arnold C, Hey J, Setz JM, Boeckler AF, Schweyen R. Retention force of removable partial dentures with different double crowns. Clin Oral Investig. 2018;22:1641–9.
Bayer S, Al-Mansour R, Grüner M, Enkling N, Stark H, Mues S. In-vitro wear simulation of retentive elements for telescopic crowns. ZWR. 2008;117:412–8.

Bayer S, Stark H, Mues S, Keilig L, Schrader A, Enkling N. Retention force measurement of telescopic crowns. Clin Oral Invest. 2010;14:607–11.

Behr M, Hofmann E, Rosentritt M, Lang R, Handel G. Technical failure rates of double crown-retained removable partial dentures. Clin Oral Investig. 2000;4:87–90.

Beschnidt SM, Chitmongkolsuk S, Prull R. Telescopic crown-retained removable partial dentures: review and case report. Compend Contin Educ Dent. 2001;22:927–8. 929-32

Bottegaga DM, Mesquita MF, Henriques GE, Vaz LG. Retention force and fatigue strength of overdenture attachment systems. J Oral Rehabil. 2004;31:884–9.

Breitman J, Nakamura S, Freedman A, Yalisove I. Telescopic retainers: an old or new solution? A second chance to have a normal dental function. J Prosthodont. 2012;21:79–83.

Burns DR, Unger JW, Elswick RK, Giglio JA. Prospective clinical evaluation of mandibular implant overdentures: Part II Patient satisfaction and preference. J Prosthet Dent. 1995;73:364–9.

Carlsson GE. Implant and root supported overdentures – a literature review and some data on bone loss in edentulous jaws. J Adv Prosthodont. 2014;6:245–52.

Carr AB, Brown DT. McCracken's removable partial prosthodontics. 13th ed. St. Louis, MO: Mosby; 2015.

Eisenburger M, Gray G, Tschernitschek H. Long-term results of telescopic crown retained dentures—a retrospective study. Eur J Prosthodont Restor Dent. 2000;8:87–91.

Emera RMK. All-zirconia double crowns for retaining complete mandibular overdenture. Clinical and microbiological evaluation of natural abutments. EDJ. 2016;62:1959–72.

Ericson A, Nilsson B, Bergman B. Clinical results in patients provided with conical crown retained dentures. Int J Prosthodont. 1990;3:513–21.

Fernandes V, Chitre V, Aras M. Prosthetic management of a case of advanced periodontitis with telescopic dentures. J Indian Prosthodont Soc. 2008;8:216–20.

Alfred GH, Kundert M, Kelsey C. Charles. complete denture and overdenture prosthetics. New York: Thieme Medical Publishers Inc.; 1993.

Grossmann AC, Hassel AJ, Schilling O, Lehmann F, Koob A, Rammelsberg P. Treatment with double crown-retained removable partial dentures and oral health-related quality of life in middle- and high-aged patients. Int J Prosthodont. 2007;20:576–8.

Güngör MA, Artunç C, Sonugelen M. Parameters affecting retentive force of conus crowns. J Oral Rehabil. 2004;31:271–7.

Güngör MA, Artunç C, Sonugelen M, Toparli M. The evaluation of the removal forces on the conus crowned telescopic prostheses with the finite element analysis (FEA). J Oral Rehabil. 2002;29:1069–75.

Hofmann E, Behr M, Handel G. Frequency and costs of technical failures of clasp- and double crown-retained removable partial dentures. Clin Oral Investig. 2002;6:104 8.

Hou GL, Tsai CC, Weisgold AS. Periodontal and prosthetic therapy in severely advanced periodontitis by the use of the crown sleeve coping telescope denture. A longitudinal case reports. Aust Dent J. 1997;42:169–74.

Igarashi Y, Goto T. Ten-year follow-up study of conical crown-retained dentures. Int J Prosthodont. 1997;10:149–55.

Isaacson GO. Telescope crown retainers for removable partial dentures. J Prosthet Dent. 1969;22:436–48.

Joda T. Combined tooth-implant–supported telescopic prostheses in a midterm follow-up of > 2 years. Int J Prosthodont. 2013;26:536–40.

Kiyama M, Shiba A. Studies on the retentive force of conical telescopic double-crown. Part 1. The retentive force of a conical telescopic double-crown is related to materials and taper angle and height of the cone and load. J Jpn Prosthodont Soc. 1994;38:1252–64.

Koller B, Att W, Strub JR. Survival rates of teeth, implants, and double crown–retained removable dental prostheses: a systematic literature review. Int J Prosthodont. 2011;24:109–17.

Korber KH. Conical crowns—a rational telescopic system (Konuskronen–Darationalele Teleskop system). Heidelberg: Hülting; 1983.

Langer A. Telescope retainers and their clinical application. J Prosthet Dent. 1980;44:516–22.

Langer Y, Langer A. Tooth-supported telescopic prostheses in compromised dentitions: a clinical report. J Prosthet Dent. 2000;84:129–32.

Lehmann KM, Armin FV. Studies on the retention capability of push-button attachments (Untersuchungen über die Retentionskräfe von Druckknopfankern). Schweiz Mschr Zanheilk. 1976;86:521–30.

Minagi S, Natsuaki N, Nishigawa G, Sato T. New telescopic crown design for removable partial dentures. J Prosthet Dent. 1999;81:684–8.

Nakagawa S, Torii K, Tanaka M. Effects of taper and space settings of telescopic Ce-TZP/A crowns on retentive force and settling. Dent Mater J. 2017;36:230–5.

Perel ML. Telescope dentures. J Prosthet Dent. 1973;29:151–6.

Pietruski JK, Pietruska MD, DDS, Sajewicz E. Long-Term follow-up of the conical crown–retained dentures fabricated using different technologies. Int J Periodont Restorative Dent. 2012;32:467–75.

Preiskel HW. Precision attachments in prosthodontics; overdentures and telescopic prostheses, vol. 2. Chicago, IL: Quintessence Publishing Co. 1973;p. 243–306.

Samra RK, Bhide SV, Goyal C, Kaur T. Tooth supported overdenture: a concept overshadowed but not yet forgotten! J Oral Res Rev. 2015;7:16–21.

Schweitzer JM, Schweitzer RD, Schweitzer J. The telescoped complete denture: a research report at the clinical level. J Prosthet Dent. 1971;26:357–72.

Schwindling FS, Lehmann F, Terebesi S, Corcodel N, Zenthöfer A, Rammelsberg P, Stober T. Electroplated telescopic retainers with zirconia primary crowns: 3-year results from a randomized clinical trial. Clin Oral Investig. 2017;21:2653–60.

Schwindling FS, Deisenhofer UK, Séché AC, Lehmann F, Rammelsberg P, Stober T. Randomized trial investigating zirconia electroplated telescopic retainers: quality of life outcomes. Clin Oral Investig. 2017;21:1157–63.

Sekiguchi Y, Kuroiwa A. Studies on pure titanium conical telescopic crown: effect of changes in taper and height of inner crown on retentive force of outer crown made by cast-on technique. J Dent Mater. 2003;22:271–82.

Shiba A. The conical double-crown telescopic removable periodontic prosthesis. Ishiyaku Euro America: St. Louis, Tokyo; 1993.

Shimakura M, Tomohisa N, Takeuchi M, Nemoto M. Retentive force of pure titanium konus telescope crowns fabricated Using CAD/CAD System. Dent Mater J. 2008;27:211–5.

Stancić I, Jelenković A. Retention of telescopic denture in elderly patients with maximum partially edentulous arch. Gerodontology. 2008;25:162–7.

Stock V, Schmidlin PR, Merk S, Wagner C, Roos M, Eichberger M, Stawarczyk B. PEEK primary crowns with cobalt-chromium, zirconia, and galvanic secondary crowns with different tapers-a comparison of retention forces. Materials (Basel). 2016;9:187.

Verma R, Joda T, Brägger U, Wittneben JG. A systematic review of the clinical performance of tooth-retained and implant-retained double crown prostheses with a follow-up of ≥ 3 years. J Prosthodont. 2013;22:2–12.

Wagner C, Stock V, Merk S, et al. Retention load of telescopic crowns with different taper angles between cobalt-chromium and polyetheretherketone made with three different manufacturing processes examined by pull-off test. J Prosthodont. 2018;27:162–8.

Wenz HJ, Hertrampf K, Lehmann KM. Clinical longevity of removable partial dentures retained by telescopic crowns: Outcome of the double crown with clearance fit. Int. J. Prosthodont. 2001;14:207–13.

Widbom T, Löfquist L, Widbom C, Söderfeldt B, Kronström M. Tooth-supported telescopic crown-retained dentures: an up to 9-year retrospective clinical follow-up study. Int J Prosthodont. 2004;17:29–34.

Wostmann B, Balkenhol M, Weber A, Ferger P, Rehmann P. Long-term analysis of telescopic crown retained removable partial dentures: Survival and need for maintenance. J Dent. 2007;35:939–45.

Wöstmann B, Balkenhol M, Weber A, Ferger P, Rehmann P. Long-term analysis of telescopic crown retained removable partial dentures: survival and need for maintenance. J Dent. 2007;35:939–45.

Yi YJ, Cho LR, Park CJ. Cause of technical failures of conical crown-retained denture (CCRD): a clinical report. J Korean Acad Prosthodont. 2003;41:714–9.

Magnetic Attachment Used in Tooth-Supported Overdentures

6

Yasemin Ozkan

6.1 Magnetic Attachments

The application of magnetic attachments in dentistry has been attempted to enhance the stability of the denture by the repulsive force of the magnet which is applied at both sides of complete dentures since 1930. Magnets are used to ensure denture stabilization in patients with advanced alveolar bone resorption. Magnetic systems are comprised of Cobalt-Samarium (Co_5Sm) magnets that are integrated into the denture base, and a "keeper" that is made of Platinum-Cobalt-Nickel alloy positioned on the root, which can be magnetized (Pictures 6.1, 6.2, and 6.3, Figs. 6.1 and 6.2).

The magnetic system is composed of the base part and a lateral wall part, a permanent magnet, a soft-magnetic shield, and a non-magnetic seal. The magnet is embedded at the mucosal surface of the denture base. A disc magnet is embedded completely, approximately at 0.2 mm depth to protect the magnet surface. Thus, the magnet force acting between the magnet and the root cap retains the overdenture itself. The attractive surface of the magnetic system and the attracted surface of the keeper are coated by the wear-resistant film, which is greater than 400 Hv of Vickers hardness.

Magnets located in the denture base are Co_5Sm magnets (Fig. 6.3), AlNiCo, Ferrite, and Cobalt-Platin (Co-Pl) magnets. The magnet attachments were used for the first time in 1967 by Winkler and Pearson when "AlNiCo" bar magnets (Aluminum, Nickel, and Cobalt alloy magnets) were used to place mutual dentures by pushing each other. However, over time Co_5Sm replaced AlNiCo magnets. Co_5Sm magnets are one of the rarely found earth elements frequently used in dental practices. It was defined at the end of the 1960s and brought a new aspect to dentistry. In the early 1980s, Neodymium-Ferrum-Boron (NdFeB) alloys were used

Y. Ozkan (✉)
Faculty of Dentistry, Department of Prosthodontics, Marmara University, Istanbul, Turkey
e-mail: ykozkan@marmara.edu.tr

Y. Özkan (ed.), *Treatment Options Before and After Edentulism*,
https://doi.org/10.1007/978-3-031-37582-8_6

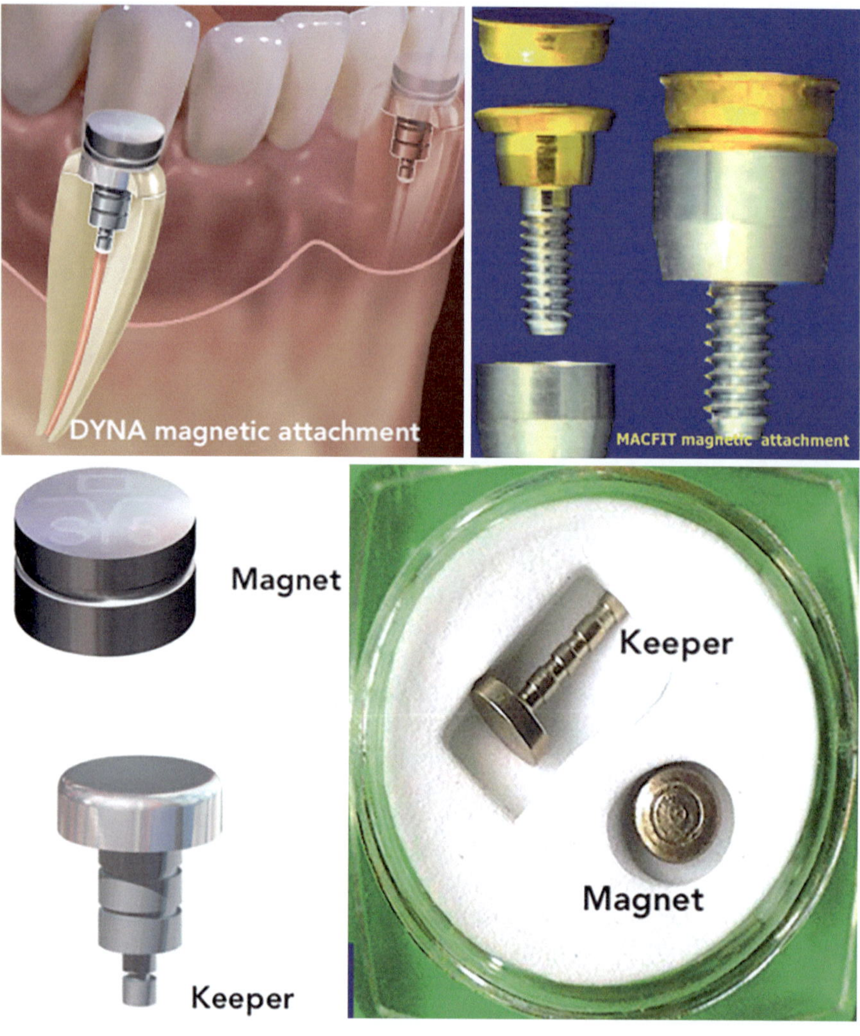

Picture 6.1 Magnet attachment in dentistry

as magnetic attachments. With the invention of the rare earth elements such as Samarium (Sm-Co) and Neodymium (NdFeB), new magnetic systems were developed in prosthodontic applications. Rare earth alloys are more retentive compared to the old ones due to high magnetism and resistance to diamagnetism features.

These magnets could be produced in dimensions small enough to be used in dental applications. Despite their size, they would provide the necessary force. Researchers reported clinically satisfying results considering using implants and magnetic attachments in patients that are unsatisfied with the existing mandibular complete denture. They are typically shorter than mechanical attachments and are particularly useful for patients with restricted interocclusal space but challenging in

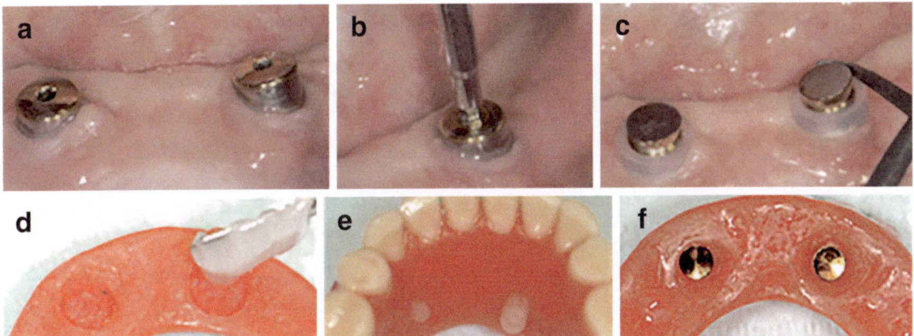

Picture 6.2 Magnet attachment application steps

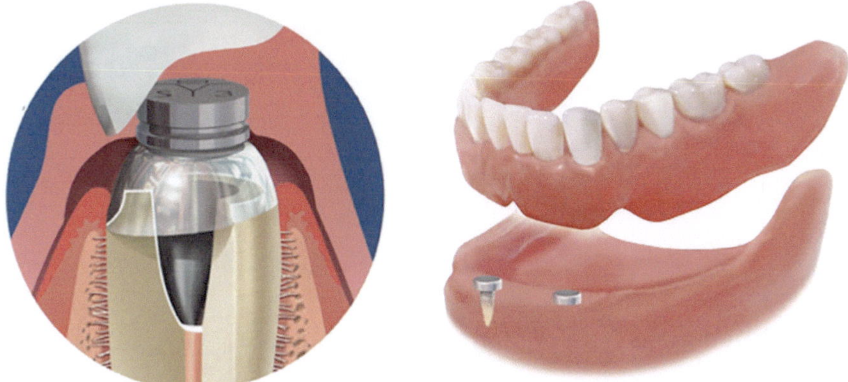

Picture 6.3 Dyna attachment system

aesthetic demands. They can also accommodate an average divergence of alignment between two or more abutments and dissipate lateral functional forces.

They are non-rigid retentive attachments, and they transmit a little shear force to the roots. Since such attachment retains overdentures by frictional force (usually friction), the attachment structure must be precise, and retention may be lost gradually due to wear. Also, magnetic attachment is easily dislodged by lateral force, which prevents damage to the implant/root (Fig. 6.4).

Clinical application of magnetic attachment has become more comfortable as several types of magnetic attachment have been introduced. Open-field and closed-field magnetic systems have been used to retain dentures for many years. Although the open-field system is the first of the magnets used for the retention of overdentures, many commercial systems now consist of the closed-field type (Figs. 6.5 and 6.6).

Fig. 6.1 Magnet attachment assembly

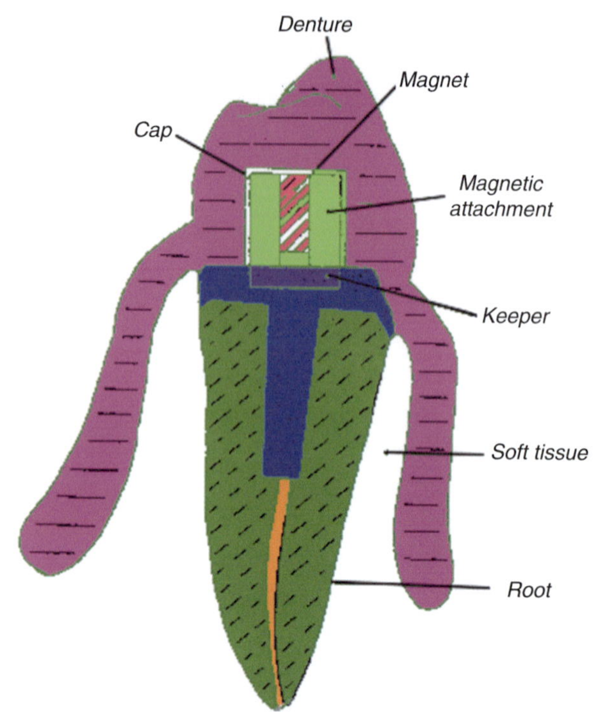

6.1.1 Open-Field Type of Magnetic Attachments

The magnetic lines of flux out of the magnet pass through not only the ferromagnetic root cap but also the nonferromagnetic materials, such as the acrylic resin base, the teeth, and the gingiva. Therefore, the magnetic path is not blocked by ferromagnetic materials only. Open-field magnets, as used in Japanese studies, managed to create a magnetic field of up to 30 mT on the root surface. The magnetic flux is created within the system when the magnets are paired with opposite poles, adjacent and fitted with ferromagnetic end plates or keepers (initially soft iron and ferromagnetic stainless steel). Therefore, this reduces the lateral field by a factor of 75–200 times, so when the magnets covered with a protective keeper get in contact, the magnetic field on the root surface only increases from 0.05 mT to 0.1 mT.

The magnet is embedded in a denture base, and a root cap cast, with the casting ferromagnetic alloy, is placed in the abutment tooth. An overdenture is retained by the magnetic force acting between the magnet and the root cap (Fig. 6.7; Pictures 6.1, 6.2, and 6.3).

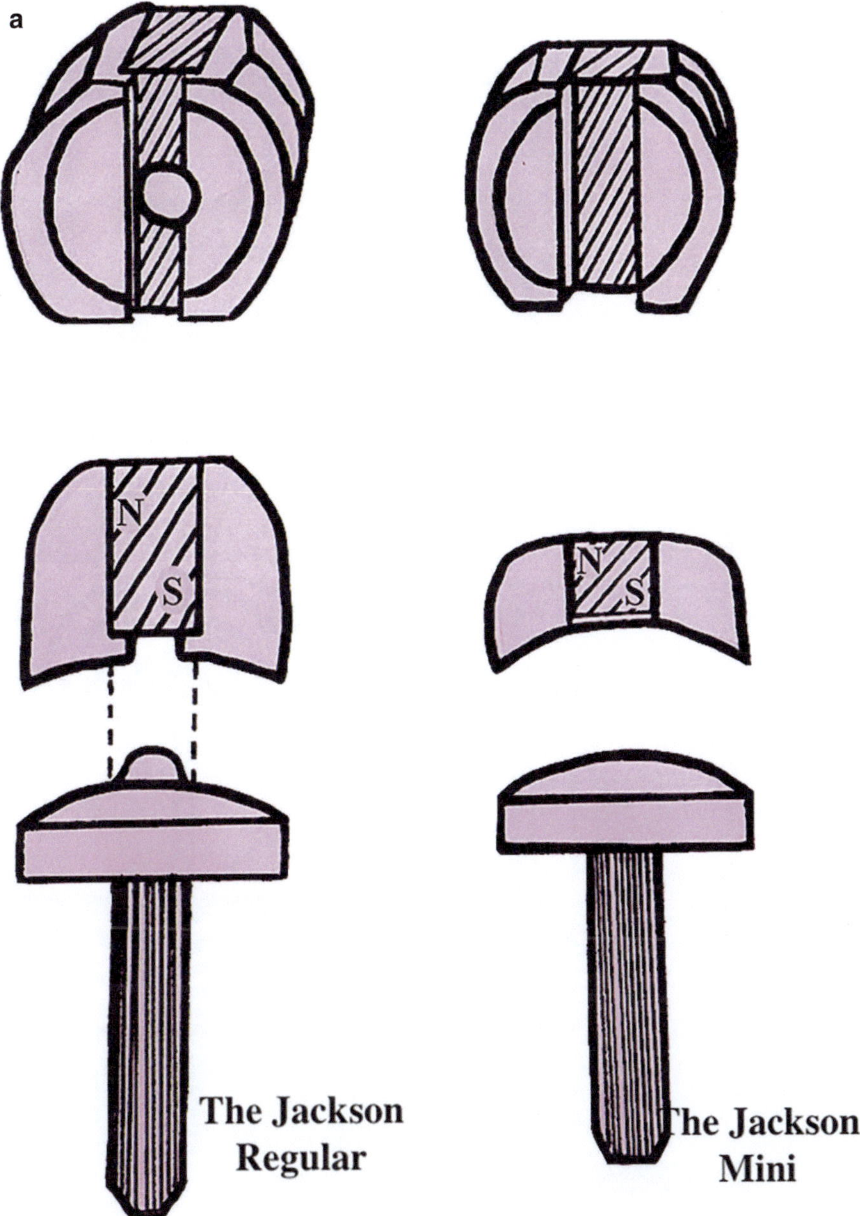

Fig. 6.2 Types of magnetic attachments: (**a**) The Jackson magnetic attachment, (**b**) the Gilling's magnet attachment, (**c**) the Dyna magnetic attachment

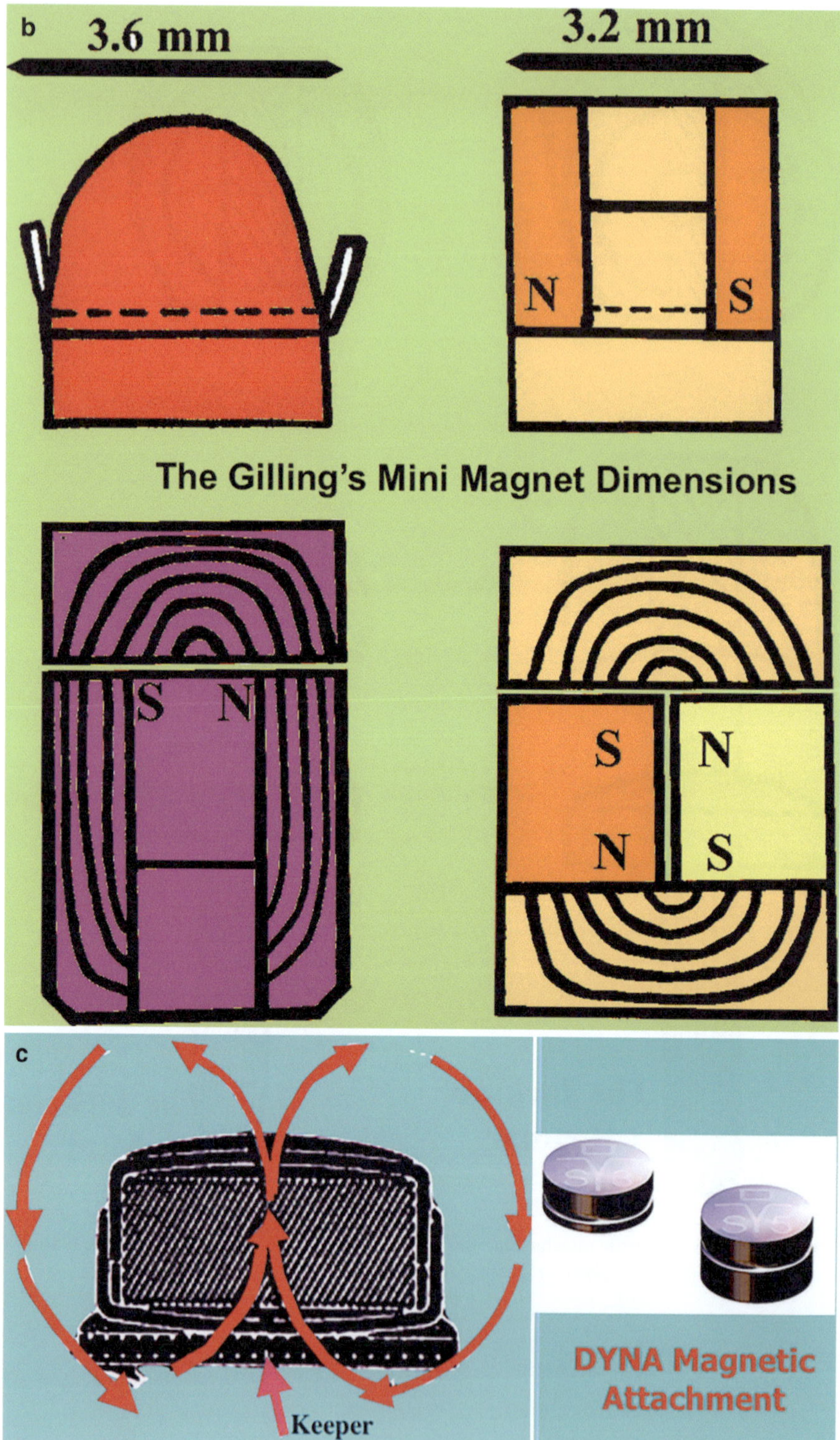

Fig. 6.2 (continued)

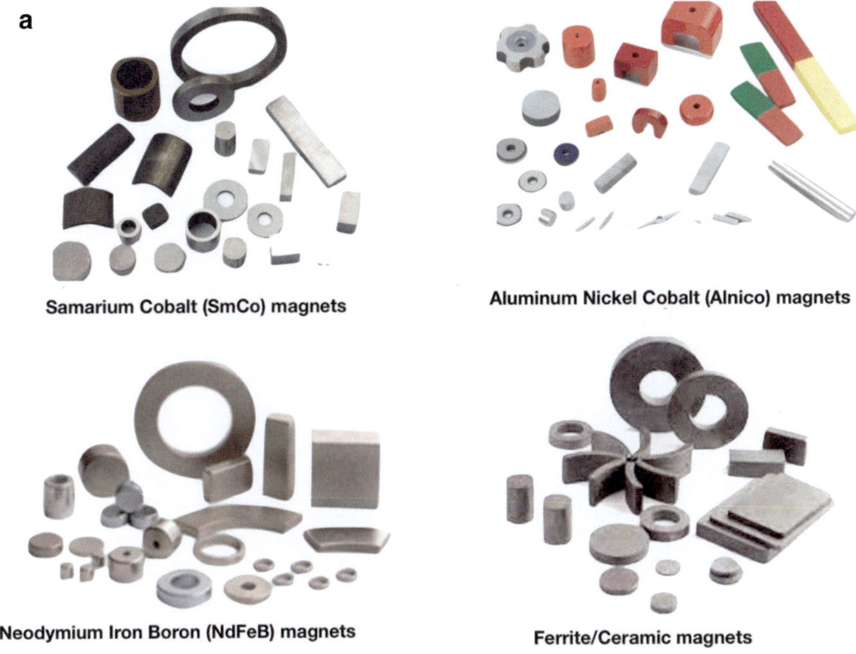

Fig. 6.3 (**a**) Different magnetic attachment materials, (**b**) Cobalt-Samarium (Co$_5$Sm) magnet attachment (open-field)

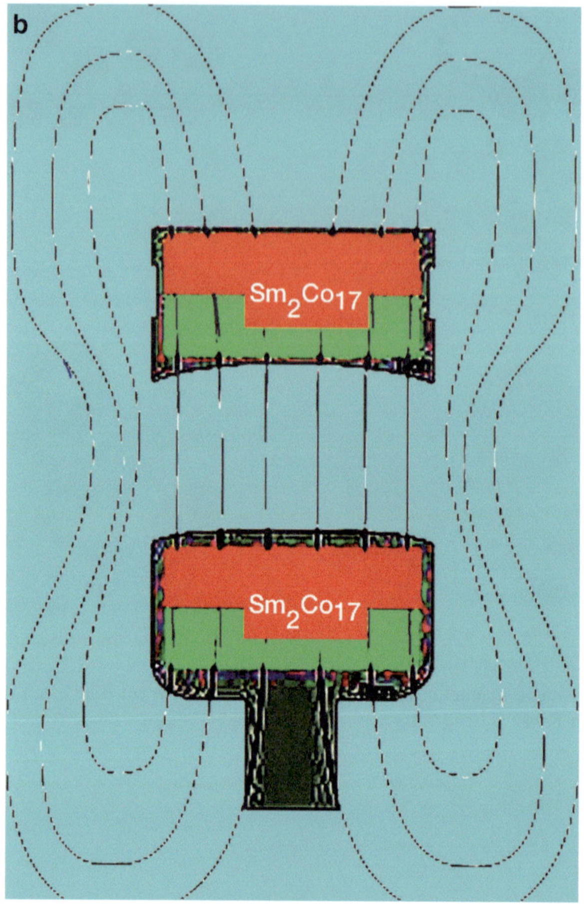

Fig. 6.3 (continued)

6.1.2 Closed-Field Type of Magnetic Attachments

If materials cover through the magnetic path which is between a magnet and a root cap, stronger magnetic forces will be obtained. In closed-field systems, the magnetic field or flux is contained within the magnet–keeper unit and yields a much higher attractive force per unit size than in open-field systems. The magnetic force permeates through the closed-field system with much less resistance than it permeates in the surrounding air. Therefore, the strength of magnetism or the "density of flux" is concentrated between the north and south poles of the magnet. Newer closed-field magnets also have a higher attractive force per unit size when the keeper and the magnet are in contact, although this force diminishes rapidly when the magnet and keeper lose contact. In closed-field systems, external magnetic flow fields are eliminated by arranging different magnetic pieces; ferromagnetic root cap and nonferromagnetic materials, such as the acrylic resin base, the teeth, and the

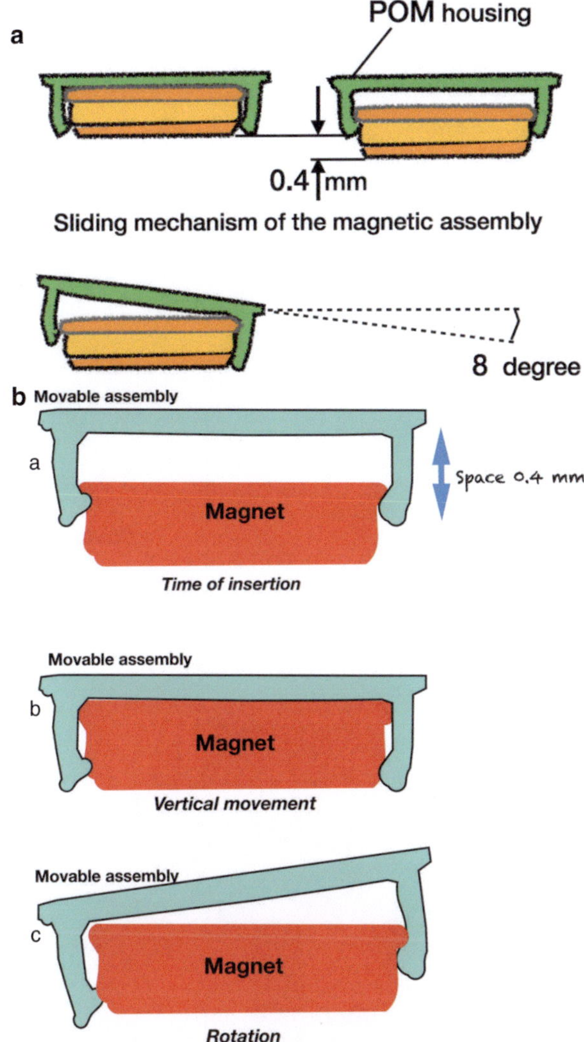

Fig. 6.4 (**a, b**) Sliding mechanism of magnetic attachment. (**c**) Single and double retainer element for magnet attachment

gingiva. The magnetic path is not closed by ferromagnetic materials only. Thus, it is not surprising that closed-field magnets have more retentive force than the others during separation. Since the nature of a closed field makes the system more biocompatible, they do not have the cytotoxic effects as open-field systems and uncoated magnets.

Overall, the magnetic circuit in a closed-field dental attachment is nearly four times stronger (mean of 5.8 N or higher; dome-type = 600 gf or 5.88 N) than older open-field circuits, and leakage of magnetic flux from the closed-circuit is

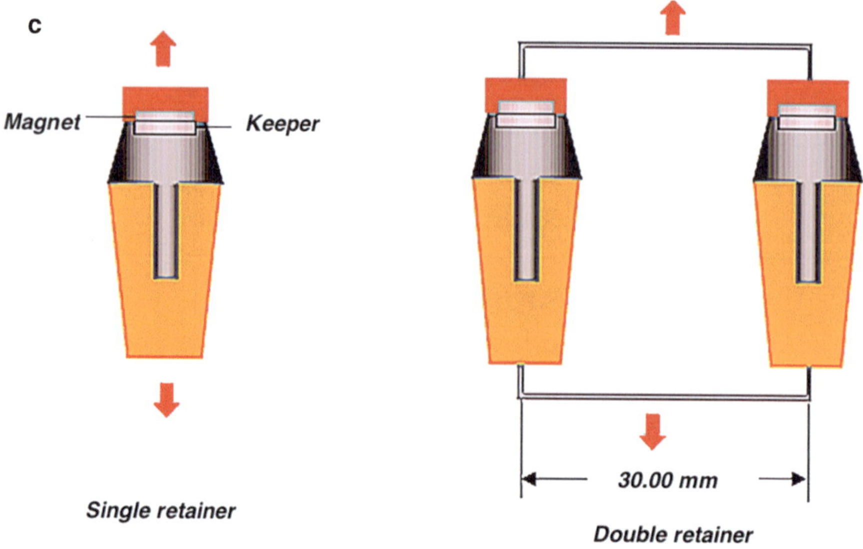

Fig. 6.4 (continued)

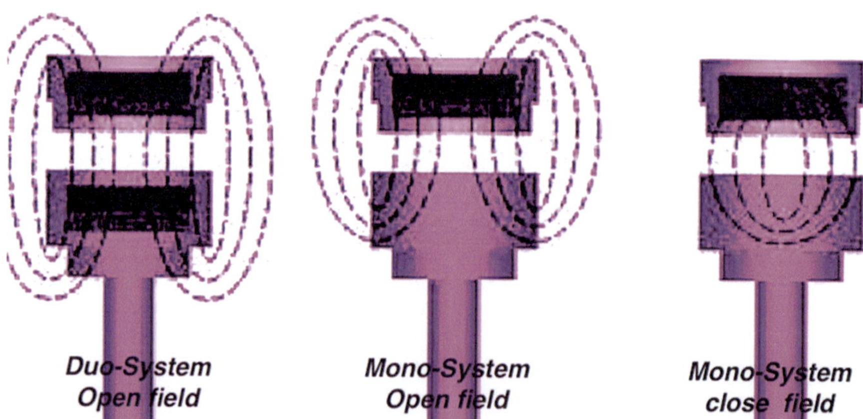

Fig. 6.5 Single and double retainer magnetic attachment

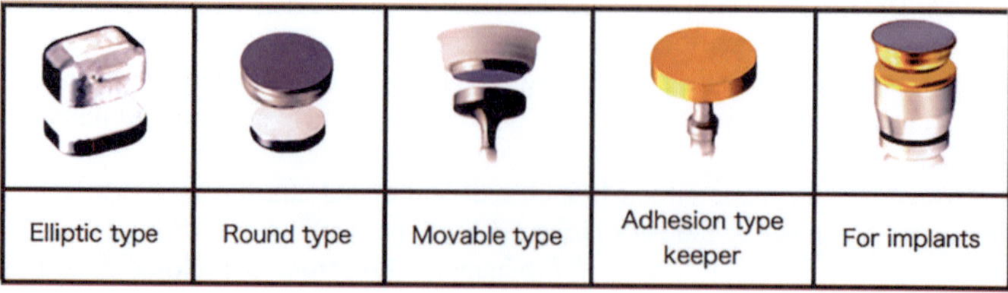

Fig. 6.6 Open- and closed-field magnetic attachments

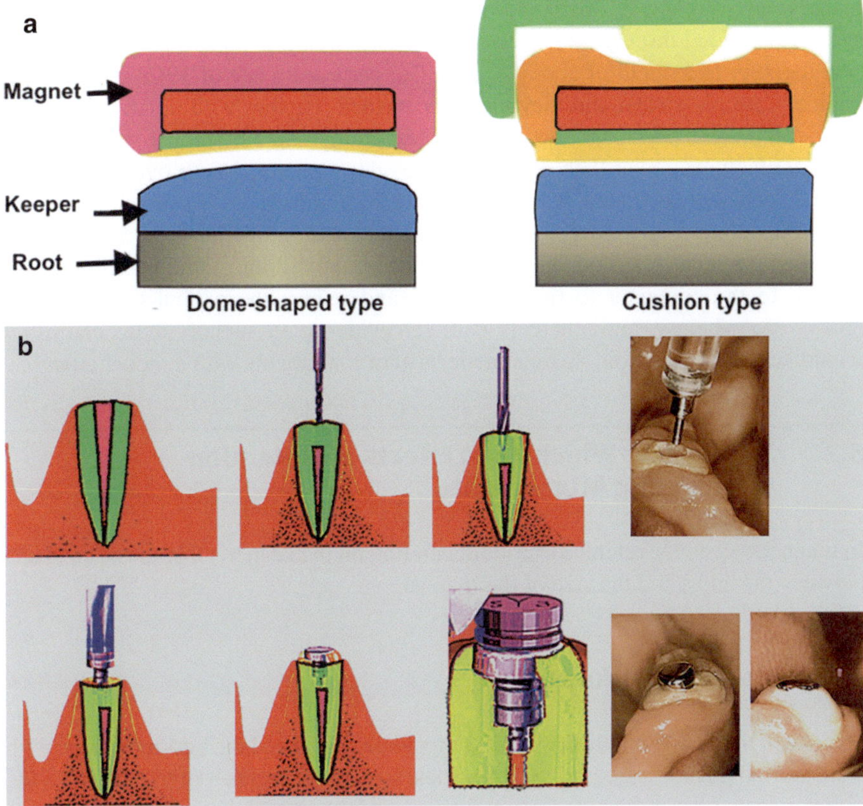

Fig. 6.7 (**a**) Dome-shaped and cushion-type magnet attachments, (**b**) magnet attachment application steps on the root

considerably less. Generally, the lifespan of a magnetic force is infinite so the retentive force of a magnetic unit should be maintained long after distortion has occurred in mechanical attachments. Moreover, the magnetic unit offers little lateral resistance to displacement, which reduces the potentially damaging lateral force directed by a denture onto a tooth or an implant.

The attractive force of a magnet is generally more resistant to the vertical forces that cause the separation compared to lateral forces. The separation force is transmitted via a resin cap, and since oblique separation forces contain lateral forces compared to vertical ones, the magnetic attachment can be chosen as a cushion-type attachment. The dislodging force of a cushion-type attachment was more laterally placed than a flat-type attachment. This is the reason for the decrease of retentive forces of a cushion-type attachment since it encounters more oblique separation force than the flat-type attachment. Cushion-type attachment can be an appropriate treatment option for the abutment that is vulnerable to lateral forces (Fig. 6.7a).

Besides, a new system has been introduced to seal the metal capsule around a magnet protecting it from corrosion within the mouth. According to the manufacturer (MAGFIT, Aichi Steel Corporation, Aichi, Japan), the integrity of the system is assured through the precise micro laser welding the two parts of the capsule together to a depth of about 70 µm. The parts are made of 19Cr–2 Mo–0.1Ti magnetic stainless steel and they are laser welded together with a narrow bead of 16Cr–12Ni–2Mo non-magnetic stainless steel containing 12% nickel. According to the manufacturer, fewer than one in ten capsules associated with overdentures on natural teeth are separated from the denture base during an 8-year clinical trial. However, interestingly there was no loss of magnetic attraction experienced. The manufacturer also reported that a 3-µm veneer of ceramic titanium nitride was applied to the container to resist abrasion and reduce the patient's exposure to nickel. Nonetheless, until there is stronger evidence to support these claims, it would be prudent to avoid this magnetic system for patients with a nickel allergy.

6.2 The Factors Which Have Effects on Retention of Magnetic Attachments

In magnetic systems, retention varies depending on the keeper's thickness, air space between the ends, and the size of the magnet.

6.2.1 Keeper's Thickness

It is stated that a 1.2 mm thick stainless-steel keeper offered the best retention. With an increased thickness, retention diminishes, and it becomes harder to place it on the root surface.

6.2.2 Air Space

The retentive force of magnetic attachments is caused by attractive forces between the N pole and S pole or by pulling forces between the magnetic structure and the keeper. The type that utilizes the former force is used in some applications. The attraction between the poles is an advantageous and commonly used method to provide a retentive force because even if there is a gap between the magnetic structure in the denture and the keeper, an attractive force will still be present. The air space between different poles of magnetic units is necessary to transmit magnetic change through keepers. It was reported that no significant increase occurred in retention after 0.8 mm detachment between the poles. This value is the accepted distance to stabilize the size of the retainer in magnetic retention.

On the other hand, there is a disadvantage in this type of attraction since more extensive space is needed, the attraction between the poles creates an open-magnetic circuit, which has a leakage of magnetic flux. In the pulling force between the structure and the keeper, the latter is set on the root, and the magnetic structure is positioned in the denture, creating a closed-magnetic circuit. However, if there is a small gap between the magnetic structure and the coping, the attractive force decreases dramatically.

Petropoulos et al. [1] analyzed the retentive force and timing of detachment of different types of attachments such as the bar, ball, and magnetic attachments. They showed that magnetic attachments have the weakest retentive force, the least variety in the retentive force, and the longest time until detachment. As such, an overdenture with magnetic attachment positions itself automatically when it comes in proximity to the proper seat position, a beneficial characteristic, especially for patients with limited dexterity. The retentive force of magnetic attachments is maximal when the insert direction is perpendicular to the keeper surface. The force decreases when the direction inclines, and it almost disappears when the direction is parallel to the keeper's surface. This characteristic tends to reduce lateral stresses to the abutment of the magnetic attachment.

6.2.3 Magnet Size and Shape

According to mean statistical measurements of root surfaces, a 5 × 3.2 mm magnetic keeper is mostly suitable for anterior and premolar teeth except for some maxillary lateral incisors and mandibular central and lateral incisors. For other teeth, cast or cemented keepers are used.

To increase the retentive force of magnetic attachments, the materials of the magnetic structure must be improved. To increase the attractive force, the size of the Sm–Co magnet must be increased. The neodymium magnet (neodymium–Ferrum–boron alloy) has a much more attractive force.

The shape of magnetic structures also affects the retentive force. The flat type with a thin disk form performed high retention force, and the cushion type with a 0.4 mm gap between the magnet assembly and resin cap showed a shock-absorbing effect on the implant fixture. Dome-type magnetic attachments have less attractive force than flat types, but dome types have a slighter decrease in non-axial-direction-attractive forces compared to flat-types. In this way, dome-type magnetic attachments have an advantage for use in the oral region where they can receive forces from various directions. Dome-shaped magnets permit lateral movement of dentures compared to flat-type magnets with cushion type. The flat-type magnet is more retentive than other types whereas the cushion type has shock-absorbing effects and permits vertical movement of dentures. When flat-type and cushion-type magnetic attachments are compared in the terms of retention and stability of the implant overdenture, the number and the type of magnetic attachment and the direction of the applied force; the cushion-type magnetic attachment was found to be less retentive in an oblique direction of the dislodging force. It is stated that the significant dimension of the cushion-type magnetic attachment is the main cause. Since cushion-type magnetic attachments contain resin caps, if the excessive self-curing resin is applied or relief of the denture is insufficient, the magnetic attachment could easily cause dislocation.

6.2.4 Corrosion

Since small parts in magnet alloys are produced by compression in a high magnetic field, they can be subject to corrosion with use. Scratches and damages at the root coping and the magnet unit that occurs during the insertion and separation of the denture can cause corrosion as well. To set the denture stably, the alloy material that is used for the keeper is required to have superior corrosion resistance in order to resist corrosion within the oral cavity. Generally, the corrosion-resistant soft magnetic materials that are used are ferrite-based stainless steel and austenite-based stainless steel. This corrosion-resistant metal material covers the permanent magnet structure except for a surface that comes in contact with the keeper, or the whole surface of the permanent magnet structure which has a thickness such that the magnetic attraction force between the permanent magnet structure and the keeper is not influenced. Therefore, 0.25 mm thick stainless-steel copings, which can be magnetized, keep the magnets in place and prevent damage and protect from corrosion for up to 10 years, and are fixed on the surfaces of the magnets. Retention does not diminish with a slight increase in the metal thickness of magnetizable alloys. The total height of the third layer of this retentive unit is about 3.00 mm. The problem of corrosion can be prevented with a stainless-steel tube that is placed inside the magnet and to the side surfaces on which they are fixed with glue.

Drago [2] reported that among the patients with magnetic attachments, 68% of the attachments became discolored and 40% corroded. These issues have created an unfavorable reputation for magnetic attachments, which, unfortunately, has lasted more than 30 years in North America.

Although the attachments used to be corrosive, this problem has been resolved, and they are now corrosion-resistant.

6.2.5 Laser-Welded Yoke Encasement

At the beginning of the 1990s, a technique was developed as a solution to protect against corrosion. In this new technique, the magnetic structure was sealed in a stainless steel housing called a "yoke" and then welded closed with a laser. Takada and Okuno [3] reported corrosion resistance of magnetic attachments with a yoke structure. Thaen et al. [4] found that magnetic attachments with a sealed yoke exhibited successful corrosion resistance during a 3-year long-term clinical study.

6.2.6 Retentive Force Following the Initial Separation

To achieve sufficient stability of the denture, the break-away force of magnetic retainers must exceed the displacing force applied to the denture. When vertical retentive force is more significant than the anterior-posterior retentive force, the stability of the denture is reported to be sufficient to maintain the denture in position on its basal seat. Gilling [5] reported that such displacing forces might be as low as

0.22 to 0.53 N. In the case of overdenture, retention of the prosthesis and retentive force of magnetic attachment are highly correlated. Gilling [5] also reported that the proper attractive force to retain overdentures is about 400–600 gf (3.91–5.88 N) and that attractive force less than 140–310 gf (1.37–3.03 N) is insufficient for retention of implant overdentures. When oblique retentive force is 53–94 gf (0.52–0.92 N), it is reported that magnetic attachment may not be able to resist the horizontal movement of the denture. The literature reported that magnetic retentive force is a continuous and permanent force between 150 and 400 gf.

It is known that magnetic attachments give a constant retention value, which is not affected by breakaway cycles. The Jackson regular attachment provides 720 g retention, the Jackson mini attachment 575 g, the Innovadent magnet 600 g, the Gilling split pole 300 g, the Magnedent 240 g, and the Dyna Magnets provide 240 g retention.

Comparing open-field matched magnet placement with different pole magnet placement, detachment of the unit and the keeper causes a sudden drop in the retentive force. Moreover, the detachment load between the magnets of the same form is double in the different pole system magnets. In conclusion, the retention force is higher between the units at a distance shorter than 0.3 mm.

In closed-field magnet systems, there is more retention at the magnet holder part or fluid field than in open-field magnets. The magnetic field in a closed magnet has less retention than surrounding air. Because of this reason, the power of the magnetism or density of the fluid is between the North and South Pole. Besides, in new magnet systems when the retainer and magnet are in contact, retentive force is very high. After separation, this force diminishes suddenly. As a result, closed-field magnets are four times more retentive than the old open-field ones (mean value: 5.8 N and more; coping type = 600 gf (gram force) or 5.88 N), and the leak of magnetic fluid is less.

Although magnetic forces decrease because of the separation of a magnet and a root cap, the descendant curve of the closed-field type is steeper than the open-field type magnets. In conclusion, the closed-field type has less stability than the open-field type. Therefore, this should be considered when magnetic attachments are used clinically.

6.3 Advantages of Magnetic Attachments

- They take a small area in overdentures.
- The magnetic force works parallelly with the denture's adhesion force and negative forces.
- It offers more stabilization and retention compared to traditional partial dentures.
- Easily applied without any unique technique.
- Offers more accessible inlet and outlet to the denture.
- Reduces lateral forces in supporting teeth.
- Simply offers better oral hygiene due to a smaller retention area for dental biofilm.
- Since it is a simple technique, it is quite useful for geriatric and disabled patients.

6.4   Disadvantages of Magnetic Attachments

- Retention loss caused by corrosion and heat exchange.
- Require lining because of inert alloys.
- Lower resistance to corrosion caused by intraoral fluids.
- Hard to repair.
- Expensive.
- Limited use of forces since the magnets only affect where they are located.
- Weak corrosive resistance of magnets within the oral fluid requires encapsulation within a relatively inert alloy such as stainless steel or titanium.
- They do not provide a positive locking device. Thus, the retention provided is generally less compared to intra-radicular retention systems.

6.5   Harmful Effects of Magnetic Attachments

The magnets could have two different types of harmful effects on tissues:

1. Magnetism-induced physical effects.
2. Corrosion-induced chemical effect.

Both Cobalt-Samarium and Neodymium-Iron-Boron magnets are used due to their small, compact lengths. They are coated with metal, but, when the coating is broken, it can rapidly be damaged due to saliva contact. Biosafety tests have shown that, although these alloys may be cytotoxic, the magnetic field has no biological effect. However, in vitro researchers have been reporting contradictory results for the biocompatibility of these materials.

Cell toxicity, cell growth, and allergic reaction were tested on the new magnets, and the results provided were compatible with international standards. Even though the toxicity studies justified magnetic alloys, biological effects including soft tissue modifications induced by long-term use of magnetic attachments led to suspicions in some researchers. In uncoated magnets, Co-Sa cytotoxic effects may be encountered. However, it is known that the uncoated Neodymium-Iron-Boron magnets have a little cytotoxic effect on cells. A model system that was created artificially containing human and rat fibroblasts has shown that both alloys were cytotoxic. Human oral mucosa fibroblasts are the most sensitive areas to the effects of rare earth magnets.

The biosafety of the rare earth magnets was investigated in detail. The effects on biological tissues were shown that the static magnetic field does not affect the dental pulp or gingival tissues. An in vitro study, made by using osteoblasts, has shown that there was no significant change in cell cultures, which were subjected to a magnetic field. Also, the magnetic field makes no change in the blood flow rate.

Therefore, in 1977, an attachment, which eliminated the magnetic field around the Gilling attachment, was developed. The safety standard of the USA is 0.02 T (Table 6.1). Although many researchers report tissue effects being between 100 and

Table 6.1 Magnetic field for countries

Countries	Arrangement		Explanations
	Electrical field (kV/m)	Magnetic field $T = A/m^2$	
Denmark, Sweden, Norway, Estonia, England, Holland	There is no regulation, but the EU is considered as a reference. National committees in some countries such as England, Holland, and Sweden make their suggestions.		
Belgium	5	–	No regulation
France, Germany, Croatia, Spain, Austria, Ireland, Lithuania, Australia	5	100	–
Greece	4	80	Coefficient of 0.8
Switzerland	5	100 (1 for some sensitive places like schools, hospitals, and old-age asylum)	The limits for sensitive places are applied only to new places
Slovenia	5 (500 V/m for sensitive places)	100 (10 for sensitive places)	The limits for sensitive places are applied only to new places
Italy	5	100 10 (mean value 4 h/day) 3 (mean value 4 h/day)	Attention value is applied to all existing institutions. The quality value is applied to all new institutions
Turkey	10	640	Determined by the Turkish Standards Institute (TSE). Also, there is one more regulation determined by BTK

1000 mT in magnet attachments, some reported tissue effects in 8 mT. The open-field magnets used in Japanese studies managed to create a magnetic field up to 30 mT on the root surface. The magnetic modification remains in the system when opposite poles are matched with each other by using a ferromagnetic posterior layer or protective outer membrane (soft iron and ferromagnetic stainless steel). Through this modification, possible side effects are reduced by 75–200 times. When contacted by the magnets covered with a protective keeper, the magnetic field on the root surface only increases from 0.05 mT to 0.1 mT.

In closed-field systems, external magnetic flow fields are eliminated by arranging magnetic pieces in order. Hence, it is not surprising that closed-field magnets have more retentive force than others during separation. Since the nature of closed-field magnetic systems makes the system more biocompatible, they do not have cytotoxic effects as open-field systems and uncoated magnets.

Nishida et al. [6] compared leak-fields between sandwich-type and open-field-type magnetic attachments and reported that the open-field type had a higher leakage-magnetic flux. The leakage level at the open-field type magnetic attachment that was detected in this study is considered unsafe by the World Health Organization

(WHO) guideline. Notably, the sandwich-type magnetic attachment had a higher leakage-magnetic flux than the cup-type magnetic attachment. Nishida et al. [6] also reported that if a magnetic structure is positioned on a keeper properly, the magnetic flux should be under 40 mT according to the WHO guideline. However, it is recommended to pay careful attention to the long-term use of implants because a gap may develop between the magnetic structure and the keeper, resulting in a leak of magnetic flux.

In the regular usage of closed-magnetic circuits, leakage of magnetic flux in the gingiva is minimal (approximately 1 mT at the most) and does not exhibit any harmful effects on the human body. It is reported that even in an open magnetic circuit if there is a 7 mm distance from the magnetic structure, leakage of magnetic flux is less than 1 mT. This minimal amount of leakage does not affect heart pacemakers.

6.6 Magnetic Resonance Imaging and Magnets

Magnets and even the ferromagnetic stainless-steel keepers may cause distortion and create artifacts during magnetic resonance imaging (MRI) of the head and neck region. Therefore, it is recommended that the patients should remove their dentures that contain magnets and have the keepers unscrewed from the implants before an MRI investigation of the region. As with most metallic dental materials, there is always a minimal risk of patient injury through the displacement of the keeper component during MRI.

New et al. [7] reported the potential hazards and artifacts of dental materials in MR imaging. Limuro (1993) [8] evaluated the effects of ferromagnetic stainless-steel devices on MR imaging artifacts. They found that there was an appearance of an MR imaging artifact at a 12 cm distance from a keeper positioned on the root, and more magnificent artifacts were produced with the increases in magnetic permeability. Additionally, the size and volume of the attachment material were reported to influence the quality of the artifact directly. To avoid these types of artifacts in MR imaging, some reports have recommended the removal of magnetic parts of magnetic attachment systems.

6.7 Modern Magnetic Attachments

6.7.1 Dyna Attachment

It is a 2.6 mm high and 4.5 mm wide open-field type of magnet. It is made of a rare earth element in a cylindrical form inside the stainless-steel covering cap. It has no control over external magnetic flux and has only fair retention for its size (Pictures 6.1, 6.2, and 6.3).

6.7.2 Magnet Attachment

There are three different sizes: The small size is 1.9 mm high and 4.5 mm wide, the medium size is 2.1 mm high and 5.00 mm wide, and the large size is 2.4 mm high and 5.7 mm wide. It is a closed system in the cylindrical form inside the stainless-steel cap. This attachment is also covered by a stainless-steel covering cap to prevent corrosion.

6.7.3 Jackson Rare Earth Attachment

There are two sizes: the regular size and the mini size. In both sizes, the $SmCo_5$ magnet is vertically compressed between two stainless steel plates and surrounded by a hemispherical protective keeper. The regular size has a diameter of 4.8 mm and a height of 3.5 mm. The height of the keeper is 1.2 mm with a 0.5 mm locating nipple which is centrally placed over the 8 mm long, 1.5 mm extensive post.

The mini size has the same design as the regular one; that is, the magnet and endplates are arranged in the same way except for the height of the magnets being 2.4 mm. The keeper is also the same but does not have a centralizing nipple. The latest Jackson magnet is placed in titanium, weighs 0.56 g, and offers 560 g retention (Fig. 6.2).

6.7.4 Gilling Mini Magnet (Keystone)

It is a sandwich-type magnet attachment with the poles placed horizontally. Flux is transferred through the endplates and completed by the keeper. In this design, the same amount of retention as the separate pole system can be provided only by using a half magnet. The magnet produced is a hemisphere of 3 mm height, 3.2 mm width, and 3.6 mm depth. It is machined to be enclosed and sealed within stainless endplates which prevent corrosion of $SmCo_5$. Neodymium, Iron, and Boron alloy magnets, which offer more retention, are still being developed (Fig. 6.2).

6.7.5 Innovadent Neo Mini

It has a similar size and weight to the Mini Magnet except for the magnet is sealed in a dome for protecting it from corrosion. It is 4.35 mm wide and offers 475 g retention. A convenient place is prepared by grinding the teeth area on the inner surface of the denture to place the magnets. The magnets are positioned in the area of retainers inside the mouth. Resin is applied to the ground area, and thereafter the denture is placed on the magnets according to the prepared occlusion. After resin sets, magnets remain in the denture. Excessive resin is eliminated by leveling and polishing. After polishing, the denture is placed inside the mouth again and occlusion, retention, and fit are checked. The patient is informed about how to make the insertion and separation of the denture and how to maintain oral hygiene and denture care.

6.7.6 Patient Satisfaction

Naert et al. [9] compared the older open-field magnetic attachment and the two types of mechanical attachment systems (ball or bar) through the follow-up of two implant-retained mandibular dentures which served for 10 years. They stated that the magnetic dentures had a mean retentive force of 3–4 N with the two implants combined (mean of less than 2 N per implant), which was significantly lower than the initial retentive force of the mechanical attachments. Besides, the magnet-retained dentures required substantially more maintenance, including the replacement of the magnets approximately twice as often (or more) as it was required for the mechanical attachments. The usual reason for replacing the magnets was wear and corrosion. However, they also stated that there was no difference in general satisfaction with an older open-field magnetic attachment compared to the ball or bar attachment systems after 10 years of service. They also reported that regardless of the attachment system used, the patients rated overall satisfaction as "excellent."

According to short-term crossover studies that used older open-field magnet systems conducted by Cune et al. [10] and Burns et al. [11], retention provided by magnets was subjectively less stable and less comfortable than mechanical attachments.

6.8 Clinical and Laboratory Procedures

There are two methods for attaching a keeper to a root cap. One is the casting method, and the other one is the direct-bonding method.

In the casting method, the magnetic keeper is usually fabricated using the cast-on technique so that it is located on the post coping. The height of the keeper is low and is easy to obtain a sufficient distance to the opposite teeth. The keeper is directly embedded in the wax pattern. Therefore, the keeper, which is fixed on a flat plate made of a soft magnetic material, is positioned inside the oral cavity, before casting with alloys or other methods. The keeper is formed to have a longitudinal section in an approximately T-shape. It is embedded and set within the root of the remaining teeth in an alveolar ridge portion in the oral cavity. However, casting shrinkage and polishing after metal casting can cause deformation in the keeper.

The casting procedure causes a contaminated layer to form on the keeper's surface. Because of this phenomenon, the surface changes from being completely flat to an uneven surface since it is sanded using abrasive paper to remove the contamination layer.

The direct-bonding method was recently developed to resolve this problem. In this technique, the keeper is bonded using resin bond cement on the cast coping where the housing patterns of the post coping are cast. Because the keeper is cemented on the root with luting cement, the attractive force keeps the original data and polishing of the keeper is easy.

Although the direct-bonding technique maintains a stable retentive force similar to a newly manufactured keeper, the height of the coping with the keeper is greater than with the cast-on technique because the housing used for direct bonding is added to the overall height. Tsuchida et al. pointed out that in the direct-bonding technique, the height of the root cap may be higher than in the casting method because this method requires space for the cement.

On the other hand, in this new technique prefabricated keepers with a post and composite resins are used, indicating that the direct-bonding method has many advantages as well.

Maeda et al. [12] reported the method of replacing a missing abutment tooth of a removable partial denture with a magnetic attachment, a prefabricated keeper containing a post and composite resin. They reported optimal support, strength, retention, and improved aesthetics in a short period by using this method.

Suminaga et al. [13] reported that the retention of the cast-on attachments was less than the direct-bonded attachments because the keeper surface using the cast-on technique was rough and required finishing and polishing for the removal of the contamination layer. Therefore, the direct-bonding technique is recommended if there is enough space between the remaining root and the opposing teeth.

To conclude, a permanent magnet structure is bonded and fixed in a retentive hole at the denture base opposing the keeper during setting a denture within the oral cavity, by using an adhesive or a self-curing resin. A magnetic attraction force acts between the keeper and the permanent magnet to set the denture not to be dislodged easily. During removal, it can easily be separated by applying a more significant force than magnetic attraction force.

Theoretically, a magnetic attachment using the direct-bonding technique can provide the amount of retentive force that the manufacturers claim because there is no alteration of the keeper surface. However, the retentive force in this study was lower than the manufacturer's data, which might have been obtained by tensile testing that exceeded a strictly perpendicular tensile direction to the magnet surface. One of the other characteristics of magnetic attachments is that the retentive force remarkably decreases even only through a slight deviation from the perpendicular direction to the magnet. Therefore, the retentive force in the patient's mouth may be lower than the retentive force obtained in this study. In contrast, the advantage of the magnetic attachment is that the retentive force is not affected by the aqueous conditions.

References

1. Petropoulos VC, Smith W, Kousvelari E. Comparison of retention and release periods for implant overdenture attachments. Int J Oral Maxillofac Implants. 1997;12:176–85.
2. Drago CJ. Tarnish and corrosion with the use of intra oral magnets. J Prosthet Dent. 1991;66:536–40.
3. Takada Y, Okuno O. Corrosion resistance of magnetic assemblies used in domestic cup yoke-type magnetic attachments. J J Mag Dent. 2008;17:13–5.
4. Thean HP, Khor SK, Loh PL. Viability of magnetic denture retainers: a 3-year case report. Quintessence Int. 2001;32:517–20.
5. Gillings BR. Magnetic retention for complete and partial overdentures. Part I. J Prosthet Dent. 1981;45:484–91.
6. Nishida M, Tegawa Y, Kinouchi Y. Evaluation of leakage flux out of a dental magnetic attachment. Annu Int Conf Proc IEEE Eng Med Biol Soc. 2007;2007:3520–3.
7. New PF, Rosen BR, Brady TJ, Buonanno FS, Kistler JP, Burt CT, et al. Potential hazards and artifacts of ferromagnetic and non-ferromagnetic surgical and dental materials and devices in nuclear magnetic resonance imaging. Radiology. 1983;147:139–48.
8. Limuro FT. Magnetic resonance imaging artifacts and the magnetic attachment system. Dent Mater J. 1994;13:76–88.
9. Naert I, Gizani S, Vuylsteke M, van Steenberghe D. A 5 year randomized clinical trial on the influence of splinted and unsplinted oral implants in the mandibular overdenture therapy. Part: peri-implant outcome. CLIN Oral Implants Res. 1998;9:170–7.
10. Cune M, van Kampen F, van der Bilt A, Bosman F. Patient satisfaction and preference with magnet, bar-clip, and ball-socket retained mandibular implant overdentures: a cross-over clinical trial. Int J Prosthodont. 2005;18:99–105.
11. Burns DR, Unger JW, Elswick RK Jr, Giglio JA. Prospective clinical evaluation of mandibular implant overdentures: Part II – Patient satisfaction and preference. J Prosthet Dent. 1995;73:364–9.
12. Maeda Y, Nakao K, Yagi K, Matsuda S. Composite resin root coping with a keeper for magnetic attachment for replacing the missing coronal portion of a removable partial denture abutment. J Prosthet Dent. 2006;96:139–42.
13. Suminaga Y, Tsuchida F, Takishin N, Hosoi T, Sugiyama K. Surface analysis of keepers on dental magnetic attachments: comparison of cast-bonding technique and direct-bonding technique. Prosthodont Res Pract. 2004;3:62–8.

Further Reading

Akaltan F, Can G. Retentive characteristics of different dental magnetic systems. J Prosthet Dent. 1995;74:422–7.

Bassi F. Comparing overdenture therapies with teeth and implant abutments. Int J Prosthodont. 2009;22:527–8.

Behrman SJ. The implantation of magnets in the jaw to aid denture retention. J Prosthet Dent. 1960;10:807–41.

Brewer AA, Morrow RM. Overdentures. 2nd ed. St Louis, MO: CV Mosby Co; 1980.

Chikunov I, Doan P, Vahidi F. Implant-retained partial overdenture with resilient attachments. J Prosthodont. 2008;17:141–8.

Connor RJ, Svare CW. Proplast-coated high-strength magnets as potential denture stabilization devices. J Prosthet Dent. 1977;37:339–43.

Crum RJ, Rooney GE Jr. Alveolar bone loss in overdentures: a 5-year study. J Prosthet Dent. 1978;40:610–3.

Dong J, Ikebe K, Gonda T, Nokubi T. Influence of abutment height on strain in a mandibular overdenture. J Oral Rehabil. 2006;33:594–9.

Fiske J, Davis DM, Frances C, Gelbier S. The emotional effects of tooth loss in edentulous people. Br Dent J. 1998;184:90–3.

Freedman H. Magnets to stabilize dentures. J Am Dent Assoc. 1953;47:288–97.

Gendusa NJ. Magnetically retained overlay dentures. Quintessence Int. 1988;19:265–71.

Gonda T, Ikebe K, Ono T, Nokubi T. Effect of magnetic attachment with stress breaker on lateral stress to abutment tooth under overdentures. J Oral Rehabil. 2004;31:1001–6.

Gonda T, Maeda Y. Why are magnetic attachments popular in Japan and other Asian countries? Jpn Dent Sci Rev. 2011;47:124–30.

Iimuro FT, Yoneyama T, Okuno O. Corrosion of coupled metals in a dental magnetic attachment system. Dent Mater J. 1993;12:136–44.

Krawczykowska H, Panek H. Applying the overdentures in the geriatric patients with residual and reduced dentition. Dent Med Probl. 2004;41:255–61.

Lewandowski JA, White KC, Moore D, Johnson C. An investigation of two rare earth magnetic systems by measuring grip force and reseating force. J Prosthet Dent. 1988;60:705–11.

Meijer HJ, Raghoebar GM, van't Hof MA, Geertman ME, van Oort RP. Implant-retained mandibular overdentures compared with complete dentures: a 5-years follow-up of clinical aspects and patient satisfaction. Clin Oral Implants Res. 1999;10:238–44.

Menicucci G, Lorenzetti M, Pera P, Preti G. Mandibular implant-retained overdentures a clinical trial of two anchorage systems. Int J Oral Maxillofac Implants. 1998;13:851–6.

Mensor MC. Removable partial overdentures with mechanical (precision) attachments. Dent Clin N Am. 1990;34:669–81.

Mericske-Stern R, Piotti M, Sirtes G. 3-D in vivo force measurements on mandibular implants supporting Overdentures. Clin Oral Implants Res. 1996;7:387–96.

Miyata T, Tanaka Y, Ishigami T, et al. Experimental observations of an effect of dental magnetic attachments on a cardiac pacemaker. J Jpn Soc Magn Appl Dent. 1993;2:11–7.

Naert I, Ghada A, Van Steenberghe D, Quirynen M. A 10-year randomized clinical trial on the influence of splinted and unsplinted oral implants retaining mandibular overdentures: peri-implant outcome. Int J Oral Maxillofac Imp. 2004;19:695–702.

Naert I, Gizani S, Vuylsteke M, Van Steenberghe D. A 5-year prospective randomized clinical trial on the influence of splinted and unsplinted oral implants retaining a mandibular overdenture: prosthetic aspects and patient satisfaction. J Oral Rehabil. 1999;26:195–202.

Pacer FJ, Bowman C. Occlusal force discrimination by denture patients. J Prosthet Dent. 1975;33:602–9.

Riley MA, Walmsley AD, Harris IR. Magnets in prosthetic dentistry. J Prosthet Dent. 2001;86:137–42.

Sagawa M, Fujimura S, Togawa M, Yamamoto H, Matsuura Y. New material for permanent magnets on a base of Nd and Fe. J Appl Phys. 1984;55:20837.

Sarnat AE. The efficiency of cobalt samarium (Co_5Sm) magnets as retention units for overdentures. J Dent. 1983;11:324–33.

Schmitz JF. Measurement of the efficiency of the platinum cobalt magnetic implant. J Prosthet Dent. 1966;16:1151–8.

Schuch C, Pinheiro de Moraes A, Onofre RS, Cenci TP, Boscato N. An alternative method for the fabrication of a root-supported overdenture: a clinical report. J Prosthet Dent. 2013;109:1–4.

Strnat KJ. The hard-magnetic properties of rare earth-transition metal alloys. IEEE Trans Magnet. 1972;8:511–6.

Takada Y, Okuno O. Effect of heat history on the corrosion of ferritic stainless steels used for dental magnetic attachments. Dent Mater J. 2005;24:391–7.

Tokuhisa M, Matsushita Y, Koyan K. In vitro study of a mandibular implant overdenture retained with the ball, magnet, or bar attachment: comparison of load transfer and denture stability. Int J Prosthodont. 2003;16:128–34.

Tsuchida F, Suminaga Y, Takishin N, Hosoi T, Maeda Y. Cast- bonding technique and direct-bonding technique on magnetic attachments. J Jpn Soc Magn Appl Dent. 2005;14:53–60. (in Japanese with English abstract)

Walmsley AD. Magnetic retention in prosthetic dentistry. Dent Update. 2002;29:428–33.

Wang X, Ohkubo C, Hosoi T, Shimpo H, Kurihara D, Murata T. Retentive forces of 3 types of attachments for root-retained overdentures. Prosthodont Res Pract. 2007;6:104–8.

Clinical Evaluation Parameters of Tooth-Supported Overdenture Treatment

7

Yılmaz Umut Aslan

7.1 Anamnesis

7.1.1 Medical and Dental Anamnesis

A detailed assessment should be made concerning the patient's medical anamnesis. Systemic and local complications should be evaluated. Medical anamnesis is followed by dental anamnesis. Some questions are directed in order to get knowledge about the dental history of the patient, and these are:

- When and how did you lose your teeth?
- What were the reasons for your unsatisfaction concerning the current denture?
- What were the reasons for your satisfaction concerning the current denture?
- What were your expectations from the current denture?
- Do you have a craniomandibular disease?
- How do you care for your denture at home?

It is easier to achieve success in the treatment of patients who previously used removable dentures and have high levels of hygiene awareness.

7.2 Extra-oral and Intra-oral Examination

1. General appearance.
2. Facial asymmetry.
3. Labial support.

Y. U. Aslan (✉)
Faculty of Dentistry, Department of Prosthodontics, Marmara University, Istanbul, Turkey
e-mail: umut.aslan@marmara.edu.tr

4. Modifications with the soft tissue.
5. Size of the tongue.
6. Condition of periodontal tissues.
7. Condition, number, and distribution of the remaining teeth.
8. Vertical and buccolingual distance.
9. Shape and size of edentulous crests.
10. Examination of edentulous areas with palpation.
11. Grading teeth mobility.
12. Measurement of free gingival depth.
13. Assessment of temporomandibular joint (TMJ) movements (any problem should be treated before applying denture).
14. Photograph evaluations.

According to the examinations, the treatment steps will be as follows. Periodontal health, the tendency for endodontic treatment, assessment of bone undercuts, support of the dental tissue, number of supporting teeth in the dental arch, localization, and cost are essential factors in planning. The prognosis of tooth-supported overdenture (TSO) treatment depends on keeping the abutment caries-free and periodontally healthy. Therefore, the following assessments need to be made before the treatment.

- Is there a caries risk and is the patient following the preventive protocol?
- How is the bone support, and has it changed?
- How is tooth mobility, and has it changed?
- What are the probing depths, and is there any attachment loss?
- How is the gingival health, and is there any inflammation?

7.2.1 Identification of the Current Problems (Decay, Extraction, Periodontal, and Endodontic Problems)

The present teeth, roots, alveolar crests, and soft tissues in the mouth should be evaluated. All these examinations will help the dentist for planning the treatment.

Clinical assessment of tooth mobility is essential. The crown/root ratio is evaluated, and insufficient teeth are extracted. The concept of "critical weight" is increasing pocket depth when the alveolar support diminishes. Essentially, 1/2 of the supporting root should be surrounded by the alveolar bone (usually apical 1/3 of the root only constitute 15–20% of the root). Roots with a good treatment prognosis are the most suitable candidates for this treatment even if there is a horizontal bone loss around the remaining roots. In case of bone loss up to this level, horizontal loads in the crest area and apical area make combined compression and tension, thus leading to hemorrhage and thrombosis in the periodontal ligament which leads to degeneration and necrosis. At last, all remaining supporting alveolar bone gets resorbed. In this case, it might be necessary to reduce the crown height and thus the crown-root ratio for the efficient periodontal treatment of the supporting teeth. Mobility solely is not considered a contra-indication due to varying crown-root ratios (Picture 7.1).

7.2.2   Assessment of Bone Undercuts

It is necessary to identify the depths, localization, and size of the undercuts around the teeth. It is essential for determining the size of the extension and the path of

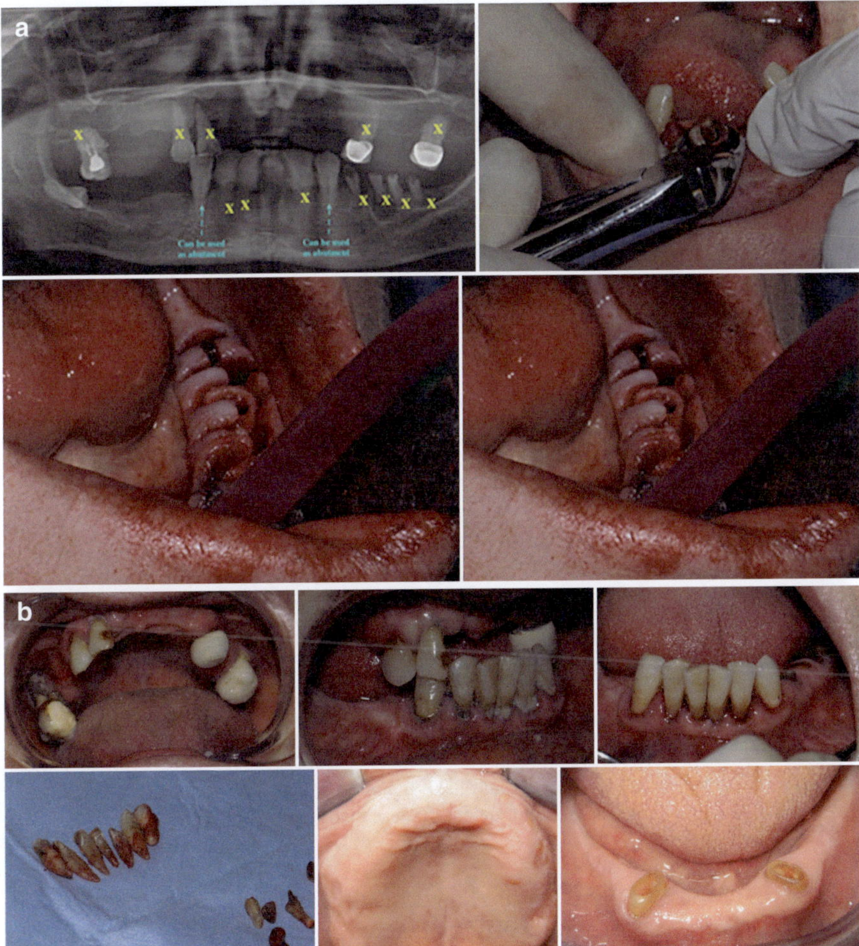

Picture 7.1 (**a, b**) According to the clinical and radiologic evaluation, hopeless teeth were extracted. For the upper jaw, all teeth were extracted and for the lower jaw, only two canine teeth were decided to use as the abutment. (**c**) *a* Preoperative situation; *b* temporary denture used to determine the esthetic appearance and vertical dimension of occlusion; *c* the preparation of two canine teeth as the abutment; *d* the final appearance of TSO; *e* the TSO intra-oral appearance; *f* attachment-retained coping and metal framework in situ

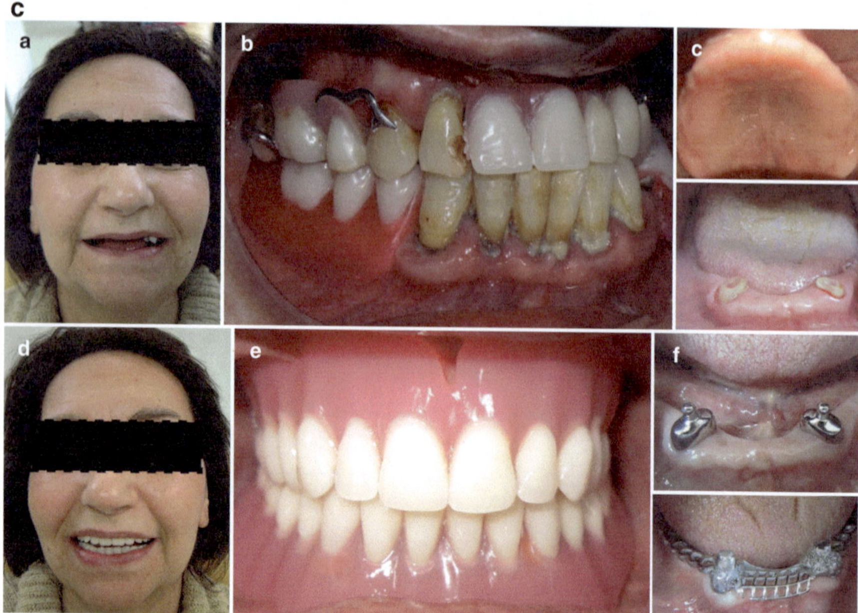

Picture. 7.1 (continued)

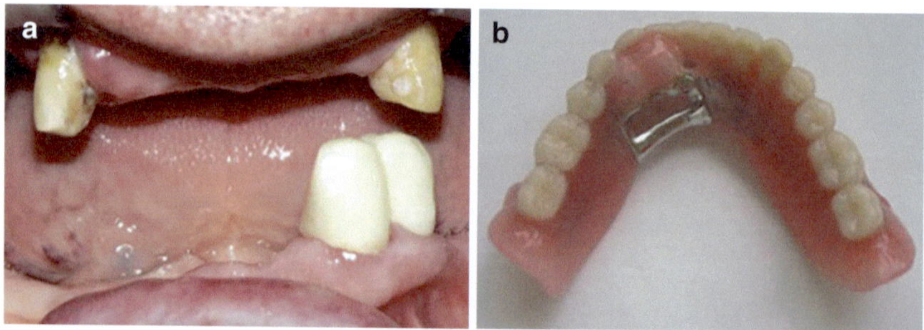

Picture 7.2 (**a**, **b**) Significant root shape of the mandibular supporting teeth will cause bulky dentures at this region (In this case, faulty planning was made)

insertion of the denture base. The bone undercuts and frenulum should be evaluated, and these anatomical structures should be corrected surgically if there is a possibility of them negatively affecting the denture retention (Picture 7.2). If there is a deep bone undercut, it might negatively affect the denture retention and relief is necessary. Furthermore, the deep undercut will also cause a bulk on the base plate, which will negatively affect the support.

7.2.3 Periodontal Surgery

Bone support and gingival health of remaining teeth are essential. The roots of the remaining supporting teeth should have a healthy periodontium.

7.2.4 Definition of Terms

Alveolar mucosa: nonkeratinized oral epithelium.

Gingiva: oral mucosa that is keratinized, described as attached or unattached.

The attached gingiva is tightly bound around teeth or implants, and it is continuous with the unattached gingiva.

Unattached gingiva, on the other hand, is defined as the gingiva that is not bound around the teeth or implants (e.g., free gingival margin, a soft-tissue wall of the sulcus or pocket).

Width of the attached gingiva: simply defined as the distance from the mucogingival junction to the free gingival margin minus the probing depth (Figs. 7.1, 7.2, and 7.3). The amount of the attached gingiva is essential for the health and long-term efficiency of the restoration.

Historically, an increased zone of keratinized tissue (KT) was presumed desirable for providing a resistant barrier against plaque-induced inflammation, for replacing nonkeratinized margins to prevent a recession, and for deepening vestibules to provide better access for toothbrushing. Furthermore, it is also necessary for dissipating functional and masticatory stress placed on the gingival margin of restoration and it improves esthetics, patient comfort, and ease of hygiene. Many researchers suggested that a lack of keratinized tissue predisposed the periodontium around teeth to deteriorate because they believed KT was more resistant to periodontal destruction

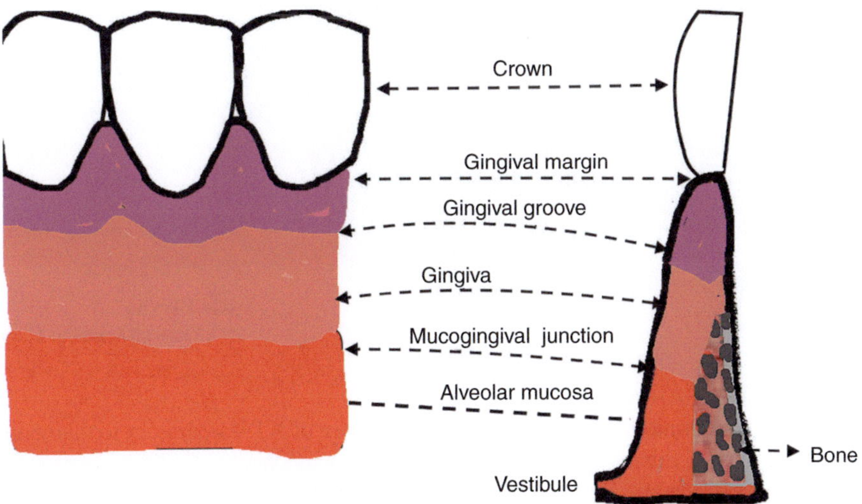

Fig. 7.1 Schematic view of the gingival structure

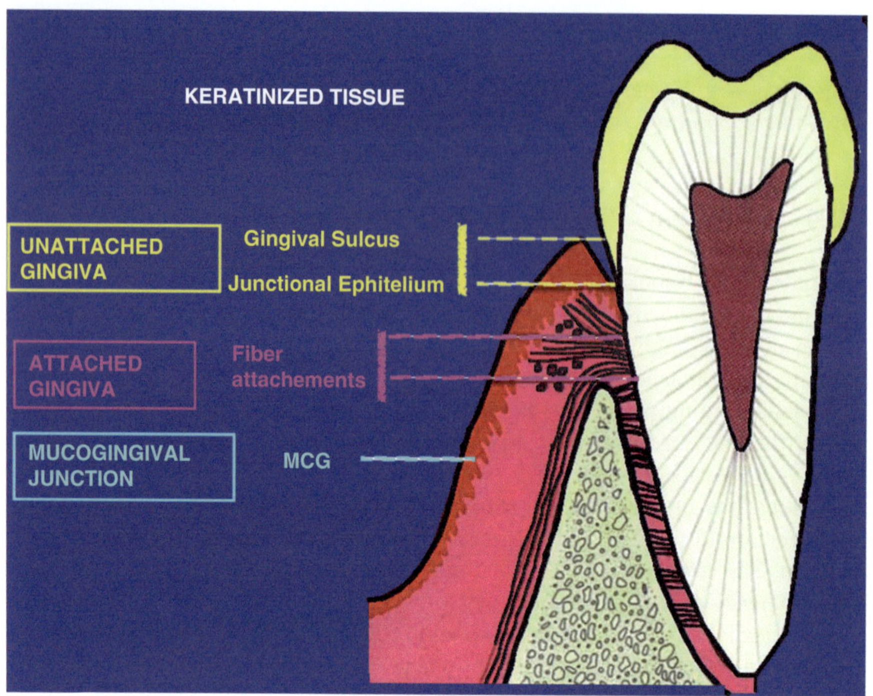

Fig. 7.2 Schematic view of keratinized tissue

Fig. 7.3 Schematic view of determining attachment loss using a periodontal probe

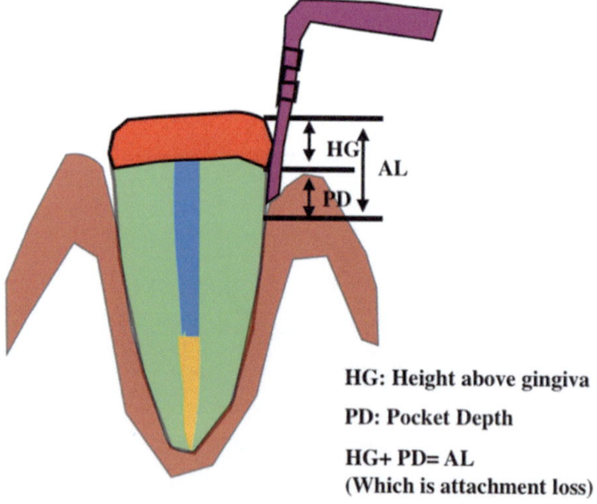

than the alveolar mucosa. It was concluded that 2 mm of KT is necessary to maintain gingival health (1 mm attached gingiva and 1 mm unattached).

Periodontal diseases are continuous risk factors for patients wearing dentures. Active periodontal diseases should be treated in the first place. Tissues should be free of inflammation, should not bleed when probed, and should be free of attachment loss (up to 3–4 mm). Generally, the reason for attachment loss is the motion of the denture and mostly the movement toward the buccolingual direction.

Essentially, the supporting teeth should not have mobility, and there should be a gingival pocket no deeper than 3 mm. Pocket elimination through periodontal therapy and attached gingiva should be formed before initiating the denture stage. The attached gingiva is obtained through a surgical operation called gingivectomy. However, the mucosa under the denture is less keratinized, and the stratum corneum is thinner. The long epithelial attachment might not work in reattachment procedures. As a surgical operation, the flap operation which replaces the apical parts of the gingiva for supporting the teeth of the denture would be considered more convenient. Following the operation, a reduced sulcus and a physiologic attachment are obtained. Obtaining the attached gingiva relates to the width of the keratinized gingiva. If sufficient, it constitutes the flap thickness which is defined as the structure that also contains the apical part and the attached gingiva. If there is less keratinized tissue, the gingival graft is necessary. The pre-operative condition of the teeth is entirely different from the post-operative condition. Stabilization of the supporting teeth can be ensured through short-term splinting, which reduces the occlusal loads.

7.2.5 Endodontic Treatment

Endodontic treatment is necessary to improve crown-root ratios (especially for weak supporting teeth) and to provide a convenient path of insertion and support for tilted or malposed teeth. It is also necessary for using hemi-section molars or root-amputated molars as abutments for overdentures.

Usually, teeth with a single root and flat or slightly inclined roots are preferred for endodontic treatment, and the root canals should be filled properly (Fig. 7.4).

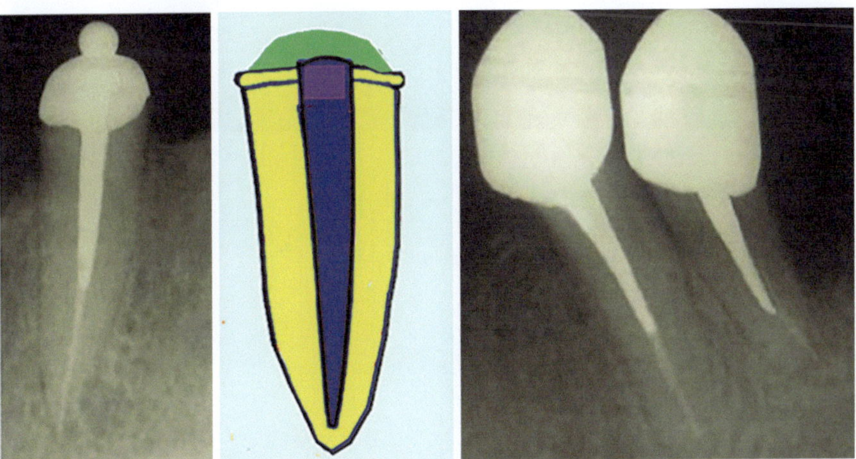

Fig. 7.4 Single root teeth should be preferred and root canals should be filled properly

7.2.6　Selection of Supporting Teeth

To distribute forces adequately to the roots, supporting teeth should ideally be positioned in an axial position and perpendicular to the direction of the occlusal forces so that the oblique group of fibers absorbs those forces. A resistant and polished surface should be obtained after the preparation of the supporting teeth. If a regular margin cannot be obtained because of the previous restoration or tooth caries, the root surface should be restored with copings (metal coping).

7.2.7　Structural Properties of the Remaining Teeth

Structural properties of the teeth should be considered before deciding to use them as abutments (Picture 7.3). Incisor teeth are generally among the first teeth

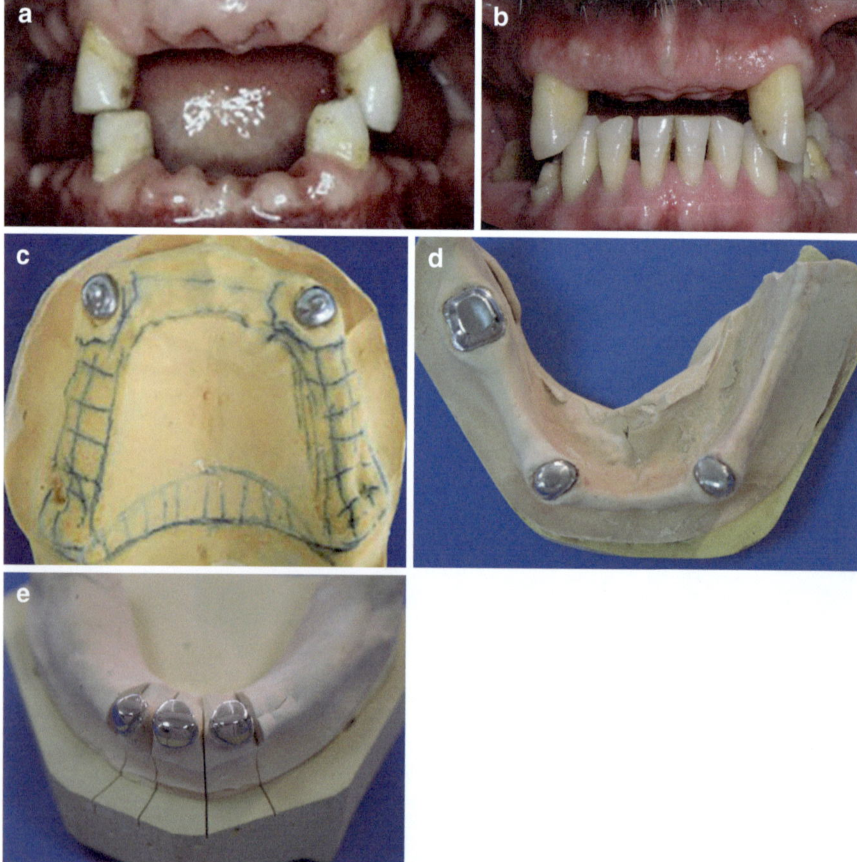

Picture 7.3 (**a**) Supporting teeth upper and lower jaw are canine teeth; (**b**) canines are mostly used for the upper jaw; (**c**) metal coping with attachment placed on the model; (**d**) canines accompanied with molars are mostly used as supporting teeth (only medium-long coping used as the retentive abutment); (**e**) incisor teeth used as a medium coping as abutments for maxillae

to be lost because of their weak conical root structures. However, premolar teeth are located in the central areas of the arch, so they offer excellent support for both the anterior and the posterior areas. On the other hand, molar teeth have a wide root surface area, but their bone loss is usually high as the bone around these teeth receives the incoming forces. Lastly, canine teeth also provide support for both the posterior and anterior segments of the denture base. From a periodontal viewpoint, canine teeth may not be the most convenient teeth since the labial surface often results in a fusion of their facial cortical plate of bone with the alveolar bone, thereby causing dehiscence of fenestration. Unfortunately, this clinical picture cannot be repaired adequately by periodontal therapy, and it breaks down easily if the tissue is traumatized. However, because of their position, the retention capacity of the tooth, less susceptibility to periodontal breakdown, and fewer anatomical and positional difficulties, canine teeth are the best choice of abutment in areas of maximum force and ridge resorption potential. So, the canines, even though they do not have a large surface area of periodontal attachment, maybe a preferable abutment since they are mostly located in the middle of the ridge. However, the prominent structure of the canine roots might negatively affect aesthetics in some cases.

Thayer (1980) [1] published an overview for stress analysis on the abutments by various attachment designs, stating that periodontal health must not only be maintained by the above considerations but also by the types of stresses applied that cause adverse pressure on the abutments and eventual periodontal breakdown during the overdenture function. The significance of loading on the periodontal vasculature is discussed by [2], and they stated that the periodontal blood flow does decrease dramatically after loading the abutment, probably due to the ischemia in the periodontal ligament. The location of the abutment tooth is also quite important for periodontal ligament recovery. The more posteriorly the abutment tooth is located, the more vasculature it will have since the vascular density of the periodontal ligament increases posteriorly, meaning that the periodontal ligament has a better chance to recover from the loading forces.

7.2.8   Location of the Supporting Teeth

- In the maxillary arch, incisors are used.
- At least one tooth per quadrant should be present.
- The ideal is two teeth per quadrant. The stress is distributed over a rectangular area.
- A tripod approach can also be used as:
  - Maxillary arch – Two central incisors and canines/premolars.
  - Ideal when opposing mandibular anterior exist.
  - When only a single incisor remains, it is still a tripod but with less mechanical advantage.

- Clinicians should consider the number of abutments when evaluating the oral cavity and suggest their influence on the attachment selection. The two canines, two premolars, or one canine/two premolars on different sides of the arch offer better support as abutments than two premolars or one canine/one premolar on the same side.
- Two adjacent teeth such as the canine and the first premolar should be not selected as the support. Since it is challenging for the patient to clean the adjacent supporting teeth, oral hygiene maybe impaired, thus the prognosis of the supporting teeth might be affected negatively. If the distance between the teeth is too limited, it is preferable to extract the weak one. Problems might occur in the placement of artificial teeth and ensuring aesthetics as the bulk under the denture increases. If adjacent roots are to be protected, the simplest solution would be to apply the copings to both surfaces separately. Connecting adjacent copings have mechanical advantages as it offers more resistance to lateral and rotational forces. However, there should be enough space for cleaning the attachment areas; at least 2–3 mm space is needed if adjacent coping is used. Furthermore, the adjacent copings complicate plaque control and overdenture construction. Only one single attachment is necessary on each side for a connected design, and it is preferred to place the attachment only to the most substantive roots.
- Four different teeth, positioned distantly from each other, offer ideal support and stability. On the other hand, increasing the number of supporting teeth causes a more complicated structure.
- When there are too many supporting teeth, the clinicians should evaluate other treatment options. In these cases, overdenture treatment should be eliminated if possible (Picture 7.4).

On the other hand, when there is a single tooth, it will be exposed to rotational forces, and it is going to be quite challenging to have a successful result.

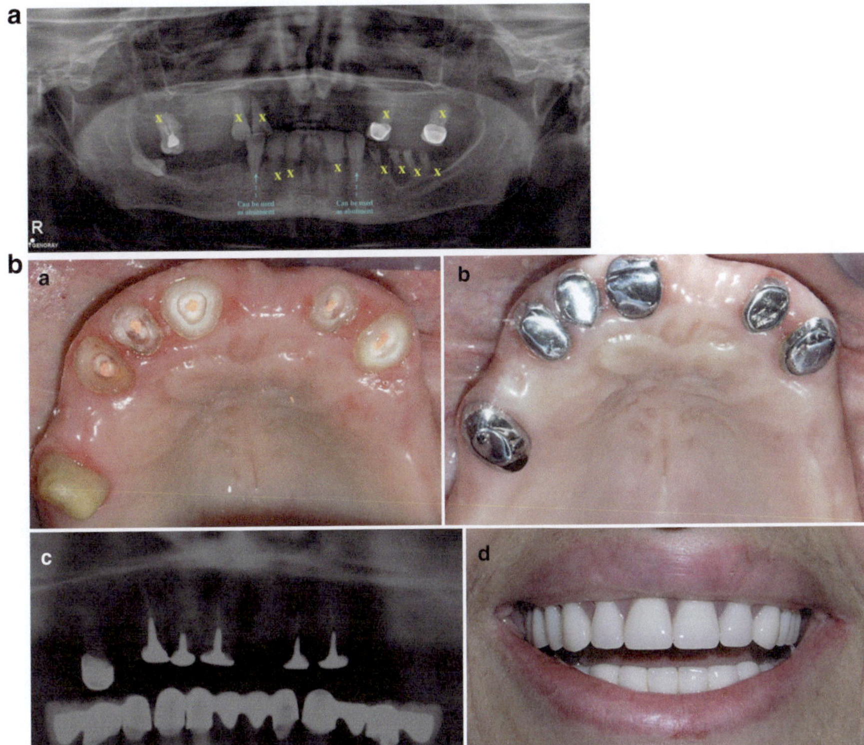

Picture 7.4 (**a**) Radiographic view of a patient. Unsuitable supporting teeth and suitable supporting teeth are marked on the panoramic X-ray. (**b**) Faulty planning (abutment numbers were used so much unnecessarily): *a* Preparation of the supporting teeth; *b* application of the metal copings; *c* radiographic view of metal coping; *d* appearance of the overdenture (wrong treatment plan may cause esthetic and phonetic problems due to too many teeth left and coping applied)

7.3 Radiographic Assessment

The panoramic and periapical X-rays should be obtained and carefully examined to get information concerning the selection of supporting teeth. Periapical radiography should investigate bone support. After the crown/root ratio is examined, weak-supported teeth should be extracted. At the radiographic examination, at least 5 mm alveolar bone support and 1/1 crown-root ratio should be observed (Pictures 7.5 and 7.6). During radiographic and clinical examination, if the periodontal health condition of the supporting teeth is not suitable, the remaining teeth are not as long as half of the length of the root embedded in the alveolar bone, and the pocket depth is more than 3 mm, extraction is recommended and realized with the consent of the patient.

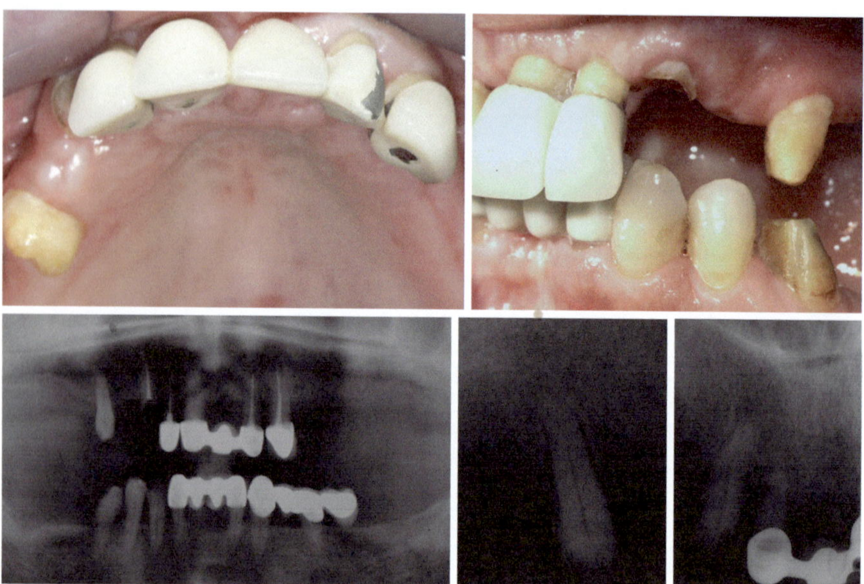

Picture 7.5 Clinical and radiographical examinations should be used to determine supporting teeth status

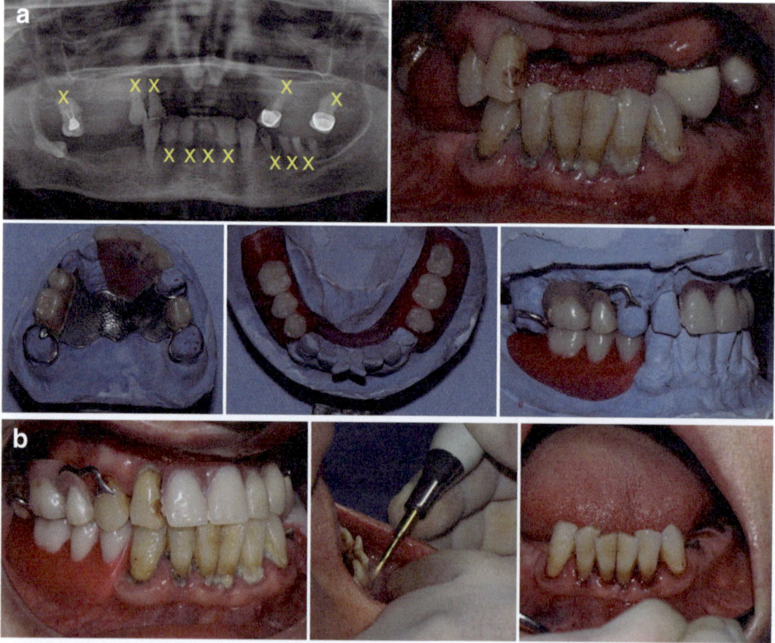

Picture 7.6 (a) Radiographical evaluations (hopeless teeth/root marked on the panoramic X-ray), clinical evaluations, and diagnostic temporary dentures for proper evaluation; (b) the temporary denture (lower jaw) and existing denture (upper jaw) were evaluated clinically, and calculus were removed mechanically to evaluate teeth properly

7.4   Examination of Diagnostic Casts on the Articulator

On the articulator, diagnostic casts are mounted in order to examine the occlusion and tooth locations. If the patient already has a denture, the vertical dimension is easily recorded. If the patient does not have dentures, a base plate and occlusal rim are constructed using diagnostic casts, and the exact vertical dimension is recorded and evaluated on the articulator. It should be mentioned that the attachment would be chosen based on the vertical dimension of occlusion, the inter-arch space, and crest width (Picture 7.7).

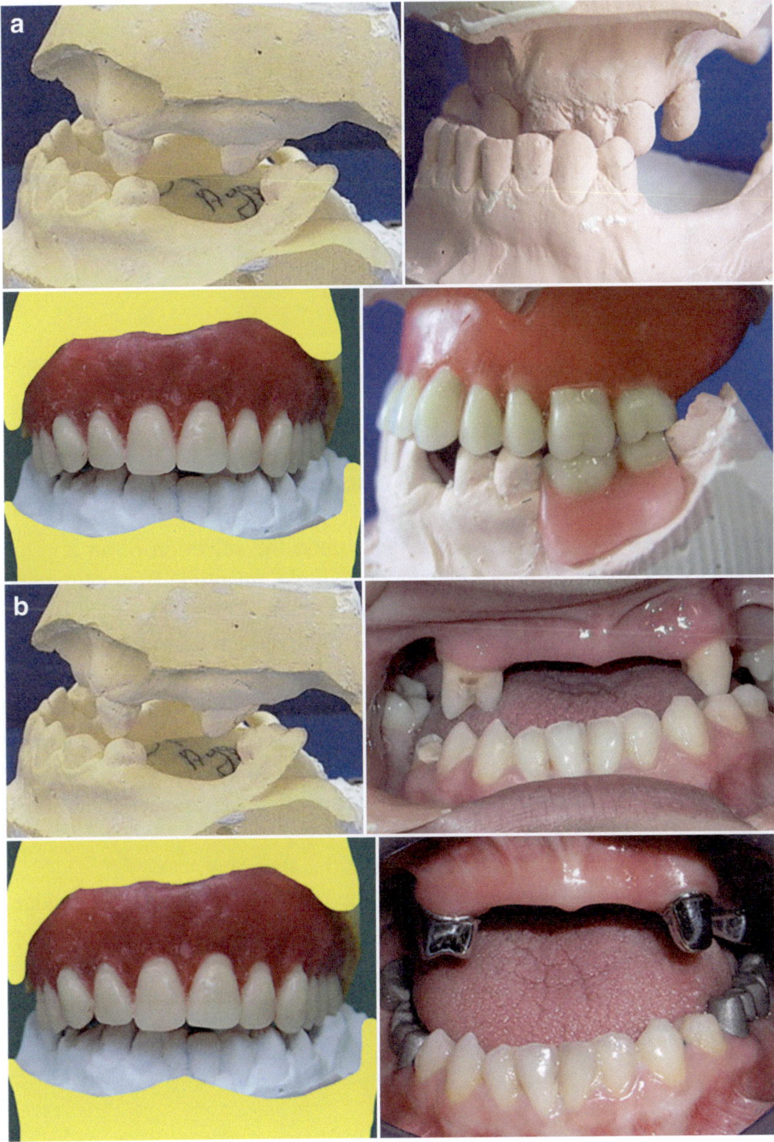

Picture 7.7   Telescope-retained overdenture (**a**) Model (**b**) Wax-up (**c**) Final

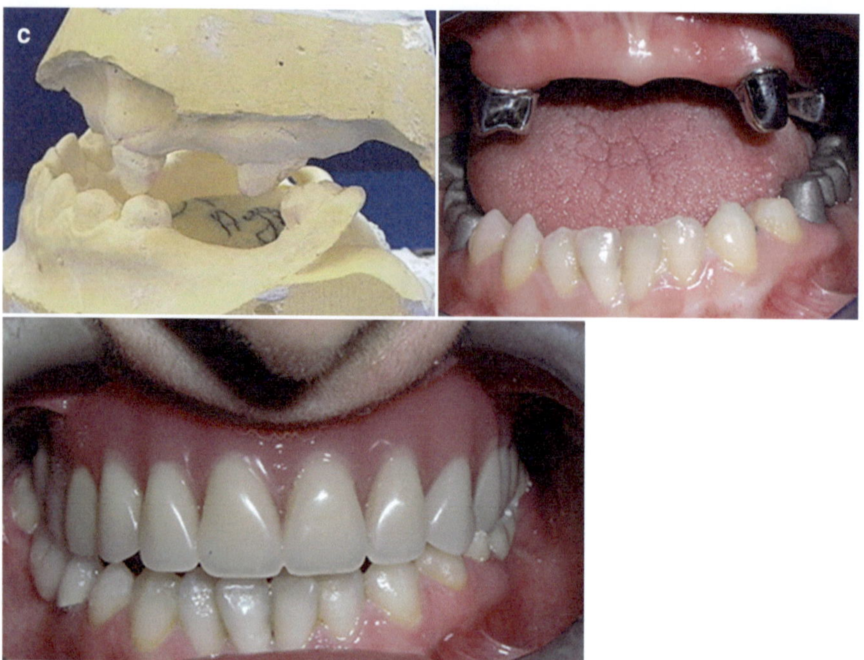

Picture. 7.7 (continued)

7.5   Selection of the Type of Attachment

The success of TSO treatment is contingent upon the selection of an appropriate attachment. TSO is treated with independent (single, unsplinted) attachments such as a ball, locator, telescope attachment, or splinted attachment. During the overdenture function, the attachment transfers forces to the remaining tooth or implant and bone, therefore the force transmission by various attachments with two different supporting structures (teeth and soft tissue) could be very important.

The following criteria should be addressed while selecting an attachment:

- The amount of support offered by the supporting tissues (teeth, edentulous ridge).
- Physiologic form of the arch.
- The quantity, placement, and orientation of the abutment.
- The maxillo-mandibular connection and the resorption of the alveolar ridge.
- Maximum occlusal force and masticatory function (evaluating the opposing arch).
- Maintenance difficulties, expense, and patients' expectations.
- Patient satisfaction.

7.5.1 The Degree of the Support by the Teeth and Edentulous Ridge

If abutments are strong and edentulous ridges are weak, *rigid attachments* must be chosen to transfer the majority of chewing forces to the supporting tooth.

If the abutments have less support and the edentulous ridge is solid, *resilient attachments* with variable levels of resilience are employed to transfer less force to the supporting tooth and the majority of the received force to the bone beneath the edentulous supporting tissues.

7.5.2 The Arch Shape

The selection of attachments is also influenced by the arch shape of the jaw. Bar attachments are appropriate for U- or square-shaped arches, but not for V-shaped arches since they leave insufficient space for the tongue. In this circumstance, the unsplinted attachment should be chosen.

7.5.3 Number, Placement, and Angle of Supporting Teeth

A telescopic attachment is utilized in symmetric teeth that give robust support on both sides of the arch. Retention and stability of the telescopic denture are directly proportional to the number and distribution of abutments along the dental arch as well as the taper of the major coping marginal walls. Individual attachments are favored when there are few teeth and the teeth or implants are parallel. The alignment of stud attachments must be 10 degrees and parallel to the denture insertion line.

When the abutments are not parallel, the bar attachments can provide parallelism. The intra-radicular attachment parallelism between roots is not required. Access posts occupy a tiny vertical space; therefore, parallelism is unnecessary for the male units on the various roots.

7.5.4 Resorption of the Alveolar Ridge and the Maxillo-Mandibular Relationship

If a vertical dimension is appropriate, bar and telescope attachments can be chosen. *Bar-clip retainers* provide superior retention and stability; they permit splinting of the teeth and are resistant to crestal bone resorption.

If the vertical dimension is insufficient, *single attachments*, such as *stud attachments* or *magnet attachments*, are recommended (considering the abutment and edentulous ridge condition). *Stud attachments* provide for adequate load transfer to the bone; they are affordable, easy to use, and simple to clean.

Magnet attachments can be used in the mandible if there is sufficient bone; however, they may not be adequate for individuals desiring improved retention.

For cases with limited inter-arch space, a small, tailored coping with an intra-radicular post (intra-radicular attachment) should be utilized.

7.6 Preparation Types of Supporting Teeth

Supporting teeth can either contribute solely to the denture's support or both support and retention. First, it should be determined whether the remaining teeth will be included in the plan to provide support or whether they will contribute to both support and retention. The incorrect indication will increase expenditures and negatively impact the treatment's prognosis.

If the clinical crown length and crown-root ratio are appropriate, the tooth should be prepared according to traditional standards (teeth can remain vital). If supporting teeth are still healthy, they are either polished and left alone or copings are placed. This preparation is suggested for telescoping and bar-retained attachments.

If the prognosis of the supporting teeth is not favorable and a future extraction is scheduled, the teeth may be used as the only support for stability. This is the easiest method of denture implantation, as it requires the least amount of space and is the simplest to organize. It does not affect the strength of the denture; however, it contributes slightly to stabilization but not retention. Typically, devitalized teeth undergo endodontic therapy.

If the crown-to-root ratio is correct, the supporting teeth serve as *retention elements*. When supporting teeth are employed as retainer components, they improve denture retention, provide periodontal support, transmit forces as vertically as possible through the denture to the periodontium, and splint or stabilize supporting teeth (Figs. 7.5 and 7.6).

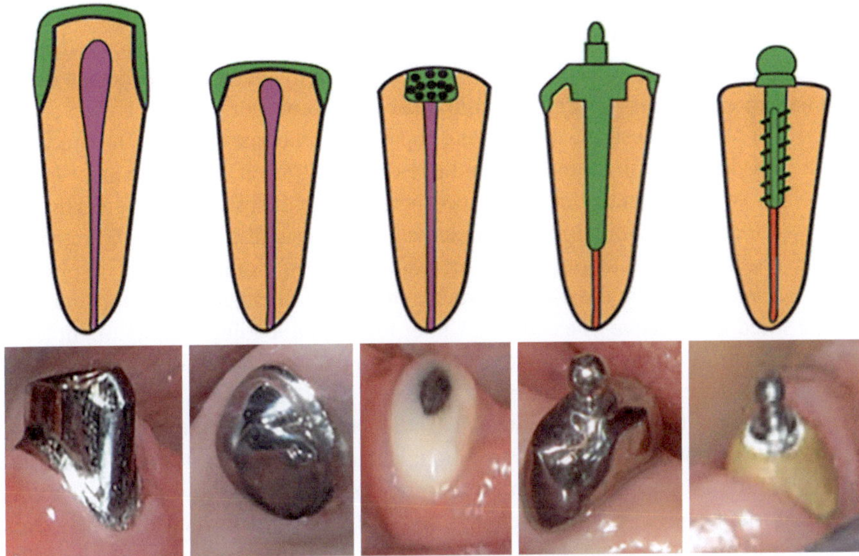

Fig. 7.5 Types of supporting and retentive teeth for TSO

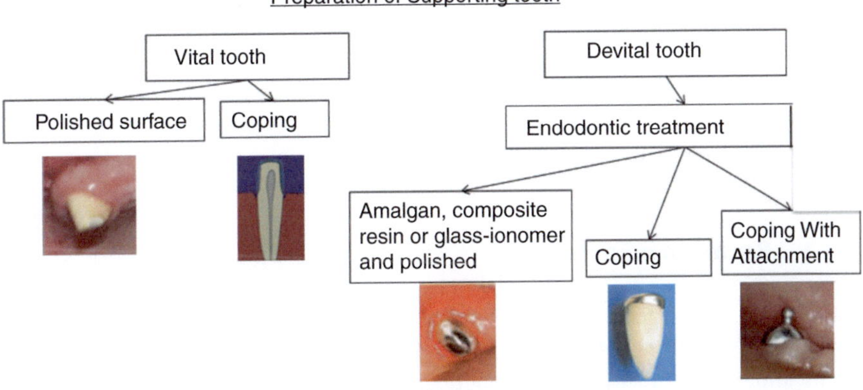

Fig. 7.6 Preparation of supporting teeth for TSO

7.7 Forces Applied to the Abutment Teeth

When choosing abutments for overdentures, the position of the tooth in the arch as well as its position between the buccal and lingual cortical plates must be carefully considered. Additionally, the angle of the tooth to be utilized as an abutment is examined. For optimal distribution of functional forces delivered to the remaining root, its axial location should be perpendicular to the direction of occlusal forces. These forces are characterized as either axial or rotary.

The direction of *axial forces* toward or away from the tooth. Axial forces are capable of both invading and extruding. Because they are the most easily tolerated, axial stresses exert the least influence on an overdenture abutment tooth. The design of the post must prevent stress concentration in order to prevent root fracture. However, the majority of root cap designs, such as long copings, short dome copings, and precision attachment designs, can withstand axial stresses of intrusion. Extrusive axial forces only occur when a retentive device is incorporated into the root cap design. The root cap must then have enough retention elements that resist the draw of the retention device. The degree of retention varies according to the type of attachment employed.

Rotational forces are the most destructive to the abutment. These factors can also be classified as intrusive or extrusive. Under functional loading, the abutment teeth are subject to intrusive forces. One or two abutments that are isolated are more sensitive to this type of load. Designs of root caps and attachments act differently in these situations, but it can be noted that non-rotational attachment designs cause torquing of the tooth root, whereas rotational attachment designs that allow rotation of the denture around the root tend to impinge on the root's supporting structures. The majority of precise attachments feature a vertical resilience factor, which is designed to provide tissue support rather than complete tooth support when the denture is in use. However, as this robust function is lost owing to tissue resorption, the aforementioned forces become more significant.

Magnetic retention is an exception to this problem in designs for retentive attachments, as it does not adhere to the same laws. The only mechanical device that offers retention without fixation is a magnet. Although abutments are always functioning as denture support components, torque forces do not apply when the root face is flat. Under functional loading of an abutment, the distal end of the saddle and the abutment exert pressure. There is no lingual impingement since there is no potential for denture movement over the keeper.

7.7.1　Rotational Forces

If rotational forces (forces away the mucosa) are applied to the denture, unsplinted attachments that allow rotation will impinge on tissues, while rigid attachments that do not allow rotation will cause the abutment to twist. If the ideal path of withdrawal is established, the patient can easily remove the denture and thus forces could be alleviated. However, forces induced by the attraction of sticky food will continue to cause rotation in this direction. The only exception to this rule is magnetic retention, which, due to the nature of magnets, provides less retention in rotational forces.

7.8　Determination of the Prosthesis Type

The position of the remaining teeth and the inter-arch space were determined based on the vertical dimension measured on the diagnostic casts. If the distance between the maxillary and mandibular arches is sufficient for the recommended treatment, the first step is to record vertical and horizontal jaw relationships.

The supporting teeth should be examined for preparation and adaptation with the primer coping, bar/stud attachments, or telescope attachment, followed by wax rims for bite registration, and the arrangement of the teeth should be evaluated with a full wax tooth setup.

After a careful planning, it should be determined that the overdenture should be used with the best suitable attachment (the treatment should be followed by a standard protocol as described in detail for each chapter for different attachments).

References

1. Thayer HH, Caputo AA. Photoelastic stess analysis of overdenture attachments. J Prosthet Dent. 1980;43:611–7. https://doi.org/10.1016/0022-3913(80)90374-1.
2. NG G, Walker TW, Zingg W, Burke PS, Effects of tooth loading on the periodontal vasculature of the mandibular fourth premolar in dogs. Arch Oral Bio. 1981;26:189–95. https://doi.org/10.1016/0003-9969(81)90129-1.

Further Reading

Basker RM, Harrison A, Ralph JP. Part II Indications for overdentures: Patient selection. In: Basker RM, Harrison A, Ralph JP. Overdentures in general dental practice. Br Dent J. 1983;155:50–4.

Beck CB, Bates JF, Basker RM, Gutteridge DL, Harrison A. A survey of the dissatisfied denture patient. Eur J Prosthodont Restor Dent. 1993;2:73–8.

Brkovic S, Stamenkovic D, Stanisic Sinobad D, Rakocevic Z, Zelic O. The influence of continuous magnetic field on periodontal tissues under overdentures. Srp Arh Celok Lek. 2009;137:363–70.

Carlsson GE. Implant and root supported overdentures-a literature review and some data on bone loss in edentulous jaws. J Adv Prosthodont. 2014;6:245–52.

Ettinger RL, Qien F. Abutment tooth loss in patients with overdentures. JADA. 2004;135:739–46.

Ettinger RL, Qien F. Postprocedural problems in an overdenture population: a longitudinal study. J Endod. 2004;30:310–4.

Laurito D, Lamazza L, De Biase A. Tissue-supported dental implant prosthesis (overdenture): the search for the ideal protocol: a literature review. Ann Stomatol. 2012;3:2–10.

Postic SD. Especially designed copings for stability of overdentures. JSM Dent. 2016;4:1061–5.

Lee MS, Su CM, Yeh JC, Wu PR, Tsai TY, Lou SL. Synthesis of composite magnetic nanoparticles Fe3O4 with alendronate for osteoporosis treatment. Int J Nanomedicine. 2016;11:4583–94.

Mascola RF. The root retained complete denture. JADA. 1976;92:586–7.

Preiskel HW. Overdentures made easy. A guide to implant and root supported prostheses, vol. 58. London: Quintessence Publish; 1996. p. 90–6.

Trock DH. Electromagnetic fields and magnets. Investigational treatment for musculoskeletal disorders. Rheum Dis Clin N Am. 2000;26:51–62.

Basker RM, Harrison A, Ralph JP. Overdentures in general dental practice. Part 2 – indications for overdentures: patient selection. Br Dent J. 1983;154:321–4.

Supporting Tooth Preparation

8

Yasemin Ozkan and Murat Feriz

8.1 Preparation of Dental Support

The preparation of abutment teeth in tooth-supported overdenture (TSO) differs based on the type of abutment teeth. Preparation is performed all around the tooth, and the prepared surface must be convex. An ideal supporting tooth preparation should be straightforward, brief, and convex, in addition to being dome-shaped with a chamfered edge finish (Fig. 8.1).

8.1.1 Simple Preparation (Preparation Supporting Teeth Barely)

This sort of formulation has the least amount of added stability with no retention. The height of the supporting tooth is decreased to 1–2 mm above the gingival level, and any residual sharp edges are softened. Preparing the gingival margin levels creates space for a suitable quantity of acrylic material for the overdenture's strength while preserving the gingival support and architecture. This form of preparation influences the insertion path of the overdenture the least. The occlusal surface of the prepared abutment should be slightly convex and well-polished, and the finish line should be chamfered just below the gingival level (Fig. 8.1).

When supporting teeth are treated endodontically, the root canal entry is sealed with amalgam, glass ionomer cement, or composite resin and shaped into a dome. Occasionally, a prefabricated post is placed during root canal therapy. To achieve stability, the occlusal portion of the prefabricated post should be left elevated. After the prefabricated post has been elevated 1–2 mm, a composite core can be added to it. Post-and-core installation utilizing prefabricated metal posts and composite resin is a standard approach in the majority of general practices. These posts are simple

Y. Ozkan (✉) · M. Feriz
Faculty of Dentistry, Department of Prosthodontics, Marmara University, Istanbul, Turkey
e-mail: ykozkan@marmara.edu.tr

Y. Özkan (ed.), *Treatment Options Before and After Edentulism*,
https://doi.org/10.1007/978-3-031-37582-8_8

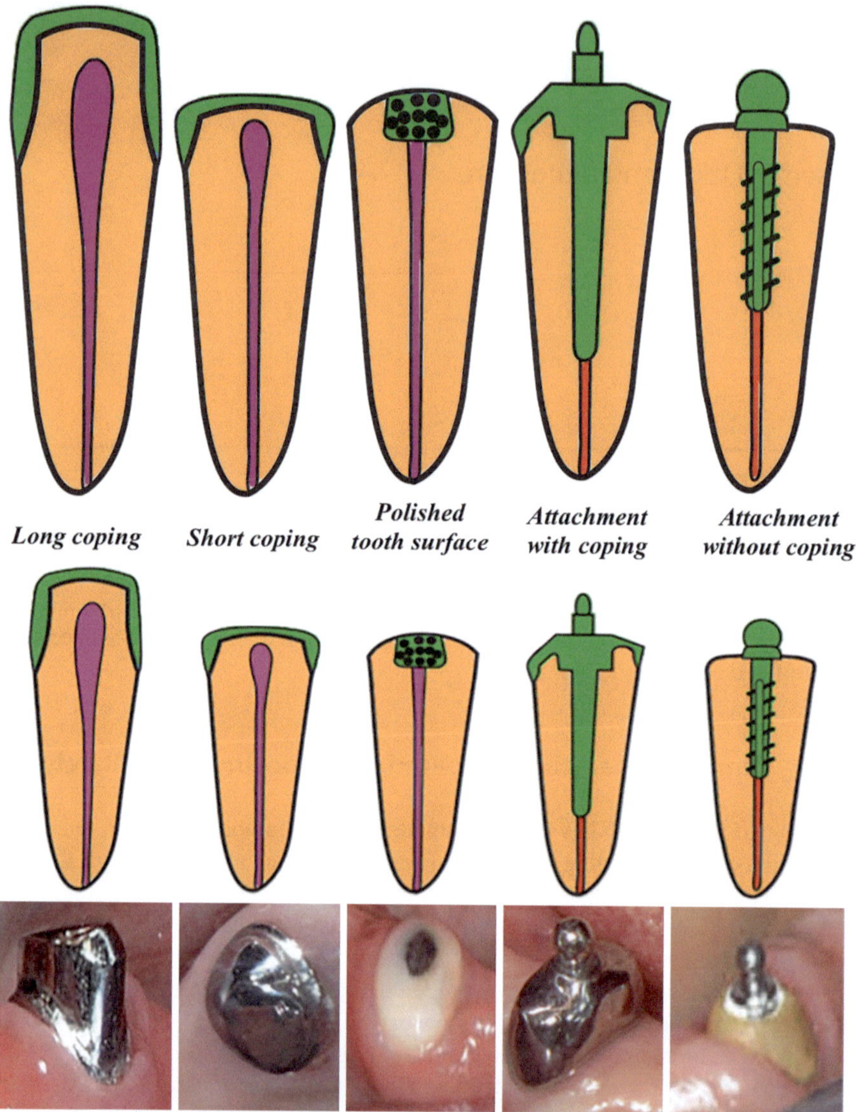

Fig. 8.1 Supporting teeth crown height of reduced by 2–3 mm and which are prepared in a convex or dome form are used

to install, robust, relatively affordable, and predictable. The prefabricated posts are available in a range of materials, designs, and sizes to accommodate specific circumstances. Post-placement and composite core buildup (also curved to provide a dome shape) can be performed in a single visit, hence decreasing fabrication time (Figs. 8.2, 8.3, and 8.4).

Dentin tubules are exposed to the oral cavity during the preparation of supporting teeth. The dentin structure closer to the pulp is less calcified than the surface of the

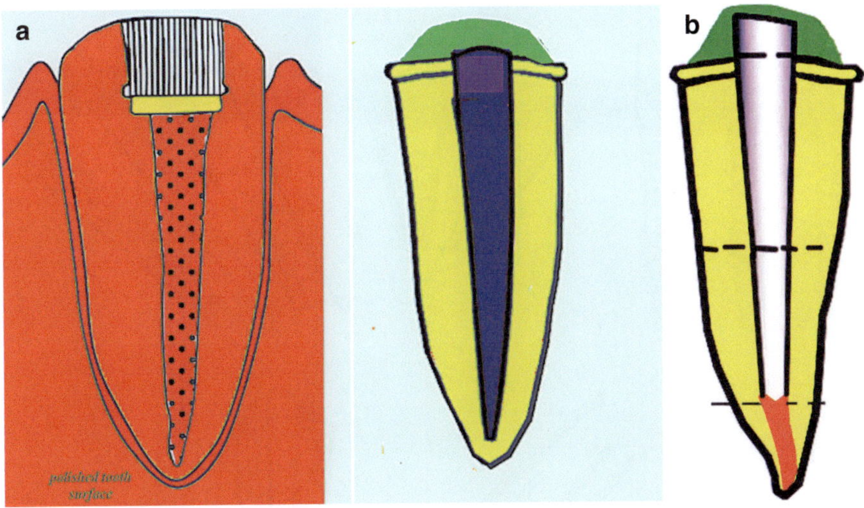

Fig. 8.2 (**a**) Preparation of tooth for simple preparation (amalgam, glass ionomer cement, or composite resin can be used to cover the root face); (**b**) the prefabricated post could be used after root canal treatment. The occlusal part of the prefabricated post should be left high and try to achieve stabilization

root dentin. Caries is the most prevalent consequence of untreated TSO. The most economical approach for sealing the dentinal tubules is to etch the surface of the prepared denture, apply a dentin bonding agent of the fourth generation, and then seal the surface with light cure. This surface will deteriorate over time, necessitating periodic maintenance. This therapy may provide temporary protection for the tooth surface. Recall visits should be scheduled 24 h following denture placement, 2 weeks later, and every 6 months.

8.1.2 Preparation Supporting Teeth for Coping

Using coping can help prevent tooth decay if the patient practices adequate dental hygiene and utilizes fluoride or chlorhexidine in high doses. If a ring-shaped coping is fabricated in the absence of secondary dentin, endodontic treatment is uniquely required. Morrow et al. considered that it was important to cover the TSO abutments with gold copings or rings to protect them against caries. Gold copings increase the cost of TSO treatment and do not prevent caries formation unless the patient maintains proper oral hygiene and uses a gel containing ideal concentrations of fluoride or chlorhexidine fluoride cannot prevent caries.

The coping that is attached to the prepared abutment is known as the "main coping" (Pictures 8.1, 8.2, 8.3, 8.4, 8.5, and 8.6). The increased coping height may risk the treatment since it needs the teeth to endure lateral and twisting forces, and the prosthesis may fracture if interocclusal space is diminished.

There are four fundamental types of coping strategies.

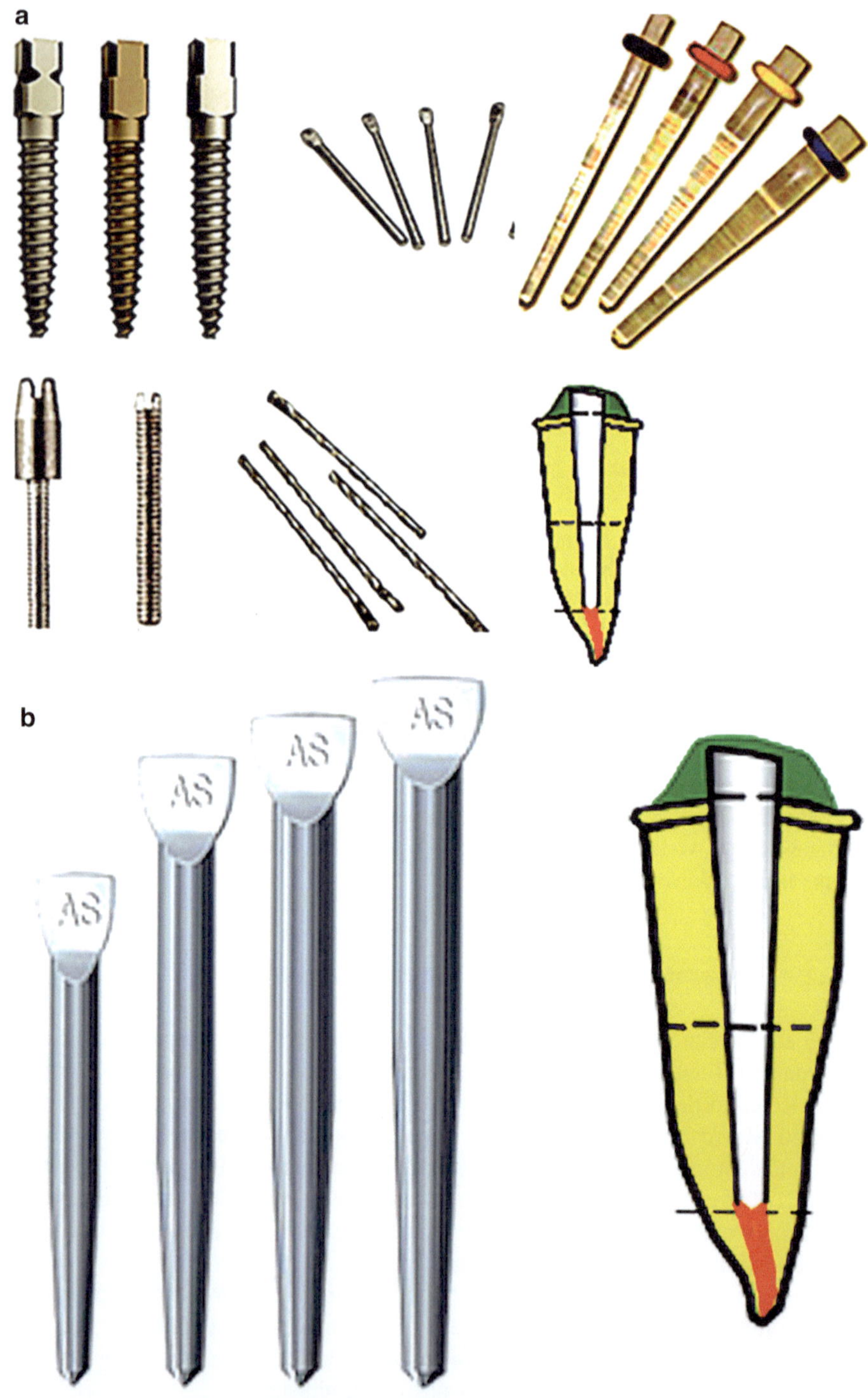

Fig. 8.3 (**a**, **b**) The prefabricated posts are available in a variety of materials, designs, and sizes to cater to the needs of the situation

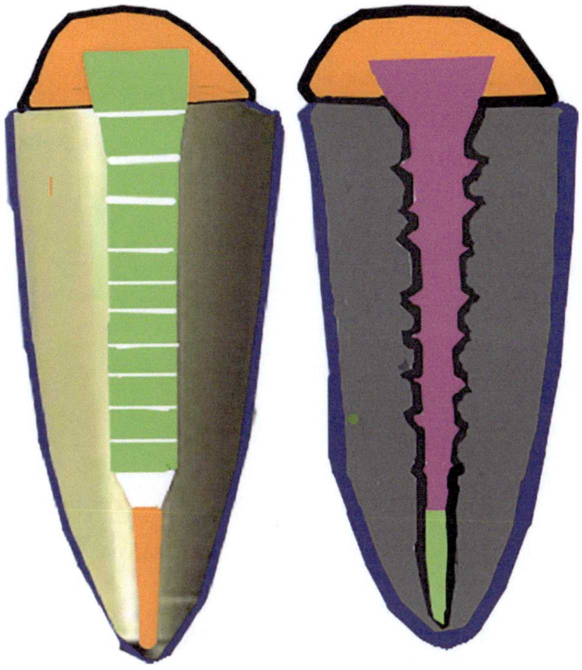

Fig. 8.4 Different types of prefabricated posts used for supporting teeth

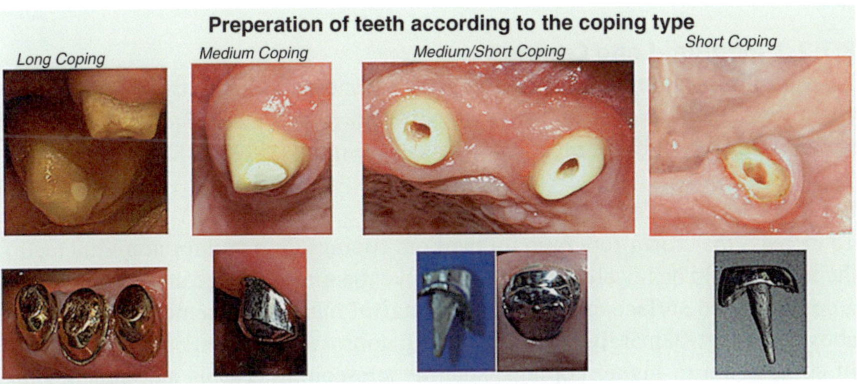

Picture 8.1 Preparation of the supporting teeth according to coping types

Long copings

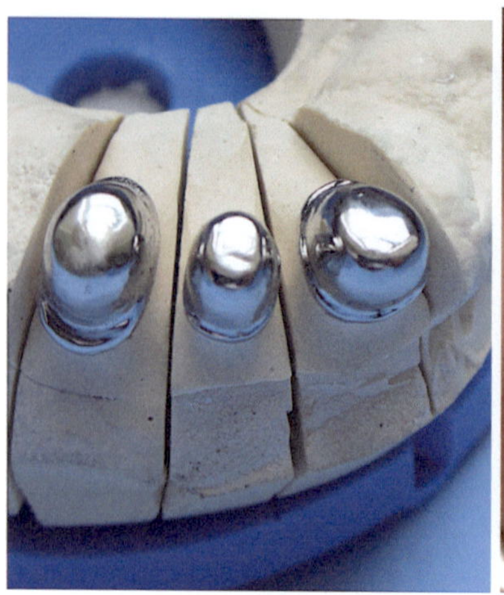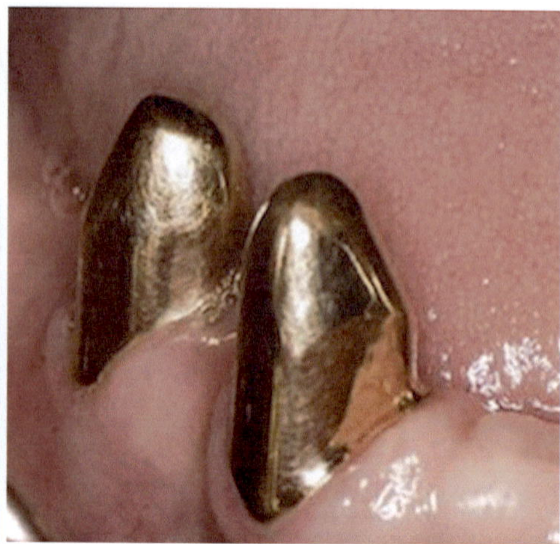

Picture 8.2 Vital teeth preparation for long coping and gold long coping

8.1.2.1 Long Copings (6–8 mm for Vital Teeth)

For the use of lengthy copings, the abutment teeth must be periodontally healthy and immobile, and there must be adequate interarch space for coping, denture base, and the arrangement of the teeth. Interarch distance or interocclusal space should be 10 mm. The teeth should be prepared using tapered walls (2–5°) with a chamfered finish line (Fig. 8.5; Pictures 8.1 and 8.2).

8.1.2.2 Medium-Long Copings

For a medium-length coping (4–6 mm for vital and non-vital teeth), the supporting teeth must be either vital or endodontically treated and tapered. Devitalization of abutments is typically required due to space constraints (Fig. 8.3).

8.1.2.3 Medium Coping

To increase the crown-root ratio for medium copings (2–4 mm for non-vital teeth), the teeth should be lowered to 2–4 mm above the gingival edge and prepared with a dome-shaped surface and chamfered gingival margin. Placement of a chamfer above the gingival margin of a metal coping improved retention of an overdenture. In comparison to higher copings, such as telescoping crowns and attachments, short copings lessen the likelihood of overdenture base fracture, and the stress distribution in the remaining teeth is also reduced, particularly in non-axial pressures (Fig. 8.6).

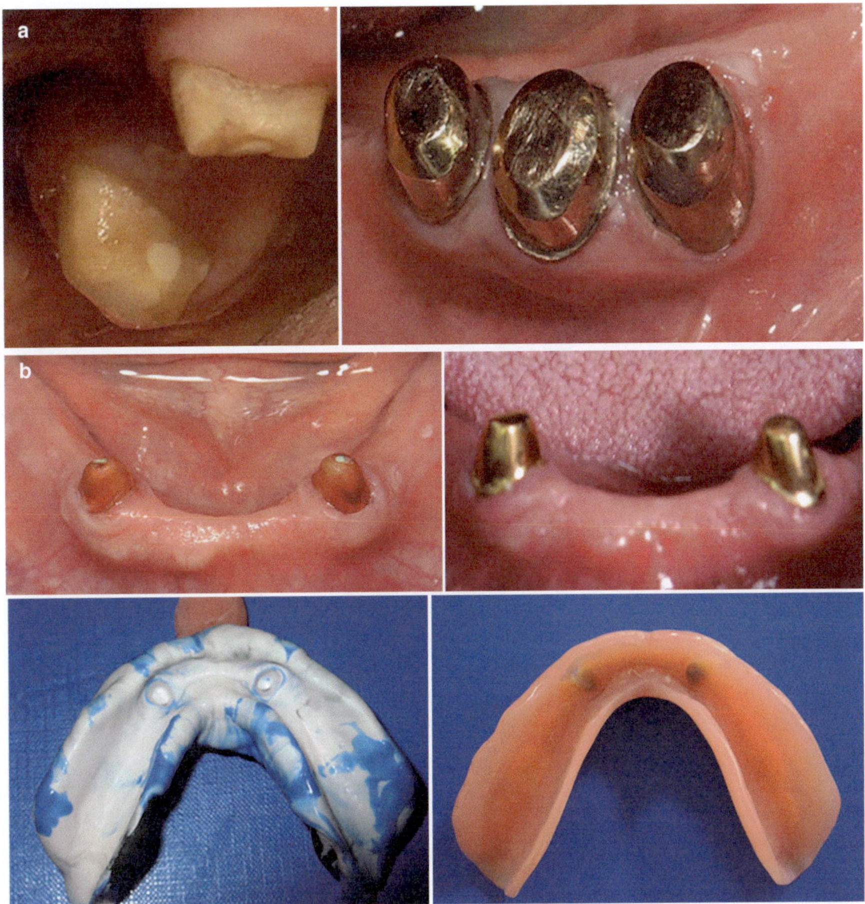

Picture 8.3 (**a**) Medium coping cast with gold metal alloys for lower canine; (**b**) after cementation impression is taken and overdenture made without a metal framework and secondary coping

8.1.2.4 Insights for Coping

After the teeth are prepared, a silicon- or polyether-based impression material is used to create an impression of the supporting tooth, which is then poured with stone to create the model. Then, the wax models are submitted for casting.

8.1.2.5 Short Copings

To accomplish retention, short metallic copings with stud attachment must be employed (Picture 8.5). The height of cast-metal coping should be between 2 and 4 mm. After attachment in the mouth, these short copings cause retention issues; consequently, it is advisable to integrate the coping with the post in the root canal.

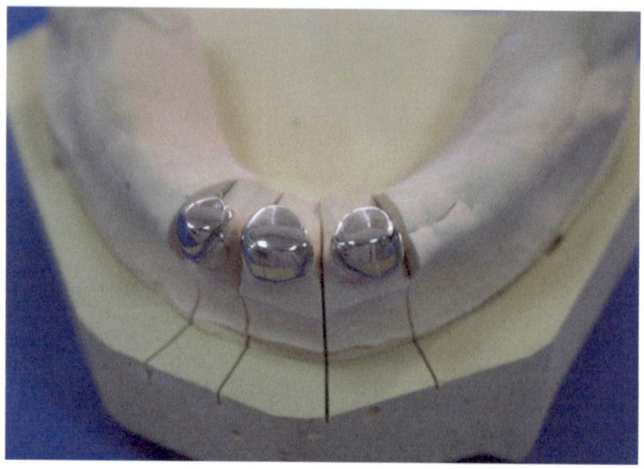

Picture 8.4 Non-vital teeth preparation with post and medium coping and medium coping cast with base metal alloys

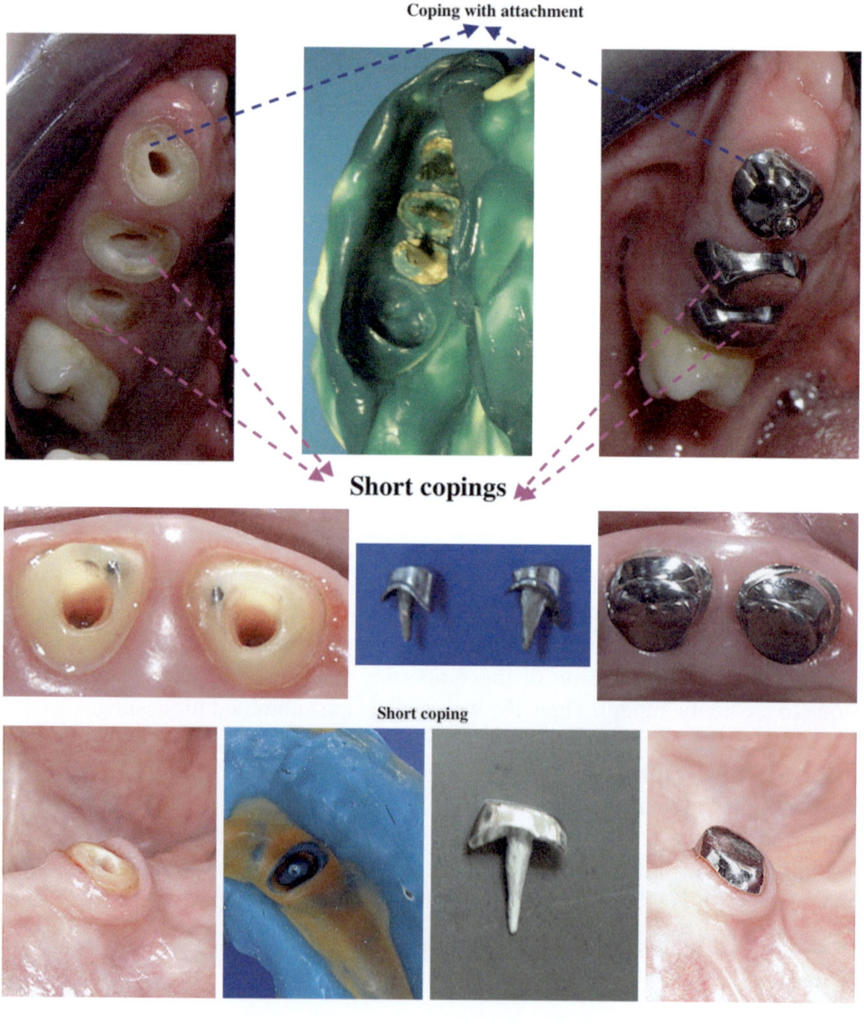

Picture 8.5 Medium copings without post cast with base metal alloys

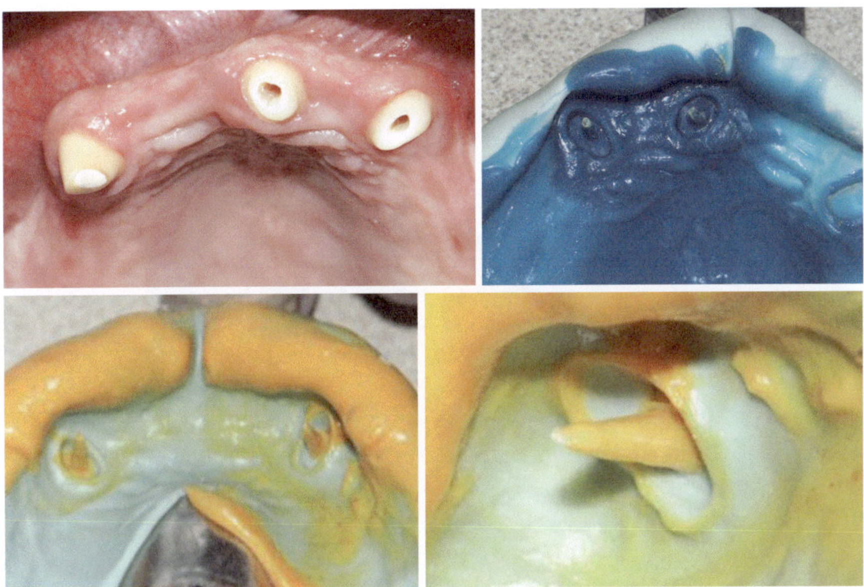

Picture 8.6 Non-vital teeth preparation with post and short coping and short coping cast with base metal alloys

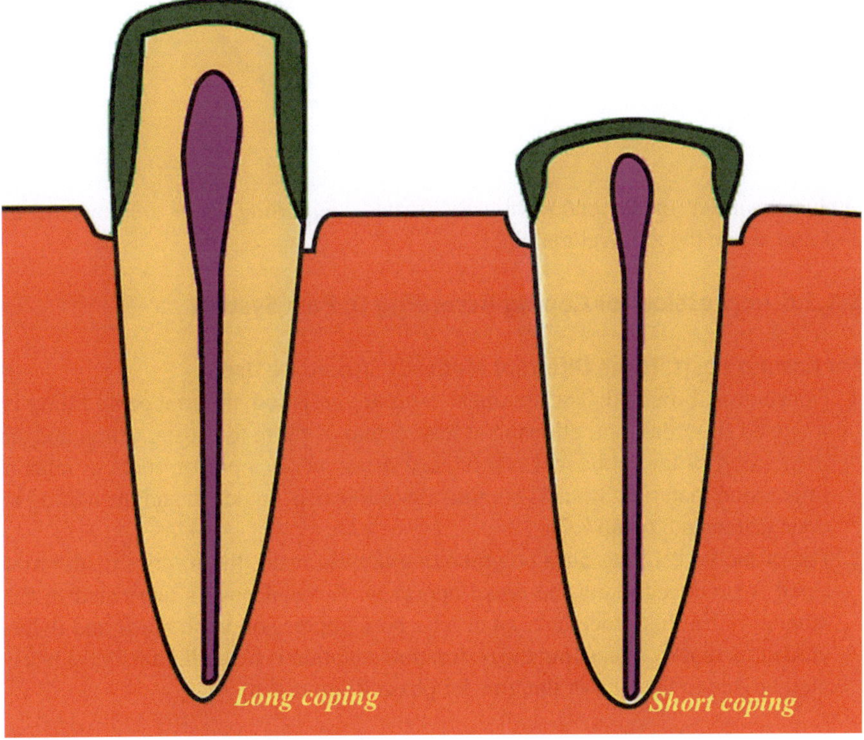

Fig. 8.5 Tooth preparation for long coping and short coping

Fig. 8.6 Dome-shaped
coping with post

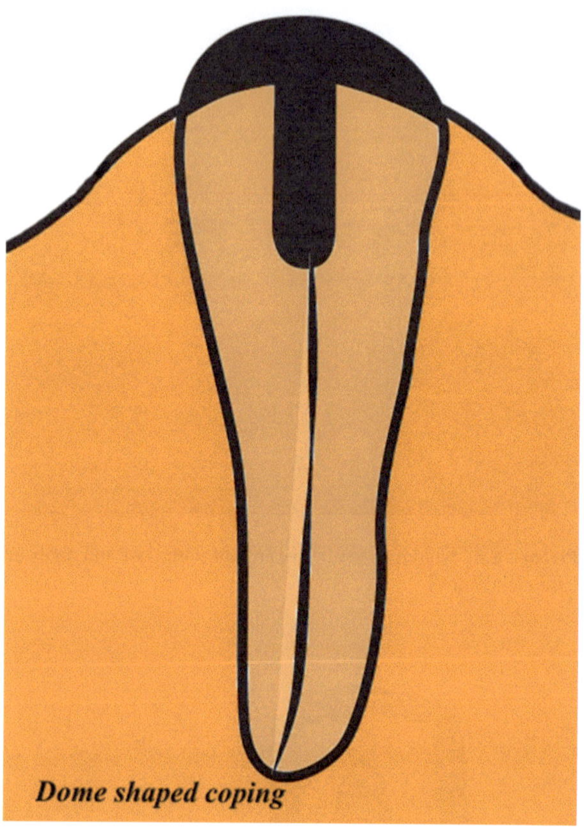

With a chamfer finish, endodontically treated supporting teeth are lowered to 1–2 mm above the gingival margin.

8.1.2.6 Impression for Coping According to Post System

For Casting Posts: Three Different Methods Should Be Used
1. Conventional method: The abutment teeth are prepared, the root canal filling is removed from the root, allowing at least 5 mm of room for post-casting, and an impression of the root canal is produced using wood, a plastic stick, or silicon impression material. Stone is put into a mold, wax is modeled, and the casting is done (Pictures 8.6 and 8.7).
2. Direct method: Using auto-polymerizing acrylic resin, the imprint of the root canal is produced using the direct approach. A metal post is fabricated in the laboratory. In this procedure, an acrylic post-impression is obtained and delivered immediately to casting; the restoration adaption is better than with the usual method due to the lack of the transfer phase (Picture 8.8).

Picture 8.7 After preparation of the supporting teeth, making an impression for post restorations and the cast model obtained

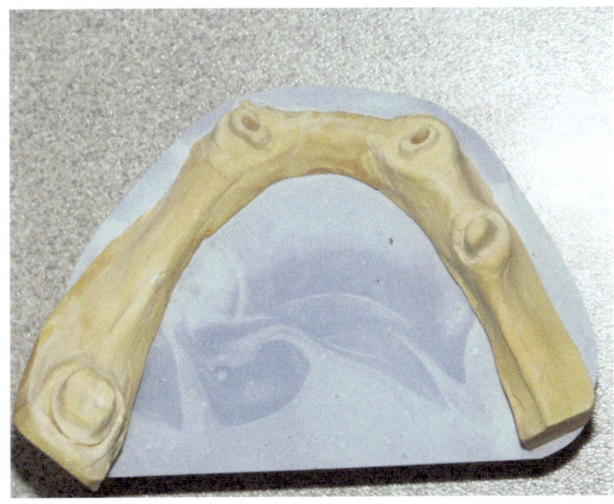

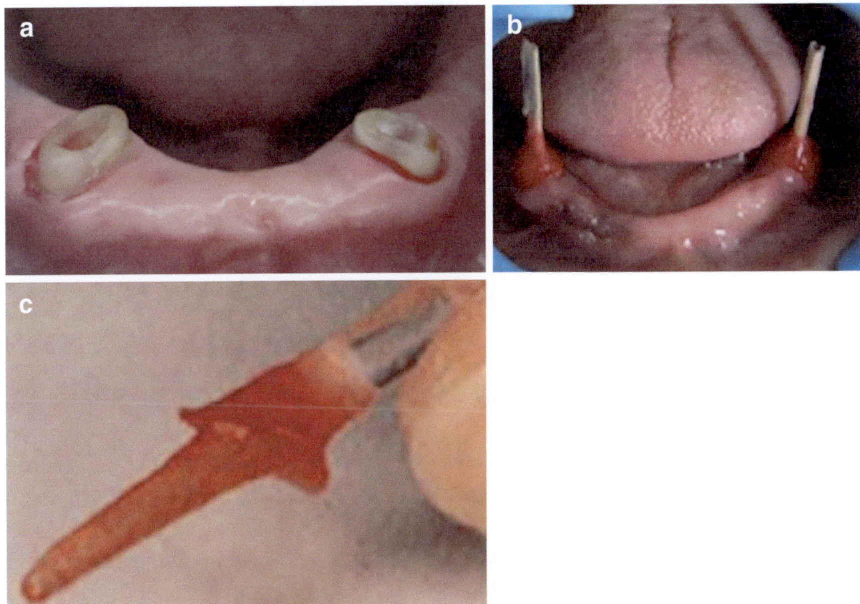

Picture 8.8 (**a**) Preparation of the supporting teeth(**b**, **c**) the impression of post coping could be taken using auto-polymerized acrylic resin (in this way post should be directly cast with metal alloys)

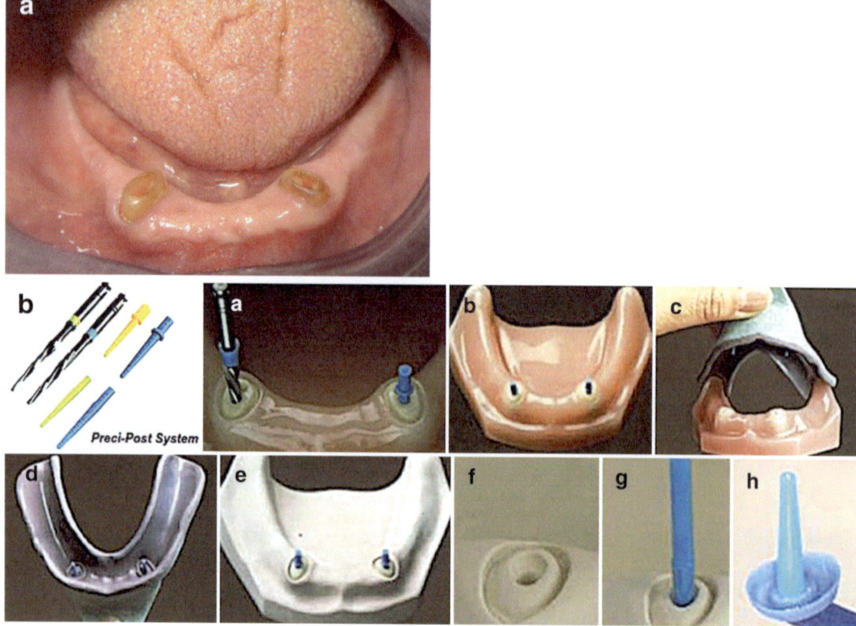

Picture 8.9 (**a**) Preparation of the root canal, (**b**) *a* Preci post plastic pattern (castable post) insert the root canal and controlled the height of the post, *b–d* Making impression of the root canal with (castable post), *e* Cast model obtained castable post in situ, *f–h* Adaptation of castable post on the model then wax coping prepared with (castable post)

3. Preci Post system: Prefabricated resin posts are utilized. Using premade resin, an impression is made and then sent to be cast (Picture 8.9). Communication between the dentist and laboratory ensures the accuracy of the casting in this approach. The "head" of impression posts is suitable with all impression materials and is bendable without breaking or distorting. Impression posts do not attach to die materials. Therefore, it is possible to create a stone casting and to remove posts from the die material without deformation. Expansion and contraction of the casting is corrected and all metal alloys, including non-precision alloys, can be cast without residue. Root canal files, impression posts, and cast posts are available in two distinct colors, depending on the extent of the root canal. After preparing the root canal with a yellow or blue root canal file, an opaque impression post is inserted into the canal. The surface of the post is roughened for retention. With post retentions, adequate adaptability to the impression material is ensured. Thus, the post and the impression are eliminated together. Molds and working molds are prepared. Cast posts replace impression posts, and wax modeling is used for coping manufacture. Then, the coping and post are cast combined, which is the most adaptable of the three techniques.

The obtained casting is retrieved with care, examined for flaws, trimmed, and polished. After being polished, metal copings with posts are set and fastened with appropriate cement.

8.1.3 Preparation of Supporting Teeth with Attachments

8.1.3.1 Tooth Preparation for Attachments Directly Placed into the Root Without a Coping

Direct screwing or cementing the prefabricated metal connection (Dalbo-Rotex Anchor, Preci-Clix Direct) into the root canal helps in simplifying the procedures. These attachments are cheaper and easier to use, but they are suitable for use when the prosthesis will be used for a short time, as they can cause tooth decay and adhesion problems (Figs. 8.7, 8.8, and 8.9; Picture 8.10).

Dalbo-Rotex Anchor and Preci-Clix Direct Attachment Preparation
The root canal housing should be 1–2 mm deeper than the length of the chosen attachment, and the root canal access should be created according to the diameter of

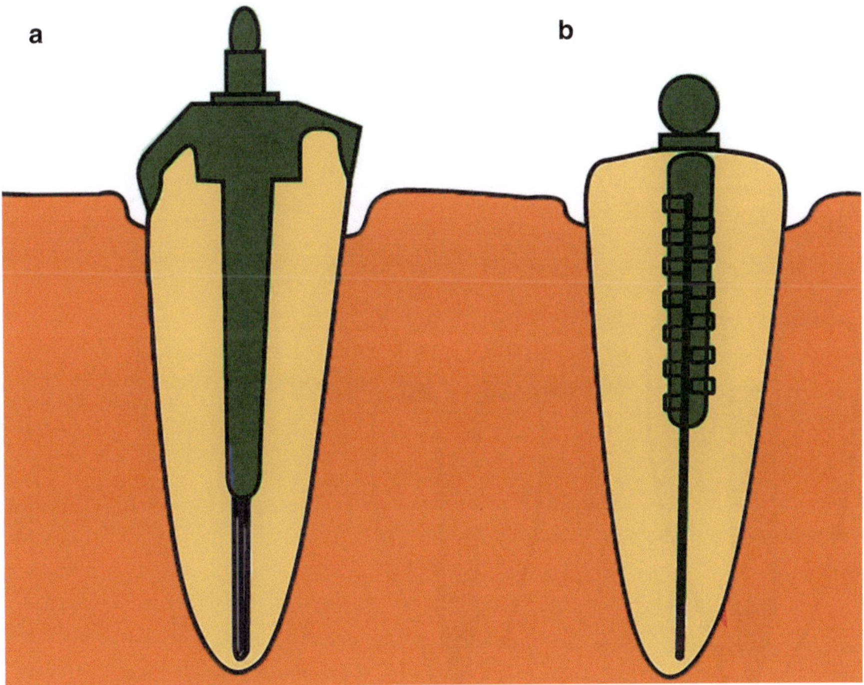

Fig. 8.7 Attachment with (**a**) and without (**b**) coping

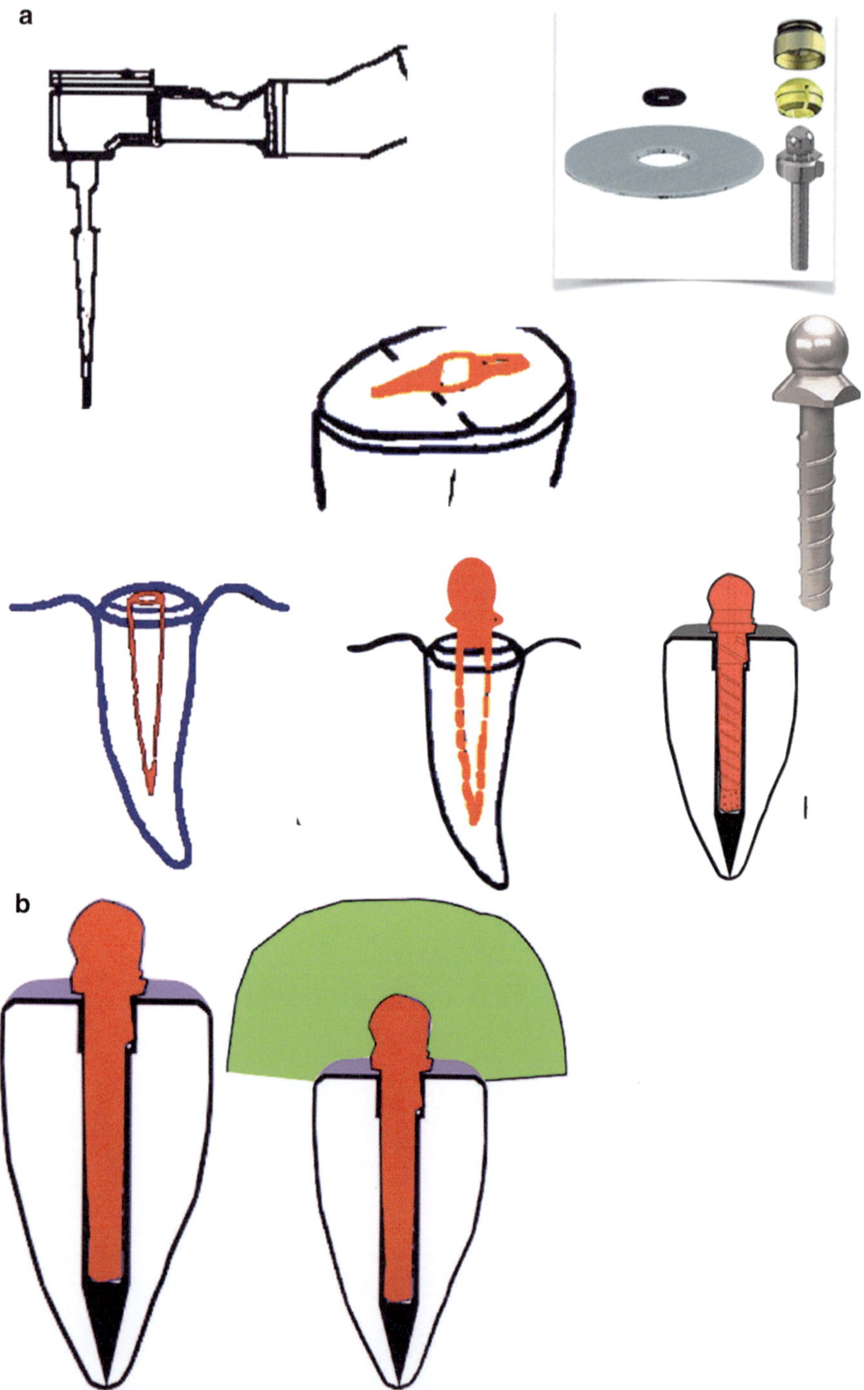

Fig. 8.8 (**a**) The attachment is directly placed inside the root cavity, (**b**) direct root attachment and the female part of the attachment with acrylic inside the denture

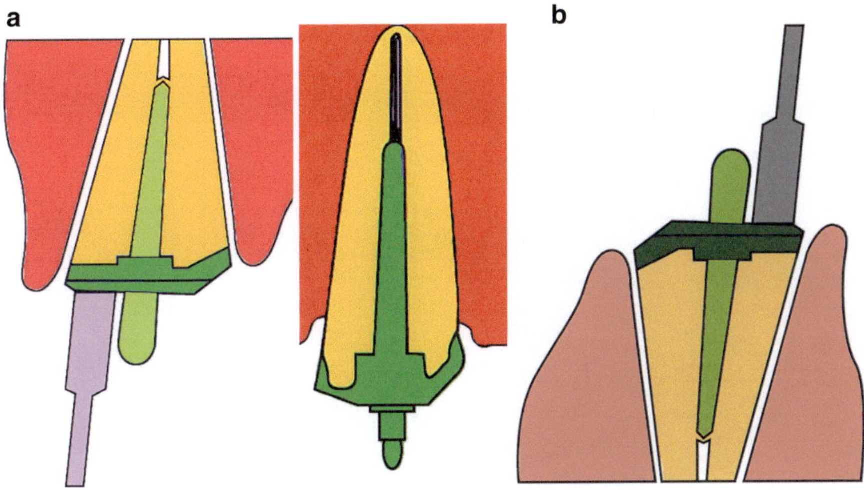

Fig. 8.9 (**a, b**) The coping should be waxed to create a thick layer for obtaining a horizontal platform and should be checked that the cast thickness should not be less than 0.5–1 mm. The flat surface is prepared for the teeth to settle on the attachment, preferably in the lingual. The attachment is placed preferably lingually using paralleling mandrel to enhance the optimum position

the chosen attachment (in the Dalbo-Rotex Anchor system, there are two attachments with a long and short neck). When the long type is utilized, the most coronal portion of the root should be prepared with 1–1.5 mm of neck space. Attachments are tested in the root, and they are cemented using the recommended procedure. The space between the attachment and the tooth is filled with composite or glass ionomer cement after cementation.

The Female Placement
The male part should be covered with wax. The female component of the denture is made as a hole, and then put within the denture using acrylic. This method provides the needed precision and retention for overdenture. When a "click" sound is heard, the female component sits totally on the male component. This connection improves retention.

8.1.3.2 Tooth Preparation for a Metal Coping with an Attachment

The short proximal walls of this sort of system should be as parallel as possible to maximize retention, and the margin is finished with a feather edge or chamfer. The coping should have the proper dimensions and contours to provide retention of the attachment, appropriately distribute stresses from the denture, and have an exact shape to protect supporting tissues. Short coping is employed because of interarch space but it must have a long post for more retention. The chamfer margin of the preparation plays a crucial role in the maintenance of the marginal seal; therefore, the margin should be chamfer, and the preparation should not follow the gingival

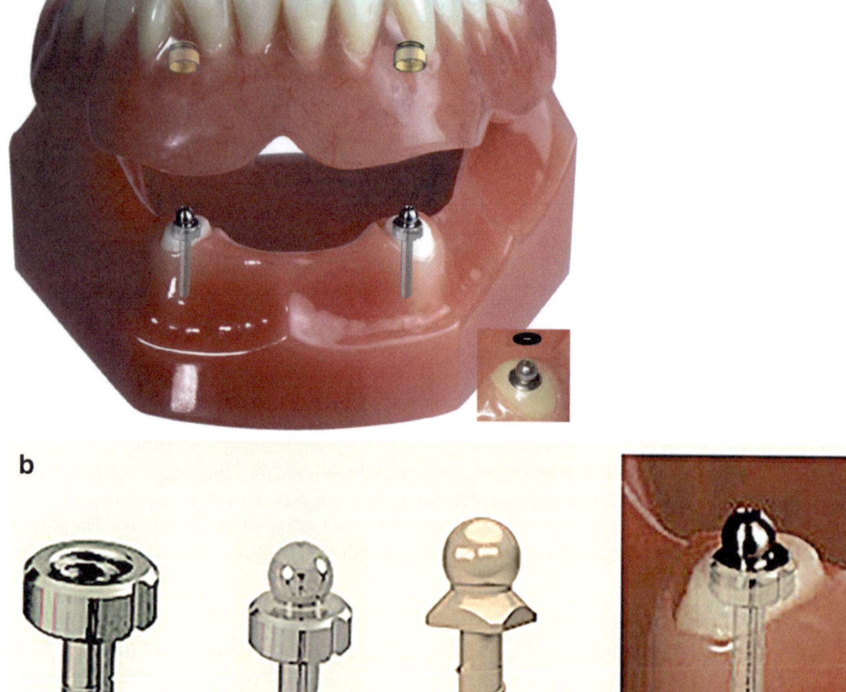

Picture 8.10 (**a**) Overdenture with direct stud attachment (without coping), (**b**) direct stud attachment types

margin if there is significant bone loss, because a reduction must be sufficient to provide space for teeth arrangement, especially in the upper anterior region.

In addition, the design of the copings is essential for attachment and aesthetic purposes. The coping must be waxed in order to produce a horizontal platform on the occlusal surface for simple attachment placement. Additionally, a horizontal plane should be provided for the correct soldering of the attachment when a prefabricated attachment is utilized. Preferably in the lingual, a flat surface is prepared for the teeth to settle on the attachment. If the flat surface is so reduced in the labial direction, the attachment housing is visible from the labial side of the denture. It is crucial to examine tooth contour while selecting the final contour of the attachment coping. Therefore, the coping can be sculpted with wax modeling to create space on the occlusal surface for the superstructure. It is necessary to calculate the vertical height and width of the copings. The optimal attachment is selected based on the height and contour of the void. When the vertical dimension is low, the acrylic base can limit the lingual tongue area, or if a large attachment is utilized, it will be visible on the occlusal plane. Attachments enable the transfer of forces to supporting teeth; if an inappropriate design is chosen, this can cause harm to supporting tissues. Depending on the design of the coping, specific modifications must be performed to prevent unintended damage and eliminate possibly dangerous forces.

Attachments are either already prepared metal cast attachments or wax resin attachments cast in a post/coping/attachment combination. In this design, stud attachments are widely employed.

A prefabricated wax male part is placed on the wax coping when a casting attachment is utilized. Using a surveyor for replacing the male part yields an occlusal surface angle of 90 degrees with respect to the insertion path. If there is an undercut along the path of insertion on the labial or lingual surface of the coping, it may cause tilting forces during the movement of the prosthesis, leading to the locking of the denture. This may cause harm to the periodontium and root, resulting in crown detachment from the root. Therefore, the coping must be designed to be compatible with the denture's insertion path.

If the attachment is to be cast using the same material as the coping, both components are invested and transferred to the casting at the same time. Check the thickness of the casting to ensure that it is between 0.5 and 1 mm. Copings should not have excessive contouring that promotes the development of soft tissue. It is recommended to gradually contour copings to protect gingiva margins. Creating embrasure gaps in the construction of copings used with bars can be problematic. Curtains should have the proper cleaning height. The gingival border should be completed above the gingiva (Figs. 8.1 and 8.7; Pictures 8.11, 8.12, 8.13, and 8.14).

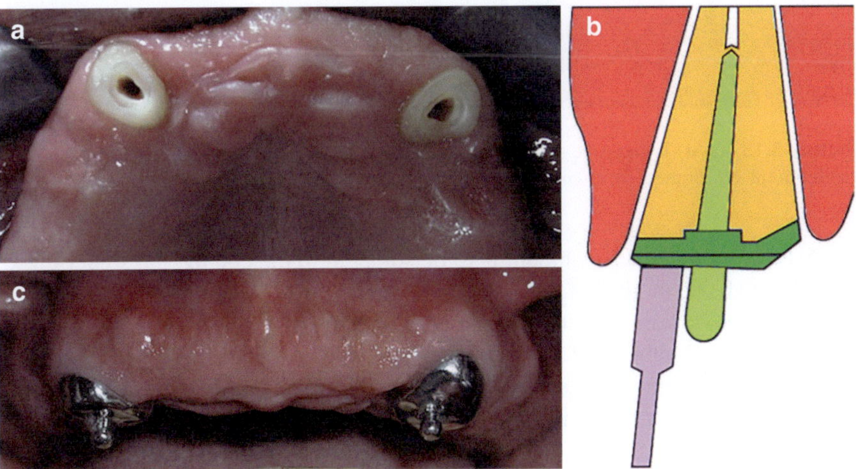

Picture 8.11 Coping using attachment: (**a**) Preparation of teeth, (**b**) placement of attachment on the waxing coping using paralleling mandrel to enhance optimum position, (**c**) attachment/coping assembly in situ

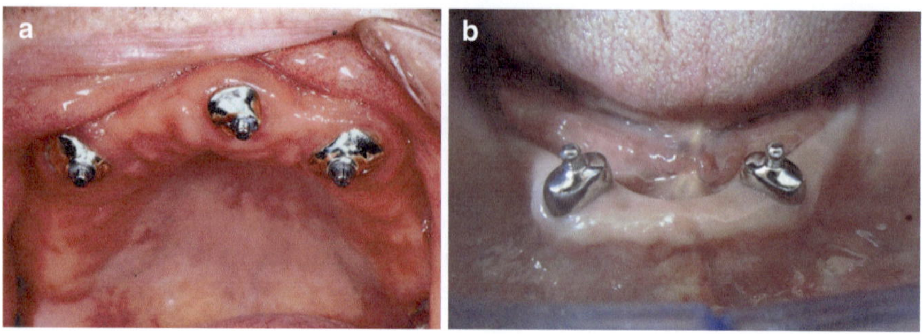

Picture 8.12 (**a**) Ceka attachment/coping assembly, (**b**) stud attachment/coping assembly

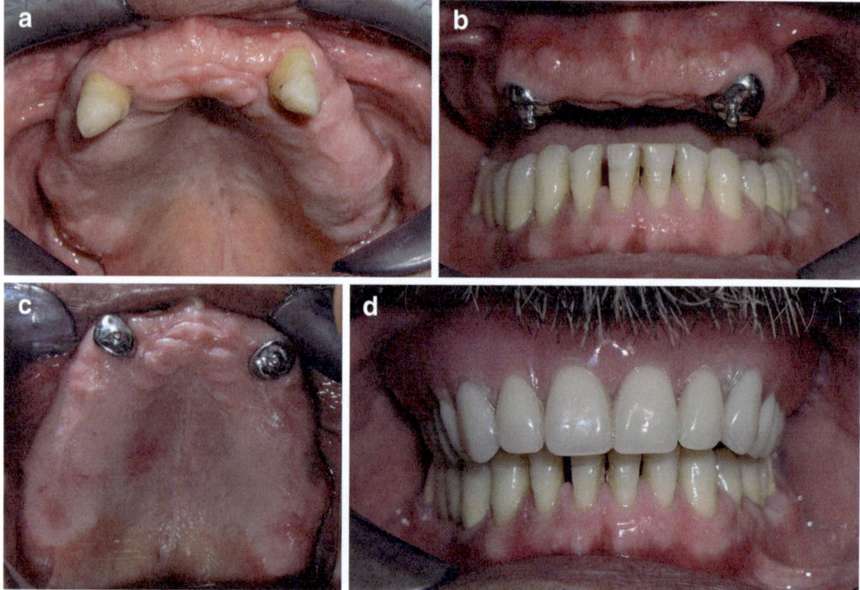

Picture 8.13 (**a–d**) Two canine-supported overdentures prepared for coping and stud attachment: (**a**) Intraoral appearance; (**b**, **c**) control of coping/attachment assembly; (**d**) overdenture in situ

If the prefabricated attachment is to be soldered to the coping, the solder thickness should be no more than 0.1 mm for maximum durability, and solder leakage on the attachment's working surface must be prevented.

The denture is fabricated immediately after the copings are cemented (optional). The clinician prefers to cement the coping during the final appointment. In the first phase, individual acrylic resin impression trays are created on diagnostic casts and checked in the mouth, the borders are corrected using impression compound, and polyvinyl siloxane impression materials are used for the final impression. Plaster type III is used to cast final models. Acrylic resin is typically required to be supported by a metal structure. After the metal framework casting, it is tried in the mouth. Using

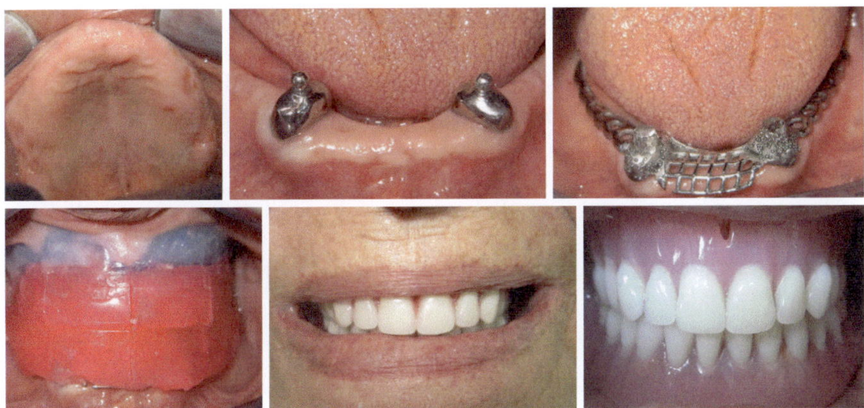

Picture 8.14 Upper complete denture lower TSO construction steps: After establishing a vertical dimension of occlusion, teeth arrangement try-in and overdenture are made

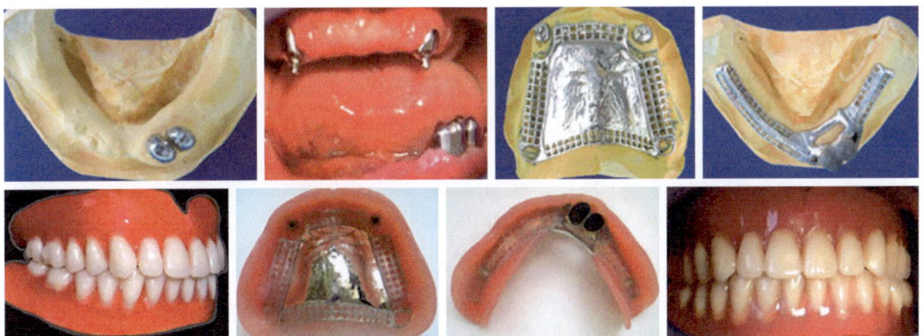

Picture 8.15 Upper complete denture - lower TSO construction steps: Mandibular primary coping controlled on the model then, try in both coping in the mouth. After impression taken with the coping the cast model obtained and the metal framework cast. Establishing a vertical dimension of occlusion, teeth arrangement try-in and overdenture made both jaws

auto-polymerized acrylic resin, a base plate is fabricated, and occlusal rims are created. Using an acrylic base plate and an occlusal rim, the following are evaluated:

1. Teeth's labial contour.
2. Vertical dimension.
3. Occlusal plane.

Intraorally, occlusal rims placed on base plates are arranged with the aid of a face-bow to record vertical and horizontal maxillo-mandibular relations. After the teeth are positioned, aesthetics, phonetics, and occlusion are evaluated during the try-in phase. After molding and polymerization, the denture is ready for polishing and finishing and is delivered to the patient (Pictures 8.14 and 8.15). After TSO therapy, all patients should get information regarding TSO wear and care.

The following should be communicated to patients:

The patient is instructed on how to insert and remove the prosthesis.

The patient is instructed to fit the prosthesis not by biting, but by feeling that the prosthesis is correctly placed on the underlying attachments.

Initially, the patient may complain about the prosthesis' bulkiness and speaking difficulty.

The patient is instructed to read aloud repeatedly until they become acclimated to the prosthesis' size.

The patient is encouraged to chew bilaterally and gently with little bits.

Further Reading

Brewer AA, Morrow RM. Overdentures. 2nd ed. St Louis, MO: CV Mosby Co; 1980.

Carlsson GE. Implant and root supported overdentures - a literature review and some data on bone loss in edentulous jaws. J Adv Prosthodont. 2014;6:245–52.

Dong J, Ikebe K, Gonda T, Nokubi T. Influence of abutment height on strain in a mandibular overdenture. J Oral Rehab. 2006;33:594–9.

Ettinger RL, Qian F. Longitudinal assessment of denture maintenance needs in an overdenture population. J Prosthodont. 2019;28:22–9.

Alfred GH, Kundert M, Charles KC. Complete denture and overdenture prosthetics. New York: Thieme Medical Publishers Inc.; 1993.

Lord JI, Teel S. The Overdentures. Dent Clin N Am. 1969;13:871–81.

Mattoo KA. Determining the need of a coping and/or its number/type in a tooth supported overdenture. J Adv Med Dent Sci. 2020;8:46–9.

Pavlatos J. Root-supported overdentures. CDS Rev. 1998;91:20–5.

Preiskel HW. Overdentures made easy: a guide to implant and root supported prostheses, vol. 1. Berlin: Quintessence Publishing; 1996. p. 38–56.

Rutkunas V, Mizutani A, Takahashi H. Wear simulation effects on overdentures stud attachments. Dent Mater J. 2011;30:845–53.

Rutkunas V, Mizutani H, Takahashi H. Evaluation of stable retentive properties of overdentures attachments. Baltic Dent Maxillofac J. 2005;7:115–20.

Samra RK, Bhide SV, Goyal C, Kaur T. Tooth supported overdenture: a concept overshadowed but not yet forgotten! J Oral Res Rev. 2015;7:16–21.

Schuch C, Pinheiro de Moraes A, Onofre RS, Cenci TP, Boscato N. An alternative method for the fabrication of a root-supported overdenture: a clinical report. J Prosthet Dent. 2013;109:1–4.

Shah FK, Gebreel A, Hamed EA, Habib AA, Porwal A. Comparison of the immediate complete denture, tooth and implant-supported overdenture on vertical dimension and muscle activity. J Adv Prosthodont. 2012;4:61–71.

Sposetti VJ, Gibbs CH, Alderson TH, Jaggers JH, Richmond A, Conlon M, Nickerson DM. Bite force and muscle activity in overdentures wearers before and after attachment placement. J Prosthet Dent. 1986;55:265–73.

Thayer HH, Caputo AA. Occlusal force transmission by overdenture attachments. J Prosthet Dent. 1979;41:266–71.

Van Waas MA, Jonkman RE, Kalk W, Van't Hof MA, Plooij J, Van Os JH. Differences two years after tooth extraction in a mandibular bone reduction in patients treated with immediate overdentures or with immediate complete dentures. J Dent Res. 1993;72:1001–4.

Wang X, Ohkubo C, Hosoi T, Shimpo H, Kurihara D, Murata T. Retentive forces of 3 types of attachments for root-retained overdentures. Prosthodont Res Pract. 2007;6:104–8.

Post-Treatment Protocol

9

Yasemin Ozkan

9.1 Maintenance and Follow-Up

All patients should be scheduled for twice-yearly technical problem monitoring following TSO treatment. The dental hygienist should undertake hygienic procedures during the delivery visit. Patients must be informed of the general directions for wearing, removing, and caring for dentures at home. Patients should remove their dentures before going to bed. Additionally, salivary replacements may be therapeutic for those with dry mouths. The necessity of maintaining the health of retained teeth was emphasized because all of the benefits of TSO were contingent on their ongoing presence. At least twice every day, the patients should be instructed to brush their teeth using fluoride toothpaste. A soft, multi-tufted toothbrush with flexible, round-tipped bristles is placed at a 45° angle and vibrated to clean the abutments during brushing. This permits the bristle tips to enter the available gingival area. Patients should not use a stiff denture brush because it may be overly abrasive, and a patient who is too vigorous may abrade the denture. Avoid toothpaste containing abrasive particles. The plastic clip becomes embedded with abrasive particles, which corrodes the metal attachments. In addition, after brushing in the morning, patients should place one drop of high-concentration neutral fluoride gel (5000 ppm) on the seating surface of the denture corresponding to the abutment and then insert the denture. To maximize the efficacy of the fluoride treatment, it has been established that the patient should abstain from eating and drinking for at least 1.5 h. The gingival sulcus between supporting teeth should be cleaned with dental floss, interdental brushes, or a toothpick affixed to the toothbrush handle. Interproximal tools clean interproximal areas and massage the gingiva to improve blood flow and tissue tone in the surrounding tissues.

Y. Ozkan (✉)
Faculty of Dentistry, Department of Prosthodontics, Marmara University, Istanbul, Turkey
e-mail: ykozkan@marmara.edu.tr

Y. Özkan (ed.), *Treatment Options Before and After Edentulism*,
https://doi.org/10.1007/978-3-031-37582-8_9

Mouthwashes containing antimicrobials, such as 0.12% chlorhexidine, are highly successful at reducing the oral bacterial population but must be used for brief periods because they disrupt the healthy mouth flora. By dipping the floss, brush, etc., into the solution and applying it topically to the desired region, staining can be minimized. Critical to the effectiveness of TSO therapy is enhanced communication between the patient and dentist regarding oral hygiene routines, as well as regular recall appointments. The major objective of protective impressions in TSO patients is to avoid the formation of plaque on the supporting teeth. Methods of protection include mechanical and chemical plaque reduction, fluoride therapy, and monitoring of poor denture use practices. As poor oral hygiene might result in the loss of the abutment, the patient should be motivated to maintain proper oral hygiene. Initial oral hygiene is the most accurate predictor of the patient's participation and prognosis for TSO in the long run. Oral hygiene should be evaluated regularly, and oral health maintenance levels should be repeated as necessary. It has been found that 5 years after the completion of prosthetic therapy, the oral hygiene of elderly patients with poor oral hygiene and periodontal disease improved to an acceptable level.

9.2 Regular Follow-Up

The majority of patients had difficulty maintaining adequate dental hygiene. It may also be the result of a poor self-image and/or other emotional issues, such as depression or alcoholism, which prohibit the patient from following the dentist's recommended preventive program. In addition, poor oral hygiene may be a result of the elderly age of TSO patients and their inability to thoroughly brush their teeth due to a loss of motor coordination or deteriorating eyesight, primarily due to cataracts. The oral health status should be evaluated at follow-up visits.

All supporting teeth, crowns, and attachments must be radiographically and clinically examined. The retention and stability of dentures should be evaluated, and occlusion should be refined. The passivity of contact between the denture and gingival region of the abutments must be investigated. Additionally, the TSO should be compared to traditional dentures delivered to other comparable participants.

Long-term tooth loss in patients with root-retained TSO is primarily caused by periodontal disease. Continued root-retained TSO abrasion can increase the plaque's virulence. Under the denture, anaerobic peripheral colonization is advancing. An increase in anaerobic bacteria may be more attributable to a decrease in saliva and buffering capacity. Therefore, proper oral hygiene is essential. Before prosthetic treatment, it is advised to surgically remove deep gingival pockets. At each recall, debris, calculus, and deep gingival pockets should be removed from supporting tissues. The success or failure of TSO is contingent upon keeping the TSO abutment teeth free of cavities and periodontal disease.

9.3 Post-prosthetic Problems

9.3.1 Abutment Problems

Tooth loss, recurrence of dental caries, recurrence of periodontal disease/periodontal attachment loss, bone loss, and tooth movement are abutment-related problems.

9.3.2 Tooth Loss

There is little evidence from longitudinal studies of TSO populations that tooth loss is a significant problem. The average tooth loss rate ranged from 1.5% to 14.3%. Brewer and Morrow connected supportive tooth loss to poor oral hygiene, arguing that periodontal illnesses and tooth decay occurred. Toolson and Smith conducted a 5-year analysis on 133 TSO abutments in 54 patients, of which 16 were withdrawn. Five of these teeth were taken due to periodontal disease, ten due to tooth decay, and one due to endodontic failure. The scientists concluded that periodontal disease was not a substantial cause of tooth loss. However, Reitz et al. examined 35 patients with 95 TSO abutments; of these teeth, 12 were extracted because of periodontal disease. In addition, research indicates that the bulk of supporting tooth loss (53.8% of cases) is due to periapical lesions caused by pulpal necrosis in crucial teeth, whereas 23.1% of instances involved recurrent decay. Moreover, despite the absence of perforation in critical teeth, problems in around 15% of patients revealed that these supporting teeth are at risk. Perforations toward the pulp in cut teeth are said to result in lesions in around 3 years. This indicates that subsequent dentin production does not result in complete closure. In other words, root fracture, endodontic failure, and pulp necrosis detected in important teeth are additional causes of loss of supporting teeth in root TSO. Routine radiographs and follow-up examinations can aid in the early diagnosis of periapical pathology.

9.3.3 Dental Caries Recurrence

Caries has been discovered as a persistent concern for TSO patients. Plaque deposition under the TSO may result in bacterial colonization, necessitating great effort on the part of the TSO wearer to prevent it. Caries should be viewed as an ongoing issue in TSO situations. Multiple longitudinal studies have recorded the rate of caries under TSO, with the annual rate for new caries ranging between 6.5% and 20%. Five years after utilizing TSO, 50% of the supporting teeth were reported to have been lost due to caries. After 3 years, 90% of abutment teeth began to exhibit periodontal deterioration. The dentinal tubules are exposed to the oral environment upon preparation of an abutment and removal of the crown. It has been noted that the dentin closer to the pulp is less calcified than the dentin closer to the root surface. Therefore, when a tooth's surface is removed, the deeper, more porous dentin is exposed, which is highly susceptible to caries-causing organisms' penetration.

9.3.4 Periodontal Disease Recurrence/Periodontal Attachment Loss

Additionally, periodontal disease has been recognized as a potential ongoing risk factor for TSO wearers. Lord and Teal wrote, "To preserve periodontal health, tissues should be free of inflammation, not bleed when probed, have an appropriate band of connected gingiva (3 to 4 mm), and a vestibular depth without undercuts." If there is less than 1 mm of connected gingiva, persistent inflammation will result, according to Lang and Loe.

Studies have shown that the significant decrease in bone height and attachment level recorded with natural teeth after a 3-year follow-up can be attributed not only to the effect of plaque pathogens but also to the fact that most of the loading during the function was transmitted to the natural tooth side, where the natural tooth is the primary recipient of occlusal stresses because the periodontal ligament of the natural tooth absorbs most of the stresses. Davis et al. and Toolson and Taylor found a considerable reduction in the width of the associated gingiva in mandibular abutments. The most significant loss was discovered on the buccal surface of the mandibular canine. This attachment loss may be the result of denture movement during function, with the majority of movement occurring in the buccal-lingual direction. In comparison to vital teeth, nonvital teeth exhibited a considerable increase in attachment loss over time.

Ramfjord, Budtz, and Thylstrup discovered that the most occlusal portion of the abutment was used to measure clinical attachment loss. Over the course of a year, the influence of TSO supporting tooth shape on plaque retention and periodontal health was assessed. One mandibular canine was repaired with a crown, while the other was reduced to a height of two millimeters above the free gingival border. After 1 year, no significant differences were seen between the contoured abutments. The lowering of the abutment tooth to 1.5– 2 mm above the gingival edge modifies the crown-root ratio and decreases the abutment's mobility by approximately 40%.

It was demonstrated that there was no statistically significant change in CAL surrounding abutment teeth in the precision attachment study group. In the semi-precision attachment control group, there was a statistically significant difference between the scores of different follow-up periods. Comparing the findings of the two groups revealed a statistically significant difference in favor of precision attachment, probably as a result of the higher CAL values observed around abutment teeth with semi-precision attachment and coping. The results demonstrated that the precise attachment with titanium flex pivot preserved extremely stable and healthy soft tissue surrounding the teeth. This may be due to improved biocompatibility and clinical hygienic behavior for precision attachment. All patients participated in a careful plaque control regimen, which may account for these results. These results agreed with those of Graser and Caton and Toolson and Smith, who concluded from their research on TSO that there was no significant change in pocket depth or attached gingiva breadth after 1 and 5 years, respectively.

9.3.5   Bone Loss

After the follow-up period, there was no statistically significant difference in the mean alveolar bone level surrounding abutment teeth in TSO patients, as determined by radiographic interpretation. Multiple papers have theorized about the proprioceptive function of periodontal ligaments in TSO-wearing patients. It is possible to hypothesize that the proprioceptive feedback mechanism, a fourth sensory input from the periodontal ligaments of the teeth, limits bone resorption by signaling against a physiologic overload of the system.

9.3.6   Tooth Mobility

According to longitudinal studies, the mobility of TSO abutments fluctuates over time. Toolson and Smith reported no significant change in mobility 5 years after the placement of the dentures; Toolson and Taylor found similar results at the 10-year TSO. Renner et al. showed, however, that 50% of the abutments had decreased mobility, whereas 50% had no changes after 4 years of observation. In addition, research has demonstrated that patients with vital abutment have less abutment tooth mobility and bone height than those with nonvital abutment. Regarding the significance of abutment teeth, however, some researchers have found that successful abutments are contingent upon the correct selection of vital or nonvital teeth, depending on the diagnosis and treatment strategy.

9.3.7   Technical Problems

These problems include attachment and coping issues, loosening coping, loss or breakage of attachment components, activation of matrices, fractures of bars and extensions, including fracture of acrylic resin denture base and denture teeth, breakage of TSO, excessive tooth wear, discoloration of denture material, and redesign or fabrication of new dentures.

Patients with TSO typically have minimal complaints. It is common for artificial teeth to become damaged. This is a technical issue since the teeth are shattered because their polymerizing surfaces are polluted, and not because the denture itself is made of a harmful substance. Before delivering a denture, clinicians should always apply pressure to ensure that the teeth are dependable and securely set. Clinicians must always maintain control over centric and non-centric movements.

The most frequent complication related to mandibular TSOs is a midline fracture. To strengthen the durability of the denture, a metal mesh was introduced during the polymerization of heat-cured acrylic. The improvement of the mechanical strength of acrylic denture base materials has been the subject of research for some time. Cobalt-chromium wires and metallic wires have been incorporated into the

PMMA matrix, resulting in a significant increase in strength. Some attachment systems (bar, telescope, and stud) are well-known for their TSO retention advantages, but nothing is known about their essential volume relative to other attachment systems (magnetic).

Consequently, their use in circumstances of limited vertical space can result in inadequate prosthetic treatment, with undesirable functional and biomechanical effects. The TSO demands a meticulous evaluation of the attachments' vertical space, that is, there must be sufficient height for roots, copings, and potential attachments, as well as an acceptable thickness of denture base material and artificial teeth, without compromising the denture's strength. It has been established that stud-retained overdentures are less sensitive and easier to clean than bar-retained overdentures. Studs and magnet attachments have achieved widespread acceptance in clinical practice due to their ease of usage. When the supported teeth are located very distally or in a diagonal arrangement, solitary attachments are recommended. Solitary attachments are neither better nor worse than bar-splinted attachments in terms of periodontal or gingival outcome, and they offer easier hygiene and fewer technical complications. Plaque accumulation was reported to be greater with magnet attachments than with stud attachments, and comfort and chewing efficiency may be diminished, reducing patient satisfaction.

A key issue is the deterioration of the elastic component, which must be replaced frequently. There are no established data available to help us determine the average lifespan of the components, the replacement time, or the repair time. Lehmann and Arnim observed that TSO stability might occur during function when attachment system retention forces ranged between 5 and 7 N; however, everyday insertion and removal in the oral environment can lead to prosthetic system degradation and loss. The retention of various attachment systems throughout the initial term of use in the oral cavity is comparable, consequently boosting patient compliance. After 1 year of use in the oral cavity, it was seen that the retention values for both attachment systems were roughly the same and comparable, but decreased with continued use as a result of fatigue. However, no component fractures were observed even after 4 years of use in the oral cavity. The retention values of both attachment methods decreased to around 35% of their initial value after 4 years of use, which can be attributed to continual wear. However, Stewart and Edwards found that the retention force of certain types of attachments decreases to 80% within a year. According to Wichmann and Kuntze, any attachment system is susceptible to constant wear due to repeated insertion and removal cycles in addition to functional loads, which are attributed to the frictional load occurring between the attachment and the base and resulting in a decrease in retention values.

With a magnetic attachment TSO, patient satisfaction was lower than with a bar attachment or stud attachment TSO, although patients preferred magnetic attachments for repeated treatments. In addition, researchers found that patients utilizing bar or ball attachments for TSO were more satisfied than those using magnetic attachments. The majority of patients favored stud attachments because of their durability. A third of the study participants favored magnetic attachments due to the comfort they provided.

9.3.8 Functional Problems

These problems include adjustments to dentures to alleviate uncomfortable places, poor retention and stability, rebasing, occlusal correction, poor esthetic rearrangement of teeth, and soft tissue hyperplasia (Pictures 9.1, 9.2, 9.3, and 9.4).

Low denture stability and discomfort in the tissue and teeth where the denture is seated are the most common complaints. One-third of patients lose the stability of their dentures within 6 years. In the correction of mandibular root-retained TSO, the lining is the most recommended prosthetic technique. Inadequate assessment of the clinical situation, particularly the adequate inter-arch space, as well as ignorance or

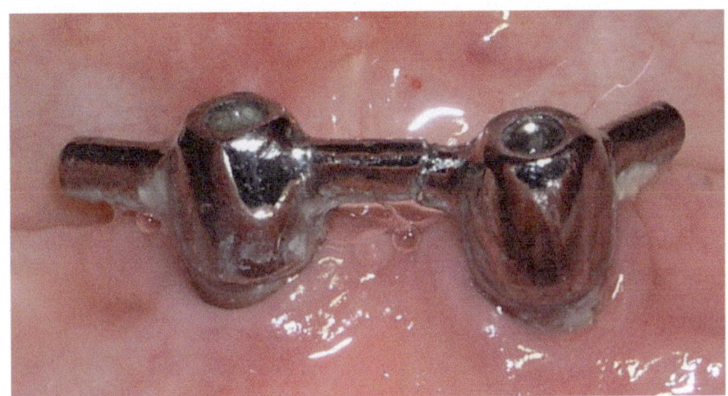

Picture 9.1 Broken bar attachment

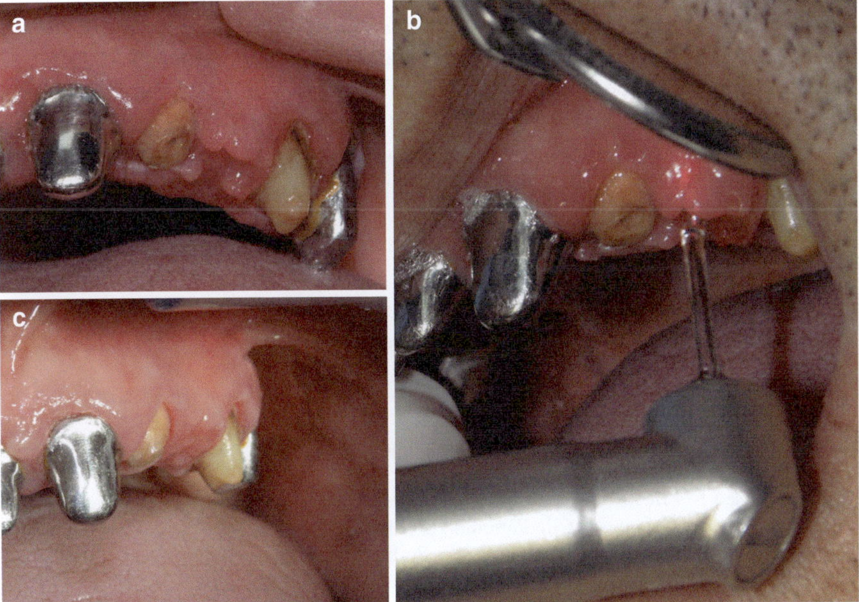

Picture 9.2 (**a**) Losing the metal coping on the tooth caused soft tissue hyperplasia, (**b**) soft tissue corrected using laser, (**c**) healed soft tissue

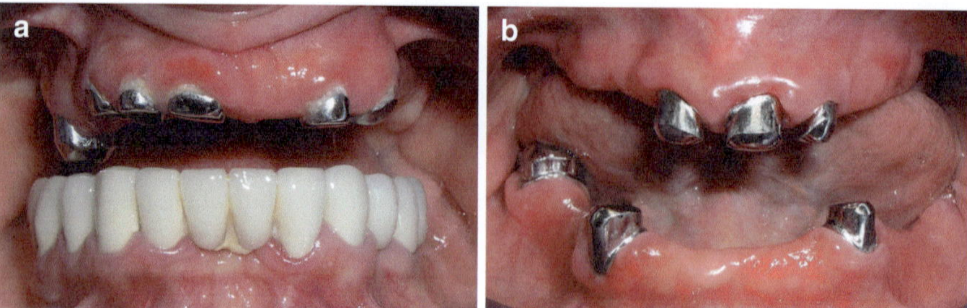

Picture 9.3 (**a**, **b**) Soft tissue problems under the overdentures

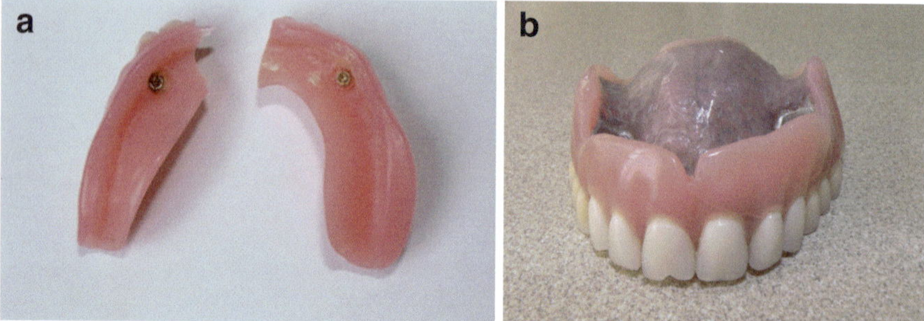

Picture 9.4 (**a**) Fracture of overdenture, (**b**) fracture of teeth

contempt for the concepts and clinical and technical procedures, result in serious denture issues [by overestimating the vertical dimension of occlusion (VDO) and improper teeth implementation]. These are followed by functional and prosthetic difficulties, such as the inability to chew, poor phonation, denture intolerance, and a greater risk of recurring fractures, which negatively affect social interactions and quality of life.

Further Reading

Basker RM, Harrison A, Ralph JP. Overdentures in general dental practice. Part 5–the use of copings and attachments. Br Dent J. 1983;155:9–13.

Dong J, Ikebe K, Gonda T, Nokubi T. Influence of abutment height on strain in a mandibular overdenture. J Oral Rehabil. 2006;33:594–9.

Budtz-Jörgensen E. Prognosis of overdenture abutments in elderly patients with controlled oral hygiene. A 5-year study. J Oral Rehabil. 1995;22:3–8.

Budtz-Jörgensen E. Effects of denture-wearing habits on periodontal health of abutment teeth in patients with overdentures. J Clin Periodontol. 1994;21:265–9.

Compagnoni MA, Souza RF, Marra J, Pero AC, Barbosa DB. Relationship between Candida and nocturnal denture wear: a quantitative study. J Oral Rehabil. 2007;34:600–5.

Crum RJ, Rooney GE. Alveolar bone loss in overdentures: a 5-year study. J Prosthet Dent. 1978;40:610–3.

Ettinger R, Qian F. Postprocedural problems in an overdenture population: a longitudinal study. J Endod. 2004;30:310–4.

Ettinger RL. Qian Abutment tooth loss in patients with overdentures. J Am Dent Assoc. 2004;135:739–46.

Fontijn-Tekamp FA, Slagter AP, Van Der Bilt A, et al. Biting and chewing in overdentures, full dentures, and natural dentitions. J Dent Res. 2000;79:1519–24.

Gonda T, Yang TC, Maeda Y. Five-year multicenter study of magnetic attachments used for natural overdenture abutments. J Oral Rehabil. 2013;40:258–62.

Kraljevic I, Glenz F, Jordi C, Zimmermann SD, Joda T, Zitzmann NU. Long-term observation of post copings retaining overdenture prostheses. Int J Prosthodont. 2020;33:169–75.

Mercouriadis-Howald A, Rollier N, Tada S, McKenna G, Igarashi K, Schimmel M. Loss of natural abutment teeth with cast copings retaining overdentures: a systematic review and meta-analysis. J Prosthodont Res. 2018;62:407–15.

Mericske-Stern R. Oral tactile sensibility recorded in overdenture wearers with implants or natural roots: a comparative study. Part 2. Int J Oral Maxillofac Implants. 1994;9:63–70.

Moldovan O, Rudolph H, Luthardt RG. Biological complications of removable dental prostheses in the moderately reduced dentition: a systematic literature review. Clin Oral Investig. 2018;22:2439–61.

Safavi KE, Grasso JE. Endodontic considerations in the restoration of partial overdenture abutments. Dent Clin N Am. 1990;34:645–52.

Stalder A, Berger CH, Buser R, Wittneben J, Chimmel M, Abou-Ayas S. Biological and technical complications in root cap–retained overdentures after 3–15 years in situ: a retrospective clinical study. Clin Oral Investig. 2021;25:2325–33.

Takahashi T, Gonda T, Mizuno Y, Fujinami Y, Maeda Y. Reinforcement in removable prosthodontics: a literature review. J Oral Rehabil. 2017;44:133–43.

Toolson LB, Smith DE. A five-year longitudinal study of patients treated with overdentures. J Prosthet Dent. 1983;49:749–56.

Toolson LB, Taylor TD. A 10-year report of a longitudinal recall of overdenture patients. J Prosthet Dent. 1989;62:179–81.

Wagner B. Kern Clinical evaluation of removable partial dentures 10 years after insertion: success rates, hygienic problems, and technical failures. Clin Oral Investig. 2000;4:74–80.

Yoshino K, Ito K, Kuroda M, Sugihara N. Survival rate of removable partial dentures with complete arch reconstruction using double crowns: a retrospective study. Clin Oral Investig. 2009;24:1543–9.